D1315898

THE SPINAL CORD INJURED PATIENT

Comprehensive Management

THE SPINAL CORD INJURED PATIENT

Comprehensive Management

BOK Y. LEE, M.D.

Professor of Surgery
New York Medical College, Valhalla
Adjunct Professor
Rensselaer Polytechnic Institute, Troy
Chief, Surgical Service
Veterans Affairs Medical Center
Castle Point, New York

LEE E. OSTRANDER, Ph.D.

Associate Professor
Biomedical Engineering Department
Rensselaer Polytechnic Institute
Troy, New York

GEORGE VAN B. COCHRAN, M.D., Sc.D.

Professor of Clinical Orthopedic Surgery
Columbia University, New York City
Adjunct Professor of Biomedical Engineering
Rensselaer Polytechnic Institute, Troy
Director, Orthopedic Engineering and Research Center
Helen Hayes Hospital
West Haverstraw, New York

WILLIAM W. SHAW, M.D.

Professor and Chief
Division of Plastic and Reconstructive Surgery
UCLA Medical Center
Los Angeles, California

W.B. SAUNDERS COMPANY
Harcourt Brace Jovanovich, Inc.

Philadelphia, London, Toronto, Montreal, Sydney, Tokyo

W. B. SAUNDERS COMPANY
Harcourt Brace Jovanovich, Inc.

The Curtis Center
Independence Square West
Philadelphia, PA 19106

Library of Congress Cataloging-in-Publication Data

The spinal cord injured patient : comprehensive
    management / Bok Y. Lee . . . [et al.].
        p.   cm.
    ISBN 0-7216-5699-4
    1. Spinal cord—Wounds and injuries—Treatment.
2. Spinal cord—Wounds and injuries—Patients—
Rehabilitation.   [1. Spinal Cord Injuries—therapy.]
I. Lee, Bok Y.
    [DNLM: WL 400 S75764]
RD594.3.S6694   1991
617.4′82044—dc20
DNLM/DLC   90-8928

Developmental Editor: Kathleen McCullough
Production Manager: Frank Polizzano
Manuscript Editor: Edna Dick
Illustration Coordinator: Joan Sinclair
Indexer: David Prout

THE SPINAL CORD INJURED PATIENT   ISBN   0-7216-5699-4
Comprehensive Management

Contributors

ROBERTA S. ABRUZZESE, Ed.D., R.N., F.A.A.N.
Adjunct Associate Professor, Marion A. Buckley School of Nursing, Adelphi University, Garden City, New York
Pressure Sores: Nursing Aspects and Prevention

JOSEPH C. ADDONIZIO, M.D. (Deceased)
Professor and Chairman, Department of Urology, New York Medical College, Valhalla, New York
Urologic Evaluation and Management of the Spinal Cord Injured Patient

NANAKRAM AGARWAL, M.D., F.R.C.S., F.A.C.S.
Associate Professor of Surgery, New York Medical College, Valhalla; Chief, Surgical ICU, Our Lady of Mercy Medical Center, Bronx, New York
Nutrition in Spinal Cord Injured Patients

MATS ASZTÉLY, M.D.
Consultant Radiologist, Department of Radiology, University of Göteborg, Sahlgrenska Sjukhuset, Göteborg, Sweden
Ultrasound Examination for the Evaluation of Spinal Cord Injured Patients

PHILLIP W. BARTH, Ph.D.
Scientific Staff, Hewlett-Packard, Palo Alto, California
Pressure Sores: Overview

WILLIAM BOND, M.D.
Department of Plastic Surgery, New York Medical College, Valhalla; Eastern Paralyzed Veterans Association Fellow, Veterans Affairs Medical Center, Castle Point, New York
Acute Abdomen in Spinal Cord Injured Patients

DANIEL A. CAPEN, M.D.
Associate Clinical Professor of Orthopedic Surgery, Rancho Los Amigos–USC, Attending Physician, Rancho Los Amigos Medical Center, Downey, California
Nonoperative Management of Cervical Instability; Surgical Stabilization in Cervical Spine Trauma

JOHN H. DAVIS, M.D.

Professor and Chairman, Department of Surgery, University of Vermont College of Medicine; Surgeon in Chief, Medical Center Hospital of Vermont, Burlington, Vermont
Management of the Patient with Multiple Injuries

LOUIS R. M. DEL GUERCIO, M.D.

Professor and Chairman, Department of Surgery, New York Medical College; Attending and Chief of Surgery, Westchester County Medical Center, Valhalla, New York
Hemodynamic Monitoring in Spinal Cord Injury Patients

FRANK J. EISMONT, M.D.

Professor of Orthopaedic and Rehabilitation and Program Director, Orthopaedic Residency Program, University of Miami Medical School; Co-Director, Acute Spinal Cord Injury Unit, Jackson Memorial Medical Center, Miami, Florida
Immediate Management of the Spinal Cord Injured Patient

HERVÉ FAVRE, M.D.

Adjunct Professor, Division of Nephrology, Hôpital Cantonal Universitaire, Geneva University, Switzerland
Body Composition and Endocrine Profile in Spinal Cord Injured Patients

GEORG D. FRISCH, M.S. (Deceased)

Department Head, Naval Air Development Center, Warminster, Pennsylvania
Human Analog Representation in Biomechanics and Biodynamics as Related to Spinal Cord Injury Management and Assessment

PAUL H. FRISCH, M.S.

Technical Director, Applied Physics Inc., Nanuet, New York
Human Analog Representation in Biomechanics and Biodynamics as Related to Spinal Cord Injury Management and Assessment

JOSEPH P. GIFFIN, M.D.

Assistant Professor of Anesthesiology, State University of New York–Downstate Medical Center; Clinical Director of Anesthesiology, Kings County Hospital Center, Brooklyn, New York
Spinal Cord Injury Treatment and the Anesthesiologist

HARRY S. GOLDSMITH, M.D.

Professor of Surgery and Adjunct Professor of Neurosurgery, Boston University School of Medicine; Attending Surgeon, University Hospital, Boston, Massachusetts
The Omentum in Spinal Cord Injury

DANIEL GRAUPE, Ph.D.

Professor of Electrical Engineering and Computer Science and Adjunct Professor of Physical Medicine and Rehabilitation, University of Illinois at Chicago; Associate Attending Staff Member (Research), Michael Reese Hospital and Medical Center, Chicago, Illinois

Patient-Responsive EMG-Controlled Electrical Stimulation to Facilitate Unbraced Walking of Paraplegics

BARTH A. GREEN, M.D.

Professor of Neurological Surgery, Orthopedics, and Rehabilitation, University of Miami School of Medicine; Director of Neurosurgery Service, and Co-Director, Acute Spinal Cord Injury Unit, Jackson Memorial Medical Center, Miami, Florida

Immediate Management of the Spinal Cord Injured Patient

KENNETH GRUSCH, M.D.

Attending Anesthesiologist, Booth Memorial Medical Center, Flushing, New York

Spinal Cord Injury Treatment and the Anesthesiologist

LINDA A. HEIER, M.D.

Assistant Professor of Radiology, Cornell University Medical College; Assistant Attending Physician, Cornell University Medical Center–The New York Hospital, New York, New York

Efficacy of Magnetic Resonance Imaging in the Diagnosis of Spinal Cord Trauma

CARL E. JOHNSON, M.D.

Clinical Assistant Professor of Radiology, SUNY Health Science Center at Brooklyn; Assistant Attending Physician, The Long Island College Hospital, Brooklyn, and Manhattan Eye, Ear, and Throat Hospital, New York, New York

Efficacy of Magnetic Resonance Imaging in the Diagnosis of Spinal Cord Trauma

K. JOHN KLOSE, Ph.D.

Research Assistant Professor of Neurological Surgery, Orthopaedics, and Rehabilitation, University of Miami School of Medicine, Miami, Florida

KATE H. KOHN, M.D.

Clinical Professor of Physical Medicine and Rehabilitation, Department of Physical Medicine and Rehabilitation, University of Illinois at Chicago; Attending Physician and Chairman Emeritus, Department of Rehabilitation Medicine, Michael Reese Hospital and Medical Center, Chicago, Illinois

Patient-Responsive EMG-Controlled Electrical Stimulation to Facilitate Unbraced Walking of Paraplegics

THOMAS A. KROUSKOP, Ph.D.

Professor, Departments of Rehabilitation and Physical Medicine, Baylor College of Medicine; Head, Rehabilitation Engineering Department, The Institute for Rehabilitation and Research, Houston, Texas

The Role of Mattresses and Beds in Preventing Pressure Sores

DOUGLAS W. LAMB, M.B., F.R.C.S.E.

Honorary Senior Lecturer, Department of Orthopaedic Surgery, University of Edinburgh; Consultant Orthopaedic Surgeon (Retired); Princess Margaret Rose Orthopaedic Hospital, Edinburgh, Scotland

Reconstructive Surgery for the Upper Limb and Hand in Traumatic Tetraplegia

BOK Y. LEE, M.D.

Professor of Surgery, New York Medical College, Valhalla; Adjunct Professor, Rensselaer Polytechnic Institute, Troy; Chief of Surgical Service, Veterans Affairs Medical Center, Castle Point, New York

Management of Peripheral Vascular Disease in the Spinal Cord Injured Patient; Deep Venous Thrombosis in Spinal Cord Injured Patients; Plastic Surgery for Pressure Sores; Paralysis Secondary to Abdominal Aortic Aneurysm; Nutrition in Spinal Cord Injured Patients

IL Y. LEE, M.D.

Chief of Rehabilitation Medicine, West Roxbury/Brockton Veterans Administration Medical Center, West Roxbury, Massachusetts

Advantages and Disadvantages of Roentgenograms in the Diagnosis of Odontoid Fractures

BERIT L. MADSEN, M.D.

Resident, Department of Radiation Oncology, Stanford University Medical Center, Stanford, California

Pressure Sores: Overview

RUSSELL W. NELSON, M.D.

Clinical Instructor in Orthopedic Surgery, Rancho Los Amigos–USC, Attending Physician, Rancho Los Amigos Medical Center, Downey, California

Nonoperative Management of Cervical Instability

JAMES T. O'HEIR

Director of Emergency Medical Services, University of Miami School of Medicine, Miami, Florida

Immediate Management of the Spinal Cord Injured Patient

GEORGE F. OWENS, M.D., F.A.C.S.

Clinical Assistant Professor of Urology, Department of Urology, New York Medical College; Attending Urologist, Westchester County Medical Center, Valhalla, Our Lady of Mercy Medical Center, Bronx, St. Agnes Hospital, White Plains, and Mount Vernon Hospital, Mount Vernon, New York

Urologic Evaluation and Management of the Spinal Cord Injured Patient

CARLETON PILSECKER, M.S.S.W.

Supervising Social Worker, Spinal Cord Injury Service, Veterans Administration Medical Center, Long Beach, California

A Changed World: Socioeconomic Problems of Spinal Cord Injured Patients

WILLIAM REINBOLD, M.D.

Assistant Clinical Professor of Psychiatry, University of California Irvine Medical School; Special Treatment Coordinator for Spinal Cord Injury, Long Beach Veterans Administration Medical Center, Long Beach, California

Management of Coping Problems in Spinal Cord Injury Rehabilitation

ALAIN B. ROSSIER, M.D.

Professor of Paraplegiology, University Orthopaedic Clinic Balgrist, Zurich University, Switzerland; Lecturer on Spinal Cord Injuries, Department of Orthopaedic Surgery, Harvard Medical School, and Adjunct Professor of Spinal Cord Rehabilitation, Department of Orthopaedic Surgery, Tufts University, Boston; Consultant (former Chief), Swiss Paraplegic Center, University Orthopaedic Clinic Balgrist, Zurich, Switzerland

Advantages and Disadvantages of Roentgenograms in the Diagnosis of Odontoid Fractures; Body Composition and Endocrine Profile in Spinal Cord Injured Patients

JOHN A. SAVINO, M.D.

Professor of Surgery, New York Medical College; Attending Physician, Chief of Trauma and Critical Care, and Director, Surgical ICU, Westchester County Medical Center, Valhalla, New York

Hemodynamic Monitoring in Spinal Cord Injury Patients

KINICHI SHIBUTANI, M.D., Ph.D.

Professor and Acting Chairman and Director of Research, Department of Anesthesia, New York Medical College; Attending Physician, Westchester County Medical Center, Valhalla, New York

Hemodynamic Monitoring in Spinal Cord Injury Patients

WILLIAM M. STAHL, M.D.

Professor and Vice Chairman, Department of Surgery, New York Medical College; Director of Surgery, Lincoln Medical and Mental Health Center, Bronx, New York

Physiologic Response to Tissue Injury

JACK STERN, M.D., Ph.D.

Attending Physician, Westchester County Medical Center, Valhalla, New York

Neurologic Evaluation and Neurologic Sequelae of the Spinal Cord Injured Patient

RUDOLPH TADDONIO, M.D.

Clinical Associate Professor of Orthopedics and Acting Vice-Chairman of Orthopedics, New York Medical College; Attending Physician, Orthopedic Surgeon, and Director, Orthopedic Surgery, Westchester County Medical Center, Valhalla, New York

Hemodynamic Monitoring in Spinal Cord Injury Patients

MICHEL B. VALLOTON, M.D.

Professor, Endocrinology Division, Hôpital Cantonal Universitaire, Geneva University; Head of the Endocrinology Division, Hôpital Cantonal Universitaire, Geneva University, Geneva, Switzerland

Body Composition and Endocrine Profile in Spinal Cord Injured Patients

N. D. VAZIRI, M.D.

Professor and Vice Chair, Department of Medicine, and Chief, Division of Nephrology, University of California, Irvine; Attending Physician, University of California, Irvine Medical Center, Orange, California

Renal Insufficiency in Patients with Spinal Cord Injury

LARS M. VISTNES, M.D.

Professor, Division of Plastic Surgery, Stanford University School of Medicine, Stanford, California

Pressure Sores: Overview

AY-MING WANG, M.D.

Clinical Associate Professor of Radiology, University of Missouri College of Medicine; Co-Chief, Division of Neuroradiology, William Beaumont Hospital, Royal Oak, Michigan

Advantages and Disadvantages of Roentgenograms in the Diagnosis of Odontoid Fractures

GARY M. YARKONY, M.D.

Assistant Professor, Rehabilitation Medicine, Northwestern University Medical School; Attending Physician and Director, Spinal Cord Injury Rehabilitation, Rehabilitation Institute of Chicago, Midwest Regional Spinal Cord Injury Care System, Chicago, Illinois

Spinal Cord Injury Rehabilitation

Preface

Spinal cord injury is a devastating physical, emotional, and financial event for the individual. This calamity happens to people of all ages and is one of the most complex and challenging of circumstances for medical/surgical management. Optimal treatment calls for the integration of a broad array of skills, a team effort, and incorporation of many diverse professional knowledge bases. Because professional participants in the care of spinal cord injured patients can best serve the patient's needs if they appreciate all aspects of treatment and support, our first goal in this book is to cover the broad issues involved in the care of the spinal cord injured patient.

The treatment of spinal cord injury is not a static field. Thus, it is necessary at relatively frequent intervals to update and describe refinements that are occurring in diagnosis and in acute and chronic care and to report advances in medical/surgical management and rehabilitation. Our second goal is to provide an evaluation of spinal cord injury by experts who are deeply involved with various aspects of spinal cord injury management.

The scope of this book includes diagnostic methods (e.g., ultrasound, magnetic resonance imaging), evaluation methods, spinal cord injury pathophysiology, medical/surgical management of complications of treatment, and issues of specialized care including electrical stimulation and pressure sore management. The table of contents shows these topics and more, all of direct relevance to the care of patients with spinal cord injury.

Of special interest in this book are the discussions of hand reconstruction essential to functional use following spinal cord injury, hemodynamic monitoring that incorporates automated patient profiling, and noninvasive assessment and prevention of deep vein thrombosis and pulmonary embolism using external pneumatic compression. A few specialized research aspects are covered, including the effective use of omentum, which may improve the spinal cord blood supply and which is transposed to the spinal cord, and the use of human analogs or manikins to test human body responses of the head and spine under simulated conditions of injury.

While no book can cover every aspect of so complex a field, this volume does provide a broad array of advice and suggestions. Reading this book is similar to listening in on practicing health experts with a broad range of expertise as they provide an impressive assemblage of experiences and insights. This book is a compendium of otherwise difficult to assemble knowledge replete with time tested methods as well as with contemporary developments in the form of new ideas, techniques, and concepts.

BOK Y. LEE, M.D.
LEE E. OSTRANDER, PH.D.
GEORGE VAN B. COCHRAN, M.D., SC.D.
WILLIAM W. SHAW, M.D.

Contents

1 Management of Peripheral Vascular Disease in the Spinal Cord Injured Patient

BOK Y. LEE, M.D. _____

The cardinal signs of peripheral arterial disease, which include intermittent claudication, rest pain, numbness, and coldness of the limbs, are absent in the spinal cord injured population. The physician thus faces the difficult challenge of identifying the patient with peripheral arterial disease at risk of development of gangrene in the absence of signs and symptoms. Additionally, the spinal cord injured patient is at high risk of development of venous disease in the form of venous thrombosis due to venous stasis. Fortunately for the physician responsible for the care of the spinal cord injured patient, a number of simple, noninvasive diagnostic techniques are available in screening for peripheral vascular disease.[1-3]

PERIPHERAL ARTERIAL DISEASE

Early detection and treatment of peripheral arterial disease often result in significant improvement of the patient's condition as well as prevention of untimely loss of a limb by amputation.

DOPPLER ULTRASOUND. When the peripheral arterial system is assessed in the spinal cord injured patient, Doppler ultrasound is typically used for the determination of two parameters: (1) segmental limb systolic pressures and (2) ankle systolic blood pressure relative to

brachial systolic blood pressure (reported as an ankle/brachial systolic pressure ratio known as the *ischemic index*).

In determination of ankle systolic blood pressure, a standard blood pressure cuff is placed proximal to the ankle with the Doppler probe over the posterior tibial or dorsalis pedis artery (Fig. 1–1). When the cuff is inflated, the

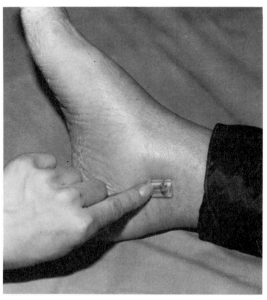

Figure 1–1. Technique of recording Doppler ultrasound waves.

From the Department of Surgery, Veterans Administration Medical Center, Castle Point, New York

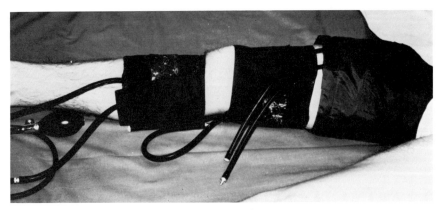

Figure 1–2. Cuffs placed for Doppler systolic blood pressure measurements.

audible blood flow signal gradually disappears; the pressure at which the audible blood flow signal returns as the cuff is slowly deflated is taken as the ankle systolic pressure. This pressure is then compared with the arm systolic pressure obtained in the standard manner with the Doppler probe replacing the stethoscope. In the absence of peripheral arterial disease, the obtained ratio (ischemic index) is 1.0 or greater; values less than 1.0 are indications of peripheral arterial disease—the lower the ischemic index, the more severe the disease. However, in the presence of severely hardened arteries associated with diabetes mellitus, the ischemic index may be greatly exaggerated.

The use of segmental limb systolic blood pressures can provide for localization and partial quantification of the arterial obstruction. Doppler systolic blood pressure is measured at the ankle with cuffs placed at the upper thigh, above the knee, at the mid-calf, and at the ankle (Fig. 1–2). Segmental systolic pressure readings at the upper thigh and above the knee are particularly important in distinguishing between aortoiliac, femoropopliteal, and combined disease. Normal thigh systolic blood pressure is about 30 mm Hg or more above the brachial systolic pressure; the above the knee, mid-calf, and ankle systolic pressures normally show a pressure gradient distally, with ankle systolic pressure approximating the brachial systolic blood pressure. The presence of extreme pressure drops between segments indicates occlusive disease between the segments.

PHOTOPLETHYSMOGRAPHY. The technique of photoplethysmography is particularly advantageous for the detection of small-vessel disease. With the placement of a standard blood pressure cuff at the ankle or metatarsal area and the photoplethysmograph probe located on the ventral surface of the toes, the point at which the pulsatile photoplethysmographic waveform returns as the cuff is slowly deflated indicates the ankle or metatarsal pressure (Fig. 1–3). The technique can be used to evaluate the blood supply of each digit and is particularly beneficial for the patient with gangrenous involvement of the toes when a decision has to be made about amputation. In the presence of a good metatarsal pressure, a surgeon could feel relatively confident of obtaining primary wound healing with amputation of the involved digit. The technique is also useful in detecting microembolization from an aneurysm or atheromatous plaque: Doppler segmental limb pressure may be normal down to the ankle, but the photoplethysmograph shows decreased metatarsal pressure caused by microembolization (Table 1–1).

IMPEDANCE PLETHYSMOGRAPHY. The technique of arterial impedance plethysmography is concerned with the detection of blood volume change in the limb. A constant high-fre-

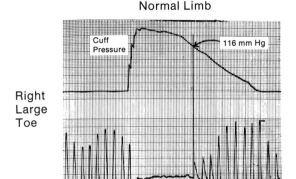

Figure 1–3. Digital blood pressure measurement on the toe with an ankle blood pressure cuff.

TABLE 1–1. Techniques for Detecting Microembolization

SEGMENTAL DOPPLER SYSTOLIC PRESSURES

	Right	Left
Brachial	122	112
High thigh	128 (1.1)	114 (1.02)
Above knee	128 (1.1)	118 (1.05)
Calf	126	90
Posterior tibial	124 (1.0)	100 (0.89)
Dorsal pedis	116 (0.95)	106 (0.95)

PHOTOPLETHYSMOGRAPHIC PRESSURES AT TOES

Toes	Right Ankle/Metatarsal	Left Ankle/Metatarsal
1	72/55	75/64
2	74/20	74/69
3	75/80	46/55
4	105/25	83/64
5	104/54	80/37

quency current is formed between two circumferential electrodes positioned on the limb (Fig. 1–4); resultant voltages are measured between two inner electrodes, and impedance waveforms are generated (Fig. 1–5). The impedance changes are due to segmental volume fluctuation. The shape of the waveform is dependent upon a number of physiologic factors such as the magnitude of ventricular contraction, blood vessel and limb tissue elasticity, and proximal and distal resistance. In the normal subject the impedance waveform is characterized by a steep systolic rise, a narrow peak, and a dicrotic notch on the diastolic down slope. In the presence of occlusive disease distal to the

measured segment, there is a prolongation of the waveform acceleration and deceleration, and a rounded peak. Proximal to an obstruction, the acceleration may be relatively normal; the peak, however, will be rounded and the deceleration portion of the curve prolonged.

ASSESSMENT OF THE MICROCIRCULATION. Increasing attention is being paid to evaluation of the microcirculation for assessments of tissue viability and wound healing potential. Two techniques that have generated considerable interest are transcutaneous oximetry and cutaneous fluorometry.

The measurement of *oxygen partial pressure transcutaneously* (TcPo$_2$), originally devised for use in pediatric intensive care, has been used primarily in assessing the optimal level of amputation. Details of the technique are available elsewhere.[4] Basically, a suitable current is applied between two polarographic electrodes composed of a platinum cathode and a silver anode immersed in an electrolyte and sealed by a semipermeable membrane. The current that results from the electrochemical reduction of oxygen in the electrolyte is proportional to the partial pressure of oxygen. A heating element in the electrode creates conditions of maximal hyperemia by local heating to temperatures within the range of 43°C to 45°C. The heat produced also alters the structure of the skin and enhances the skin's permeability to gases.[5] These factors produce a TcPo$_2$ value that approximates the partial pressure of oxygen in arterial blood. A number of additional factors influence the measurement of the TcPo$_2$ reading: blood perfusion, skin metabolism, the struc-

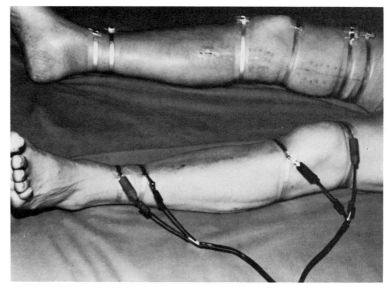

Figure 1–4. Electrode placement for impedance plethysmography.

Peripheral Impedance

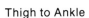

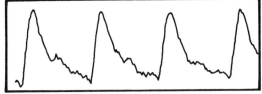

Thigh to Ankle

ACCELERATION = 3.61 OHM/SEC
ACCEL TIME = 136 MSEC
DECELERATION = 2.04 OHM/SEC
DECEL TIME = 181 MSEC
PEAK HEIGHT = 307.3 MOHMS

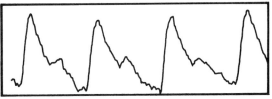

Below Knee

ACCELERATION = 1.94 OHM/SEC
ACCEL TIME = 136 MSEC
DECELERATION = 0.94 OHM/SEC
DECEL TIME = 209 MSEC
PEAK HEIGHT = 171.2 MOHMS

Figure 1–5. Impedance plethysmographic waveforms.

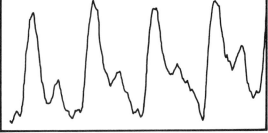

Popliteal Area

ACCELERATION = 0.68 OHM/SEC
ACCEL TIME = 158 MSEC
DECELERATION = 0.502 OHM/SEC
DECEL TIME = 185 MSEC
PEAK HEIGHT = 69.2 MOHMS

ture of the microcirculation, the consumption of oxygen by the electrode, the response time of the electrode, the tissue temperature profile, and the physiologic effects of hyperthermia.

In normal adult skin, $TcPo_2$ measurements are subject to considerable variation: at a level of 10 cm below the knee, $TcPo_2$ measurements have been reported to vary from 40 mm Hg[7] to 100 mm Hg.[8] In elderly subjects, a normal $TcPo_2$ below the knee is about 60 ± 10 mm Hg and should be about 10 mm Hg higher above the knee and about 10 mm Hg lower at the foot; in young subjects, $TcPo_2$ should be

about 5 mm Hg to 15 mm Hg higher than seen in elderly subjects.[5]

In patients with vascular disease, a significant gradient in $TcPo_2$ is seen as one measures distally on the leg, similar to the gradient seen in segmental Doppler systolic blood pressure measurements. The presence of mild ischemia may produce a $TcPo_2$ gradient similar to that seen in normal individuals, but in the presence of severe ischemia, an above-knee-to-foot $TcPo_2$ gradient of greater than 30 mm Hg has been reported.[2] The reduced $TcPo_2$ in ischemic limbs results primarily from the reduced arterial blood pressure and not a reduction in tissue $TcPo_2$.[9]

The transcutaneous measurement of oxygen partial pressure is simple and convenient, and, in contrast to segmental Doppler systolic blood pressure measurements, the measurement is not influenced by the calcification of arteries seen in diabetic patients.[10,11]

Cutaneous fluorometry has been shown to be useful in predicting viability of skin flaps[12] and assessing ischemia.[13] Administered intravenously, fluorescein is delivered to all perfused areas and diffuses into the extracellular fluid. When illuminated with ultraviolet light or blue light, adequately perfused areas fluoresce yellow-green. Originally judged qualitatively, the advent of quantitative measurements with a fluorometer has enhanced the usefulness of the technique. The device transmits blue light to excite the fluorescein and monitors the fluorescence from the fluorescein-stained tissue via a fiberoptic light guide. The instrumentation provides a quantitative measurement both of dye uptake and elimination by the perfused areas. Serial documentation is possible by subtracting residual fluorescence existing from a previous injection. The distribution of fluorescein dye correlates highly with gradations of skin perfusion and, ultimately, skin viability.[14]

Perfusion is determined by analysis on the basis of the kinetics of dye wash-in and wash-out from body tissues. Wash-in provides a more rapid measurement of perfusion provided that the readings are compensated for skin color. This is done by normalizing all fluorometric readings with those readings before dye infusion. Although the wash-out method provides absolute perfusion data unaffected by color, measurements are obtained more slowly, and the results can be distorted by poor kidney function.

The quantitative wash-in measurement, expressed in dye fluorescence units, is commonly reported as a percentage of the value obtained from a well-perfused region. In normal persons, a mean dye fluorescence index of about 77 is obtained. There is a trend to increasing index values as one proceeds distally from above the knee to the toes.[15] This gradient, however, has not been found to be significant. Discriminant analysis has established a dye fluorescence index of 40 for predicting skin viability: indexes greater than 42 accurately predict viability and indexes less than 38 accurately predict failure of an amputation to heal.[15]

The use of fluorescein can be relatively safe. Slow administration of a relatively low concentration dilute dose in resting patients is associated with fewer side effects than are seen following a more rapid injection or a larger dose or both.[15]

An additional technique that has recently been used is *cutaneous pressure photoplethysmography*.[16,17] The technique is based on localized perfusion pressure in cutaneous tissue. The instrumentation incorporates both pressure and photoplethysmographic monitoring devices within a hand-held probe. An infrared light source in the probe illuminates the surface of the skin, and light reflected back to the probe is modulated by changes in the volume of blood within the illuminated region. With increasing pressure, a level is reached at which pulsations cease. As pressure is reduced, the pressure at which pulsation returns is taken as the cutaneous perfusion pressure. It has been established that patients with cutaneous photoplethysmography pressures over 50 mm Hg at the dorsum of the foot achieve primary healing of their amputations.[17]

PERIPHERAL VENOUS DISEASE

The spinal cord injured patient is at particularly high risk of development of venous thrombosis of the lower extremity. Loss of movement in the lower extremity produces venous stasis because calf muscle movement no longer pumps venous blood proximally. Undetected and untreated, venous thrombosis can precipitate pulmonary emboli, an event associated with a high mortality rate.

COAGULATION DYNAMICS. The role of blood coagulation is being given increasing attention as a factor in peripheral vascular disease. Hypercoagulability, particularly when associated with the venous stasis characteristic of the spinal cord injured patient, is a major causative factor in the development of deep venous thrombosis. Monitoring coagulation dynamics has become a necessity. The technique of thromboelastography provides a measurement of dynamic changes in viscosity and elastic properties of a blood clot. The thromboelastogram provides a permanent graphic documentation of the various phases of the coagulation process.

Two types of instrumentation are available. In both, a piston is lowered into the patient's blood that has been placed in a rotating cuvette

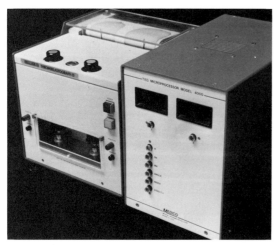

Figure 1-6. The thromboelastograph for measuring blood coagulation dynamics.

(Fig. 1-6). Initially, the blood is liquid and does not move the piston. The piston begins to rotate with the cuvette as the first fibrin strands begin to form. In the mechanical-optical system, the moving piston deflects a light source directed at light-sensitive film that begins to show a divergence of the original straight line into two curved lines corresponding to the oscillation of the cuvette. In the direct-writing system, the oscillations of the cuvette are transferred to a stylus that prints the thromboelastogram on heat-sensitive paper.

In the native whole blood thromboelastogram (Fig. 1-7), the first value obtained is the r time, or reaction time, in minutes (30 sec = 1 mm). This is the initial straight line of the tracing and represents the time from the initial drawing of the blood to the formation of the first fibrin strands. A normal r time is 8 to 12 minutes (16 to 24 mm). Alterations of production of plasma thromboplastin constituents or clotting factors XII, XI, IX, and VIII (first-stage factors of the intrinsic pathway) affect the r time. A shortened r time indicates hypercoagulability that can be associated with thrombosis, postoperative trauma, shock, or first-stage disseminated intravascular coagulation. A prolonged r time can be associated with an inherited defect in thromboplastin production such as hemophilia or an acquired defect such as seen during anticoagulation therapy.

The second value is the k value, which is the time from the initiation of the clot (the end of the r time) to a predefined level of clot strength, the point at which the diverging curved lines are 20 mm apart. The k value is a measure of the rapidity of clot development; a normal value is 4 to 8 minutes. The k value responds to intrinsic plasma and platelet factors, is nonresponsive to prothrombin complex factors, is prolonged in association with coagulation defects such as intrinsic factor deficiency, circulating anticoagulants, thrombocytopenia, and qualitative platelet defects, and is shortened in association with hypercoagulability.

The maximum amplitude, ma, which is the maximum distance between the two diverging lines, is a direct function of the maximum dynamic properties of fibrin and platelets; it is representative of the stiffness or strength of the clot. A normal ma value is approximately 50 mm. The maximum amplitude is affected by the dynamic properties of fibrin calcium, fibrin stabilizing factor, and platelet formation. A decreased ma is associated with thrombocytopenia, dextran therapy, anticoagulation therapy, qualitative platelet defects, and decreased fibrinogen levels. An increased ma is seen in hypercoagulability.

With celite-activated thromboelastography, the patient's blood is "activated" with celite, a chemical additive. Celite-activated thromboelastography (Fig. 1-8) involves a comparison between two simultaneous tracings: one nor-

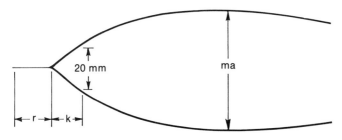

Figure 1-7. The native whole blood thromboelastogram.

r = reaction time (8 - 12 minutes)
k = coagulation time (4 - 8 minutes)
ma = maximum amplitude (50 mm)

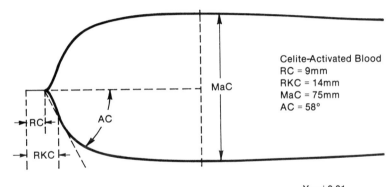

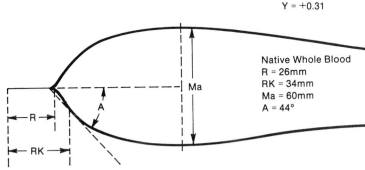

Celite-Activated Blood
RC = 9mm
RKC = 14mm
MaC = 75mm
AC = 58°

Y = +0.31

Native Whole Blood
R = 26mm
RK = 34mm
Ma = 60mm
A = 44°

Figure 1–8. The comparison of simultaneous tracings for celite-activated thromboelastography.

mal and one celite-activated sample. The first two measurements obtained are the R and RC values expressed in millimeters as the distance from the first mark to a point where the diverging lines are 2 mm apart. RK and RKC values are a combination of the r and k values of native whole blood thromboelastography. Ma and MaC are identical to the maximum amplitude of the native whole blood thromboelastography. The angle, a parameter unique to the celite-activated technique, is indicative of the rate of clot stiffening and reflects the rate and quality of developing fibrin and platelet aggregates. The measurements obtained from celite-activated thromboelastography are analyzed using the following equation:

$$Y = A_1 + A_2 + R + A_3RK + A_4Ma$$
$$+ A_5A + A_6RC + A_7RKC$$
$$+ A_8MaC + A_9AC$$

where:

$A_1 = -55.55$ $A_4 = -0.03816$ $A_7 = +1.966$
$A_2 = +0.386$ $A_5 = -0.1639$ $A_8 = +0.17321$
$A_3 = -0.508$ $A_6 = -2.088$ $A_9 = +0.877$

A Y value between -5 and $+1.5$ is normal; greater than $+2$ is indicative of hypercoagulability, and less than -5 is indicative of hypocoagulability. In native whole blood thromboelastography, hypercoagulability is characterized by a shortened r time and k value and an increased ma. This is indicative of a rapidly forming clot that develops a high degree of stiffness. Hypocoagulability is characterized by a prolonged r time and k value and a decreased ma indicative of a slow-forming clot that attains a low degree of stiffness. Such a tracing would be obtained during heparin therapy.

IMPEDANCE PLETHYSMOGRAPHY. This noninvasive test measures the changes in the electrical conductivity of the leg caused by obstruction of venous outflow. The technique noninvasively quantitates venous capacitance and venous outflow. From the impedance plethysmogram (Fig. 1–9) one can measure the increase in venous volume following inflation of a pneumatic cuff placed around the lower thigh. The maximum venous outflow is measured as the decrease in volume during the first 3 seconds following release of the occluding cuff. Alternatively, the venous capacitance can be calculated and used with the maximum venous outflow to score the patient's venous hemodynamics (Fig. 1–9). The mathematical relationships for impedance plethysmography are:[18]

$$Z_0 = \frac{\rho L}{A} = \frac{\rho L^2}{V}$$

$$\Delta Z_0 = \frac{-\rho L^2}{V^2} \Delta V$$

Venous Impedance Plethysmography

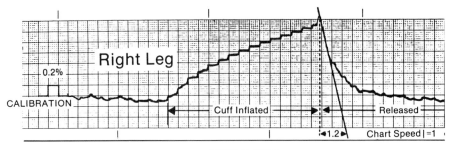

IPG Calculation

$$\frac{(\text{Rise}) \ (\text{Chart Speed})}{\text{Run}} \quad \text{X Calibration} = \% \text{ Volume Change/Sec.}$$

$$\frac{(50\text{mm}) \ (1 \text{ cm/Sec})}{1.2 \text{ cm}} \quad \text{X} \quad \frac{0.2\%}{5\text{mm}} \quad = 1.66\%/\text{Sec.}$$

Figure 1–9. Tracings and calculations for venous impedance plethysmography.

where:

Z_0 = baseline impedance (ohms),
ΔZ_0 = change in impedance with V,
ΔV = change in volume (cc),
ρ = resistivity of limb (150 ohm cm),
L = distance between measuring electrodes (cm),
A = cross-sectional area of limb (cm²),
V = A·L (cc).

Dividing the above equation for ΔZ_0 by that for Z_0, and by the time interval ΔT, yields the change in blood volume per unit time and per unit volume of tissue:

$$\frac{\Delta V/\Delta T}{V} = \frac{-\Delta Z_0/Z_0}{\Delta T} \text{ ml/sec/cc tissue.}$$

Multiplying by 6000 converts to the conventional reflux units of ml/min/100 cc tissue.

If the initial test results are abnormal or equivocal, the test should be repeated three times in succession with the best result of the tests being used for interpretation. This test will not detect the presence of hemodynamically insignificant thrombi or small isolated calf thrombi. The presence of extensive collateral formation or recanalization of a long-standing clot may lead to a false-negative result.

Impedance plethysmography can also be used to differentiate primary from secondary varicose veins and to quantitate venous reflux. We can consider the venous system as two separate venous reservoirs, one within the calf muscle and the other within the subcutaneous tissue (Fig. 1–10). These reservoirs communicate through numerous perforating veins, in-

cluding the long and short saphenous veins. The saphenous veins however are unique in that they empty directly into the major deep veins with no direct communication with the veins within the calf muscle pump. The outflow tract of the calf muscle is the popliteal vein.

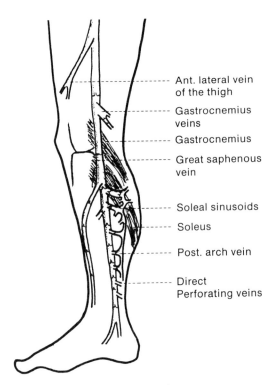

Ant. lateral vein of the thigh
Gastrocnemius veins
Gastrocnemius
Great saphenous vein
Soleal sinusoids
Soleus
Post. arch vein
Direct Perforating veins

Figure 1–10. The venous system has two separate reservoirs, one within the calf muscle and the other within the subcutaneous tissue.

Contraction of the calf muscle normally forces blood into the popliteal/femoral vein only. Upon relaxation, the pressure is higher and blood is forced into the deep system through communicating veins.

In the case of valvular incompetency of the long saphenous vein there is retrograde blood flow during exercise, while the valves in the communicating veins and the pump outflow tract within the calf muscles are normal. The calf pump can compensate for the superficial reservoir with only a minor degree of insufficiency. Clinically this is reflected as varicose veins, mild aching pain in the legs, and slight edema of the ankle.

In the case of incompetent valves in the communicating veins, blood is forced directly into the superficial veins during muscle contraction. Thus the pressure in the superficial veins does not fall during exercise, and the symptoms are more serious: ankle edema, skin pigmentation, eczema, and sometimes ulceration of the skin overlying the incompetent communicating veins.

With stenosis or valvular incompetence in the outflow tract, the calf pump is unable to empty during calf muscle contraction. The high pressure generated within the pump causes dilation of the communicating veins and secondary valvular incompetence. If there is obstruction in the outflow tract, pressures may rise during exercise, producing severe symptoms: constant aching pain, venous claudication, skin pigmentation, eczema, lipodermatosclerosis, ulceration, and, in rare cases, fibrous ankylosis of the ankle joint.

To differentiate primary from secondary varicose veins, the patient's legs are placed in a dependent position with impedence electrodes attached to the calf; a pneumatic boot is placed over the calf, inflated to 60 mm Hg, allowed to stabilize, and then rapidly released. The test is repeated with a tourniquet placed above the knee to occlude the superficial venous system. The initial test done without the tourniquet provides a measure of total venous reflux; the second with the tourniquet in place provides a measure of deep venous reflux. By subtracting the deep venous reflux value from the value for total venous reflux, one obtains a measure of the superficial venous reflux. Normal venous reflux refilling time is less than 20.0 ml/100 cc. A patient's varicosities would be designated as primary if application of the tourniquet reduced the reflux to within normal range (less than 20 ml/min/100 cc) and designated as secondary if the reflux value was abnormal

(greater than 20 ml/min/100 cc) both with and without the tourniquet.

PHLEBORHEOGRAPHY. This technique is based on the fact that rhythmic respiration will cause variations in venous pressure and volume and that such variations can be recorded from the lower extremity. Air-filled cuffs are placed around the thorax and at several levels of the lower extremity to apply compression and record transmitted impulses. An absence of significant reduction in the waveform size indicates the presence of an acute episode of deep vein thrombosis. In the presence of a long-standing thrombus, the waveforms are present but are typically smaller and have a rounded peak as opposed to normal. Distal compression will give momentary pooling of the blood in the presence of deep venous thrombosis. By examination of the baseline for recordings taken at different levels, the location of a thrombus can be identified. In normal persons, calf compression will cause a fall in the baseline. The technique is highly sensitive for detecting proximal vein thrombosis.

RADIOACTIVE FIBRINOGEN UPTAKE. This technique is perhaps the most sensitive test for the detection of a developing thrombus or one that is extending or lysing. Briefly, radio-labeled fibrin is injected into a peripheral vein and is then incorporated into the developing thrombosis. The radioactive fibrin thus incorporated into the developing clot can be detected noninvasively. After administration, the first screening is done at 2 hours to allow for the removal of any denatured fibrinogen and for equilibrium between intravascular and extravascular fibrinogen. The screening can then be done every 24 hours. Radioactivity counts from the lower extremities are expressed as a percentage of the radioactivity count obtained over the heart. The percentage should remain relatively constant as radioactivity should be washed out of the heart and lower extremities at the same rate. Realistically, however, there is a slight increase that should not exceed 2 per cent per day as a result of the greater rates of extravascular fibrinogen in the leg than in the heart. Deep venous thrombosis is determined to be present if there is a 20 per cent or more increase in radioactivity at the same position on two different days.

This technique is not specific for the presence of deep venous thrombosis. Increased radioactivity counts are also seen in the presence of superficial thrombophlebitis, hematoma, ulceration, arthritis, cellulitis, or fractures and wounds. The technique will not detect the presence of thrombus in the groin or pelvic areas due to the high background radioactivity of the bladder.

DOPPLER ULTRASOUND. This technique monitors the velocity of blood flow in the veins. A spontaneous signal should be obtained from all patent deep veins of the leg. The technique's accuracy depends heavily on the skill and experience of the technician.

The velocity patterns of the lower extremity's veins reflect the periodic changes in intra-abdominal pressure due to breathing. Velocity flow signals that vary with breathing and are interrupted by a deep breath indicate vein patency proximal to the probe. When the flow is unchanged by a deep inspiration, the vein proximal to the probe is obstructed. Deep venous occlusion can cause the flow velocity signal in the superficial veins to be greatly increased compared with the contralateral limb.

In the normal, patent vein, compression of the extremity distal to the probe produces an increased velocity signal. An increased flow signal is seen with release of the compression. With placement of the Doppler probe over the popliteal vein, compression proximal to the probe causes blood flow toward the probe if the venous valves are incompetent. With the probe positioned over the posterior tibial vein during compression of the calf muscles, a back-and-forth flow velocity signal will be seen with compression and release in the presence of incompetent venous valves. Flow reversal in the femoral vein can be detected during quiet respiration when the patient is tilted to the head-up position; with the probe over the saphenous vein, back-and-forth reflux sounds can be detected in the presence of incompetent valves by running the finger distally over the course of the vein.

The Compartment Syndrome and Pressure Measurement

In the compartment syndrome, swelling within a limb due to hemorrhage, edema, or other pathology of soft tissue is constrained within an anatomic space whose walls consist of fascia. The ischemia resulting from the pressure creates a progressive cycle of swelling, further ischemia, and tissue damage. Diagnosis and monitoring of pressures in the compartment is frequently done by insertion of a Wich or Stryker catheter directly into the compartment, because clinical signs are unreliable in predicting catastrophic tissue damage.

The compartment syndrome is encountered in traumatic injuries of the limbs and in surgical treatment of large-vessel disease utilizing vascular grafts (i.e., the revascularization compartment syndrome). It can also be induced by strenuous training in young adults. Permanent neuromuscular damage and possible loss of a limb can occur when diagnosis and treatment are delayed. Surgical fasciotomy is a treatment that requires accurate diagnosis because the treatment poses risks of infection and healing problems.

Direct pressure measurements are invasive and add to patient risk and discomfort. A non-invasive approach to monitoring the compartment syndrome consists of observing changes in the bulk viscoelastic properties of the limb that will occur with the compartment syndrome. A platform of large surface area rests lightly on the surface of the skin and serves as a reference for tissue displacement. A centrally located indenter is used to apply pressure, and both pressure and displacement are recorded directly above a limb compartment. The observed pressure-volume displacement relationship shows both elastic and viscous components. The increase in compartmental pressure becomes higher, and the bulk limb tissue becomes more nearly pure elastic. The use of matched sites provides controls by which to account for differences among subjects in fat content and muscle tone.

REFERENCES

1. Rutherford RB: Vascular Surgery, 2nd ed.. Philadelphia, W.B. Saunders, 1984.
2. Greenhalgh RM: Diagnostic Techniques and Assessment Procedures in Vascular Surgery. Orlando, Grune & Stratton, 1985.
3. Bernstein EF: Noninvasive Diagnostic Techniques in Vascular Disease. St. Louis, C.V. Mosby, 1985.
4. Hebrank DR: Noninvasive transcutaneous oxygen monitoring, a review. J Clin Eng 6:41, 1981.
5. Spence VA, McCollum PT: Evaluation of the ischemic limb by transcutaneous oximetry. *In* McGreenhalgh RM (ed): Diagnostic Techniques and Assessment Procedures in Vascular Surgery. Orlando, Grune and Stratton, 1985, pp 331–341.
6. Eberhard P, Mindt W, Kreuger R: Cutaneous oxygen monitoring in the newborn. Pediatrician 5:335, 1976.
7. Franyeck UK, Talke P, Bernstein EF, et al: Transcutaneous PO_2 measurements in health and peripheral arterial occlusive disease. Surgery 91:156–163, 1982.
8. Mustapha NM, Redhead RG, Jain SK, et al: Transcutaneous partial oxygen pressure assessment of the ischemic lower limb. Surg Gynecol Obstet 156:582–584, 1983.

9. Eickoff JH, Engell HC: Transcutaneous oxygen tension (TcPO$_2$) measurements on the foot in normal subjects and in patients with peripheral vascular disease admitted for vascular surgery. Scand J Clin Lab Invest 41:743–748, 1981.

10. Wyss CR, Masten FS, Simmins CW, Burgess EM: Transcutaneous oxygen tension measurements on limbs of diabetic and nondiabetic patients with peripheral vascular disease. Surgery 95:339–346, 1984.

11. Karanfiliam RG, Lynch TG, Zirul VT, et al: The value of laser Doppler velocimetry and transcutaneous oxygen tension determination in predicting healing of ischemic forefoot ulcerations and amputations in diabetic and nondiabetic patients. J Vasc Surg 4:511–516, 1986.

12. McCraw JD, Meyers B, Shanklin KD: The value of fluorescein in predicting the viability of arterialized flaps. Plast Reconstr Surg 60:710–719, 1977.

13. Lowry K: Evaluation of peripheral vascular disease using intraarterial fluorescein. Am Surg 30:35–39, 1964.

14. Silverman DG, Noran KJ, Brousseau DA: Serial fluorometric documentation of flourescein dye delivery. Surgery 97:185–192, 1985.

15. Silverman DG, Roberts A, Reilly CA, et al: Fluorometric quantification of low-dose fluorescein delivery to predict amputation site healing. Surgery 101:335–341, 1987.

16. Lee BY, Thoden WR, Madden JL, McCann WJ: Cutaneous pressure photoplethysmography: A new technique for noninvasive evaluation of peripheral arterial disease. Cont Surg 25:39–43, 1984.

17. Lee BY, Ostrander L, Thoden WR, Madden JL: Use of cutaneous pressure plethysmography in managing peripheral vascular occlusive disease. Cont Surg 30:58–67, 1987.

18. Webster, JG: Measurement of flow and volume of blood. In Medical Instrumentation. Boston, Houghton-Mifflin, 1978, p. 421.

Deep Venous Thrombosis in Spinal Cord Injured Patients

2

BOK Y. LEE, M.D.

Deep venous thrombosis and pulmonary embolism are major health problems and result in significant mortality and morbidity. In the United States it has been estimated that deep venous thrombosis and pulmonary embolism are associated with 300,000 to 600,000 hospitalizations yearly and up to 50,000 deaths each year.[1] The spinal cord injured patient is at particularly high risk for the development of deep venous thrombosis.[2-6] In these patients, the loss of the active calf muscle pump in the paralyzed limbs significantly reduces blood flow velocity. Additionally, blood flow and volume is unsteady, vascular tone is abnormal and directly dependent upon local and regional stimulation, and the capability of the vascular system to adjust to such conditions as muscular exercise and thermoregulation is lost.[7] The consequent sluggishness of venous return is further exacerbated by hypercoagulability associated with spinal cord injury.[3] When coupled with the pressure exerted by the bed on the calf muscles, this sluggishness puts the bedridden spinal cord injured patient at high risk for the development of deep venous thrombosis.

Reports on the incidence of deep venous thrombosis in the spinal cord injured patient during the first few weeks following injury vary widely. Similar variance is seen with the incidence of pulmonary embolism. Just as reports in the literature differ as to the incidence of deep venous thrombosis from the particular institution, the incidence also varies among patients at any one study site. Watson[5] found an 81 per cent incidence of deep venous thrombosis in 431 spinal cord injured patients with complete lesions versus 8 per cent in patients with incomplete lesions. Similarly, patients with dorsal lesions had a 23 per cent incidence of deep venous thrombosis compared with 12 per cent in patients with cervical lesions. It is of interest to note that Watson[5] found that the time to onset of deep venous thrombosis was one month following the injury to the spinal cord in a large majority of patients (72 per cent); the incidence dropped off precipitously after one month to 12 per cent at two months after injury and 14 per cent at three months after injury. More importantly, Watson[5] found pulmonary embolism to occur at the same time as the deep vein thrombosis (i.e., the pulmonary embolism occurred without warning) in 45 per cent of patients. At 1, 2, 4, and 8 weeks after the diagnosis of the deep vein thrombosis, the incidence of pulmonary embolism was 14, 18, 14, and 9 per cent, respectively.

A significant reduction in mortality from pulmonary embolism has not been seen in spite of available therapy. As shown by Watson,[5] 45 per cent of pulmonary emboli in a series of spinal cord injured patients occurred without warning. It is readily apparent that the best treatment of pulmonary embolism is prophylaxis—that is, prevention of deep venous thrombosis.[1]

PATHOGENESIS OF DEEP VENOUS THROMBOSIS

Three factors contribute to the development of deep venous thrombosis: venous stasis, hypercoagulability, and vessel injury.

12

Venous Stasis

A natural antithrombotic effect is exerted by the flow of blood through a vessel. The natural flow of blood accomplishes several objectives: (1) it dilutes locally activated clotting factors; (2) in areas of clotting factor activation, the normal flow of blood renews circulating inhibitors of the clotting mechanism; and (3) the normal flow of blood, by means of its limitation of red blood cell aggregation, maintains normal blood viscosity.[9] In the presence of venous stasis, both volume and velocity of blood flow are decreased. Although the precise mechanism of the formation of a thrombus due to venous stasis is uncertain,[9] it is clear that once thrombus formation is initiated, the thrombus develops rapidly and grows and may extend into the lumen of the vessel, promoting further stasis.

Immobility is the most common precipitating factor in the development of venous thrombosis. In patients undergoing surgery, clearance times for the leg veins have been shown to be significantly slower in anesthetized patients than those in awake patients.[10] The parallel to the spinal cord injured patient is obvious.

In the lower limbs, the deep paired veins are embedded in the thick calf muscles, which, in turn, are surrounded by the strong crural fascia. This arrangement enables the calf to function as a pump during contraction of the calf muscles. The contraction of the calf muscles compresses the veins, emptying them proximally. Repetitive contraction results in an emptying of the deep veins. Thus, in an immobile patient, the absence of the calf muscle pump promotes the development of venous stasis.

Hypercoagulability

The concept of hypercoagulability, i.e., a state of circulating blood that is more readily coagulable than normal,[8] is not well understood. In patients undergoing surgical procedures, postoperative changes in platelets, coagulation proteins, and fibrinolytic activity have been identified as factors that may lead to thrombosis.[11] Similar changes have been noted in nonsurgical patients with thrombosis, but a cause-and-effect relationship has not been established.[9]

Functionally, hypercoagulability can be divided into two categories: tissue injury and impaired defense mechanism.[8] Tissue injury is an initiator of thrombosis in activating the coagulation sequence, and an impaired defense mechanism facilitates thrombosis. This includes deficiencies of antithrombin III, proteins C and S, and heparin cofactor II; the presence of a high concentration of inhibitors of plasminogen activator; presence of defective plasminogen or a low fibrinolytic response; the administration of estrogen; and impaired blood flow.[8]

Vessel Injury

The endothelium of the blood vessel is important in preventing thrombus formation because it contains several antithrombotic substances such as tissue plasminogen activator and prostacyclin and a number of glycosaminoglycans.[9] Damage to the endothelium resulting in the exposure of the subendothelium may provide a stimulus for thrombus formation as platelets adhere, aggregate, and release the contents of their secretory granules, leading to thrombin formation, local activation of coagulation factors, and clot formation.[12]

PREVENTION OF DEEP VENOUS THROMBOSIS

A number of modalities are available for prevention of deep venous thrombosis, including adjusted-dose heparin, low-dose heparin, warfarin, dextran, external pneumatic compression, and pressure-gradient elastic stockings. The recent National Institutes of Health Consensus Development Conference on the Prevention of Venous Thrombosis and Pulmonary Embolism, however, reported that external pneumatic compression and pressure-gradient elastic stockings are "the methods of choice" for prophylaxis in patients with head injury and acute spinal cord injury.[1] External pneumatic compression is recommended over stockings, however, as pressure-gradient stockings have not been adequately studied and "must be carefully fitted if they are to have prophylactic merit."[1] Indeed, external pneumatic compression is recommended for use in most high-risk patient groups.

Our own work using external pneumatic compression[13–16] has shown it to be most effective in preventing postoperative deep venous thrombosis in general surgical patients[13–15] as well as the recognized high-risk group of patients undergoing hip replacement or hip fracture repair.[16]

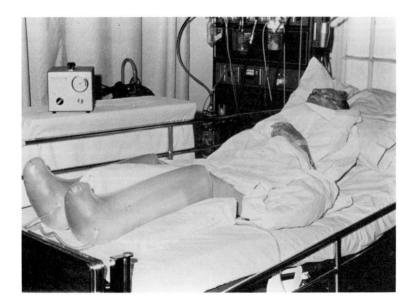

Figure 2–1. The external pneumatic compression system in use. The system is fitted to the patient by a technician, who ensures the proper functioning of the system.

Protocol for Use of External Pneumatic Compression

Before the use of external intermittent pneumatic compression, the patient is screened using venous impedence plethysmography to determine the patency of the venous system. (The procedure for this test is discussed elsewhere in this text.) The recording of a positive impedance plethysmogram, indicating the possible presence of pre-existing thrombosis, is a contraindication to the use of the system. Resolution of the pre-existing thrombosis is required before use of external pneumatic compression. The external pneumatic compression system is fitted to the patient (Fig. 2–1) by a

technician, who ensures the proper functioning of the system. The system can then be used continuously. During continuous use, the nursing staff can remove the system for routine skin care. If the system is discontinued for a period exceeding 30 minutes, an impedance plethysmogram should be obtained before the system is replaced.

Operation of the System

The external pneumatic compression system is completely noninvasive and designed to reduce the risk of deep venous thrombosis by simulating calf muscle contraction. The system (Fig. 2–2) consists of an easily portable pneu-

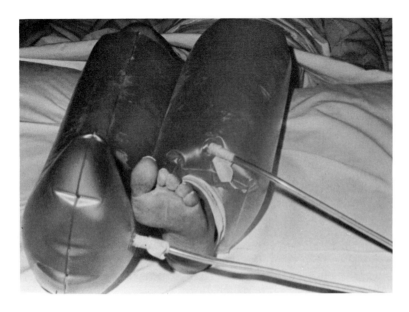

Figure 2–2. The external pneumatic compression system consists of an easily portable pneumatic compressor and paired, double-walled inflatable plastic boots or sleeves.

Canine Study — Augmentation of
Venous Flow during Boot Inflation

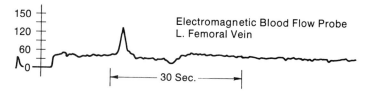

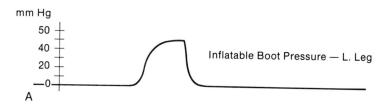

Figure 2–3. Experimental studies in the canine (A), primate (B), and human (C) using intraoperative electromagnetic flowmetry have shown external pneumatic compression to impart a pulsatile component to venous blood flow.

A

Primate Study — Augmentation of
Venous Flow during Boot Inflation

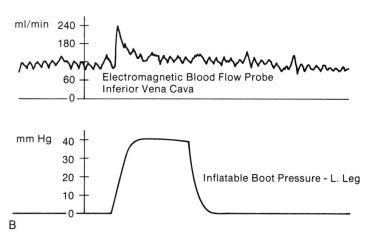

B

Augmentation of Venous Flow during Surgical Boot Inflation

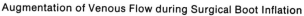

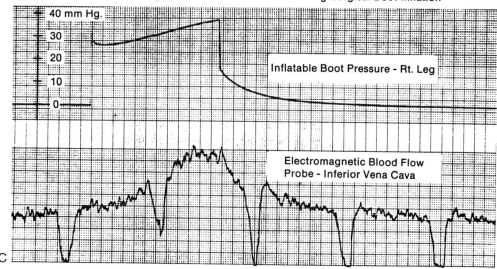

C

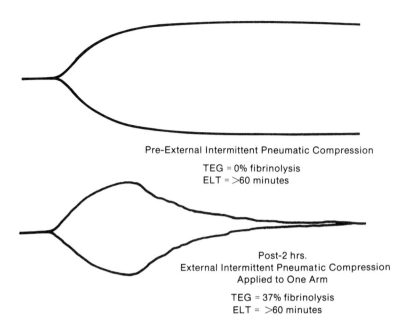

Pre-External Intermittent Pneumatic Compression

TEG = 0% fibrinolysis
ELT = >60 minutes

Post-2 hrs.
External Intermittent Pneumatic Compression
Applied to One Arm

TEG = 37% fibrinolysis
ELT = >60 minutes

Figure 2–4. Studies using thromboelastography have shown external pneumatic compression to enhance the naturally occurring fibrinolytic activity of the venous system.

matic compressor and paired, double-walled inflatable plastic boots or sleeves. The system's pneumatic compressor provides a rhythmic cycle of inflation and deflation that yields an intermittent compression of the calf muscle. While the system is inflated, the patient's legs float comfortably on an evenly distributed cushion of air.

The controls of the system's pneumatic compressor consist of a single on-off switch and a dial for control of the inflation pressure. During operation, there is a standard 12 sec compression and 48 sec decompression cycle. An inflation pressure of 40 to 45 mm Hg has been found to produce sufficient emptying of the calf veins. The system operates with any air source of 35 to 136 psig. The effectiveness of the system is due to both mechanical and biomechanical effects.

Mechanical Effect of External Pneumatic Compression

We have shown external intermittent pneumatic compression to impart a pulsatile component to venous blood flow in mimicking calf muscle contraction.[13] In studies on canines and primates, intraoperative electromagnetic flowmeter studies have shown pulsatile flow in the canine femoral vein (Fig. 2–3A) and primate inferior vena cava (Fig. 2–3B) that coincided with the 12 sec compression phase of the cycle. Similar results have been recorded in humans (Fig. 2–3C). During a major abdominal surgi-

cal procedure, an electromagnetic flow probe placed around the inferior vena cava (with the external pneumatic compression system on the lower extremities) recorded a pulsatile component in the venous flow with little or no net increase in mean venous return.

Biochemical Effect of External Pneumatic Compression

A study by Hills et al.[17] found that the protection against deep venous thrombosis afforded by external pneumatic compression was not apparent in patients with malignancies. This suggested a factor other than the mechanical effects of mimicking calf muscle contraction contributes to the system's prophylactic effect. A subsequent study by Allenby et al.[18] found an increase in fibrinolytic activity to be associated with the use of external pneumatic compression. Using thromboelastography (Fig. 2–4), we have quantitatively demonstrated enhanced fibrinolytic activity with external pneumatic compression.[19] In 50 patients who had external pneumatic compression applied to one arm for two hours, 62 per cent showed a quantitative increase in fibrinolytic activity ranging from 8 to 116 per cent (mean ± s.d. = 245 ± 286 per cent). It is possible that external pneumatic compression, by means of its producing a transient period of venous occlusion and/or simulating calf muscle exercise, causes a release of plasminogen activators into the blood stream.[18,19]

REFERENCES

1. Consensus Conference: Prevention of venous thrombosis and pulmonary embolism. JAMA 256:744–749, 1986.
2. Perkash A, Perkash V, Perkash I: Experience with management of thromboembolism in patients with spinal cord injury. Part I. Incidence, diagnosis and rate of some risk factors. Paraplegia 16:322–331, 1978–1979.
3. Todd JW, Frisbie JH, Rossier AB, et al: Deep venous thrombosis in acute spinal cord injury: Comparison of ^{125}I fibrinogen leg scanning, impedance plethysmography and venography. Paraplegia 14:50–57, 1976.
4. Van Hove E: Prevention of thrombophlebitis in spinal cord injury patients. Paraplegia 16:332–335, 1978–1979.
5. Watson N: Venous thrombosis and pulmonary embolism in spinal cord injury. Paraplegia 16:113–121, 1978–1979.
6. Watson N: Anticoagulant therapy in prevention of venous thrombosis and pulmonary embolism in spinal cord injury. Paraplegia 16:265–269, 1978–1979.
7. Bidart Y, Maury M: The circulatory behaviour in complete chronic paraplegia. Paraplegia 11:1–24, 1973.
8. Wessler S: Prevention of venous thromboembolism: rationale, practice, and problems. Prevention of Venous Thrombosis and Pulmonary Embolism, National Institutes of Health Consensus Development Conference, March 24–26, 1986, pp. 15–18.
9. Peterson CW: Venous thrombosis: An overview. Pharmacotherapy 6 (Suppl.):12S–17S, 1986.
10. Lewis CE, Mueller C, Edwards SW: Venous stasis on the operating table. Am J Surg 124:780–784, 1972.
11. Bergquist D: Postoperative thromboembolism: Frequency, etiology, prophylaxis. New York, Springer-Verlag, 1983, pp. 35–50.
12. Baumgartner HR, Muggli R, Tschopp TB, Turritto VT: Platelet adhesion, release and aggregation in flowing blood—effects of surface properties and platelet function. Thromb Haemost 35:124–138, 1976.
13. Lee BY, Madden J, Trainor FS, et al: Detection and prevention of deep vein thrombosis in the general surgical patient. In Madden JL, Hume M (eds): Venous Thromboembolism: Prevention and Treatment. Appleton-Century-Crofts, 1976, pp. 61–90.
14. Lee BY, Thoden WR, Trainor FS, Kavner D: Non-invasive detection and prevention of deep vein thrombosis in the geriatric patient. J Am Geriatr Soc 28:171–175, 1980.
15. Lee BY, Trainor FS, Kavner D, et al: Noninvasive prevention of thrombosis of deep veins of the thigh using intermittent pneumatic compression. Surg Gynecol Obstet 142:705–714, 1976.
16. Lee BY, Sarabu MR, Thoden WR, et al: Intermittent pneumatic compression in the prevention of deep vein thrombosis following hip replacement or fracture. Contemp Orthoped 2:585–588, 1980.
17. Hills NH, Pflug JJ, Jeyashingh K, et al: Prevention of deep vein thrombosis by intermittent pneumatic compression of the calf. Br Med J 1:131–135, 1972.
18. Allenby F, Boardman L, Pflug JJ, Calnan JS: Effects of external pneumatic compression of fibrinolysis in man. Lancet 2:1412–1414, 1975.
19. Lee BY, Thoden WR, Sarabu MR, et al: Fibrinolytic activity of intermittent pneumatic compression. Contemp Surg 18:77–79, 82, 86, 1981.
20. Gore RM, Mintzer RA, Calenoff L: Gastrointestinal complications of spinal cord injury. Spine 6:538–544, 1981.
21. Miller LS, Staas WE, Herbison GJ: Abdominal problems in patients with spinal cord lesions. Arch Phys Med Rehabil 56:405–408, 1975.

Acute Abdomen in Spinal Cord Injured Patients

3

WILLIAM BOND, M.D.

A great challenge exists in the diagnosis of an acute abdomen in the spinal cord injured patient. Typical findings may be missing or misleading. Because of delayed diagnosis and misdiagnosis, the mortality rates for an acute abdomen in these patients still stands at 10 to 15 per cent.[1] Timely diagnosis and management is based on an understanding of the level of spinal cord injury and whether this is complete (no movement or sensation below the level of injury) or incomplete. By way of example, we shall present 20 cases from our last 20 years of experience of abdominal surgery in spinal cord injury patients.

LEVEL OF INJURY

There are three major levels of injury to the spinal cord. Within these regions there may be variations of somatic and autonomic innervations. Completeness or incompleteness of the injury may mean that typical findings are absent or modified; incomplete lesions usually produce a response more likely to lead to localization and a timely diagnosis.

Lesions below T11 and T12 spare the splanchnic outflow tract, with the abdominal wall skin and musculature innervations usually left intact. In such patients, the presentation of abdominal disease is the same as in the patient with an intact spinal cord.[2] Lesions of the lower thoracic cord from T10 to T12 interrupt somatic sensation below the level of injury. Visceral sensations, however, may enter the posterior root and travel several levels above this cord injury, using the sympathetic chain, or they may travel an accessory vagal pathway.

Usually, innervations of the abdominal wall, bladder, and distal colon[3] undergo extensive alterations. High cord lesions above T5 block both the splanchnic outflow tract and impulses involving the abdominal wall muscles and skin.

SIGNS AND SYMPTOMS

In the initial injury period, spinal shock causes an absence of reflexive activity below the cord lesion. There can be a paucity of signs and symptoms: flaccid paralysis of the abdominal wall muscles may completely mask peritonitis; shock is often the initial presentation of perforated or gangrenous lesions.[1] A high index of suspicion must be maintained during the period of spinal shock to avoid the high mortality associated with a delay in diagnosis.

After the period of spinal shock, reflexive arcs are re-established below the level of injury. A number of signs and symptoms must be borne in mind, especially for high cord lesions above T5. Anorexia, nausea, and a vague feeling of being unwell are early clues of possible abdominal involvement. The patient feels "restless."[1,2] Abdominal pain is described as dull and not localized. This is believed to be due to slow conduction velocities of unmyelinated class C fibers of distal-to-injury reflex area. In contrast, pain associated with radiculopathy is described as sharp, burning, and often bilateral, with pinprick hypersensitivity. Referred pain may be based on innervations that share a common or similar embryologic origin: the diaphragm can refer pain to the neck and shoulder (Fig. 3–1), the stomach to the intra-

18

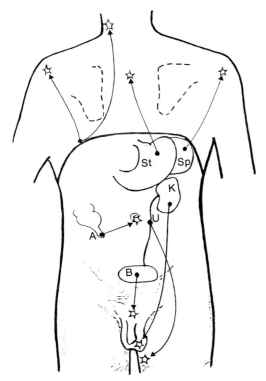

Figure 3–1. Examples of referred pain locations.

out bradycardia is caused by bladder, bowel, and peritoneal reflexive arcs. Patients usually complain of a severe headache. Although a nonsurgical cause such as distended bladder is more common, this can be an important clue if other symptoms and signs are present.

Fever may simply be a response to ambient conditions, such as a thermostat-controlled airbed. A high, spiking fever above 39°C usually indicates a genitourinary infection, while lower ranges of fever may be associated with abdominal events.[5,6] "Quadriplegic fever" almost always has a definite cause.[1,5]

Initial laboratory studies of the spinal cord injured patient with a possible acute abdomen usually include CBC with differential, serum chemistries, and urine studies. These are most helpful if baseline studies are available. Chest x-ray, flat plate of the abdomen, and intravenous pyelogram (IVP) have also proven to be quite useful as part of the initial work-up[3] allowing differentiation among abdominal, genitourinary, or supradiaphragmatic pathology.[7]

Cleansing of the bowel using cathartics or enemas is not needed before initial IVP studies. Chronic constipation and impaction makes evaluation difficult and sometimes dangerous.

scapular area, the spleen to the shoulder, the appendix to the umbilicus, the kidney to the testes, the ureter to the inner thigh, and the bladder to the perineum.[8]

Abdominal distention with dilated loops of bowel is common in spinal cord injured patients. Unless there is progression or other signs and symptoms, it alone may not be of great significance. Increased spasticity of the abdominal wall muscles may make palpation of the abdomen difficult or impossible. Although tenderness is usually absent, it may herald a perforated bladder or viscus or other emergency event. Abdominal masses, when palpable, may be due to chronic constipation. Even neurogenic bowel dysfunction can cause problems involving distention and discomfort that mimic an acute abdomen.

Diarrhea and urinary incontinence may be reflexive activity of an abdominal process, via reflexive arcs to the bladder and distal colon. Reflexive activity causes a rise in pulse, respiration rate and blood pressure. These alone are frequently seen in the stabilized spinal cord injured patient without surgical pathology. Autonomic hyperreflexia is mostly associated with abdominal emergencies in patients with high cord lesions above the splanchnic outflow tract.[1] The transient hypertension with or with-

ILLUSTRATIVE CASES

CASE 1.

This 30-year-old male incomplete quadriplegic at the C6 level presented with a one-day history of nausea. Bowel sounds were hyperactive, the abdomen was distended, and a dull pain was localized to the right lower quadrant. Vital signs included pulse rate of 80 to 90 bpm, temperature of 99.4°F, and blood pressure of 124/84 mm Hg (the patient's usual blood pressure was 105/70 mm Hg). An ilioconduit procedure had been performed several years earlier. That night the patient vomited his supper and complained of a very severe headache. Digital disimpaction was unproductive for stool. A flat plate x-ray of the abdomen was ordered and showed small bowel obstruction. An emergency exploratory laparotomy with lysis of adhesions was performed. The postoperative course was unremarkable.

CASE 2.

This 54-year-old male complete paraplegic at the level of T8 presented with flaccid paralysis in the lower extremities. During the night he had a temperature spike to 104°F and he complained of back pain radiating to the right lower inguinal area. On physical examination, the left flank was tender to percussion. The white blood count was 31,000 per/cm³, urinalysis found more than 100,000 organisms of proteus, and x-ray revealed left ureteral and renal calculi. Retrograde studies confirmed left ureteral obstruction. An emergency ureterolithotomy was performed. The postoperative course was uncomplicated.

CASE 3.

This 52-year-old male complete paraplegic at the level of T7 had been followed for several months for ischemic colitis. He suffered from loose bowel movements, abdominal pain, and rectal bleeding. Although a diversionary transverse colostomy was performed, it did not solve these problems. Follow-up barium enema studies showed a persistent "thumbprint" pattern in the left colon. A left hemicolectomy was performed with an uneventful recovery.

CASE 4.

This 53-year-old man had incomplete paraplegia at the level of L2 with severe peripheral vascular disease. Primarily he had had a left above-knee amputation for gangrene, axillofemoral bypass, and right above-knee amputation. An aortogram at that time demonstrated occlusion of the distal aorta with a meandering artery (Fig. 3–2). Two nights postoperatively, his temperature had risen to 102°F with a pulse of 120 bpm. He complained of diffuse abdominal pain without localization; bowel sounds were hyperactive; there was no nausea, vomiting, or diarrhea. Plain abdominal x-rays showed dilated loops of

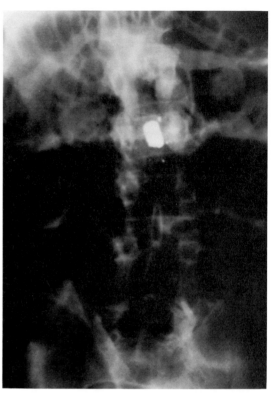

Figure 3–3. Abdominal x-rays of the same patient as Figure 3–2, showing dilated loops of the small bowel.

small bowel. The left colon was not visualized (Fig. 3–3).

Laboratory studies were significant for a mild elevation in CK enzyme. (A drug screen was positive for cocaine.) The white blood count was 6,100/cm³ with an unremarkable differential. The urinalysis showed no acute infection. On the third postoperative night he became hypothermic to 96.6°F and hypotensive with blood pressure down to 90/40 mm Hg from his usual 150/90 mm Hg. The pulse was 80 bpm and described as irregular.

Initial treatment consisted of nasogastric suction and intravenous fluid replacement. Differential diagnosis included postoperative ileus, small or large bowel obstruction, or mesenteric vascular thrombosis. With decreasing return of gastric secretions, a trial clamping of the gastric tube was done. Air had appeared in the left colon on x-ray by this time. The patient tolerated this well and the tube was removed. Two days later, his abdomen was again distended and even tympanatic. Gastric suction was reinstated.

Although a barium enema was attempted, it was unsuccessful as a result of fecal impaction. Colonoscopy was performed; large amounts of stool were visualized but no obstruction was seen. Flatus reappeared after this. The abdominal pain resolved and enemas finally yielded positive results. Several days later the gastric suction was discontinued. A regular diet was tolerated thereafter and his usual bowel care was re-

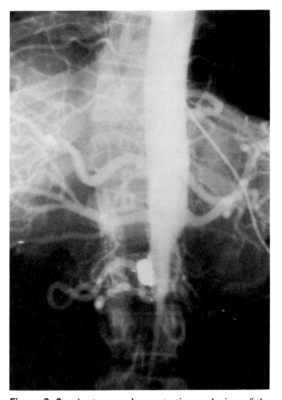

Figure 3–2. Aortogram demonstrating occlusion of the distal aorta with a meandering artery.

sumed. At this time gallbladder series and upper GI series were obtained with normal findings.

CASE 5.

This 66-year-old male incomplete paraplegic at the level of T10 was admitted for surgical reconstruction of a right ischial pressure sore. A superiorly based gluteus maximus myocutaneous flap was used to close the defect under general anesthesia.

On the second postoperative night the patient's temperature rose to 103.4°F. Panculturing identified Proteus in the urine, and the same species was found in preoperative cultures. Rapid defervescence came about with selected postoperative antibiotic treatment.

By the third postoperative day the patient complained of general malaise. The fourth postoperative day saw the onset of mild left lower quadrant pain. For the next three days the patient's abdomen became progressively distended with hyperactive bowel sounds. However, there was never guarding or rebound or episodes of nausea or vomiting. Concurrent with this was postoperative atelectasis. Although the breath sounds were diminished, the lungs sounded clear. Chest x-ray of the sixth postoperative day revealed pleural effusion requiring thoracentesis. The effusions did not recur and with intense respiratory therapy the patient's postoperative atelectasis quickly improved.

Laboratory studies during this time showed a white blood count between 9.8 and 9.6 thousand per cubic mm. Repeated sputum and blood cultures were negative. Vital signs were consistent with preoperative baseline values, except for mild tachypnea and the fever.

Bowel care and enema were given on the seventh postoperative day in the face of the progressive abdominal distention. This produced evacuation of large amounts of stool with abdominal decompression.

DISCUSSION

A total of 20 spinal cord injury patients requiring abdominal surgery have been reviewed for this study. Acute cholecystitis occurred most commonly, followed by perforated viscus and bowel obstruction (Table 3–1).

Cholecystitis has been reported without any presenting symptoms or signs.[1,2,5] Because of this, cholelithiasis in the spinal cord injured patient is an acceptable indication for cholecystectomy. If the procedure is uncomplicated, appendectomy may be done simultaneously.[6] All of our four patients with cholecystitis presented with abdominal pain. For three patients this was a chronic problem of up to several months' duration. The diagnosis of cholecystitis was made when gallbladder study was in-

TABLE 3–1. Acute Abdominal Procedures in Spinal Cord Injured Patients: A 20-Year Experience

LESIONS	NO. OF PATIENTS
Acute cholecystitis	4
Perforated viscus	3
Bowel obstruction	2
Lower GI bleeding	2
Bowel volvulus	1
Abdominal aortic aneurysm	1
Pyelonephritis	1
Ureterolithiasis	2
Ischemic colitis	1
Dolichocolon	2
Metastatic carcinoid tumor	1
	Total 20

cluded as part of the radiologic examination of the gastrointestinal tract. The fourth patient presented with right upper quadrant pain of sudden, acute onset. He was a T8 complete paraplegic whose abdominal wall spasm made physical examination very difficult. However, rebound tenderness was believed to have been elicited over the gallbladder. A sonogram showed gallstones and an uneventful cholecystectomy was performed.

Abdominal adhesions remain the most common cause of small bowel obstruction in patients with previous abdominal surgery. This is also true for spinal cord injured patients. This population additionally undergoes procedures for the diversion of urine and stool in dealing with complex decubitus ulcer problems. This was the presentation in Case 1. The severe headache he complained of probably represented an autonomic disreflexia crisis secondary to intestinal obstruction. A prompt work-up indicated the need for exploratory laparotomy and lysis of adhesions. The other patient with small bowel obstruction in our series also underwent a lysis of adhesions; diverting colostomy and ilioconduit had been performed previously to aid in healing severe decubitus ulcers.

No hernias were seen in this series. Elective repair is thought to be indicated to avoid the risk of overlooked strangulation.

Appendicitis did not occur in our series. However, Charney et al.[1] reported five cases of acute appendicitis. All patients had perforations with abscess formation and had high cord injuries. Delay in diagnosis in this series ranged from three days to three weeks.[1] Dollfus et al.[8] reported one abscess (5000 ml) from a perforated appendix. A high index of suspicion helped arrive at early intervention in four other cases.[8] The one appendectomy performed in our series was done incidentally in the course of an exploratory laparotomy. This patient had severe abdominal pain and rectal bleeding necessitating multiple transfusions. Although barium enema and upper GI series suggested regional enteritis, no significant pathology was found at the time of surgery. The patient, a T10 incomplete paraplegic, recovered uneventfully.

Urologic surgical case presentations, as represented by Case 2, were consistent with those in the literature previously cited. All these patients had high spiking fevers suggesting genitourinary pathology. Intravenous pyelograms demonstrated ureteral calculi. Lithotomies were performed in two cases. In the third case, perinephric and periureteral abscesses were found in addition to a ureteral stone, requiring additional drainage.

Bowel obstruction in the spinal cord injured patient is frequently due to fecal impaction. The signs and symptoms of abdominal distention warrant a surgical consultation. Colon pathology in this series ranged from ischemic colitis (Case 3) to sigmoid volvulus, perforated diverticulum, and dolichocolon. Surgical management in these cases was straightforward after the pathology was defined and documented. More frequently, the colon may be obstructed by feces. Case 4 illustrates an extensive work-up that stopped just short of exploratory laparotomy.

In the postoperative period of myocutaneous flap reconstruction it is desirable to put the bowel at rest. This is done through diet and enemas preoperatively, then diet and an anticathartic regimen postoperatively. Because of this, some abdominal distention is usually seen after surgery. The patient in Case 5 presented with a rapid onset of abdominal distention in such a postoperative period. Also, this patient had had previous abdominal exploration, putting him at risk of adhesions.

The management of fecal impaction in such a postoperative period is further complicated by the fact that the patient is on an airbed. Colonoscopy and radiologic studies are usually not bedside procedures. Transferring the patient out of the airbed places the flap at risk for dehiscence, infection, and pressure necrosis.

In Case 5, a high spiking fever provided the clue to a urologic source. An entire genitourinary work-up in the month before the patient's admission, including cystoscopy and intravenous pyelogram, had demonstrated normal upper and lower tracts. Urinalysis with culture

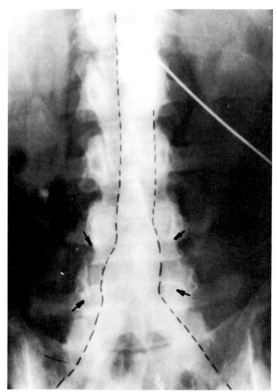

Figure 3–4. An arteriogram demonstrating possible leakage of an abdominal aortic aneurism.

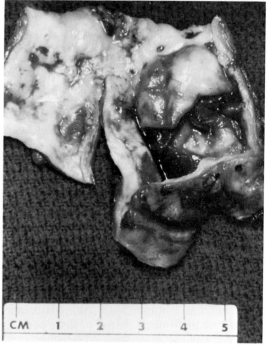

Figure 3–5. Gross specimen of the posterior wall in the same case as Figure 3–4.

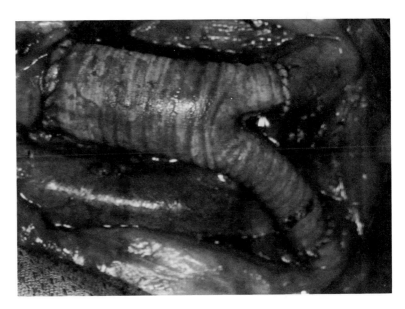

Figure 3–6. The resected aorta for the same case as Figure 3–4.

identified the urinary tract infection. This was treated with appropriate antibiotics.

With colonoscopic decompression of the colon, bowel function returned and the patient's condition improved. In contrast, another 23-year-old C7 quadriplegic, still in spinal shock three weeks after his initial injury, presented with distention but with no other signs or symptoms. Abdominal x-ray showed free air. At emergency laparotomy, the stomach was found to be perforated. An omental patch was used to close the defect and the patient recovered uneventfully.

Another quadriplegic was admitted in septic shock with abdominal distention. Rapid workup showed a bowel obstruction. At laparotomy an internal hernia and anterior cecal wall perforation were found and repaired with reduction and cecostomy. He died three weeks postoperatively of septic complications.

Another consultation for abdominal pain and distention demonstrated a pulsatile abdominal mass. A lumbar arteriogram demonstrated possible leakage of an abdominal aortic aneurysm (Fig. 3–4). The specimen shows the leak in the posterior wall (Fig. 3–5). This was resected uneventfully (Fig. 3–6).

SUMMARY

A total of 20 cases of acute abdomen in spinal cord injured patients seen over the past 20 years is presented. One patient admitted in septic shock died postoperatively of multisystem organ failure. The mortality rate of 5 per cent is consistent with other reported rates of 10 to 15 per cent. Types of surgery included biliary, aorta, gastric, colonic, genitourinary, and lysis of adhesions. In the stabilized spinal cord injured patient, delay in surgery is to be avoided. Early clues of fever, pain, anorexia, and dysreflexia deserve work-up. Laboratory values are best interpreted against baselines. Genitourinary problems may not only mimic the acute abdomen but may also be coexistent with it.[4]

Finally, it is imperative to know the level of spinal cord injury and whether it is complete or not. These patients will tolerate early exploratory laparotomy much better than they will a delayed diagnosis with catastrophic sequelae.[1–8]

REFERENCES

1. Charney KJ, Juler GL, Comarr AE: General surgery problems in patients with spinal cord injuries. Arch Surg 110:1083–1088, 1975.
2. Juler GL, Eltorai IM: The acute abdomen in spinal cord injury patients. Paraplegia 23:118–123, 1985.
3. Miller LS, Stass WE Jr, Herbison GJ: Abdominal problems in patients with spinal cord lesions. Arch Phys Med Rehabil 56:405–408, 1975.
4. O'Hare JM: The acute abdomen in spinal cord injury patients. Proceedings, Annual Clinical and Spinal Cord Injury Conference, 15:113–117, 1966.
5. Sugarman B, Brown D, Musher D: Fever and infection in spinal cord injury patients. JAMA 248:66–70, 1982.
6. Greenfield J: Abdominal operations on patients with chronic paraplegia. Arch Surg 1077–1087, 1949.
7. Ingberg HO, Prust FW: The diagnosis of abdominal emergencies in patients with spinal cord lesions. Arch Phys Med Rehabil 49:343–348, 1968.
8. Dollfus P, Holderback GL, Husser JM, Jacob-Chia D: Must appendicitis be still considered as a rare complication in paraplegia? Paraplegia II:306–309, 1974.

Immediate Management of the Spinal Cord Injured Patient

BARTH A. GREEN, M.D., K. JOHN KLOSE, Ph.D.,
FRANK J. EISMONT, M.D., and JAMES T. O'HEIR

Spinal cord injury, like all forms of trauma, is a disease mainly of young people, with most injuries occurring in the second and third decades and mostly in young males. The majority of such injuries occur in the early hours of the morning and are often associated with alcohol or drug use, although not necessarily by the victims of paralysis. Vehicular accidents—particularly automobile and motorcycle accidents—are the most common causes of spinal cord injury. After vehicle accidents, the approximate ranking of frequency is falls and industrial, agricultural, and sporting accidents. However, in many metropolitan areas, gunshot wounds are at or near the top of the causal list. A significant portion of spinal cord injuries are associated with multisystem trauma; this is a factor leading to increased morbidity and mortality and plays an important role in determining early treatment priorities.

There is an approximately equal distribution of patients with quadriplegic and paraplegic, i.e., cervical and thoracolumbar, injuries in this country.[1,2] Similarly, complete and incomplete lesions are distributed equally, although the trend nationally seems to be shifting toward more incomplete and more cervical injuries. The mid and low cervical regions represent the most mobile levels of the spinal column and therefore are the most frequently injured. The thoracolumbar junction is the second most mobile level and the second most commonly injured.

In terms of cost and demands on the health care delivery system, spinal cord injuries are considered catastrophic. This form of trauma has an associated high morbidity incidence as evidenced by the development of at least one systemic complication in most patients. The overall mortality is estimated to be about 10 per cent during the first year, although our center and other large centers have experienced a less than 5 per cent mortality during the year after injury. Most of these early deaths occur in the first two weeks following injury and are associated with cardiopulmonary complications. Although systemic morbidity is higher in the early postinjury period, it continues to be a problem throughout the life of the paralysis victim, especially with regard to urinary tract and skin infections, soft tissue contractures, heterotopic bone, autonomic dysreflexia, pain, and spasticity problems.

IMPORTANCE OF A SYSTEMS APPROACH

We advocate a systems approach as optimal for spinal cord injury treatment. This approach is based on the philosophy that a specialized group of physicians, nurses, and allied health professionals can provide optimal care in this unusual but devastating form of trauma because of the volume of experience characteristic of a center setting and the group's commitment and capability in providing continuity of care from the accident scene through the life of

24

the paralysis victim. The systems approach consists of five components: prevention, prehospital care, acute care, rehabilitation, and lifelong medical follow-up.[3–5] We believe that this approach translates into decreased morbidity, mortality, and costs. This has been substantiated to some degree by reports of the national Model Systems Demonstration Projects for Spinal Cord Injury and the State of Florida Spinal Cord Injury System.

The system must include prevention programs aimed at the population at highest risk, teenagers. One cannot deny the logic of preventing an injury or disease rather than bearing the costs of treating it and the associated consequences. The "front end," or the initial care phase, involves prehospital management based on emergency medical services (EMS). It is essential for the staff of the spinal cord injury center to become intimately involved in both prevention and emergency medical services activities within their geographic area of responsibility, including education programs and research activity. The acute in-hospital care phase follows and includes the definitive diagnosis and early medical and surgical management of the injury and its associated systemic complications. This stage includes the emergency room triage, imaging, and surgical and intensive care management as well as intermediate floor care.

Whereas the rehabilitation phase formally begins at the transfer from the acute floor to the rehabilitation center, this phase should be initiated in the intensive care unit immediately after the paralyzing injury. The acute phase can vary from one to two weeks to months or even years, depending on the degree of deficit and the systemic complications associated with the injury. The average time spent in rehabilitation ranges from three to six months, with the higher level injuries often requiring prolonged in-patient stays. Finally, rounding out this system's care is the lifelong follow-up care phase. This has placed an increasingly important demand on the health care system because of the number of acute trauma victims who survive their initial hospitalization. Biannual outpatient spinal cord injury clinic visits are instrumental in minimizing the long-term morbidity and associated costs.

PREHOSPITAL MANAGEMENT

In the 1970s, the majority of paralysis victims arrived at the hospital with what was defined as *complete* lesions, i.e., no movement or sensation below the level of injury, and with a very poor prognosis for any functional recovery. In the 1980s, the majority of victims arrived with incomplete lesions, i.e., some evidence of movement or sensation distal to their level of injury indicating a better prognosis for at least some degree of motor and/or sensory recovery. While the velocity insult impact or type of injury has not significantly changed during the last couple of decades, one factor that has changed is the role of the first responder at the accident scene. In most instances the well-meaning "Good Samaritan" or highway patrolman has been replaced by the highly sophisticated and well-trained emergency medical technician (EMT) or paramedic. These technicians are trained in advanced life support and are capable of administering intravenous medications and initiating advanced forms of cardiopulmonary resuscitation, including defibrillation, intubation, and the use of wireless ECG telemetry monitoring. The modern paramedic has the training and equipment to provide optimal prehospital care to ensure the expedient arrival of trauma victims to the emergency department with maximal preservation of neurologic function and a better chance for recovery.[6] These well-trained personnel also offer the intriguing possibility of providing an accident scene baseline neurologic assessment, which could allow initiation of pharmacologic treatment in the first minutes, rather than hours or days, following injury.

Once the injury is identified as potential spinal cord trauma, the priorities at the accident scene include respiratory and cardiovascular stabilization followed by spinal column immobilization on a spine board or splint in a neutral supine position. Although the spine board remains a simple and effective means of immobilization, more sophisticated stretchers that facilitate x-ray and magnetic resonance imaging (MRI) are now available. These have the added advantage of being compatible with the hospital-based diagnostic and therapeutic equipment. All spinal cord injury victims should have two large intravenous lines, a Foley catheter, and a nasogastric tube inserted and maintained (the stomach and bladder emptied at the accident scene) before and during transport. We recommend the Trendelenburg position for transportation as a means of minimizing the possibilities of aspiration and shock, which represent the two major causes of death in the prehospital phase. Special orthoses have been developed that allow the effective maintenance of cervical traction during transportation, and telemetry monitoring allows for direct visual monitoring of the cardiovascular system by the emergency department physician during the prehospital and transport phase of care.

The modified University of Miami Neurospinal Index (UMNI) can be used by paramedics to aid in performing an effective neurologic assessment in seconds at the accident scene without delaying transport or implementation of definitive treatment.[7] Communication from the paramedic to the physician in the emergency department of a local hospital or spinal cord injury center provides critical lead time for the receiving facility to prepare special resources to optimize the patient's triage and management. Today, paramedics are able to intubate and defibrillate and administer intravenous medications to acutely injured patients but are not usually allowed to insert Foley catheters or nasogastric tubes. As of this writing tremendous controversy rages over the issue of patient delivery to the nearest hospital. Should an acute accident victim—spinal cord injury or otherwise—be transported to the nearest local hospital, which may not have the optimal resources to stabilize and manage the injuries? Unfortunately, this issue is being settled in courts of law, and the fate of the EMS system is being determined by juries of lay persons who are not knowledgeable in the management of accident victims, rather than by groups of physicians, nurses, and allied health professionals experienced in the care of trauma victims.

EMERGENCY DEPARTMENT CARE PROTOCOL

The emergency department represents the first component of the systems approach wherein the full team of physicians, nurses, and allied health professionals begin to interact directly with individuals sustaining spinal cord injury. The basic priorities established at the accident scene continue to be the focus of attention in the emergency department, including cardiopulmonary stabilization and spinal column immobilization. A detailed but rapid history, physical, and neurologic assessment is performed as blood, urine, and arterial oxygen samples are obtained and more sophisticated monitoring instrumentation is inserted and

calibrated. Systemic stabilization is directed at preventing hypoxia and hypotension, either or both of which can be devastating to the spinal cord parenchyma, creating an evolving secondary injury. A multisystem assessment is performed by either an emergency department physician or trauma surgeon, who immediately obtains neurosurgic and orthopedic surgical consultations. At our center, neurosurgic and orthopedic surgeons comprise an integrated spinal cord injury team with protocols and shared responsibilities for medical and surgical management. In the emergency department, life-threatening systemic injuries, closed or penetrating, take priority over a spinal cord injury. However, whenever possible, both of these factors are dealt with simultaneously.

When acute life-threatening situations have been resolved, the primary focus of care centers on preservation and restoration of function. The immediate care management of spinal cord injury victims remains a controversial topic. If one questioned 12 neurosurgeons, 12 orthopedic surgeons, and 12 physiatrists, one would probably get as many different early management plans for the same patient. There have not been any credible prospective, randomized, well-controlled clinical trials to justify the choice of one mode of treatment over another. This is surprising considering the tremendous socioeconomic impact that this paralyzed population has on the United States as well as other nations of the world.

Generally, in North America, the emphasis is on the early stabilization and rapid mobilization of spinal cord injury victims, with the majority of these patients undergoing some type of surgical procedure or having external immobilization technique to stabilize the spine in the acute stage. This approach allows rapid mobilization and the early institution of rehabilitation in this patient population. However, in many parts of the world, especially in Europe and Australia, most physicians follow the philosophies and standards established almost 40 years ago by Sir Ludwig Guttman at Stoke Mandeville Spinal Injury Centre in England. Patients in that system are nonsurgically immobilized and stabilized during a prolonged initial period of bedrest and conservative fracture management. This is followed by a comprehensive rehabilitation approach stressing reentry into society as well as vocational training.

Both philosophies, although differing in their basic approach, emphasize attempts to limit the neurologic deficit. The controversy lies not with that goal but rather with the aspirations of certain clinical groups, including our own, to attempt to reverse or prevent permanence of some or all of the neurologic deficit that has occurred, utilizing what had previously been mainly laboratory research strategies. Contemporary approaches toward this goal, in appropriate cases, include the early (within the first several hours) administration of intravenous agents such as neuropeptides, neuropeptide analogs, and new-generation steroids. In spite of the fact that there is not a good comprehensive historical data bank relating to outcome of spinal cord injuries, certain factors that can influence outcome are accepted and recognized by most clinicians. These include the probability that high-velocity injuries will result in poorer outcome than low-velocity injuries and of open injuries having a less positive prognosis than closed injuries. Other factors include age and level of lesion, with older patients having a higher morbidity and mortality and patients with a higher level of paralysis suffering a higher number of complications and a higher mortality.

Clinical trials performed cooperatively between centers or within centers in this country and elsewhere have failed to extrapolate "laboratory cures" achieved in acutely paralyzed animals to human spinal cord injury victims.[8,9] One must recognize that a possible reason for this failure is not so much the lack of effectiveness of the pharmaceutic agents as the inability of clinicians to apply those therapies to appropriate populations of spinal cord injuries. An injury that is the result of a 90 mile per hour car crash into a telephone pole with severe disruption of the spinal column and spinal cord or a similar injury caused by a gunshot wound slamming through the spinal cord are much less likely to respond to an intravenous neuropeptide or steroid dose than the lower impact diving or sports injury associated with minimal spinal column and spinal cord parenchymal disruption. Unfortunately, none of the previous clinical studies have taken such practical issues into consideration. This situation further emphasizes the need for a better profile analysis of the human spinal cord injury victim and the detailed characterization of spinal cord lesions with regard to diagnosis, optimal treatment, and prognosis. If one accepts the fact that the primary injury is related to the velocity and mechanism of injury, which is not within the clinician's control (but which may be preventable), then the emphasis of management

obviously must be placed on minimizing or reversing secondary consequences to the spinal cord parenchyma. One study could be devised involving management of systemic complications such as hypotension, hypoxia, and sepsis and another with more localized issues such as spinal cord blood flow, swelling, and metabolic alterations. These issues are further compounded by the tremendous biological variability of human paralysis victims.

POSTEMERGENCY PROTOCOL

When immediate life-threatening situations have been resolved, a comprehensive neurologic assessment is performed and should include a thorough motor and sensory examination including a multimodality breakdown of sensory function with separate attention paid to dorsal and lateral column assessments. The rectal examination is essential in all spinal cord injury victims because of the significance of sacral sparing of voluntary motor (sphincter contraction) or sensory (pinprick) function in the perianal region, which classifies a patient as having an incomplete lesion and is significant in the prognosis and treatment plan. Motor and sensory examinations are much more reliable than reflexes, especially with regard to prediction of outcome or differentiation between complete and incomplete lesions. Voluntary motor function, as opposed to reflex withdrawal, is a more important part of the neurologic examination. The sensory component of the neurologic test should include pain and temperature perception, which represent the lateral columns. This has more significant prognostic value regarding the return of motor function than does preservation of touch, vibration, or position sense representing the dorsal columns.[7]

Following neurologic assessment, routine chest and abdomen films are taken, as well as an AP and lateral survey of the entire spinal column, since 15 to 20 per cent of spinal injuries occur at multiple levels. If neurologic deficit is present that is compatible with a cervical spinal cord injury, Gardner Wells tongs or halo rings are used, and traction is applied depending on the level of injury and degree of spinal element disruption. This traction is usually applied in neck injuries with a starting level of 5 lb per interspace; a C4–C5 injury, for example, would necessitate between 20 and 25 lb of traction. In cases of obviously severely disrupted spinal column or ligaments, the initial traction level is lowered to 3 to 5 lb until follow-up x-rays are obtained to prevent overdistraction and further damage to the spinal cord and/or nerve roots. If adequate alignment is not achieved with the initial level of traction, the weights are increased until a maximum of about twice the baseline level, i.e., at the most, 50 or 60 lb for a low cervical injury. Intravenous diazepam is used as a supplement for muscle relaxation.

It is well recognized that traction is not a sound physiologic maneuver because muscle reacts to pulling by shortening and an increase in spasms. Therefore, if a total reduction and alignment cannot be achieved within the first hour of injury, we advocate elective nasotracheal intubation and the use of a short-acting systemic paralyzing agent such as d-tubocurare with ventilating support in order to expedite manual manipulation and reduction of the fracture dislocation and immediate decompression and realignment of the spinal canal.[10,11] In the cervical area this can be achieved in most cases in a closed fashion without surgery. The exception to this rule includes the rare cervical burst fracture or herniated disc or devastating cases of ankylosing spondylitis associated with a fracture dislocation. These cases are best treated with early surgical intervention in our experience. When realignment has been achieved following intravenous medication, the systemic paralysis can be reversed and the patient extubated except in the case of high quadriplegics. In these patients elective intubation is often a reasonable course with ventilatory support as a prophylaxis against atelectasis or pneumothorax for the first several days.

In thoracic and lumbar spinal levels, unfortunately, traction and manipulation are not effective means of reduction and maintenance of alignment in cases of fracture dislocations. In cases with injury below T12 through the sacrum, realignment and decompression are simultaneously achieved in the surgical suite. A less aggressive approach is taken in patients with complete injuries below T1 and above T12. The patients with incomplete lesions at those levels are treated with an equally aggressive surgical protocol of open reduction and stabilization. To further investigate the bony and neural elements involved in the spinal cord injury, immediately after x-rays are done, high resolution image CT scans are taken through the area of injury. More recently, we

have utilized imaging; sagittal and transverse T1 and T2 images are obtained. Early evaluation of the capabilities of MR scanning in the acute spinal cord injured patient has revealed that a significant number have soft tissue problems, and also herniated discs, which were not fully appreciated even with high resolution CT scanning.[11] This was unexpected in that we had abandoned myelogram/CT several years ago because of an increased confidence in high resolution CT imaging. It appears that our standard protocol will include MR imaging in the future.

PATIENT TRIAGE

Following the emergency room assessments and treatment, patients are triaged into one of the following therapeutic pathways: (1) Paralyzed patients with no imaging evidence of neural element compression and no evidence of spinal fractures or instability are transferred directly to the ICU for standard acute care treatment without any surgical indication or indication for orthosis. (2) Patients with extrinsic neural element compression but with spinal column instability are transferred to the ICU for immobilization and standard treatment and taken to the operating room within 7 to 10 days for elective stabilization or placement in halo orthosis or both. These are most often cervical level injuries. (3) Patients with imaging evidence of neural element compression intractable to closed manipulations and who arrive at the center within the first 24 hours are taken immediately to the operating room for open decompression and stabilization. These patients most often have thoracic and lumbar—rarely cervical—injuries. (4) Patients with penetrating wounds of the neck, chest, or abdomen, with life-threatening multisystem involvement taking priority over their neurologic injury, are taken to the operating room for exploration and primary treatment of their visceral damage. When they are stabilized, they are triaged according to the principles described above. (5) Patients suffering penetrating wounds primarily involving the spinal column without significant systemic injuries have surgical exploration, decompression, and debridement if they present with incomplete neurologic deficits with intractable neural element compression as in the case of closed injuries. Some decompressions of complete cervical or lumbar injuries are delayed for reasons of intractable pain or potential lower motor neuron nerve root recovery or because of intractable CSF fistula, infection, or cysts.

SURGICAL PROTOCOL

Although is is not possible within this chapter to present a detailed protocol for surgical management of all spinal cord injuries, it is probably appropriate to present some basic principles of surgical triage and management. Indications for surgical treatment include spinal cord and/or nerve root compression or spinal column instability that is not amenable to nonsurgical management, i.e., such devices as halo orthosis, and thoracolumbar support orthosis (TLSO). Surgical patients are further subcategorized into those needing immediate procedures or procedures delayed as described above.

A basic principle for the surgical treatment of spinal cord injuries is that no surgical procedures to decompress neural elements should be performed unless equal attention is paid to stabilization of the bony and soft tissue spinal elements—i.e., decompression should always be combined with stabilization. Philosophically, our surgical goals are directed toward neural element decompression and early spinal stabilization to expedite rapid mobilization while minimizing the systemic consequences of prolonged immobility. The term *spinal fusion* is often mistakenly thought to be synonymous with immediate postoperative stability when, in fact, spinal fusion is an internal splinting allowing early mobilization of a patient as long as appropriate external support, such as a halo apparatus, rigid collar, or thoracolumbar orthosis, is utilized. Bony fusion may take from 8 to 12 weeks and sometimes as long as 16 to 24 weeks to mature, during which time the patient should be actively participating in a full rehabilitation program while being protected by external bracing. Certain fractures can be primarily treated with halo or TLSO type orthosis and do not require surgical intervention. Each case should be considered individually with regard to clinical management, with many factors taken into consideration, including the patient's age, general medical status, level of injury, type of bony injury, neurologic deficit, and the results of imaging and physiologic assessments.

A standard protocol has been developed in our institution for the surgical management of injuries from the foramen magnum down through the sacrum. This protocol includes anterior, posterior, lateral, and, in certain cases, combined approaches to the cervical, thoracic, and lumbosacral spines, depending on the type of bony disruption, ligamentous injury, and neurologic deficit. Each approach takes into consideration the basic principles of simultaneous decompression and stabilization. In the acutely paralyzed person, the anterior or lateral approach to the thoracic or lumbosacral spine is rarely indicated, with the posterior and posterolateral approaches being adequate to achieve the goals described. However, in the cervical area, although the anterior and posterior approaches are rarely indicated, they probably are equally utilized to accomplish surgical goals depending on the individual characteristics of the spinal cord injury.

New generations of surgical instrumentation are now available for all spinal levels, including various new plates and screws as well as rod instruments. Instrumentation with or without wiring should never be used alone but always supplemented with autologous or heterologous bone graft. The same is true when acrylic is used to strengthen the construction. It is our opinion that acrylic has little, if any, place in the surgical management of the acute trauma patient; however, this represents an area of controversy.

The protocol developed for postoperative monitoring includes somatosensory evoked potentials (SEPs) and realtime electromyography (EMG) along with the experimental use of electromagnetically generated motor-evoked responses. Other monitoring devices include the use of realtime spinal ultrasonography for visualizing the spinal cord and nerve roots during and after decompression and stabilization procedures are performed. Utilization of this technology has eliminated the need for intraoperative myelography and postoperative myelograms and CT scans and has almost totally eliminated the need for follow-up surgical procedures to correct inadequacies in the initial operation.

In addition to those for monitoring, protocols are established for utilization of perioperative intravenous antibiotics and steroids, patient positioning, and use of anesthetic agents. Many patients are nasotracheally intubated and positioned awake to record their neural status after positioning and before induction of a general anesthetic—nitrous narcotic combinations are preferred over general inhalation agents to optimize electrophysiologic monitoring. Technology including loupe magnification and headlight illumination is routinely utilized, and, in special cases, the magnification illumination of the operating microscope can be of benefit. Hemostasis has become an increasingly important surgical consideration and presently, use of the cell saver, which recycles the patient's blood and returns approximately 25 to 50 per cent of the patient's lost volume intraoperatively, is complemented by use of agents such as powdered thrombinated Gelfoam and Avitene.

Spinal cord injury surgical management is best implemented by a team including neurologic and orthopedic surgeons, as well as anesthesiologists, technicians monitoring the evoked responses, the radiologic technician, and the ultrasonographic technician. It is not uncommon, however, to consult with a general or thoracic surgeon or neuroradiologist to enhance the effectiveness of our surgical therapies.

When the surgical procedure is completed, it is essential for the patient to be awake; a complete neurologic examination must be repeated and the results compared with those of the preoperative assessments. In addition, plain x-ray imaging of the surgical sites should be accomplished as a postoperative baseline. Most patients should be placed on the Roto-Rest treatment table for kinetic therapy initiated immediately in the recovery room or ICU (see below) to avoid the devastating effects of the prolonged immobilization often necessary for the surgical procedure.[5] It is important for the surgical team to report on the patient's neurologic and skeletal status to other spinal cord injury team members responsible for care in the ICU or on the floor after the recovery room period of observation. Spinal cord injured patients, because of their neurologic deficit and systemic involvement, are more susceptible to complications or sudden changes in status than is the general postsurgical patient population and must be observed and monitored carefully.

INTENSIVE CARE MANAGEMENT PROTOCOL

After the emergency room triage and imaging protocols and necessary surgery are completed, patients are taken to the ICU. The priorities in the ICU include systemic stabilization with establishment of more sophisti-

cated monitoring systems (such as a Swan-Ganz catheter) as indicated, and immobilization of the spinal column. Ideally, while the spinal column is splinted and immobilized to prevent secondary injury, the patient's body should be at least physiologically mobilized to minimize the devastating systemic effects of paralysis and immobility. This is accomplished by placing acutely injured patients on a kinetic Roto-Rest treatment table following their arrival in the ICU. According to protocol, each patient is rotated 20 out of 24 hours with rotation interrupted only for feeding, hygiene, physical or respiratory therapy, diagnostic tests, and x-rays. The kinetic Roto-Rest treatment table represents the most effective equipment for management of acute spinal cord injury patients in the ICU setting. It provides a system of hatches and flaps, permitting access to all areas of the body without compromising spinal stability. Alternative devices utilized in the past (including the Stryker frame, Circoelectric bed, air beds, and/or water beds) are neither safe nor effective in treatment of this patient population because of their inability to maintain spinal stability as well as the compromise of respiratory function, especially in patients maintained in the prone position. The Stoke-Eggerton bed adequately stabilizes the spine; however, as in the other aforementioned equipment, patients remain in a static position for at least two hours at a time, exposing them to the hazards of prolonged immobility. The Roto-Rest table can also be used to transport the patient to the operating room; it can be utilized as an operating table and permits restarting kinetic therapy following arrival into the recovery room or back to the ICU. While this treatment table does not replace good nursing care, it allows nursing personnel to concentrate on more skilled nursing interventions and assessments rather than spending the majority of their time turning or lifting the patient or caring for potentially preventable complications.

The highest morbidity and mortality in the spinal cord injured population occurs in the first two weeks following injury and is most commonly associated with cardiopulmonary complications. However, every system of the human body is affected by immobility; atelectasis and respiratory secretion stasis can lead to pneumonia as well as other respiratory complications. Vascular system stasis accounts for the high frequency of deep vein thrombosis, which translates into fatal pulmonary emboli in between 3 and 13 per cent of the cases reported.

Pressure on insensitive skin can lead to decubitus ulcers, and extremity immobilization compounded by the severe catabolic state results in rapid muscle atrophy and the evolution of contractures of the soft tissues around the joints. Skeletal system immobility is also associated with a massive mobilization of calcium into the blood and urinary systems. Its presence is associated with urinary tract stones, heterotopic bone formation, and severe osteoporosis as well as pathologic fractures. Urinary tract stasis is frequently associated with infections and calculus formation. Gastrointestinal paralysis combined with a state of relative ischemia of the gut can result in gastrointestinal stress ulcerations and hemorrhages as well as chronic constipation and obstruction. Pancreatitis is commonly associated with paralytic ileus.

Considering the multisystem consequences of paralysis which are compounded by immobility, it seems logical to implement a kinetic therapy protocol as quickly as possible after the patient's arrival into the ICU.[12] In addition to the kinetic therapy protocol, specific systemic protocols have been developed for every major cardiac index in patients suffering multitrauma or other high-risk patients. Prophylactic intubation is utilized in patients with significant chest wall injuries or with a high level of quadriplegia and potential compromise of the diaphragm or accessory respiratory muscles. This manuever minimizes the potential hazard of sudden atelectasis or pneumothorax. These patients are kept on a mechanical ventilator with nasotracheal intubation and are slowly weaned from the respirator when they are more physiologically and nutritionally stable. Intubation with a soft tube can be prolonged for a period of three to four weeks before a tracheostomy may be needed.

The high risk of gastrointestinal bleeding (stress ulcer) is offset by maintenance of a large sump tube in the stomach from the time of admission to the ICU. The tube is attached to low constant suction to keep acid out of the stomach. Every four hours the suction is interrupted and pH is measured. If it is less than four, antacids are added and titrated until the pH is neutralized. Another major GI complication is paralytic ileus, which may or may not be associated with pancreatitis. All patients are started on intravenous hyperalimentation within 24 hours of admission and this is maintained until bowel sounds return and enteral feeding is appropriate. This counteracts the massive catabolic changes which are inevitable following trauma and are further exacerbated by the paralysis associated with spinal cord injury.

The genitourinary system is monitored with an indwelling Foley catheter for several days until the patient's condition is physiologically stabilized, at which time intermittent catheterization is initiated every four hours with a careful balance of intake and output to prevent overdistention of the bladder. Urinary tract cultures are obtained on a weekly basis, as are other invasive line cultures and sensitivities because sepsis represents a major source of ICU morbidity in this patient population. This potentially devastating complication can be best controlled with the implementation of rigid sterile techniques for dressings and line changes and careful monitoring of the results of the culture and sensitivities, temperature, and white blood cell count. Although many quadriplegics and paraplegics have asymptomatic urinary infection on a chronic basis following their spinal cord injury, a culture with greater than 1000 organisms indicates that infection should be treated aggressively in the ICU because of the patient's acute physiologic compromise and multiple invasive lines.

An essential component of the ICU protocol for these patients in the acute phase is early interaction with various members of the rehabilitative center staff, including a primary rehabilitation physician, physical and occupational therapists, rehabilitation psychologist, and social service personnel. It is essential that the full-time intensive care staff as well as part-time allied health professionals fully understand not only the physiologic consequences of paralysis but also the psychologic ones. Shortly after arrival in the ICU, each patient should be carefully informed (as also should have been done in the emergency department when possible), of the diagnosis and prognosis, with family and close friends being an integral part of these discussions.

Patients arriving with complete lesions are told that they have approximately a 5 per cent chance of naturally recovering some distal function and that they have less than a 1 per cent chance of further deterioration. Each of these possibilities is carefully explained. Patients arriving with incomplete lesions with some distal sparing of motor and sensory function are told that they have a good chance of recovering at least some degree of function, but the exact extent is unpredictable with the present state-of-the-art knowledge regarding prognosis of their injury. At the same time they are given a sensitive but factual description of their injury and outlook. They are also informed of the status of spinal cord injury research with regard to the potential reversal of at least some part of their paralysis. It is emphasized that although today there is no cure for their crippling injury, investigators the world over are actively researching such treatments as cellular and tissue transplantation in an attempt to re-establish functional connection of the traumatized spinal cord and peripheral nerves. All victims of paralysis undergo a predictable psychological sequence, including initial "denial," followed by "anger," "depression," and ultimately a "coping" stage. Their families or significant others experience the same emotional stages, although often not at the same time.

All of the allied health professionals dealing with acutely paralyzed patients and their families have an important responsibility; they serve as intermediaries between what was a short time before a healthy, active person and the strange and frightening environment where that person now lies dependent. When the responsible physician and allied health professional team determine that the patient is a suitable candidate for transfer to the intermediate floor level of care, a conference should be scheduled with the patient's family and members of both the ICU and floor staff. At this conference, both short- and long-term goals should be established and agreed upon by all involved. The bonding of a paralyzed person to his family or significant others is just as critical a consideration as the bonding of a newborn to its mother. This involvement should begin early and be maintained throughout the ICU and intermediate care phases as it is an integral part of the rehabilitation center activities.

Each step in the progression of care from ICU to floor and then to the rehabilitation center represents a decrease in intensity of care and dependence and an increase in individual patients' responsibilities and participation in their care. On the acute treatment floor it is possible for allied health professionals from the rehabilitation team to more actively participate and indoctrinate the spinal cord injured patient into a more routine schedule, including the activities which will become an integral part of the rehabilitation process. Mobilization into a wheelchair is accomplished as quickly as possible and the patient, if capable, is taught such important skills as self-catheterization

and digital evacuation of the bowels. Training the bowel and bladder are priorities initiated in the ICU but more effectively implemented in the intermediate floor care phase. Patients are started on combination stool softener and laxative on a daily basis and on an every other day suppository program. Later during rehabilitation this regimen may be replaced with a more natural combination of prune juice with bran powder and digital stimulation. As soon as feasible, the patient is transferred for day therapy to the rehabilitation center, especially if it is located within the same complex as the acute care spinal cord injury ward. This process smooths the transition from intermediate floor care to the rehabilitation center.

Ideally, patients suffering a spinal cord injury without significant multisystem trauma should be stabilized and transferred to the rehabilitation center within the first two to three weeks following injury. This goal of rapid stabilization and mobilization is not practical in cases of higher levels of neurologic deficit, especially with respirator dependence, or in patients with significant systemic injuries and complications. The faster the mobilization, the less opportunity for a significant morbidity to occur. The spinal cord injury team develops a unique esprit de corps associated with the pride with which they carry out their skilled responsibilities in guiding the acute paralysis victim through the various phases of hospitalization and reintegration into society. Physicians and allied health professionals committed to victims of this type of trauma universally report a high level of gratification in dealing with patients who initially are totally helpless and dependent and become, in many cases, remarkable achievers in spite of their physical disabilities. As important as is the knowledge of research results to these patients, it is equally significant to the physicians and allied health professionals providing them with daily care. It is not unusual for these team members to be involved with some form of clinical or basic laboratory research in addition to their primary hospital-based responsibilities. In many cases, yesterday's patients tomorrow become lifelong friends of the physicians and allied health professionals, a unique situation in health care.

REFERENCES

1. Bracken MB, Collins WF, Freeman DF, et al: Efficacy of methylprednisolone in acute spinal cord injury. JAMA 251:45, 1984.
2. Green BA, Eismont FJ: Acute spinal cord injury: A

systems approach. Cent Nerv Syst Trauma 1:173, 1984.

3. Green BA, Klose KJ: Acute spinal cord injury, Part I. *In* Sheinberg P (ed): Neurology and Neurosurgery Update Series, Vol II, Lesson 27, Princeton, N.J., Continuing Professional Education Center, Inc., 1981.

4. Green BA, Magana IA: Spinal Cord Trauma: Clinical Aspects. *In* Davidoff M (ed): Handbook of the Spinal Cord, Vols IV and V. New York, Dekker, 1987, pp 63–92.

5. Green BA, Green KL, Klose, KJ: Kinetic nursing for acute spinal cord injury patients. Paraplegia 18:181, 1980.

6. Green BA, Kahn T, Klose, KJ: A comparative study of steroid therapy in acute experimental spinal cord injury. Surg Neurol 13:91, 1980.

7. Green BA, Khan T, Klose KJ, De La Torre J: Acute spinal cord injury: Current Concepts Clin Orthop 154:125, 1981.

8. Green BA, Klose KJ, Goldberg ML: Clinical and re-search considerations in spinal cord injury. *In* Becker DP, Povlishock JT (eds): Central Nervous System Trauma Status Report. Bethesda, NINCDS, NIH, 1985, pp 341–368.

9. Hall WJ, Green BA, Colodonato JP: Spinal cord injury: Emergency Management. Emer Med Serv 5:28, 1976.

10. Klose KJ, Green BA, Smith RS, et al: University of Miami Neuro-spinal Index (UMNI): A quantitative method for determining spinal cord function. Paraplegia 18:331, 1980.

11. Mesard L, Carmody A, Mannarino E, Ruge D: Survival after spinal cord trauma. Arch Neurol 35:78, 1978.

12. Stover SL, Fine PR (ed): Spinal Cord Injury: The Facts and Figures. Birmingham, University of Alabama at Birmingham, 1986.

13. Young JS, Northrup NE: Statistical information pertaining to some of the most commonly asked questions about spinal cord injury. SCI Digest 1:11, 1979.

Management of the Patient with Multiple Injuries

JOHN H. DAVIS, M.D.

In the patient who has multiple injuries a high probability of a spinal cord injury exists. Since the care of the patient with spinal cord injuries is covered elsewhere in this text, this chapter will deal with multiple injuries exclusive of spinal cord injury. The latter will be mentioned only when it is germane to the management of other injuries.

Management of the patient with multiple injuries provides a unique clinical challenge for the physician. Treatment must be prioritized according to physiologic parameters necessary for survival; these include the ABCs—that is, *A*irway, *B*reathing, and *C*irculation. Another factor in management of the patient with multiple injuries is that treatment often must be started before all diagnostic tests are accomplished as resuscitation proceeds.

The prehospital management of patients with multiple injuries must be guided by the principle of avoiding further injury. To accomplish this, the patient may require neck splinting or placement on a spine board before movement even though no definitive diagnosis of injury in these areas has been made. When possible, radio communication with the base hospital should be established, protocols should be instituted if they exist.

Management at the scene includes extrication of persons who are trapped in a vehicle, maintenance of a patent airway and assisting ventilation when indicated, protection of the spine following blunt trauma, control of external hemorrhage with direct pressure bandaging, and stabilization of long bone fractures when they exist. Intravenous fluid administration, intubation, and other rususcitative measures may be necessary when transport time will exceed 15 minutes and when the emergency crew is equipped to carry out these procedures.[1-3]

Rapid transportation to the appropriate facility should be undertaken. This is usually effectively accomplished by means of ground vehicles such as properly equipped ambulances. If the distance that the patient must be moved is greater than 25 miles, or when a great deal of time will be lost in ground transportation (as with heavy traffic congestion), helicopter transport may be more efficient if it is available. Although helicopters are usually efficient for covering a distance up to about 100 miles, for distances beyond this, fixed-wing aircraft are more suitable.

TABLE 5–1. Triage—Setting Priorities

TOP PRIORITY
Establish a patent airway
Maintain adequate ventilation
Tamponade external hemorrhage
Replace lost blood volume
Immobilize cervical spine (blunt trauma)
TRIAGE DECISION-MAKING
Initiate and maintain a flow sheet
Conduct rapid, complete examination
Splint fractures and dislocations
Identify sources of blood loss
    Abdomen–peritoneal lavage
    Pelvis–roentgenogram
    Chest–roentgenogram
Lateral C spine film (blunt trauma)
Decompress stomach
Catheterize bladder
Get baseline lab values, blood cross-match
Consider antibiotics and tetanus prophylaxis

Once the patient has reached definitive care, that is, the emergency department, triage is the first step in management (Table 5–1). Vital signs should be taken and a quick assessment of any obvious injuries should be carried out. When it is known, information concerning the type of accident, time of injury, and any known pre-existing medical conditions may be helpful in treatment.

LIFE-SUSTAINING MEASURES

Initial resuscitation consists of correcting any physiologic abnormalities which exist. The most important goal is to maintain adequate oxygen flow to the peripheral tissues. Thus, the airway must be clear and adequate ventilation must be present. In the latter, the chest cage must be intact and the lungs must be functioning adequately. If air is being exchanged in the lung, the next step is to ensure that oxygen delivery to peripheral tissues is continuing. This depends upon an adequate volume within the circulatory tree, and a pump (heart) that is working satisfactorily. In most instances, we can assume that the pump is working satisfactorily and can turn our attention to the maintenance of blood volume. Diminished blood volume due to hemorrhage is a common denominator of major injuries, and restoration of volume takes a high priority in resuscitation.

External hemorrhage, as mentioned earlier, should be tamponaded with manual compression followed by a pressure dressing. Volume restitution then depends upon the rapid administration of crystalloid solution through two large-caliber intravenous catheters. If there is no response in the blood pressure to two liters of Ringer's lactated solution administered rapidly, one must consider the possibility that the pump mechanism is not functioning properly. While ongoing massive hemorrhage can dampen the response to the Ringer's lactate solution, in most patients some response will be seen with the rapid administration of fluid volumes. However, in the event that the pressure does not seem to respond, one must look for distended neck veins to suggest myocardial dysfunction. Probably the most common cause of myocardial dysfunction is cardiac contusion in blunt trauma and pericardial tamponade secondary to hemorrhage in penetrating wounds.

Patients should not be moved during initial treatment measures; those who have been placed on a spine board should remain there,

and the neck should be immobilized until further evaluation can take place.

With the breathing at least temporarily under control and with fluid resuscitation under way, the next step is a rapid physical examination. The patient must be completely disrobed but should not be moved until spinal injury has been ruled out. A quick palpation of the spine from the base of the skull to the coccyx is important, looking for either physical abnormalities or tenderness. If this examination is negative, it may be safe to roll the patient over for inspection of the flanks and the back. It is imperative that this initial assessment include a rectal examination and inspection of the perineum and the axillae and a check of neurologic function and peripheral pulses. Upon completion of the inspection for obvious abnormalities, if none are seen, further studies can be undertaken. This includes the splinting of long bone fractures to alleviate pain and minimize additional blood loss. A nasogastric tube should be inserted to decompress the stomach and eliminate the risk of pulmonary aspiration. Blood in the gastric aspirate may indicate the possiblity of an injury to the stomach or the duodenum. A Foley catheter is also inserted to empty the bladder in preparation for peritoneal lavage and also to determine whether hematuria is present. Urinary output is used in the evaluation of effective fluid resuscitation.

Ongoing blood loss is usually indicated by a failure of the blood pressure to return to normal levels following a fluid load or a response and then a softening of the pressure. The presence of bleeding into the chest can be determined by means of a chest roentgenogram; this will dictate the need for the placement of a thoracotomy tube for drainage of fluid or trapped air.

Identification of abdominal injury is most difficult by clinical examination; the most satisfactory diagnostic test is the immediate use of peritoneal lavage. This is carried out by inserting a plastic catheter through a small stab wound in the infraumbilical position after the peritoneum has been grasped and opened under direct vision. The return of bloody fluid after the installation of a liter of Ringer's lactated solution is a reliable indication that intraperitoneal hemorrhage has occurred.[4] Once this rapid examination of the patient and the institution of emergency measures has taken place, a more detailed examination and treatment plan can be developed.[5]

Tetanus prophylaxis should be carried out in

any patient with a contaminated injury, and routine laboratory tests should be done; including a complete blood count and urinalysis. In addition, blood gases and baseline chemistries should be obtained. A blood sample should be sent to the blood bank for typing and crossmatching so the blood will be available if needed immediately.

Airway and Breathing

The prevention of hypoxia by establishment of an adequate patent airway and by maintenance of adequate ventilation may be a lifesaving step in the management of the critically injured patient. Hypoxia is most often caused by either airway obstruction or by hypoventilation. The latter may be compounded by ventilation-perfusion mismatching, alveolar-capillary diffusion abnormalities, or right-to-left pulmonary shunting.

Hypoxia is suggested by anxiety, restlessness, and mental confusion. Hypoxia may be caused by airway obstruction as a result of foreign bodies such as blood, teeth, or bony fragments within the airway, by soft tissue collapse of the pharynx due to extensive facial injuries, or by direct trauma to the tracheal laryngeal structures. These patients usually are hoarse, they may be snoring, or they may have stridor and supraclavicular and intercostal retraction as accessory muscles are used for breathing.

Hypoxia can also be caused by hypoventilation secondary to a blunted ventilatory drive, which results from intracranial injury.[6] Failure of the negative intropleural pressure secondary to hemopneumothorax, a flail chest wall, or an open thoracic wound may also restrict mechanical ability to ventilate. Finally, spinal trauma causing respiratory muscle weakness may also lead to hypoventilation. Clinically, one must suspect hypoventilation in the presence of diminished breath sounds and decreased chest wall movement. The addition of distended neck veins and a deviated trachea suggest a tension pneumothorax, which must be corrected rapidly before it leads to death.

Airway management in the critically injured patient often requires endotracheal intubation. Factors that may influence the decision to intubate include the patency of the airway, a satisfactory ventilatory drive, severe thoracic injury compromising the ventilatory effectiveness, a cervical spine injury that may paralyze the respiratory muscles, and finally serious maxillofacial injury that may eventually compromise the airway.

The first step in airway management is to quickly inspect the mouth and remove any foreign bodies and suction out blood and secretions that may be obstructing the airway. This is followed by elevation of the angle of the mandible to prevent pharyngeal obstruction, and then either an oropharyngeal or nasopharyngeal tube should be placed to maintain the airway. During these maneuvers traction should be kept on the head to prevent hyperextension of the neck in case an unstable cervical spine injury exists.[7] A reservoir mask should probably be utilized at this time, since it can deliver a 90 per cent oxygen concentration at 12 liters per minute.[8] If there is a suspicion of hemopneumothorax, a tube thoracostomy should be placed immediately. This is usually done in either the fourth or fifth intercostal space because the diaphragm may rise to the fourth intercostal space with full expiration.

In the patient who has sustained blunt injury, the physician must assume that an unstable cervical spine fracture exists until it can be ruled out by roentgenography. Although the actual incidence of cervical injury in vehicular trauma is unknown, it has been reported to be as high as 24 per cent.[9] Most neck injuries occur at C5–C6 or C6–C7 level. A crosstable lateral cervical spine (CTLCS) roentgenogram will demonstrate 98 per cent of unstable cervical fractures. It is most important that C7 be visualized in order to rule out a fracture at this level.

Patients who may need operative airway control include those who have severe maxillofacial injury or a suspected cervical spine injury. Cricothyrotomy with the insertion of a 6 mm internal diameter endotracheal tube is probably the preferred approach for adults.[10,11] This has largely replaced tracheostomy; however, if the surgeon is more comfortable with tracheostomy and has wider experience in that area, it is a perfectly satisfactory approach in operative airway intervention. Treatment of patients who have direct laryngeal trauma or tracheal disruption[12] demands emergency tracheostomy; this injury cannot be managed by cricothyrotomy.

For most patients, nasotracheal intubation is the method of choice for the establishment of an airway; however, it is not a satisfactory approach in the patient who is apneic. It is quite satisfactory for the patient with a potential cervical spine injury who has no major facial trauma. Intubation can be carried out with the patient awake, it can be accomplished without moving the neck, it is relatively easy to perform, and with it the endotracheal tube may be removed from the mouth. While it is a "blind" procedure, the success rate exceeds 90 per cent in experienced hands.[13,14] Major complications of nasal bleeding and retropharyngeal tears[15] may be avoided by use of careful technique.

Nasotracheal intubation is the method of choice in the conscious patient with an intact cervical spine. It can be performed in these patients without the need of sedation or muscle relaxation and it can be used to avoid the so-called *crash intubation*. When the physician is unable to successfully carry out nasotracheal intubation, orotracheal intubation is the next step. In most awake critically injured patients, it is necessary to induce muscle paralysis in order to open the mouth adequately and facilitate the positioning of the head for this approach. We prefer to use succinylcholine (0.5 to 2.0 mg/kg of body weight) intravenously for the muscle relaxant. It has a rapid onset—usually less than one minute—and has a relatively brief duration of about 2 to 10 minutes.[16] Whenever this approach is used, personnel must anticipate the possibility of operative airway intubation and be prepared to carry this out and have the necessary equipment standing by.

Finally, in the unconscious patient who has no spinal injury, orotracheal intubation is probably the preferred approach. It is a quick, safe maneuver that permits direct visualization of the trachea, therefore ensuring that the tube is in the proper place. Proper position of the tube should be confirmed by roentgenography as soon as possible after its placement.

Treatment of Hypovolemia

When the aforementioned maneuvers have provided adequate oxygen delivery to the alveoli, it is essential to verify that adequate volume is available to carry the oxygen to the peripheral tissues. Shock may be caused, in the postinjury state, by inadequate circulating blood volume, which is the most common cause. Shock can also be brought about by impaired myocardial function or by altered vascular resistance or a combination of these. Hypovolemia secondary to external blood loss should be controlled with manual pressure and a pressure bandage over the bleeding point. Internal bleeding, which may not immediately be controlled, can be compensated for by the administration of fluid volumes.

The patient in shock may have a temporary increase in volume by the simple maneuver of raising the legs. This maneuver is just as satisfactory as the use of MAST trousers.

Two large-caliber intravenous lines should be started, usually in the antecubital space, and crystalloid solution (in the form of Ringer's lactated solution) should be run wide open into both intravenous lines. The aim here is to re-establish volume as quickly as possible; salt solutions are just as effective as colloid-containing solutions in restoring tissue perfusion.[17,18]

In most patients, short 14-guage catheters can be inserted into each antecubital space; these provide a quick access route that in most cases does not lead to serious complications. When the patient is in such severe shock that venous access cannot be obtained by the percutaneous route, access is most easily accomplished through a venous cutdown. Although the access is usually provided via the saphenous vein at the ankle, the access procedure can also be carried out through the antecubital fossa. With two large-caliber catheters in place and Ringer's lactated solution flowing wide open into each of these, adequate volume can be administered.

As mentioned earlier, when the first IV line is placed, blood should be obtained for type and cross-matching, for hematocrit determination, and for other baseline laboratory tests. The goal in the administration of crystalloid solution is to return the patient's systolic blood pressure to as close to normal as possible. It must be remembered that a minimum of 3 ml of crystalloid solution is required to match 1 ml of blood lost, and in some instances the ratio is even higher, depending on the volume deficit. If the systolic blood pressure persists below 80 mm Hg, the patient has probably sustained an acute blood loss in excess of one third of the blood volume. The systemic blood pressure, pulse rate, and urinary output plus the overall appearance of the patient are practical guides to of the effectiveness of hypovolemia treatment.

When time permits, a central venous pressure line (CVP) should be inserted to help differentiate hypovolemic shock from cardiogenic shock. A CVP less than 5 cm of water implies hypovolemia whereas a CVP greater than 15 cm suggests that volume replacement has been adequate. In both instances the CVP serves as a guide only and should be utilized in conjunction with clinical evaluation of the patient.

Crystalloid solution is a satisfactory early replacement for blood that has been lost because it repletes the extracellular as well as the intracellular deficits, the hemodilution created enhances perfusion by reducing blood viscosity, and the increase in cardiac output provides adequate tissue oxygenation.[19,20] The use of crystalloid solution, of course, cannot be continued indefinitely because circulating red cells will become depleted. Blood should be added to the resuscitation fluid when the crystalloid infusion exceeds 50 ml/kg. If cross-matched blood is not yet available, uncross-matched, type-specific whole blood should be used and is rarely associated with serious complications.[21,22] While micropore filters are generally placed in the infusion line for banked blood, they should not be used under emergency situations because they impede infusion capabilities.

A major complication of massive blood and fluid resuscitation is a bleeding diathesis[7,23] The cause, which has not been clearly defined, is probably multifactorial. Banked blood is deficient in Factors V and VIII, as well as in platelets, and at the same time is replete with fibrinsplit products and vasoactive substances. These factors become important when approximately 15 units of blood have been administered. While autotransfused blood is somewhat safer than banked blood,[24] its use in large quantities is associated with the same problem. The use of fresh frozen plasma and fresh platelets minimize the rise of coagulopathy after massive transfusion.[25] It is our general policy to administer fresh frozen plasma after the tenth unit of banked blood or autotransfused blood has been administered and then with each subsequent four units of blood. Platelets are usually added after 15 units of blood transfusion and after that are replaced empirically with each additional five units of transfused blood. Coagulation profiles are obtained, consisting of the prothrombin time, activated partial thromboplastin time, and platelet counts. We try to ensure that the platelet count remains in excess of 50,000 per cubic mm in the acute trauma patient.

Other problems that may occur during massive blood transfusion include hypocalcemia, acidosis, and hypothermia. Hypocalcemia results from citrate in the blood but does not occur until the transfusion rate exceeds one unit per every five minutes. In addition, decreased serum-ionized calcium depresses myocardial function[26,27] before it affects the coagu-

lation cascade. Calcium gluconate (10 mg/kg intravenously) is therefore given to patients having changes in the ST interval on the electrocardiogram rather than being given on the basis of volumes transfused.

Hypothermia is associated with decreased survival in experimental hemorrhagic shock.[28] Moderate hypothermia (32°C or 90°F) causes platelet sequestration and inhibits the intrinsic clotting pathway. The core temperature of injured patients can decrease rather insidiously when they experience exposure at the scene of the accident and while in the emergency department and when cold resuscitation fluids are given. Therefore, resuscitation fluids in trauma units should be prewarmed to 40°C and the blood should be infused with a heat exchanger in the line to warm it. In addition, heating and aerosolizing the oxygen in a ventilator is a very efficient method of preventing hypothermia.[29]

Acidosis is another common complication of hypovolemic shock; the administration of bicarbonate would seem logical as a preventive measure. Moderate acidosis (a pH of 7.20) impairs coagulation,[29,30] myocardial contractility,[31] and oxidative metabolism,[32] presenting a lifethreatening situation. Acidosis usually occurs as a result of a rise in lactic acid production secondary to hypovolemia; however, it is automatically corrected when volume has been replaced. Therefore, the use of sodium bicarbonate in the treatment of shock is not indicated, except in patients who suffer a protracted period of shock.

Therapy in Carodiogenic Shock

The patient who remains hypotensive, despite an adequate airway and vigorous fluid administration, must be considered to be in cardiogenic shock. Clinically, this is suggested by distended neck veins and a central venous pressure elevated in excess of 15 cm of water. Cardiogenic shock is usually the result of (1) tension pneumothorax, (2) pericardial tamponade, (3) myocardial contusion and/or infarction, or (4) air embolism.

Tension pneumothorax results from a tear in the pleura or a bronchus, allowing a progressive accumulation of air in the pleural space. As the pressure builds up, the ipsilateral lung collapses and the mediastinum begins to shift to the contralateral side; this results in compression of the opposite lung. There is a resultant restriction in air exchange and a ventilation-perfusion mismatch, resulting in hypoxemia. Venous return to the heart is impaired because of the rising pleural pericardial pressure so that myocardial performance begins to decrease. The clinical signs of tension pneumothorax are a tracheal deviation and a shift of the cardiac impulse to the contralateral side. There is increased resonance to percussion and breath sounds are diminished on the involved side.

Because these clinical signs are often difficult to ascertain during rapid early treatment in a busy emergency department, any patient who remains in shock following adequate fluid resuscitation and who has suffered a penetrating thoracic wound or blunt chest trauma should have venting of the injured hemithorax. As a test and a temporizing measure, a large-caliber needle may be inserted into the anterior second intercostal space; this should be followed by the rapid placement of a large (at least 36 French) chest tube through the lateral fifth intercostal space.[33] Once the tube has been placed, the presence of a massive air leak suggests a disruption of the bronchus so that immediate bronchoscopy and possible thoracotomy are indicated.[34]

Traumatic cardiac tamponade occurs when there is an accumulation of blood or air within the pericardial sac of sufficient volume to compromise myocardial function. Under chronic conditions the pericardial sac may contain a liter or more of fluid and the heart still functions reasonably well. In the acute situation, accumulation of 150 ml of blood may cause severe hemodynamic instability and can lead to death if not rapidly corrected. The pathophysiology consists of impaired diastolic ventricular filling secondary to the elevated intrapericardial pressure,[35] which leads to depressed myocardial contractility secondary to coronary arterial insufficiency.[36]

The classic physical signs of cardiac tamponade are known as *Beck's triad* and consist of arterial hypotension, central venous hypertension, and distant heart sounds. When present, this triad is diagnostic, but it is absent in more than one third of the patients with postinjury tamponade.[37] The best diagnostic tool is a high index of suspicion, particularly in patients with penetrating injuries in the region of the heart. It can also result from blunt trauma but this cause is less common. It must be remembered that the pericardial sac can be injured with wounds that occur in the axilla, back, and supraclavicular and subxyphoid regions. Wounds in any of these areas should arouse suspicion of tamponade, particularly if there is failure of the blood pressure to rise in the face of what appears to be adequate resuscitation. If a central venous pressure line has been inserted, it usually will read above 20 cm when tamponade exists.

The management of pericardial tamponade consists of immediate pericardiocentesis either in the emergency department or in an operating room if that is available. The latter is preferred because of the availability of good illumination, adequate instruments and surgical assistance as well as facilities for cardiopulmonary bypass, intra-aortic balloon assist devices, and autotransfusion. However, if the hemodynamic status is such that movement to the operating room may jeopardize the patient's life, immediate decompression of the pericardial sac is mandatory. This is carried out using an 18 cardiac needle, which is inserted in the left xyphoid-costal angle and directed toward the posterior aspect of the left shoulder. Although an electrocardiographic lead connected to the needle is helpful as a guide, it is not absolutely necessary if the time factor is critically important. Aspiration of as little as 15 ml of blood may improve the cardiac output enormously and thus permit safe transport to the operating room for a more definitive procedure. There is a false-negative aspiration rate of about 15 per cent in patients because the blood in the pericardial sac has clotted.[37,38] When possible the patient should be taken to the operating suite so that the cardiac wound itself can be satisfactorily managed. The pericardium is opened widely anterior to the phrenic nerve and cardiorrhaphy is carried out with pledgeted sutures.[39]

Cardiogenic shock may also result from myocardial contusion, which is present in about 20 per cent of patients who have sustained blunt chest trauma.[40] As one might guess, the right ventricle is the most often injured because of its anterior position. An impact such as a steering wheel against the sternum may drive it against the heart, causing direct myocardial damage. Ventricular arrhythmias seem to be the major acute complication of myocardial contusion.

Diagnosis of this condition is difficult because ECG changes are nonspecific or may be lacking altogether. Use of creatinine phosphokinase isoenzyme (CPK-MB) is inconclusive as a diagnostic test, as is technetium pyrophosphate scintigraphy. Other tests are more accurate, but they are not generally available for routine use in an emergency department. These include ECG-gated, blood pool radionuclide angiography, and two-dimensional endocardiography. Therefore, the diagnosis depends upon a high index of suspicion, the presence of cardiogenic shock, and injury to the anterior chest either noted by history or by physical signs of precordial trauma.

Management is similar to that of acute myocardial infarction. Adequate oxygenation should be carried out, and fluid administration should be carefully controlled while serum electrolytes are being monitored. If arrhythmias occur, pharmacologic management of these is mandatory. It should be remembered that left ventricular contractility can be diminished when right ventricular overload has occurred. This is brought about by a reduction in the filling volume of the left ventricle. If the damage is severe and cardiogenic shock continues, emergency intraaortic balloon counter pulsation may be effective. The balloon can be inserted in the emergency department by means of the percutaneous technique.

A subtle but potentially rapidly lethal complication of chest trauma is air embolism. Although in most instances it follows penetrating trauma, it can occur with blunt injury.[41,42] When the lung is injured and air is able to flow into an injured pulmonary vein, it may embolize to the coronary arterial system. Patients with this complication may remain hemodynamically stable until active airway control is instituted. At that point, positive airway pressure and reduced pulmonary venous pressure secondary to the associated shock may cause air to move from the lung into the venous system. These patients must be managed by emergency thoracotomy with a cross-clamping of the pulmonary hilar region and aspiration of the air from the left ventricle. Open cardiac massage is then instituted, and if there is extensive damage to the lung, pulmonary resection may be required.[43]

The use of emergency thoracotomy in the emergency department continues to be a controversial issue. It may well be justified in the patient whose condition suddenly deteriorates into a cardiac arrest after arrival in the emergency department. The cause of the arrest is often not determined, and continued external cardiac massage is usually not effective in these patients.[44,45] The purpose of open thoracotomy under these conditions is to quickly determine whether there is pericardial tamponade and release it if it is present, to control any intrathoracic blood loss that may be rather massive, to undertake direct cardiac massage, and finally to clamp the descending thoracic aorta just as

it goes through the diaphragm in order to increase the perfusion to the coronaries and the cerebral circulation and to diminish further blood loss below the diaphragm.

The approach is usually through the left fifth intercostal space; this provides rapid access to the heart and the descending thoracic aorta as well as the left lung. If necessary, the incision can be extended across the sternum in order to increase the exposure of the heart and the right lung.

Survival depends to a large extent on the type of injury and is most probable in patients with stab wounds to the right side of the heart. In this situation the mechanism is cardiac tamponade, and suture of the stab wound with release of the tamponade will allow a rapid recovery. The use of open thoracotomy to attempt to resuscitate the patient who has suffered a cardiac arrest due to exsanguinating blood loss from multiple injuries is rarely successful. The reason for this is that even though the heart has continued to beat, it has been so ischemic over a period of time that irreversible damage has probably occurred.

DEFINITIVE EVALUATION

Once the primarily life-saving measures are under way, a more definitive assessment must be made of the patient with multiple injuries. This is best accomplished by starting at the head and carefully examining the patient from the head to the toes.

Head and Upper Spine

Careful inspection of the scalp for lacerations, for ongoing blood loss, and for a possible depression injury should be done. The signs of a possible basal skull fracture consist of bleeding in the ear, ecchymosis over the mastoid process (Battle's sign), and periorbital blood staining (raccoon eyes). Cerebral spinal fluid leaks, such as otorrhea or rhinorrhea, suggest a dural tear. When severe facial injury exists so that the bones of the face are unstable, an anterior basilar skull fracture is a possibility. Patients with such injuries should never have a nasogastric tube placed through the nose, since it may enter the cranial vault. It should always be placed through the mouth.

The patient's cerebral function needs to be noted at the time of admission; this evaluation should be repeated at reasonably frequent intervals in order to detect any signs of deterio-

TABLE 5–2. Glasgow Coma Scale

1. Eye Opening
   Spontaneous ———4
   To Voice ———3
   To Pain ———2
   None ———1

2. Verbal Response
   Oriented ———5
   Confused ———4
   Inappropriate words ———3
   Incomprehensible words ———2
   None ———1

3. Motor Response
   Obeys commands ———6
   Purposeful movement (pain) ———5
   Withdraw (pain) ———4
   Flexion (pain) ———3
   Extension (pain) ———3
   None ———1
   Total GCS Points ————
   (1 + 2 + 3)

ration. The Glasgow coma scale (Table 5–2) is the most widely used method of evaluation and is reproducible from individual to individual; a score of less that 8 indicates serious head injury. In addition, one should ascertain the pupillary reflexes, motor and sensory symmetry, deep tendon reflexes, and rectal sphincter tone. When abnormalities are found, neurosurgical consultation should be obtained as quickly as possible.

The cervical, thoracic, and lumbar spine must be palpated for any evidence of deformity or any tenderness. In any patient who has had blunt trauma, a spine injury must be considered present until eventually ruled out by x-ray. Evaluation of physical signs alone will not eliminate this possibility.

Injuries to the Neck Produced by Blunt Trauma

One of the most serious injuries following blunt trauma to the neck is laryngotracheal disruption. This injury usually occurs following compression of the chest between the steering wheel and the vertebral column or if the patient strikes a wire fence while riding a snowmobile or bicycle or even while sled riding. The signs and symptoms include airway distress, dysphonia, dysphagia, stridor, hoarseness, and hemoptysis. Usually there is a contusion on the neck and often subcutaneous emphysema with crepitus, and the laryngeal anatomy may be markedly distorted. Although provision of adequate ventilation is the top priority, one must be aware that there may be an unstable cervical fracture, and that must be excluded.

This is a difficult situation to manage and its treatment is best accomplished in the operating room. When the patient's condition is stable, treatment should take place in an operating room where optimal lighting, equipment, and adequate personnel are available. Attempts at intubation may extend the injury or may prove impossible and create airway decompensation. Emergency cricothyrotomy may worsen the ventilation and be difficult to accomplish because of the anatomic distortion. Tracheostomy may be dangerous since the distal trachea may retract down into the superior mediastinum, making control of the airway almost impossible. With the patient in the operating room and with adequate assistance and equipment, a systematic approach can be used and the incision can be extended as far as necessary in order for retraction of the distal trachea to be controlled.[12]

VASCULAR INJURIES. Injury to the carotid or vertebral arteries is extremely rare in blunt trauma and usually results from an intimal tear with dissection and secondary thrombosis. When this injury does occur, there may be no history of a direct blow to the neck because rotation or hyperextension or both of the cervical spine can also cause the injury. When injury is suspected, four-vessel angiography is necessary to not only identify the level of the injury but to help determine whether or not repair is feasible.

Penetrating Neck Injury

While penetrating injuries to the neck are not common, they can be extremely dangerous if not managed in a propitious manner. Following clinical evaluation, a cross table lateral (C spine) cervical spine film is often helpful before endotracheal intubation takes place. If the patient's neurologic function is intact, it is reasonable to assume that one can proceed with intubation. Cricothyrotomy may be necessary when the patient has severe oropharyngeal bleeding that can make oral or nasal intubation almost impossible.

There is considerable controversy regarding the indications for exploration of the neck, but generally most investigators believe that if the platysma muscle has been penetrated exploration should be carried out. The expanding hematoma and/or external hemorrhage are indications along with either severe hemoptysis and/or dysphagia. Stridor, hoarseness, and difficulty in speaking are also indications for exploration. In the hemodynamically stable patient, angiography should be carried out if there is any suggestion that the wound is in the region of the various vascular structures within the neck. Whenever a pharyngoesophageal injury is suspected, endoscopy should be carried out, usually at the time of operation.[46]

Blunt Chest Trauma

Most of the injuries that occur within the chest following blunt trauma are due to rapid deceleration following high-speed vehicular accidents. The impact of the chest against the steering wheel or dashboard is often the cause of these injuries. They can also occur as a result of a fall or direct blows to the chest in other circumstances. The chest injuries can be subtle and often are overshadowed by serious injuries to the abdomen, the head, or the extremities. A high index of suspicion based upon the cause of the trauma should prevent the physician from overlooking these injuries.

PULMONARY CONTUSION. Bruising of the lung or pulmonary contusion is found in one third to one half of all severely injured patients.[47,48] A sudden severe blow to the chest may lead to overdistention of the alveoli and a shearing of alveolar tissue as it swings around within the chest. Alveolar gas exchange becomes diminished secondary to increased capillary membrane permeability, edema formation, local hemorrhage from the tearing of some of the vessels, and eventually an elevated pulmonary vascular resistance. The hemorrhage in contusion is rarely severe because it represents a bruising rather than major hemorrhage. As already mentioned, these injuries can be extremely subtle and an initial chest roentgenogram may show nothing or perhaps only a small localized infiltrate. By 24 to 36 hours, however, there may be overt consolidation of an area of the lung.[47,49] Hemopneumothorax complicates pulmonary contusion in up to half of the patients; in some cases hemorrhage may be great enough to create hemoptysis and a compromised airway.[50]

The initial management is to maintain oxygenation of the patient while avoiding fluid overloading. Formerly most of these patients were intubated as a matter of course, but now many clinicians think that intercostal nerve blocks will alleviate the chest wall pain and allow for adequate gas exchange.[48,51] If the patient must be intubated and placed on mechanical ventilation, the early use of positive end expiratory pressure may be beneficial.[52,53]

The use of prophylactic antibiotics remains unproven and is usually the surgeon's choice. There is no good evidence that this measure is beneficial.

RUPTURE OF THE TRACHEOBRONCHIAL TREE. A sudden rise in intraluminal pressure against a closed glottis may cause a rupture of the tracheobronchial tree. This usually occurs with a shearing force resulting from the airway being compressed against the spine.[34] The tears may be complete or partial and may be classified as type I or type II. In type I rupture, the right main or distal left bronchus beyond the parietal pleural reflection is torn and thus the patient has a pneumothorax with a continued air leak. Type II injury occurs in either the trachea or the proximal left bronchus (that is, within the mediastinum) and usually is indicated by mediastinal emphysema. As soon as such a lesion is suspected, bronchoscopy should be carried out to make the diagnosis. While minor tears may be treated nonsurgically, most of the major disruptions will require immediate thoracotomy.[54]

TEAR OF THE THORACIC AORTA. One of the major complications that can result from blunt chest trauma, only recognized in recent years, is that of a tear of the thoracic aorta. If the aorta is transected, most of the patients (probably 80 per cent) who exsanguinate at the accident scene will die almost immediately.[55] Those patients that we see in the emergency department, and this is probably 20 per cent of the cases, are alive because the aortic adventitial tissue and the pleura have contained the hemorrhage and prevented a free intrathoracic hemorrhage.

We have demonstrated in the monkey that intra-aortic pressure may rise as high as 1800 mm Hg for a few milliseconds during compression of the sternum against the vertebral column. With sudden deceleration the heart and aorta move forward and twist on the relatively fixed descending aorta at a time when intraluminal aortic pressure is quite high.[56] The aortic tear usually occurs just distal to the left subclavian artery in those patients who survive. The ascending aortic route may be damaged by acute lengthening stress such as results from a fall from a great height.[57,58]

Those patients who survive the immediate tear and arrive alive in the emergency department may show little or no evidence of the catastrophic injury that has occurred.[58] Of those patients who survive one hour after the injury, 15 per cent have rupture into the thorax within 6 hours and 25 per cent have this within 24 hours.[55] Thus, there is a period of time during which those patients reaching the emergency department may have definitive therapy carried out—in many instances, a lifesaving procedure. Most of these patients will have sustained multisystem injury, and the symptoms of the torn thoracic aorta are often minimal. Thus, if on an early chest film a widened mediastinum is seen, one should be suspicious that a possible thoracic aortic tear has occurred and aortography and surgical intervention will be necessary as soon as possible. Hypertension secondary to stretching of the sympathetic nerves around the aortic isthmus has been seen in approximately half of the patients with this injury.[59] There are a number of other signs and symptoms that may occur but none of them are definitive for aortic injury. In the case of patients who have sustained an injury to the sternum suggesting compression of the thoracic contents, or who have fallen from a great height, the physician should suspect the possibility of a thoracic aortic tear.

The most classic sign of an aortic tear is a widening of the mediastinum on the initial chest roentgenogram. Superior mediastinal widening beyond 8 cm is considered pathognomonic until aortic tear is ruled out by aortography. Other changes on the roentgenogram are shown in Table 5–3. Any patient with a mediastinum widened beyond 8 cm must undergo aortography at some point in the course of their immediate work-up. It must be remembered that a widened mediastinum may be brought about by venous bleeding, but this is rarely fatal.[60,61] Unfortunately, approximately one fourth of the patients with acute thoracic aortic tears have a normal initial chest roentgenogram.[62]

The management of these patients is difficult and often requires major triage decisions in the

TABLE 5–3.   Roentgenographic Changes Indicating Aortic Tear

1. Widened superior mediastinum
2. Ill-defined aortic knob
3. Obliterated aorticopulmonary window
4. Left pleural apical cap
5. Nasogastric tube deviated to the right
6. Tracheal deviation to the right
7. Caudad displacement on the left main bronchus
8. Abnormal descending aortic contour
9. Obliterated paraspinus strip
10. Left hemothorax

emergency department. Imagine the patient with a severe head injury, a widened mediastinum, and a grossly positive peritoneal lavage.[57,63] If the patient is hemodynamically unstable, immediate laparotomy should be carried out because the abdomen is the most likely site of the hemodynamic instability. In the patient who is stable, head CT scan followed by arteriography before laparotomy would be the most logical approach. This is obviously a multiteam approach, and surgical management must be prioritized. When necessary, the aortic isthmus can be approached via a left posteriolateral thoracotomy at the same time that a second team explores the abdomen.[57]

Penetrating Chest Trauma

It is surprising how few patients with penetrating injury of the chest actually require surgical intervention. About 15 per cent of all these patients will require thoracotomy.[64] Continuing hemorrhage, cardiac tamponade, and air embolism are the indications for immediate exploration of the chest. Although continued bleeding into the chest is not easily defined, a practical guideline that we use is as follows: when the inital blood loss from the thoracotomy tube is between 1200 and 1500 ml, immediate surgery is indicated. If the bleeding is somewhat less than this but continues at a rate of more than 250 ml per hour for 3 consecutive hours, surgical intervention is indicated. In most instances, with injury to the lung and bleeding, the insertion of the thoracotomy tube will allow the injured lung to press against the rigid chest wall and thus stop the bleeding in the low pressure system of the lung. These guidelines for surgical intervention must be tempered by evaluation of the patient's general condition. For example, if 1200 ml of blood is found to be escaping from the initially placed thoracotomy tube while the patient remains stable and some time has elapsed since the injury occurred, it may be advisable to delay surgical intervention. If on the other hand the thoracotomy tube is inserted shortly after injury and blood is flowing from the tube at the rate of 1200 to 1500 ml, the patient should be prepared for immediate operation.

A group of patients with particularly dangerous injuries includes those in whom a bullet has traversed the mediastinum. Because of the many structures that could be affected, the likelihood of serious injury is great. However, selective management of these patients, with angiography and esophagoscopy as diagnostic indicators of injury in the mediastinum, can be used.[65,66]

It is important to recognize that abdominal injury may occur with what appears to be a thoracic injury. One must remember that the diaphragm rises to the mid chest with full expiration.[65,67] The lower thorax, which may contain abdominal viscera under the diaphragm, is defined as superiorly the nipple line anteriorly (the fourth intercostal space) and the tip of the scapula posteriorly. It is easy with these landmarks to see how a penetrating missile in the lower chest may actually enter the abdomen after traversing the diaphragm and injure the intraabdominal viscera. If the injury to the diaphragm is great, the abdominal viscera may herniate into the chest. This may lead to strangulation of the intestine. It is difficult to diagnose such injuries by physical examination; therefore, peritoneal lavage is the diagnostic method of greatest value.

Blunt Abdominal Trauma

Injury to the abdominal viscera following blunt trauma is easily missed and is a frequent cause of preventable death. Physical signs may be misleading; the peritoneal signs are subtle and frequently overshadowed by pain resulting from associated injuries such as fractures. Many of these patients are unconscious because of associated head injury. It has been estimated that up to one third of patients who will require emergency laparotomy have an initial benign abdominal examination.[68] Blood loss into the peritoneal cavity, which can occur following injury, may be relatively massive without producing major abdominal distention.

The use of diagnostic peritoneal lavage therefore is recommended early in the evaluation of the patient with multiple injuries; it was first described by Root and associates in 1965.[69] It has been proven to have a sensitivity of 98 per cent and is a valuable diagnostic tool. Indications for lavage in the emergency department include the patient who is in coma from a head injury, the patient who is severely intoxicated or paralyzed, a physical examination which is equivocal in the patient who is hypovolemic, and the patient who must be anesthetized in order to manage associated injuries. We use the semi-open method, in which a small incision is made just below the umbilicus and then carried through the fascia to the peritoneum. The peritoneum is then grasped and the catheter inserted as the peritoneum is opened.[4] If the patient has had a previous midline abdominal incision, we will usually make the approach along the lateral margin of the rectus muscle. When the catheter is inserted, aspiration of more than 10 ml of blood from the peritoneal cavity constitutes an indication for laparotomy. If gross blood is not withdrawn at the time of insertion of the catheter, a liter of saline is introduced into the peritoneal cavity and then allowed to run out by gravity. If the red blood count in this fluid exceeds 100,000 cells per cubic millimeter, this result is an indication for laparotomy. The clinical test that can be used involves adding some of the return fluid to a test tube and seeing if a newspaper can be read through the tube. This is a crude index but is satisfactory; however, we believe that doing a count on the fluid is a more satisfactory way of making the determination. A white blood count in excess of 500 per cubic millimeter or an increase in certain enzymes such as the amylase and the alkaline phosphatase in the peritoneal fluid may indicate injury that is not indicated by gross bleeding.

Unfortunately, approximately 2 per cent of patients have a false-negative peritoneal lavage. In these patients the injury is usually to the duodenum, pancreas, jejunum, bladder, diaphragm, or renal pedicle. The surgeon must have a high index of suspicion for a possible injury to the abdominal viscera following blunt trauma. If the automobile accident victim has been held in his seat by a lap type of seatbelt, the possibility of these rather subtle lesions must be suspected.[70] In these cases additional diagnostic tests may be of value, including serum amylase determination for the possibility of pancreatic injury, a Gastrografin study to evaluate the stomach and the duodenum, cystography for possible bladder injury, and intravenous pyelography to assess renal function. CT scan may be of help in these patients if it is readily available in the emergency department.

Although the routine role of intravenous pyelography is somewhat controversial,[71,72] it does serve as a useful test of renal function. It demonstrates that two kidneys are present and that both are functioning; this information may be of help at the time of a laparotomy. When gross hematuria is present, an intravenous pyelogram is essential, whereas with microscopic hematuria it should be carried out if the mechanism of injury was rapid deceleration. An intravenous pyelogram can be performed in the operating room at the time of laparotomy if a urologic injury is noted.

Pelvic Fracture

While most pelvic fractures occur following blunt injury, they can also occur as a result of penetrating injury. The mortality rate in pelvic fractures can be very high and often exceeds 50 per cent in patients with open pelvic fractures. Uncontrollable hemorrhage accounts for a major portion of the morbidity in these cases. The large series of venous channels on the posterior pelvic wall are often disrupted with major pelvic fractures, and because tamponade of these is not possible, blood loss may be enormous. Blood may fill the pelvis and dissect up retroperitoneally as far as the diaphragm.

The initial physical examination in patients with multiple trauma should include a careful examination of the pelvis. Manual compression of the pelvis will often give evidence of instability and much of the bony pelvis can be felt on a careful rectal and/or pelvic examination. In those patients in whom a fracture is suspected, pelvic roentgenograms are enormously helpful. These patients are probably helped by the application of a MAST garment if they are in severe shock. The MAST garment allows a partial fixation of the pelvic bones and thus reduces associated venous bleeding. The temporary stabilization then can be made permanent by means of external or internal fixation.[73,74]

In patients who have a fractured pelvis, but also demonstrate ongoing signs of hypovolemia, additional sources of bleeding must be sought. Because these are usually in the peritoneal cavity, peritoneal lavage is mandatory. The catheter should be inserted immediately above the umbilicus to avoid the pelvic hematoma. A negative lavage is a reliable sign that there is no serious intraperitoneal blood loss. A positive lavage may be false in as high as 15 per cent of cases because the pelvic hematoma has ruptured into the peritoneal cavity. If readily available, a CT scan may help in differentiating these problems.

Those patients who have the MAST garment in place, and who have a known pelvic fracture and a grossly positive peritoneal tap, should undergo laparotomy because of the likelihood of intraperitoneal bleeding as the source of the hypotension. If on the other hand the patient seems to be relatively stable but has a minimal positive peritoneal lavage, pelvic and abdominal arteriography[75] may be of great help. Bleeding from branches of the internal iliac system may be amenable to percutaneous embolization.

Patients with pelvic fractures usually have a relatively high incidence of rectal and/or genitourinary injuries. Digital rectal examination is extremely important to identify bony fragment penetration of the bowel. The prostate may be located very high and be difficult to reach; this suggests that there has been urethral injury. When gross blood is present at the urethral meatus, this is confirmatory evidence of urethral injury. If urethral disruption is suggested, a retrograde urethrogram should be obtained to determine whether or not there is a urethral tear or a bladder rupture or both. When such an injury is manifested on urethrogram, catheterization should be avoided and a suprapubic cystotomy carried out.

Penetrating Abdominal Trauma

When a penetrating injury of the abdomen occurs, the loss of bowel sounds, involuntary guarding, diffuse tenderness, and acute bleeding are indications for laparotomy (Fig. 5–1). False-positive and false-negative results of examination are not uncommon, and the need for laparotomy depends somewhat upon the mechanism of injury.

Gunshot wounds are usually more serious than stab wounds and more frequently cause major visceral damage. Although most civilian gunshot wounds are of the low velocity type, about 80 per cent actually enter the peritoneal cavity, and visceral damage is significant in approximately 95 per cent of the injuries.[76] I believe that all gunshot wounds of the abdomen should be explored if biplane abdominal roentgenograms indicate that the bullet has traversed the abdomen. Those few patients in whom the bullet track is tangential and the missile appears to be lodged in the abdominal wall can be observed if peritoneal lavage is negative.

If one is fairly certain that the bullet has entered the abdominal cavity and diagnostic tests are to be undertaken, they should be based on the suspected tract of the bullet. It should be borne in mind, as mentioned earlier, that bullets in the upper abdomen may have traversed the chest as well as the peritoneum. In most instances the patient will need surgical exploration relatively quickly, with little time available to carry out a battery of diagnostic studies. These patients should have a broad-spectrum antibiotic started at the time of initial exami-

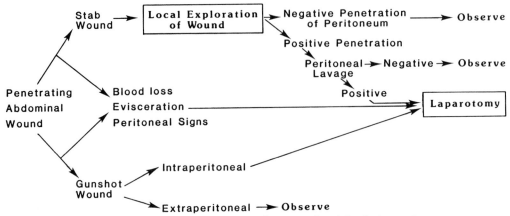

Figure 5–1. Selective management for penetrating abdominal wounds.

nation because of the high likelihood of perforation of the bowel.

STAB WOUNDS. Stab wounds may be managed selectively as seen in the diagram in Figure 5–1. Although most stab wounds of the abdomen actually enter the peritoneal cavity, less than half produce severe visceral injury requiring operation.[77] Formal wound exploration should be carried out under local anesthesia to verify that the stab wound has actually penetrated the posterior fascia and peritoneum. One cannot determine this by looking at the wound or by blind probing. If evisceration exists, penetration of course has occurred and no further evaluation need be undertaken because the patient will require laparotomy.

In those patients undergoing local exploration in whom there is no evisceration but in whom perforation of the peritoneum seems to have occurred, peritoneal lavage should be carried out. Peritoneal lavage in these instances may have a higher false-negative rate because of the possibility of the stab wound injuring the bowel while producing only minimal bleeding. If lavage in such patients yields negative results, they should be observed closely for at least 24 hours to rule out perforation of the intestine. If abdominal signs occur during this period of observation, immediate laparotomy should be carried out.

Extremity Injury

A complete neurovascular assessment of all four extremities should be carried out while the patient is being examined in the emergency department. All findings should be carefully recorded because they may assume major importance at a later date when the more acute injuries have been treated. Each limb should be examined for deformities, swelling, ecchymosis, and penetrating injuries of the skin. Pulses should be palpated and identified and gross motor function should be recorded.

An expanding hematoma or an open wound that is spurting bright red blood indicates that there is probable arterial injury. Manual pressure should be applied, followed by a dressing to control the hemorrhage; blind clamping should never be carried out. Whenever an injury or a fracture has occurred close to a major artery, the possibility of vascular injury should be considered. Classic signs of distal ischemia are pain, pallor, paresthesia, paralysis, and pulselessness. However, a palpable pulse does not always indicate that the arterial tree is intact. It is also frequently difficult to evaluate the peripheral pulses in the patient who is in shock and has severe vasoconstriction. One should always compare one limb with the other under any set of circumstances to ascertain at least some clue as to whether or not a difference is present in the arterial inflow. Fortunately, a little more time is available before the major vascular injury must be repaired so that life-threatening injuries in the chest and abdomen can be managed before the vascular injury. While six hours is usually considered a safe interval of ischemia in the extremity, these injuries should be repaired more expeditiously if possible.

A particularly vexing injury is one involving the popliteal artery, which may occur as a result of a posterior dislocation of the knee. The artery may be intact or disrupted, there may or may not be a peripheral pulse, or there may be an intimal tear which will evolve into occlusion of the artery in a reasonably short time if it did not occur at the time of the accident. These injuries are easily missed and require a high index of suspicion in any patient who has sustained knee injury. If there is any question about the peripheral circulation in the injured extremity, the patient should undergo arteriography as quickly as possible. This can be done by inserting a needle into the femoral artery and injecting dye and taking x-rays of the distal extremity. This can be carried out in the operating room if the patient has had to undergo life-saving surgery for injuries in the abdomen or chest. Since examination of the extremity may be more difficult under these circumstances, angiography should be carried out in any case in which distal ischemia is suspected.

If there is major arterial injury that will need repair, the concomitant venous system should be carefully examined; repair should be undertaken of any disruption that is found.[78]

DEFINITIVE SURGICAL CARE

While not all patients with multiple injury will require surgical treatment, the great majority of them will at some point in early management. It is the responsibility of the surgeon in charge to make the decision as to when operative intervention should be carried out. The decision must be based upon the patient's status, the rapidity with which this is changing, and the availability of a well-equipped, well-staffed operating room and adequate personnel to maintain resuscitative efforts as the operative procedure is carried out.

The operating suite that will be utilized for care of these patients should have extra equipment usually not found in suites intended for elective surgery. This equipment includes strong lighting, multiple instruments for procedures involving any area of the body and, blood warming and fluid warming devices used to protect the patient against hypothermia. There should be monitoring devices which can be displayed on an easily visible screen for the operating team, and extra personnel should be available who can measure output through thoracotomy tubes and urinary catheters as well as help with infusion of large volumes of fluids.

Head and Spinal Injury

Closed head injury is one of the most common injuries seen in patients with blunt trauma. The use of the CT scan in the preoperative diagnostic evaluation of a patient with head injury has made the management of head injuries much more effective. Craniotomy is usually carried out to evacuate a clot—either epidural, subdural, or intracerebral—and also to elevate depressed skull fractures for the purpose of relieving pressure on the brain. Brain function can be protected by the prompt evacuation of a hematoma and the control of intracranial bleeding. Penetrating injuries to the cranium are explored in order to remove bone fragments, to debride the damaged brain, and to provide for decompression. Additionally, the placement of an intracranial pressure switch, a device to monitor intracranial pressure, has become an almost routine part of the management of acute head injuries.

In the patient with multiple injuries, it may be necessary that the neurosurgical team carry out some of these procedures at the same time that either chest or abdomen or both are being explored for major hemorrhage.

Blunt Cervical Trauma

Injuries within the neck following blunt trauma may be extremely difficult to diagnose. A high index of suspicion is necessary following blunt trauma, and a very careful physical examination is important in order to detect indications which would suggest that injury has occurred.

CAROTID ARTERY INJURY. When blunt trauma has occurred in the region of the carotid arteries, careful evaluation of neurologic function is mandatory and early angiography should be undertaken. A CT scan, which usually precedes angiography, is used to rule out intracranial hemorrhage, particularly in the patient who is unconscious. Similar to trauma involving the popliteal arteries, severe blunt trauma to the neck may cause an intimal tear at the carotid bifurcation. Blood flow may be satisfactory for a period of time so that the symptoms may be delayed in onset.[79] The intimal flap may cause thrombosis a few hours after its onset and produce sudden and catastrophic neurologic symptoms. Intracranial embolization of material from the carotid injury may also occur and create serious neurologic dysfunction. If at the time of angiography the lesion is at the base of the skull and thus inaccessible via the neck incision, a neurosurgeon should be consulted to consider an extracranial-intracranial arterial bypass.[80]

There has been some controversy concerning the operative management of blunt and penetrating carotid artery injuries. It is my belief that those patients who are asymptomatic but have a carotid arterial injury or those who have neurologic deficits but are not in coma should have revascularization. When the patient is comatose it is probably unnecessary to carry out carotid artery repair, and simple ligation may be all that is needed. However, if the injury is more than six hours old at the time of possible surgical intervention, revascularization could produce a hemorrhagic infarction in the brain. I do not believe this has been clearly documented in the acute postinjury patient; I would advise that repair of the carotid be carried out under these circumstances.[81,82]

The carotid artery is exposed through an oblique incision along the anterior border of the sternocleidomastoid muscle. This incision may be extended up behind the ear if the lesion is high, and subluxation of the mandible may be carried out to give the operating surgeon additional exposure. Use of an internal carotid shunt under these circumstances is not clearly defined but it probably would be helpful when an interposition graft is necessary. If simple suture of the intimal flap or a simple end-to-end anastomosis is to be done, an internal shunt is probably not necessary. However, when the surgeon is unsure of the amount of time that might be required for the repair, a shunt is a good safety mechanism. These patients must be given heparin during the operative procedure unless it is contraindicated because of serious injuries elsewhere. Most of these injuries can be repaired by simple suture or by direct anastomosis; however, occasionally an interposition vein graft must be used when the lesion is more extensive. Angiography at the completion of the procedure is mandatory in order to determine clearly the situation within the artery following the repair. Unfortunately, the results of most repair procedures of blunt carotid injuries are not good, most likely because of delay in recognition and because of the associated injuries. Only about one third of these patients regain normal cerebral function.[79,83]

LARYNGOTRACHEAL INJURY. When a severe blow is struck to the anterior neck, frequently the structures of the neck are compressed against the spine, producing severe injury. There may be fracture, avulsion, or dislocation of laryngotracheal structures accompanied by intraluminal soft tissue damage.[84] If the airway has been secured while the patient is in the emergency department, no further evaluation need be done until the patient undergoes operation. If the patient is relatively asymptom-

atic, definitive study may be carried out at operation. It is important in these injuries to have an otolaryngologist involved early in the diagnosis and management because many of these injuries are rather subtle and require special knowledge in proper management. When injury is suspected or known to have occurred, CT of the larynx is important in order to define the extent of the injury and help plan the surgical approach.

At operation indirect laryngoscopy is the first step in evaluation; the surgeon can then evaluate vocal cord mobility and search for tears in the mucosal lining of the larynx or for hematomas. If severe injury has occurred that will threaten the airway in time, a planned tracheostomy should be carried out in order to provide adequate ventilation as swelling and hemorrhage occurs. When a severe disruption of the laryngotracheal complex has occurred, an otolaryngologic surgeon should undertake operative repair.

PHARYNGOESOPHAGEAL LACERATION. While blunt injury to the pharynx and/or esophagus in the neck is unusual, it must be carefully searched for when the trachea has been injured. Because of the anatomic location of the esophagus behind the trachea, a blow serious enough to injure the trachea may well have also injured the esophagus. Oral contrast studies, usually preceded by endoscopy, should be used in order to identify tears in the esophagus. Neither of these modalities is completely reliable, because the esophagus can easily collapse and the tear in the esophageal wall falls together so that no hole is obvious. It is sometimes necessary to use an injection of methylene blue through a catheter in the esophagus in order to test for an injury, particularly when the suspected area is surrounded by hematoma.

Tears in the pharynx may be successfully treated nonsurgically, and some that are never recognized may heal spontaneously. However, it is best to explore all injuries and carry out primary repair and external drainage of the involved neck compartment. Full-thickness lacerations should be closed in two layers, the mucosa being approximated with an absorbable suture and the muscle with a nonabsorbable suture. Drainage of the prevertebral space should be carried out with multiple Penrose drains; the drains must not lie against the anastomotic line because of the increased risk of breakdown at that point.

PENETRATING NECK INJURIES. As mentioned earlier, exploration of anterior neck wounds should be carried out if the platysma muscle has been penetrated. Preoperative evaluation of these patients depends to some degree on the judgment of the surgeon regarding the location and type of the injury. When it is suspected that the esophagus has been injured, contrast injection and then endoscopy should be carried out. Preoperative angiography should be used in the patient with multiple wounds, with hematomas over the vessels, or a level 1 or 3 trauma with possible arterial injury.

CAROTID AND VERTEBRAL ARTERY INJURY. Exploration of the neck is usually carried out through an oblique incision along the anterior border of the sternocleidomastoid muscle. This is the route of choice when arterial injury is suspected. A collar incision may be used if the injuries appear to be bilateral, as in the case of a missile traversing the anterior aspect of the neck. If carotid artery injury is suspected and if a hematoma is present, proximal control of the artery should be obtained before the hematoma is unroofed. I prefer to explore the carotid artery and repair it under almost all circumstances, although this has been discussed further in the section under blunt carotid injury. The argument has been made that if there is a carotid stump pressure in excess of 70 mm Hg, ligation of the carotid can be carried out with minimal neurologic deficit.[85]

A direct surgical approach to repair the artery is usually carried out without the use of a shunt. When the reconstruction will take an increased amount of time, or when an interposition graft must be used, a shunt should be inserted. Most wounds can be repaired by arteriorrhaphy following appropriate debridement. Some will require the use of an autogenous vein patch or even a graft interposition when the damage is more extensive.[83] Many options exist in the repair of the carotid artery; the experienced vascular surgeon will choose the one that seems most appropriate for the extent of injury.

Injury to the vertebral arteries following penetrating trauma is not only rare but may be missed because of the vessels' deep location and the fact that interruption of the vessel will usually not cause major neurologic symptoms.[86] Generally speaking, ligation is the treatment of choice in acute vertebral injury unless angiography suggests that collateral circulation—particularly from the opposite vertebral artery—is inadequate.

PENETRATING LARYNGO/TRACHEO/ESOPHAGEAL INJURIES. Penetrating injury in the neck in the region of either the larynx, trachea, or the esophagus must be evaluated with awareness of the possibility that perforation has occurred. Assessment will require indirect and direct laryngoscopy and possibly bronchoscopy and esophagoscopy. In addition to these, contrast studies may be necessary to define any perforation. Although consultation with an experienced otolaryngologist is invaluable in repair of lesions of the larynx, the principles of repair are those identified with blunt trauma to this region. The operative exposure for perforating injuries is similar to that for blunt injury and usually involves use of an incision parallel to the sternocleidomastoid muscle.

In the repair of an esophageal injury, a two-layered closure using absorbable sutures in the mucosa and a nonabsorbable suture to the muscle layers should be carried out. Although good drainage should be established, the drains should not be positioned next to the suture line. A temporary esophageal fistula is not uncommon following such a repair, but these will close spontaneously if adequate drainage is present.

Blunt Chest Trauma

Although injury to the thorax is extremely common in trauma, less than 5 per cent of patients who sustain blunt injury require surgical intervention.[23,47,64] In some cases immediate thoracotomy in the emergency department is necessary because of massive hemorrhage into the chest or because of air embolism. Although these occur extremely rarely, they should be kept in mind when this type of injury is present.

RUPTURE OF THE HEART. Whereas most patients who have had blunt cardiac rupture die at the scene of the accident, those who do reach the hospital usually have pericardial tamponade as the major finding. If such patients can be stabilized with pericardiocentesis, they must be taken to operation, during which a median sternotomy can be performed to treat the lesion.

In most patients, a standard left anteriolateral thoracotomy should be carried out and if necessary extended across the sternum into the right side of the chest. Patients who have survived to reach the hospital usually have an atrial tear, at least two-thirds of which occur on the right side.[87] Acute bleeding is usually controlled with a vascular clamp; however, balloon catheters may be helpful during the resuscitation of these patients. Simple suture repair is adequate for most atrial wounds. A ventricular wound usually will require digital compression for temporary hemostasis and then repair with interrupted sutures using Teflon pledgets.

When traumatic rupture of the pericardium without cardiac injury has occurred, the pericardium should be surgically repaired in order to prevent herniation of the heart or of the abdominal viscera in the event of an adjacent diaphragmatic tear.[88]

INJURY TO THE AORTA AND GREAT VESSELS. A tear of the thoracic aorta is usually diagnosed because of a high index of suspicion based on the type of injury that has occurred and the presence of a widened mediastinum on a routine chest roentgenogram. About 95 per cent of these lesions are at the isthmus just distal to the left subclavian artery.[57,89] With a high index of suspicion and with a widened mediastinum, preoperative angiography is the gold standard of diagnostic methods. Whereas far more angiograms will be obtained than transected aortas will be found, this is necessary to make the diagnosis in those patients whose lives can be saved.

Once the diagnosis is made, a left posteriolateral thoracotomy is performed which gives excellent access to the descending aorta. If the injury has occurred to the ascending aorta as demonstrated on the angiogram, a sternal splitting incision will provide better exposure. Cardiopulmonary bypass may be required for lesions in the proximal aorta. When the major branches of the aorta have sustained injury, various incisions must be used to provide the maximum exposure. These injuries can vary from a small laceration to a complete circumferential separation of the aorta. Usually the hemorrhage is contained by the adventitia so that the patient has not exsanguinated before reaching the hospital. The question arises as to the need for cardiopulmonary bypass or distal perfusion during aortic cross clamping. If the repair can be made by direct clamping and either lateral suture or a repair that can be carried out in less than 30 minutes, distal perfusion is probably not that important. However, if there is any question that the repair will take longer than 30 minutes or will require the insertion of a graft or other delaying techniques, an external shunt[90] should be prepared. The majority of these injuries require a short interposition graft; we usually use a Dacron graft for this purpose.[57]

RUPTURED ESOPHAGUS. Blunt trauma causing injury to the esophagus is rare and is frequently accompanied by tracheal injury.[91] A tear in the esophagus is usually located longitudinally and above the pulmonary hilum. A right posterior lateral thoracotomy is utilized and the esophagus repaired as would be the case in a penetrating wound. Two-layer closure with a mucosal layer of absorbable sutures and a nonabsorbable suture closure of the muscular layer are generally utilized. A parietal pleural flap is brought up against the suture line and used to reinforce the repair. A nasogastric tube is inserted and brought down past the point of repair to decompress the stomach; the mediastinum is drained through the adjacent pleural space with large-caliber thoracostomy tubes. If the perforation is not recognized until a later period of time, more complex procedures including esophageal diversion and pedicle flaps may be necessary.

TRACHEOBRONCHIAL TEAR. Injury to the tracheobronchial tree following blunt trauma usually involves the main stem bronchus within 2.5 cm of the carina.[34] Early diagnosis is essential and brochoscopy is valuable in making the diagnosis. It should be repeated if there is a persistent air leak or lobar atelectasis. Minor tears may be managed nonsurgically if the leak can be controlled; however, most of these injuries require immediate thoracotomy. A posteriolateral thoracotomy in the fifth intercostal space on the side of the injury is carried out. A standard endotracheal tube should have been inserted and it can be advanced beyond the injury into the uninvolved bronchus where it can serve as a stent. A split-function endotracheal tube may also be inserted and is useful in repairing rather extensive injuries. Primarly suture repair is the treatment of choice and is usually feasible in most instances. On rare occasions reimplantation of the bronchus is necessary; if the damage is quite extensive, a pneumonectomy may be required.

Penetrating Chest Wounds

Most penetrating chest wounds heal quite successfully with conservative management, but about 15 per cent require urgent thoracotomy, usually for cardiac tamponade or continuing massive hemorrhage.[92,93]

CARDIAC INJURY. Penetrating wounds of the heart usually require immediate surgery. While the blood pressure may remain normal, there is usually an increase in the heart rate and an increase in the peripheral vascular resistance while subendocardial ischemia develops.[94] Losses of blood volume should be compensated for as quickly as possible, and when the lesion is suspected because of the nature of the penetrating wound, pericardiocentesis should be carried out promptly. If pericardiocentesis fails to produce liquid blood, usually because the blood within the pericardium has clotted, a subxyphoid window may be made, with a window in the pericardium providing a temporizing measure.[38] However, the patient should be taken to the operating suite soon for planned repair of the cardiac injury and correction of the instability due to cardiac tamponade.

If the patient's condition is seriously unstable, immediate anteriolateral thoracotomy done in the emergency department can be lifesaving. The pericardium is evacuated, and digital control of the bleeding site in the heart is accomplished. Suture of the hole is then carried out using pledgeted sutures, with care taken to avoid the coronary arteries.

For the patient who is hemodynamically stable but in whom a cardiac wound is suspected, a median sternotomy is usually the approach that will provide the best exposure. The pericardium is opened widely and the contained blood is evacuated. Wounds of the vena cava or the atria are usually controlled with partial occlusion clamps, and direct suturing is carried out. Wounds of the ventricles are controlled with direct finger pressure and then pledgeted sutures are used to close the wound. The sutures should be placed deep to the coronary arteries when the wound is close to one of the coronary arteries.

If coronary arteries have been transected, ligation is carried out. In cases of severe cardiac dysfunction, immediate reconstruction of the damaged coronaries should be accomplished.[95] Injuries to the septum or the valves of the heart are generally treated at a later date under elective conditions provided that the patient is hemodynamically stable. Patients who have sustained direct wounds of the heart should have assessment at a later date for such possible injuries because they may have been missed at the initial operation.[96]

INJURY TO THE GREAT VESSELS. Serious bleeding may occur with a penetrating wound to the thorax because of damage to the great vessels. Immediate exsanguination is not uncommon but if the patient survives to reach operation it is usually because the bleeding has been contained within the mediastinum. The operative approach is similar to that utilized for blunt trauma: median sternotomy with the neck extension for right-sided injuries and a high left anterolateral thoracotomy with an extension into the neck for left-sided lesions.[97] Generally, the most versatile incision is a bilateral anterolateral thoracotomy crossing the sternum. Intrathoracic bleeding should be controlled by digital pressure when possible or with partial occlusion vascular clamps. Hematomas, as in the vascular system elsewhere, should not be entered until proximal and distal arterial isolation has been established. Although repair is best accomplished by lateral arteriorrhaphy when that is possible, insertion of an interposition graft may be necessary.

PERFORATION OF THE ESOPHAGUS. This injury can be quite subtle and is easily missed because of the inadequacies of contrast studies and endoscopy in diagnosing a perforating lesion.[98,99] When injury to the esophagus does occur, contamination of the periesophageal spaces with acid digestive juices and partly digested food particles may lead to serious infection. Perforations of the lower portion of the esophagus are best approached through a left-sided thoracotomy, whereas higher lesions are best approached through a right-sided thoracotomy. If massive tissue destruction has not occurred, such as with stab injuries and low-energy gunshot wounds, primary repair is the treatment of choice. The suture line is reinforced with a parietal pleural flap[99] or a viable muscle flap.[98] A nasogastric tube is inserted through the repair site into the stomach for decompression and enteral feeding.

When the diagnosis has been delayed, the management of the wound becomes much more complex. Some form of esophageal exclusion and diversion in continuity is the accepted standard. Following the thoracotomy, the esophageal wound is sutured and mediastinal and pleural drainage is established. The esophagus is ligated distal to the injury with heavy chromic catgut, which will lyse within about two weeks. This prevents reflux of the gastric juices up into the site of repair. A gastrostomy or needle jejunostomy is then placed in order to provide access for enteral feedings. The procedure is completed with diversion of the cervical esophagus to allow oral secretions to egress from the esophagus. Adequate mediastinal drainage is the major need in repair of late esophageal lesions.

Pulmonary and Tracheobronchial Injury

Continuing hemorrhage is the major reason for early thoracotomy in noncardiac penetrating trauma.[64,97] Massive air leak is occasionally a cause for surgical intervention but its occurrence is infrequent. Exposure is usually obtained by a posteriolateral thoracotomy on the injured side or with bilateral trans-sternal anterior thoracotomies when injury to both pleural cavities is suspected.

A penetrating wound may involve the esophagus or the trachea or both; both of these organs lie in close proximity to the great vessels. When the esophagus is perforated, the problem of contamination of the periesophageal spaces must be addressed, and the diagnosis may be delayed because contrast studies and endoscopy may be misleading.[98,99] If the lower third of the esophagus has been perforated, a left-sided thoracotomy is used; a right-sided thoracotomy is utilized for lesions of the upper two-thirds of the esophagus. If the injury is acute, but not a destructive type of injury, primary repair is the method of choice. Minimal debridement of the wound edges is required and direct suture is carried out. A parietal pleural flap is usually placed over the primary repair to reinforce it, and a nasogastric tube is inserted through the point of repair into the stomach for gastric decompression and to allow for the possibility of early feeding.[100]

When the diagnosis of an esophageal injury is delayed, a more extensive procedure is necessary. The esophageal injury should be repaired and mediastinal and pleural drainage established. The area of esophagus that is distal to the injury is ligated to prevent gastric reflux, and the proximal portion of the esophagus is brought out through the neck as a cervical esophagostomy. This allows emission of the oral secretions so that the patient will not experience the sensation of constant choking. Closure of the distal esophagus is carried out with large-caliber chromic sutures which usually will lyse within approximately two weeks. Adequate mediastinal drainage is a necessary element in good treatment because breakdown of the anastomosis with an esophageal fistula is common in the case of injuries which go unrecognized.

Most penetrating injuries involving the lung will respond satisfactorily to tube thoracostomy. As the lung undergoes expansion with respiration, the bleeding usually is tamponaded; the air leak can be managed by a thoracostomy tube. On rare occasions, severe bleeding will occur following a penetrating wound to the pulmonary hilum that necessitates direct surgical treatment. Thus unrelenting bleeding in the chest is the primary reason for surgical exploration.

The management of penetrating tracheal injuries is similar to that already described for blunt trauma. Usually, penetrating injuries can be managed by interrupted suture repair following debridement. Generally speaking, these injuries are approached through a posterolateral thoracotomy on the injured side; the sternum is crossed into the opposite pleural cavity if injury on both sides is suspected.[41]

Abdominal Trauma

Blunt abdominal injury requires surgical exploration in approximately 20 per cent of patients, whereas stab wounds may require exploration in up to 35 per cent and exploration is required in about 90 per cent of patients following gunshot wounds. The physical signs and/or positive peritoneal lavage are usually the most clear-cut indications for immediate surgical intervention. While the various types of injury differ somewhat, management of wounds involving the abdominal organs is fairly similar for all types of injury. As mentioned earlier, the patient should be fully resuscitated and preferably in rather stable condition at the time surgical therapy is undertaken. Occasionally, it is necessary to operate on a patient who is in shock, considering the cross clamping of major vessels to stop hemorrhage as a part of the resuscitation procedure. Whether this should be done through the chest with clamping of the descending thoracic aorta or whether the aorta can be controlled in the upper abdomen and the arterial inflow decreased by this means is the surgeon's decision. There is no good evidence that one is superior to the other. I believe that most surgeons would choose to attempt control of the bleeding within the abdomen rather than approaching it through cross clamping of the descending thoracic aorta. Whereas the latter approach has the disadvantage of requiring a chest incision in an already seriously ill patient, it has the advantage of being one of the fastest ways to gain control of the arterial inflow into the abdomen.

The abdomen is explored through a midline incision extending from the xyphoid to the pubis. The bleeding is rapidly controlled by packing and applying pressure as the free blood is removed from the abdomen to allow the surgeon the opportunity of determining the source of bleeding. As mentioned, if the bleeding is profuse the abdominal aorta should be compressed as it traverses the diaphragm. While the aorta is being compressed, the volume status should be restored as quickly as possible.

The next step is to quickly explore the right upper quadrant and the left upper quadrant. The liver and the great vessels surrounding it may be the source of bleeding. On the left side, possible injury to the spleen should be quickly ruled out. These organs should then be packed tightly if bleeding is occurring there and the rest of the abdomen explored for other sources of bleeding. Once the bleeding has been controlled with packs and appropriately applied vascular clamps, other injuries can be identified and their treatment undertaken. For example, wounds of the gastrointestinal tract should be temporarily closed with noncrushing clamps and packed off with moist pads for subsequent repair.[101]

LIVER INJURY. The liver is the largest and heaviest intraperitoneal organ and therefore is the one most frequently injured. The majority of injuries to the liver are minor wounds which can be managed by simple suture techniques; in many of them bleeding has ceased by the time laparotomy is carried out.[102,103] Superficial wounds which are still bleeding at the time of laparotomy can usually be controlled by simple gauze packing.[104] In many of these injuries the bleeding will stop promptly and the abdomen may be closed without further drainage. If oozing continues, perihepatic drainage may be necessary.

When more serious liver injury has occurred and bleeding is quite active, partial control can be obtained by carrying out the Pringle maneuver, which involves temporary occlusion of the porta hepatis, including the portal vein, hepatic artery, and common bile duct. A soft clamp across these structures so as not to injure them and then packing of the injured area with large tight packs will usually stem the acute hemorrhage. The surgeon probably has up to an hour in which to work on the ischemic liver.[105] If the Pringle maneuver fails to slow the bleeding, a torn hepatic vein or an actual tear in the retrohepatic vena cava may be the cause. An aberrant left hepatic artery usually arising from the left gastric artery may be the source of bleeding in some of these injuries. A right hepatic artery may originate from the superior mesenteric artery and may also be a source of major hemorrhage. These aberrant right and left hepatic arteries do not lie within the porta hepatis; therefore, when a clamp is placed across the porta, bleeding may continue.

Once the bleeding has been partially controlled, then the direct suture ligation of the bleeding vessels within the damaged liver sub-

stance is the next step. When there is moderately extensive damage to liver parenchyma, bleeding will well up from the crevice within the injured tissue. It is necessary in these cases to expand the crevice and carry out direct suture ligation of the vessels and the bile ducts in the region.[106] Using either the finger fracture technique or the knife handle fracture technique, the liver must be thoroughly explored and all bleeding controlled under direct vision.

In those rare instances in which direct vessel ligation does not achieve hemostasis, selective hepatic artery ligation may be necessary. In most instances, ligation of the hepatic artery is a safe procedure because the portal vein provides sufficient oxyen to the hepatic tissue until collaterals are functional.

When bleeding continues despite all of the aforementioned maneuvers, the surgeon is faced with the alternative of packing the liver to control the hemorrhage and reoperating in 24 hours or carrying out a complete hepatic lobectomy. The latter should be carried out only by a surgeon with experience in the field and never attempted without adequate blood for transfusion in reserve. If the liver is packed tightly and the bleeding can be controlled, the patient should be scheduled for reoperation in 24 hours for removal of the packs and an attempt to control the bleeding under direct vision. If the surgeon has had limited experience with procedures in this area, the packing will provide time to transport the patient to a center in which more adequate treatment may be available for this serious injury.[107,108]

One of the most difficult sources of hemorrhage to control in abdominal trauma is injury to the retrohepatic vena cava or the hepatic veins as they enter the vena cava. These injuries usually follow blunt trauma; the right or left hepatic vein is torn out of the wall of the cava, leaving a rather large hole that bleeds briskly. When the Pringle maneuver has failed to slow the bleeding, and blood seems to be coming up around the liver regardless of the surgeon's attempts control it, retrophepatic bleeding is probably occurring. The abdominal incision should be extended immediately into a median sternotomy incision or over into the right chest depending on the surgeon's preference. The liver can then be elevated and the retrohepatic area visualized and control of the hemorrhage attempted. We have used the Pilcher shunt[109] placed through the saphenofemoral junction to bypass this area and reduce the amount of blood loss. Mortality for this injury continues to be approximately 80 per cent in adults, and it is difficult to know whether the shunt has made a major difference.

BILIARY TRACT INJURY. Fortunately, injury to the biliary tract is quite uncommon and is usually combined with other intraperitoneal injuries. The gallbladder may be perforated by a penetrating injury and blunt trauma may avulse the gallbladder from the liver.[110] The management of gallbladder injury usually consists of cholecystectomy carried out in the standard fashion. One may resort to cholecystostomy in the unstable patient with multisystem trauma and in whose treatment speed is of a major importance.

Injury to the common bile duct is managed in a manner that is dependent upon the lesion. For example, a simple wound of the common bile duct is managed by debridement and primary repair over a T tube. If there is extensive damage to the common duct, it is probably necessary to use a biliary-enteric bypass.[36,111] The usual method of making the bypass is to use a Roux-en-Y limb of jejunum because there is concomitant damage to the duodenum and pancreas in most cases when the common bile duct is injured.

TRAUMA TO THE SPLEEN. In the past, any injury to the spleen has been a reason to remove it. In recent years, however, the spleen has become recognized as an important immunologic organ and has been shown to play a major role as a reticuloendothelial filter.[112] It has been demonstrated that postsplenectomy sepsis may be a major complication, and while the risk of infection is greatest in the child under two years of age, the adult is also a potential candidate for fatal infection.[113,114] The demonstration that the splenectomized individual has an increased incidence of fatal infection has spurred the surgeon to attempt to salvage the spleen whenever possible.[115] The enthusiasm for splenic repair, however, should not overshadow the need for splenectomy when it may be a life-saving procedure. To take an extra hour or so to repair a spleen when the patient's life is in jeopardy from other injuries is inexcusable. Splenic repair is best attempted if the patient is hemodynamically stable with no other life-threatening injuries. In addition, the surgeon should be familiar with the methods available for salvaging the spleen and the spleen should be amenable to repair.

When the spleen is to be removed, it is necessary to mobilize it completely by incision of its phrenicolienal and lienorenal peritoneal attachments. These ligaments are usually avas-cular and can be mobilized by cutting them without direct visualization. Occasionally a large vessel may run through the lateral ligament; it must be divided and ligated to provide for complete mobility of the spleen. When these ligaments are divided, the spleen can be freed from its posterior attachments by blunt dissection. It is rotated medially up into the abdominal wound for complete inspection. Large packs are usually placed in the gutter where the spleen has been mobilized in order to control any bleeding that may occur and to provide a support for the spleen.

If the injury to the spleen is simply small capsular tears, electrocautery plus use of a topical hemostatic agent may be all that is necessary. If there are deep lacerations in the spleen, these must be repaired similarly to those in the liver—that is, individual vessel ligation should be carried out and interlocking mattress sutures then are placed to help compress the area and prevent further bleeding. When a major splenic fracture has occurred, this portion of the spleen is removed and the capsule is closed over the resected area once the individual vessels have been ligated. Finally, it may be necessary to identify the splenic artery and its lobar branches. Ligation of a lobar branch will devascularize a segment of spleen, and this will usually demarcate the line of resection. Once the ischemic portion is amputated, bleeding of the cut end is controlled with sutures and the use of topical agents when indicated.

If the patient is not stable, and if the spleen is severely injured, splenectomy is the treatment of choice. The splenic artery and vein are ligated individually and the spleen is removed. Many surgeons then salvage sections of the spleen that have been removed and place these in an omental pouch. Although there is no question that some splenic function is retained with this technique, whether or not adequate immunologic function is produced remains to be proven.

Patients who have lost more than 50 per cent of the spleen should be given polypneumococcal vaccine in the postoperative period.

INJURIES TO THE DUODENUM AND PANCREAS. Blunt duodenal injury is usually caused by crushing of the duodenum against the spine or on occasion a blowout of an air-filled closed duodenal loop occurs. Blunt trauma to the pancreas is also usually due to compression of the pancreas against the vertebral column. A variety of techniques have been developed for the management of injuries to the duodenum and pancreas; these must be tailored to fit the type of injury that has occurred.[116,117]

In most instances, the injuries can be identified at the time of laparotomy for intra-abdominal hemorrhage. Any history of a compression type injury such as hitting the steering wheel, blood in the nasogastric tube, blood or bile staining of the retroperitoneal area in this region, or wounds that have penetrated the upper mid abdomen are all indications for careful and complete exploration of these structures. A Kocher maneuver is performed to expose the pancreatic head and the first two portions of the duodenum. The lesser sac is entered through the gastrocolic omentum, which permits examination of the body and tail of the pancreas and the third portion of the duodenum. The fourth portion of the duodenum is usually visualized by division of Treitz's ligament.

If at the time of exploration a duodenal contusion is discovered, it usually does not require any treatment. Most of these hematomas are absorbed within one to two weeks and allow the duodenum to open completely. Simple lacerations of the duodenum or a minimal perforation usually can be controlled by primary closure using a two-layer closure. For large rents in the duodenum, closure utilizing a Roux-en-Y coverage of the defect may be satisfactory. Extremely severe injuries of the duodenum are probably best managed using a pyloric exclusion procedure.[118] A gastrostomy is made on the greater curvature of the antrum and the pylorus is delivered into that wound. The pylorus is then closed with an 0 polyglycolic purse string suture. This suture will usually lyse in about two weeks and allow the pylorus to reopen. A side-to-side gastrojejunostomy is then performed using the gastrostomy made to deliver the pylorus. Pancreaticoduodenectomy is rarely indicated and must be reserved for massive disruption of the duodenum and the head of the pancreas.[119] Placement of a needle catheter jejunostomy for early postoperative enteral feeding in all patients with high-risk duodenal wounds must be carried out at the time of repair.[120]

The management of pancreatic trauma largely depends on the site of injury, the status of the ductal system, and the amount of crushing that has occurred. Since most injuries occur with the pancreas being compressed against the vertebral column, distal pancreatectomy is usually the treatment of choice. This leaves the head of the pancreas intact and with adequate pancreatic gland to provide normal pancreatic function. If the pancreas has contusions but it is believed that the duct is still intact, simple drainage of the area is all that is necessary. Some drains are placed and any pancreatic fistulas that do occur will usually resolve spontaneously.[116] When the head of the pancreas has been severely damaged, the treatment depends to some degree on the amount of damage to the duodenum and perhaps the common bile duct. If all of these are seriously injured, pancreaticoduodenectomy becomes the treatment of choice.

Needle catheter jejunostomy is again an important adjunct to the management of severe pancreatic injury.[100,120]

INJURY TO THE STOMACH AND SMALL BOWEL. Perforation of the stomach and small bowel are second in incidence only to liver injury following penetrating abdominal wounds. Although blunt rupture of the stomach is uncommon, high jejunal and distal ileal disruptions may occur after severe deceleration with lap belt restraint.[121] It is extremely important at the time of laparotomy to carefully inspect the entire gastrointestinal tract, particularly the posterior surface of the stomach and duodenum. If penetrating injury has occurred and there is a hole in the intestinal tract, one should always look for the second hole. Although occasionally a tangential wound occurs, most often when a hole is seen another hole can be found on the posterior aspect of the intestine.

Primary repair of the stomach and or small bowel is usually accomplished rather satisfactorily because of a rich blood supply and a relatively low bacterial count that occurs at this level. When there is a questionable area of viability of the small bowel as a result of severe contusion or multiple perforations, the segment should be resected and an end-to-end anastomosis accomplished.

TRAUMA TO THE COLON AND RECTUM. Injury to the large intestine usually results from penetrating wounds, although high speed vehicular trauma may result in blunt disruption. Primary repair of the colon is satisfactory if certain criteria can be met. These are (1) less than six-hour interval from the time of injury; (2) clean wound without mesenteric involvement; (3) minimal fecal contamination; (4) fewer than two associated intraperitoneal injuries; (5) absence of shock or major intraoperative blood loss; and (6) an otherwise stable patient. If these criteria cannot be met, primary closure should not be carried out. The axiom that right-sided colon injuries are less serious and can be treated more aggressively than left-sided ones has not been proven in clinical practice.[122]

If primary repair cannot be carried out within the peritoneal cavity, exteriorization of the sutured colon provides an alternative to colostomy.[122,123] In the majority of instances, the exteriorized segment will heal and the added morbidity of colostomy closure will be avoided.

In those instances in which the primary closure or exteriorization of the colon does not appear to be a satisfactory alternative, colostomy is the treatment of choice. A distal mucous fistula provides management for the distal segment of the large intestine.

Trauma to the rectum usually results from penetrating wounds, usually gunshot wounds, or bone fragment penetration following major pelvic fracture. These wounds involve high risk for infection because of the contaminated hematoma that occurs. A proximal defunctioning colostomy must be carried out for all full-thickness rectal defects.[124,125] With the patient in a lithotomy position following the abdominal exploration and creation of the colostomy, the remainder of the operation is carried out through the perineal approach. The retrorectal space is opened to the level of the coccyx, all devitalized tissue is removed, and adequate drainage is established. The rectal wound is sutured in two layers when possible, although the unrepaired injury will often heal quite adequately. We prefer to evacuate the rectal contents and irrigate the rectum with copious amounts of saline at this time to reduce the fecal contamination as much as possible.

Injuries to the Abdominal Vasculature

Most deaths that occur immediately following abdominal injury are secondary to major bleeding. The most lethal of these are injury to the retrohepatic vena cava, the visceral aorta, and the main portal vein.[126] Most of these injuries cause the patient to arrive at the hospital in severe shock and require major resuscitative efforts, necessitating that the patient be taken to the operating suite rather rapidly as a part of the resuscitation. Occasionally, a major vascular injury will be rather subtle because of retroperitoneal tamponade, as may occur with hepatic vein injury.

The abdomen is opened through a long midline incision; a copious amount of blood usually is found in the peritoneal cavity. This is rapidly evacuated, and with at least two suckers in active use, the location of the bleeding can generally be determined. Packing of the area is then carried out. By this time the bleeding usually will have slowed enough to allow the surgeon to plan a next maneuver and to fairly precisely locate the source of the bleeding. Right or left rotation of the viscera is often critical to expose the major intra-abdominal vascular system.[127,128] Mobilization of the left side is carried out in a search for hematomas and bleeding from the diaphragmatic aorta to its bifurcation. The aorta and all the aortic branches are well exposed through this approach. A right-sided reflection is carried out to provide good visualization of the infrahepatic vena cava, the portal venous system, and the right renal vessels. Repair of injury to the great vessels within the abdomen should be accomplished by lateral suture when possible. If a portion of the vessel has been removed, a vein patch may be utilized to make up the deficit. When complete transection has occurred, end-to-end anastomosis following debridement of the edges of the injury is preferable. However, this is often not feasible because of the amount of tissue that has been destroyed. Therefore, an interposition vein graft is the treatment of choice and if this is not possible an interposition of synthetic material such as Gortex may be satisfactory. In instances of heavy contamination, ligation of the damaged vessel and the placement of an extra-anatomic bypass may be the treatment of choice.

Injury to the great veins is directly repaired when possible. If the lumen diameter appears to be severely compromised by the injury, a vein patch may be added to provide normal luminal size.[129] If the vena cava is severely injured below the renal veins, ligation can be carried out. Above the renal veins, an interposition graft made up of a panel of pieces of saphenous vein may be satisfactory. Synthetic grafting can be used but would be the last choice.[130]

The portal vein is particularly difficult to manage because of its anatomic location. Although portal vein ligation can be carried out and is tolerated in most patients, repair is the treatment of choice.[131] If ligation is carried out, then a second-look procedure should be carried out 24 hours later with the necessity of a portosystemic shunt kept in mind.

The iliac vessels, because of their lack of stabilization within the pelvis, may cause serious hemorrhage when injury has occurred. These arteries should be repaired whenever possible, as should the veins. Although ligation of the iliac veins can be carried out if necessary, repair or grafting is preferred when other conditions are controlled.

Injury to the Genitourinary System

Injury to the kidney is not uncommon and usually consists of contusion and shallow lacerations. Intravenous pyelography carried out before laparotomy can demonstrate that the kidneys are intact and that they are present bilaterally. Some contrast extravasation may occur, indicating a laceration of the kidney, but usually this does not require surgical intervention. When a major injury to the kidney has occurred that involves massive tissue disruption, exploration and possible repair should be carried out. When a portion of the kidney can be removed, or when the multiple lacerations can be repaired, this is the treatment of choice. If the parenchymal injury is so severe as to prevent any type of repair, the kidney should be removed.

Injury to the renal vessels is often subtle, and results of attempts at kidney salvage can be disappointing. The reason for this is that the injury is often not discovered if an IVP is not done at the time of admission to the emergency department or soon after. While salvage has been reported in cases as late as 12 hours after injury, in general the limit of ischemia to the kidney is approximately four hours. Either thrombectomy or an aortorenal bypass graft should be carried out, depending upon the type of injury to the vessels.

Disruption of the ureter is an unusual injury and occurs primarily with a penetrating wound. If there is a question of an injury in the region of the ureter, an injection of indigo carmine or methyline blue may be given intravenously and the area under suspicion observed for the possibility of a leak of bluish urine. Ureteral repair is carried out using a variety of techniques selected on the basis of the type and extent of the injury.

Perforation of the bladder may be intraperitoneal or extraperitoneal. Intraperitoneal injury is usually at the dome of the bladder; these injuries are repaired in two layers and drainage is provided by a suprapubic cystotomy. Extraperitoneal bladder injuries are usually secondary to pelvic fractures. The treatment may consist of open repair or in some instances it may be managed by urethral drainage.[132]

Urethral tears usually occur in men and are classified according to their location in reference to the urogenital diaphragm. Management of these injuries is best carried out by the urologic specialist. While the management has a low priority in the patient with multiple injuries, injuries to the urethra may be quite debilitating. Anterior tears that usually follow a straddle injury should be repaired as soon as possible, whereas posterior injuries that usually follow a pelvic fracture are managed by delayed repair.

Injuries to the Peripheral Vessels

It is important to minimize the time lag from injury to the peripheral vascular system to the time of definitive repair. The "golden period" of six to eight hours that is usually suggested may be compromised by a variety of factors such as shock, disruption of collateral blood vessels, venous occlusion, and elevated compartment pressures. One of the most discouraging phenomena, which occurs on occasion, is thrombosis of small peripheral vessels, so that a satisfactory repair of a major artery still leads to gangrene with pulses present in the extremity.

The need to plan the operative approach carefully would include the following: The first step is preoperative angiography and the second involves timing of bony stabilization in the event of long bone fracture. Bony stabilization should occur before repair of the vessel. However, if this will prolong the time to vascular repair, a vascular shunt may be inserted to maintain circulation while the bony repair is taking place. A third consideration is positioning of the patient on the operating table and selection of a proper incision, and a fourth is the need for immediate fasciotomy.

With the patient positioned, the type of incision is chosen on the basis of the particular injury. Proximal arterial control is mandatory and is the first maneuver that is carried out. Distal control of the vessel is then accomplished before the attempt is made to repair the injury. Once the vessel has been isolated and controlled, a Fogarty catheter is passed down the distal arterial tree in order to remove any clots that have formed and to provide an access for heparin solution infusion. The proximal segment is then cleaned out of clots by insertion of a Fogarty catheter up the proximal artery. Arterial repair is carried out with standard techniques utilizing direct repair when possible. Venous patching or end-to-end anastomosis are useful when they can be satisfactorily accomplished without undue tension. An interposition graft, which can be useful, is usually taken from a nearby vein. For cases in which the major veins of the extremity with the arterial injury have been damaged, the venous bypass graft should be removed from the opposite limb. If for some reason the construction of a venous interposition graft is not possible, the use of Gortex as an interposition graft may be acceptable.

The role of postoperative anticoagulation remains controversial. Many of these patients have such severe injuries that anticoagulation may be contraindicated. If injury has occurred only to the arterial system and repair has taken place, the use of anticoagulation may make more sense. If the repair is satisfactory, however, and the distal pulses appear strong at the completion of the procedure, anticoagulation is probably not necessary.

REFERENCES

1. Copass MK, Oreskovich MR, Baldergroen MR, et al: Pre-hospital cardiopulmonary resuscitation of the critically injured patient. Am J Surg 148:20, 1984.
2. Jacobs LW, Sinclair A, Beiser A, et al: Prehospital advanced life support—benefits in trauma. J Trauma 24:8, 1984.
3. Jorden RC: Multiple trauma. *In* Rosen P (ed): Emergency Medicine: Concepts and Clinical Practice. St. Louis, C.V. Mosby Co, 1983.
4. Moore JB, Moore EE, Markovchick VC, et al: Diagnostic peritoneal lavage for abdominal trauma: superiority of the open technique at the infraumbilical ring. J Trauma 21:570, 1981.
5. Davis JH: Initial evaluation and triage of the multiply injured patient. *In* Najarian JS, Delaney JP, (eds): Emergency Medicine—Trauma—Shock—Sepsis—Burns. Chicago, Year Book Medical Publishers, 1982.
6. Vicario SJ, Coleman R, Cooper MA, et al: Ventilatory status early after head injury. Ann Emerg Med 12:145, 1983.
7. Aprahamian C, Thompson BM, Finger WA, et al: Experimental cervical spine injury model—evaluation of airway management and splinting techniques. Ann Emerg Med 13:584, 1984.
8. White RD, Goldberg AH, and Montgomery WA: Adjuncts for airway management and control. *In* McIntyre KM, Lewis AC (eds): Advanced Cardiac Life Support. Dallas, American Heart Association, 1981.
9. Bucholz RW, Burkhead WZ, Graham W, et al: Occult cervical spine injuries in fatal traffic accidents. J Trauma 19:768, 1979.
10. Boyd AD, Romita MC, Conlan AA, et al: A clinical evaluation of cricothyroidotomy. Surg Gynecol Obstet 149:365, 1979.
11. Brantigan CO, Grow JB: Cricothyroidotomy: Elective use in respiratory problems requiring tracheostomy. J Thorac Cardiovasc Surg 71:72, 1976.
12. Sofferman RA: Management of laryngotracheal trauma. Am J Surg 141:412, 1961.
13. Danzl DF, Thomas DM: Nasotracheal intubations in the emergency department. Crit Care Med 8:677, 1980.
14. Iserson KV: Blind nasotracheal intubation. Ann Emerg Med 10:468, 1981.
15. Tintinalli JE, Claffey J: Complications of nasotracheal intubation. Ann Emerg Med 10:142, 1981.
16. Jorden RC, Rosen P: Airway management in the acutely injured. *In* Moore EE, Eiseman B, and Van Way CW (eds): Critical Decisions in Trauma. St. Louis, C.V. Mosby Co., 1984.
17. Carrico CJ, Canizaro PC, Shires GT: Fluid resuscitation following injury. Rationale for use of balanced salt solution. Crit Care Med 4:46, 1976.
18. Moss GS, Lowe RJ, Jilek J, et al: Colloid or crystalloid in the resuscitation of hemorrhagic shock: A controlled clinical trial. Surgery 89:434, 1981.
19. Moore FD, Dagher FJ, Boyden CM, et al: Hemorrhage in normal man. I. Distribution and dispensal of saline infusions following acute blood loss: Clinical kinetics of blood volume support. Ann Surg 163:485, 1966.
20. Moss, GS: An argument in favor of electrolyte solution for early resuscitation. Surg Clin North Am 52:3, 1972.
21. Blumberg N, Bove JR: Uncrossmatched blood for emergency transfusions: one year's experience in a civilian setting. JAMA 240:2057, 1978.
22. Gervin AS, Fischer RP: Resuscitation of trauma patients with type-specific uncrossmatched blood. J Trauma 24:327, 1984.
23. Ashbaugh DG, Peters GM, Halgrimson CG, et al: Chest trauma—analysis of 685 patients. Surgery 95:546, 1977.
24. Mattox KL, Walker LD, Beall AC, et al: Blood availability for the trauma patient: Autotransfusion. J Trauma 15:663, 1975.
25. Galloway WB: Coagulation problems in the trauma patient. In Moore EE, Eiseman B, and Van Way CW (eds): Critical decisions in trauma. St. Louis, C.V. Mosby Co., 1984.
26. Stulz PM, Scheidegger D, Drop CJ, et al: Ventricular pump performance during hypocalcemia: Clinical and experimental studies. J Thorac Cardiovasc Surg 78:185, 1979.
27. Trunkey D, Holcroft J, Carpenter, MA: Calcium flux during hemorrhagic shock in baboons. J Trauma 16:633, 1976.
28. Wilson JN, Marshall SB, Beresford V, et al: Experimental hemorrhage on survival and a comparative evaluation of plasma volume changes. Ann Surg 144:696, 1958.
29. Miller JW, Danzl DF, Thoma DM: Urban accidental hypothermia: 13 cases. Ann Emerg Med 9:456, 1980.
30. Dunn EL, Moore EE, Breslich DJ, et al: Acidosis-induced coagulopathy. Surg Forum 30:471, 1979.
31. Collins JA: Problems associated with the massive transfusion of stored blood. Surgery 75:274, 1974.
32. Fry DE, Ratciffe DJ, and Yates JR: The effects of acidosis on canine hepatic and renal oxidative phosphorylation. Surgery 88:296, 1980.
33. Millikan JS, Moore EE, Steiner E, et al: Complications of tube thoracostomy for acute trauma. Am J Surg 140:738, 1980.
34. Grover FL, Ellestad C, Avom KV, et al: Diagnosis and management of major tracheobronchial injuries. Ann Thorac Surg 328:384, 1979.
35. Frank MJ, Nadimi M, Lesniak LJ, et al: Effects of cardiac tamponade on myocardial performance,

blood flow and metabolism. Am J Physiol 220:179, 1971.

36. Kitahama A, Elliot LF, Overby JL, et al: The extrahepatic biliary tract injury—perspectives in diagnosis and treatment. Ann Surg 196:536, 1982.

37. Evans J, Gray LA, Rayner A, et al: Principles for the management of penetrating cardiac wounds. Ann Surg 189:777, 1979.

38. Trinkle JK, Toon RS, Franz JL, et al: Affairs of the wounded heart: penetrating cardiac wounds. J Trauma 19:467, 1979.

39. Mattox KL, Beall AC, Jordan GL, et al: Cardiorrhaphy in the emergency center. J Thorac Cardiovasc Surg 68:886, 1974.

40. Jones JW, Hewitt RL, and Drapanas T: Cardiac contusion: a capricious syndrome. Ann Surg 181:567, 1975.

41. Graham JM, Mattox KL, and Beall AC: Penetrating trauma of the lung. J Trauma 19:665, 1979.

42. King, MW, Aitchinson JM, Nel JP: Fatal air embolism following penetrating lung trauma: An autopsy study. J Trauma 24:753, 1984.

43. Davis JH, Jackson RS: Chest trauma. In Cherniak RM (ed): Current therapy of respiratory disease, 2nd ed., Philadelphia, B.C. Decker, 1986.

44. Baker CC, Thomas AM, Trunkey DD: The role of emergency room thoracotomy in trauma. J Trauma 20:848, 1980.

45. Cogbill, TH, Moore, EE, Millikan, JS, et al: Rationale for selective application of emergency department thoracotomy in trauma. J Trauma 123:453,1983.

46. Narrod JA, Moore EE: Selective management of penetrating neck wounds: A prospective study. Arch Surg 119:574, 1984.

47. Blair E, Cemalettin T, Davis JH: Delayed or missed diagnosis in blunt chest trauma. J Trauma 11:129, 1971.

48. Richardson JD, Adams L, Flint LM: Selective management of flail chest and pulmonary contusion. Ann Surg 196:481, 1982.

49. Pepe PE, Potkin RT, Reus DH, et al: Clinical predictors of the adult respiratory distress syndrome. Am J Surg 144:124, 1982.

50. Shin B, McAslan TC, Hankins JR, et al: Management of lung contusion. Ann Surg 45:168, 1979.

51. Trinkle JK, Richardson JD, Franz JL, et al: Management of flail chest without mechanical ventilation. Ann Thorac Surg 19:355, 1975.

52. Lucas CE, Ledgerwood AM: Pulmonary response of massive steroids in seriously injured patients. Ann Surg 194:256, 1981.

53. Weigelt JA, Mitchell RA, Snyder WH: Early positive end-expiratory pressure in adult respiratory distress syndrome. Arch Surg 114:497, 1979.

54. Kirsh MM, Orringer MB, Behrendt DM, et al: Management of trachobronchial disruption secondary to nonpenetrating trauma. Ann Thorac Surg 22:93, 1976.

55. Parmley LF, Mattingly TW, Maneon WC: Nonpenetrating traumatic injury of the aorta. Circulation 17:1089, 1958.

56. Erickson DR, Blair E, Davis JH, Dwyer E: Pathodynamics of blunt chest trauma: A preliminary report. Am Surg 36:717, 1970.

57. Kirsh MM, Behrendt DM, Orringer MB, et al: The treatment of acute traumatic rupture of the aorta: A 10-year experience. Ann Surg 184:308, 1976.

58. Rittenhouse EA, Dillard DH, Winterscheid LC, et al: Traumatic rupture of the thoracic aorta: A review of the literature and a report of five cases with attention to special problems in early surgical management. Ann Surg 170:87, 1969.

59. Fox S, Pierce WS, Waldhausen JA: Acute hypertension: Its significance in traumatic aortic rupture. J Thorac Cardiovasc Surg 77:622, 1970.

60. Gundry SR, Williams S, Burney RE, et al: Indications for aortography in blunt thoracic trauma: A reassessment. J Trauma 22:664, 1982.

61. Marsh DG, Sturn JT: Traumatic aortic rupture: roentgenographic indications for angiography. Ann Thorac Surg 21:337, 1976.

62. Applebaum A, Karp RB, Kirklin JW: Surgical treatment for closed thoracic aortic injuries. J Thorac Cardiovasc Surg 71:458, 1976.

63. Borman KR, Aurbakken CM, Weigelt JA: Treatment priorities of combined blunt abdominal and aortic trauma. Am J Surg 144:728, 1982.

64. Jurkovich GJ, Moore EE: Traumatic hemothorax. In Edlich RE (ed): Emergency Medical Therapy—1984. New York, Appleton-Century-Crofts, 1984.

65. Arnoff RJ, Reynolds J, Thal ER: Evaluation of diaphragmatic injuries. Am J Surg 144:671, 1982.

66. Richardson JD, Flint LM, Snow NJ, et al: Management of transmediastinal gunshot wounds. Surgery 90:671, 1981.

67. Moore JB, Moore EE, Thompson JS: Abdominal injuries associated with penetrating trauma in the lower chest. Am J Surg 140:724, 1980.

68. Davis D, Bohlman H, Walker E, et al: The pathological findings in fatal craniospinal injuries. J Neurosurg 34:603, 1971.

69. Root HD, Hauser CW, McKinley CR, et al: Diagnostic peritoneal lavage. Surgery 57:633, 1965.

70. Williams JS, Kirkpatrick JR: The nature of seat belt injuries. J Trauma 11:207, 1971.

71. Griffen WO, Belin RP, Ernst CB, et al: Intravenous pyelography in abdominal trauma. J Trauma 18:387, 1978.

72. Guice K, Oldhma K, Eide B, et al: Hematuria after blunt trauma: When is pyelography useful? J Trauma 23:305, 1983.

73. Flint LM, Brown A, Richardson JD, et al: Definitive control of bleeding from severe pelvic fractures. Ann Surg 189:709, 1979.

74. Slatis P, Karaharju FO: External fixation of unstable pelvic fractures. Clin Orthop 151:73, 1980.

75. Gilliland MG, Ward RE, Flynn TC, et al: Peritoneal lavage and angiography in the management of patients with pelvic fracture. Am J Surg 144:744, 1982.

76. Moore JB, Moore EE: Changing trends in the management of combined pancreaticoduodenal injuries. World J Surg 8:791, 1984.

77. Thompson JS, Moore EE, Van Duzer-Moore S, et al: The evaluation of abdominal stab wound management. J Trauma 20:478, 1980.

78. Rich NM, Metz CW, Hutton JE, et al: Internal versus external fixation of fractures with concomitant vascular injuries in Vietnam. J Trauma 11:463, 1971.

79. Krajewski LP, Hertzer, NR: Blunt carotid artery trauma—report of two cases and review of the literature. Ann Surg 191:341, 1979.

80. Fry RE, Fry WJ: Extracranial carotid artery injuries. Surgery 88:581, 1980.

81. Brown MF, Graham JM, Feliciano DV, et al: Carotid artery injuries. Am J Surg 144:748, 1982.

82. Ledgerwood AM, Mullins RJ, Lucas CE: Primary repair versus ligation for carotid artery injuries. Arch Surg 115:488, 1980.

83. Perry MO, Snyder WH, Thal ER: Carotid artery injuries caused by blunt trauma. Ann Surg 192:74, 1980.

84. Newman TS, Bockman MA, Moody P, et al: An autopsy study of traumatic deaths: San Diego, 1979. Am J Surg 144:722, 1982.

85. Ehrenfeld WK, Stoney RJ, Wylie EJ: Relation of carotid stump pressure to safety of carotid artery ligation. Surgery 93:299, 1983.

86. Meier DE, Brink BE, Fry WJ: Vertebral artery trauma—acute recognition and treatment. Arch Surg 116:236, 1981.

87. Martin TD, Flynn TC, Rowlands BJ, et al: Blunt cardiac rupture. J Trauma 24:287, 1984.

88. Clark DE, Wiles CS, Lim MK, et al: Traumatic rupture of the pericardium. Surgery 93:495, 1983.

89. Kirsh MM, Orringer MB, Behrendt DM: Management of unusual traumatic ruptures of the aorta. Surg Gynecol Obstet 146:365, 1978.

90. Stavens B, Hashim SW, Hammond GL, et al: Optimal methods of repair of descending thoracic aortic transections and aneurysms. Am J Surg 145:508, 1983.

91. Stothert JC, Buttorff J, Kaminski DL: Thoracic esophageal and tracheal injury following blunt trauma. J Trauma 20:992, 1980.

92. Borlase B, Metcalf RK, Moore EE, Manart FD: Penetrating wounds to the anterior chest. Am J Surg 152:649, 1986.

93. Breaux EP, Dupont JB, Albert HM, et al: Cardiac tamponade following penetrating mediastinal injuries: Improved survival with early pericardiocentesis. J Trauma 19:461, 1979.

94. Wechsler AS, Auerback BJ, Graham TC, et al: Distribution of intramyocardial blood flow during pericardial tamponade: Correlation with microscopic anatomy and intrinsic myocardial contractility. J Thorac Cardiovasc Surg 189:717, 1979.

95. Espada R, Whisennand HH, Mattox KL, et al: Surgical management of penetrating injuries to the coronary arteries. Surgery 78:755, 1975.

96. Fallahnejad M, Kutty ACK, Wallace HW: Secondary lesions of penetrating cardiac injuries—a frequent complication. Ann Surg 191:228, 1980.

97. Graham JM, Feliciano DV, Mattox KL, et al: Management of subclavian vascular injuries. J Trauma 20:537, 1980.

98. Cheadle W, Richardson JD: Options in management of trauma to the esophagus. Surg Gynecol Obstet 155:380, 1982.

99. Michael L, Grillo HC, and Malt RA: Esophageal perforation. Ann Thorac Surg 33:203, 1982.

100. Moore EE, Jones TN: Nutritional assessment and preliminary report on early support of the trauma patient. J Am Coll Nutr 2:45, 1984.

101. Davis JH: Initial operative management of multiple abdominal organ injury. *In* Najarian JS, Delaney, JP (eds): Emergency Medicine—Trauma—Shock—Sepsis—Burns. Chicago, Year Book Medical Publishers, 1982.

102. Defore WW, Mattox KL, Jordan GL, Beall AC: Management of 1,590 consecutive cases of liver trauma. Arch Surg 111:493, 1976.

103. Levin A, Gover P, and Nance FC: Surgical restraint in the management of hepatic injury: A review of Charity Hospital experience. J Trauma 18:399, 1978.

104. Lucas CE, Ledgerwood AM: Prospective evaluation of hemostatic techniques for liver injuries. J Trauma 16:422, 1976.

105. Huguet C, Nordlinger B, Block P, Conard J: Tolerance of the human liver to prolonged normothermic ischemia. Arch Surg 113:1448, 1978.

106. Pachter HL, Spencer FC, Jofstetter SR, Coppa GF: Experience with the finger fracture technique to achieve intrahepatic hemostasis in 75 patients with severe injuries of the liver. Ann Surg 197:771, 1983.

107. Feliciano DV, Mattox KL, Jordan GL: Intra-abdominal packing for control of hemorrhage: A reappraisal. J Trauma 21:285, 1981.

108. Svoboda JA, Peter ET, Dang CV, et al: Severe liver trauma in the face of coagulopathy. Am J Surg 144:717, 1982.

109. Pilcher DB, Harman PK, Moore EE: Retrohepatic vena cava balloon injuries—a continuing challenge. J Trauma 17:837, 1977.

110. Soderstrom CA, Maekawa K, DuPriest RW, et al: Gallbladder injuries resulting from blunt abdominal trauma. Ann Surg 193:60, 1981.

111. Busuttil RW, Kitahama A, Cerise E, et al: Management of blunt and penetrating injuries to the porta hepatis. Ann Surg 191:641, 1980.

112. Sherman R: Perspective in management of trauma to the spleen: 1979 Presidential Address, American Association for the Surgery of Trauma. J Trauma 20:1, 1980.

113. O'Neal BJ, McDonald JC: The risk of sepsis in the asplenic adult. Ann Surg 194:775, 1981.

114. Upadhyaya P, Simpson JS: Splenic trauma in children. Surg Gynecol Obstet 127:781, 1968.

115. Millikan JS, Moore EE, Moore GE, Stevens RE: Alternatives to splenectomy in adults after trauma. Am J Surg 144:711, 1982.

116. Cogbill TH, Moore EE, Kashuk JL: Changing trends in the management of pancreatic trauma. Arch Surg 177:722, 1982.

117. Kashuk JL, Moore EE, Cogbill TH: Management of the intermediary severity duodenal injury. Surgery 92:758, 1982.

118. Vaughan GD, Frazier OH, Graham DY, et al: The use of pyloric exclusion in the management of severe duodenal injuries. Am J Surg 134:785, 1977.

119. Lowe RJ, Saletta JD, Moss, GS: Pancreaticoduodenectomy for penetrating pancreatic trauma. J Trauma 17:731, 1977.

120. Moore EE, Dunn EL, Jones TN: Immediate jejunostomy feeding—its use after major abdominal trauma. Arch Surg 116:681, 1981.

121. Denis R, Allad M, Atlas H, et al: Changing trends with abdominal injury in seat belt wearers. J Trauma 23:1007, 1983.

122. Stone HH, Fabian TC: Management of perforating colon trauma—randomization between primary closure and exteriorization. Ann Surg 190:430, 1979.

123. Shannon FL, Moore EE: Primary colon repair—a safe alternative. Surgery 95:851, 1985.

124. Rothenberger D, Velasco R, Strate R, et al: Open pelvic fracture: A lethal injury. J Trauma 18:184, 1978.

125. Trunkey D, Hays RJ, Shires GT: Management of rectal trauma. J Trauma 13:411, 1973.

126. Davis JH: Vascular injuries to the abdomen. *In* Kerstein M (ed): Management of Vascular Trauma. Baltimore, University Park Press, 1984.

127. Bascaglia LC, Blaisdell WF, Lim RC: Penetrating abdominal vascular injuries. Arch Surg 99:764, 1969.

128. Mattox KL, McCollum WB, Jorden GL, et al: Management of upper abdominal vascular trauma. Am J Surg 128:823, 1974.

129. Millikan JS, Moore EE, Cogbill TH, et al: Inferior vena cava injuries. A continuing challenge. J Trauma 23:207, 1983.

130. Peterson NE, Millikan JS, Moore EE: Combined renal and caval trauma—a review of personal and recorded experience. J Urol 33:567, 1985.

131. Pachter HL, Drager S, Godfrey N, et al: Traumatic injuries of the portal vein—the role of acute ligation. Ann Surg 189:383, 1979.

132. Richardson JR, Leadbetter GW: Nonoperative treatment of the ruptured bladder. J Urol 114:213, 1975.

Hemodynamic Monitoring in Spinal Cord Injured Patients

JOHN A. SAVINO, M.D., KINICHI SHIBUTANI, M.D., Ph.D.,
RUDOLPH TADDONIO, M.D., and LOUIS R. M. DEL GUERCIO, M.D.

The multiple trauma patient in general, and the patient with spinal cord injury in particular, presents the clinician with a variety of clinical diagnostic dilemmas and therapeutic challenges in hemodynamic management. Trauma patients exist in a hormonal milieu of increased catecholamines and corticosteroids and other catabolic hormones which predispose them to a hypercatabolic nutritional state, as well as a hyperdynamic circulatory state.

Most patients after sustaining multiple injuries require resuscitation in the emergency department, and inherent in the resuscitation of hemodynamic instability are diagnostic physical, laboratory, and radiologic examinations. A significant percentage of these patients will proceed to recovery, and an integral aspect of that result will entail one or more operative interventions. There are, however, a proportion of these patients who will develop marked deterioration of various organ systems, and the underlying pathophysiologic abnormalities will be sepsis and malnutrition.

The pulmonary function, reflected by oxygenation, ventilation, mechanics, and perfusion, may deteriorate into a clinical syndrome frequently referred to as the adult respiratory distress syndrome (ARDS). The renal function may decline rapidly, as reflected by depression in the urinary output and clearance of creatinine and urea, until a state of acute renal failure ensues. Likewise, the gastrointestinal tract may sustain the effects of sepsis with bleeding from the stomach and the duodenum, as well as biliary (acalculous cholecystitis) and hepatic decompensation.

Inherent in the management of the trauma victim is the capability on the part of the intensive care physician and the traumatologist to manage the various aspects of hemodynamic instability created by the failure of one or more of the organs mentioned in order to avoid the clinical state of multiple organ failure which inevitably leads to death.

This chapter describes a variety of hemodynamic states that frequently are characteristic of the spinal cord injury patient. The hyperdynamic state typical of the multiple trauma patient and burn victim are described. The frequently encountered hypovolemic state which may be attributed to either internal or external fluid losses is elaborated upon, as well as the effects of fluid overload. Severe head injury patients with related hemodynamic effects secondary to the severity of injury, and the negative effects on hemodynamics from therapeutic maneuvers to decrease intracranial hypertension, are also discussed.

The classic presentation of the cervical cord injured patient in "spinal shock" is discussed with the associated effects on pulmonary, circulatory, and other related organ function. Commonly, in the postresuscitation phase of management trauma patients who have associated neurologic injuries of the brain and cord develop infectious complications, which precipitate decline of circulatory dynamics frequently described as "septic shock." These cardiopulmonary abnormalities can be divided into an early and late stage and will similarly be elaborated upon along with some of the detrimental effects of therapy.

PHYSIOLOGIC MONITORING TECHNIQUES

In the trauma patient the sine qua non of resuscitation entails in most cases rapid infusion of large volumes of crystalloid solutions and blood products. However, a proportion of these severely injured patients sustain concomitant neurologic (head and spine), thoracic, abdominal, and extremity injuries that mitigate against simplified monitoring techniques and therapeutic interventions. Although the monitoring of heart rate, arterial blood pressure, and central venous pressure has been a useful guide, these values do not provide a sufficient basis for accurate diagnosis and proper management, especially when complications occur or during prolonged complex operative procedures. The value of the central venous pressure is limited by the fact that it basically reflects the functional state of the right ventricle, which does not parallel that of the left ventricle. Information about the function of the left heart is often essential for proper evaluation. In recent years, use of the Swan-Ganz catheter technique has allowed easy monitoring and analysis continuously of both ventricles, and utilization of the data obtained influences therapeutic maneuvers in the management of multiple trauma patients.

These catheters are easily inserted under local anesthesia percutaneously via the internal jugular or subclavian vein. Serial pressure measurements via the right atrium, right ventricle, and pulmonary artery are recorded, and a mixed venous blood sample is obtained simultaneously with an arterial sample only after position of the catheter is documented by x-ray. Cardiac outputs are then measured by thermal dilution with automated calibration accomplished by a programmable calculator. Blood samples are analyzed for pH, gas tensions, carboxyhemoglobin saturation, hemoglobin, hematocrit, and lactate values. Primary and derived data of ventricular function include cardiac index, pulse rate, stroke index, left and right ventricular stroke work, as well as total and pulmonary vascular resistance. Arteriovenous oxygen content difference, oxygen consumption, and venoarterial admixture are calculated as indicators of oxygen transport and respiratory function. The adequacy of oxygen transport in meeting metabolic requirements is reflected by the blood lactate level and calculated base deficits. All of these variables are analogue-plotted on a preprinted logical format previously described as the automated physiologic profile (APP).[1] The normal values for the APP represent one standard deviation from mean for healthy young male adults in the resting state (Fig. 6–1).

The advantage to the use of these sophisticated monitoring techniques is that they provide the clinician with a cardiopulmonary physiologic assessment that permits rapid determination of myocardial performance and oxygen delivery and ultimately reduces mortality. Recently, Shoemaker[2] et al. developed a predictive or severity index from a large series of shock patients and found that these indices were highly accurate in predicting survival or death after acute life-threatening surgical problems. Furthermore, they found that the therapeutic goal to maintain blood volume, cardiac index, oxygen delivery, and oxygen consumption at "optimal" values in critically ill patients was associated with a reduction in mortality. In clinical practice when critically ill surgical patients are managed, physiologic monitoring and therapy start only after the patient has developed the shock syndrome and sometimes after cardiac arrest. Optimization of oxygen delivery and cardiac performance should ideally begin before the occurrence of these disastrous problems.

A brief review of the physiologic concepts will facilitate understanding of the physiologic profile described. Oxygen delivery is a direct function of the cardiac output and the arterial oxygen content, which actually represents the oxygen bound to hemoglobin (1.34 ml/gm). The cardiac output, the amount of blood ejected from the heart into the systemic circulation each minute, is a reflection of preload, afterload, myocardial contractility, and heart rate.

The preload is the degree of muscle fiber stretch imposed by filling of the ventricles during diastole. According to Starling's law of the heart, this varies directly with the cardiac output and can be approximated by the pulmonary capillary wedge pressure (PCWP). This pressure can be obtained with the use of a pulmonary artery catheter when the balloon is inflated and the catheter tip progresses into a more distal branch of the pulmonary artery. This pressure measurement reflects the pressures of the left ventricle in cases in which there is no mechanical obstruction between the balloon tip and the left ventricle, i.e., mitral stenosis, left atrial tumor, or pulmonary vein obstruction (normal 5 to 15 mm Hg). Also obtained from the use of this catheter are the pulmonary artery systolic and diastolic pres-

Automated Physiologic Profile

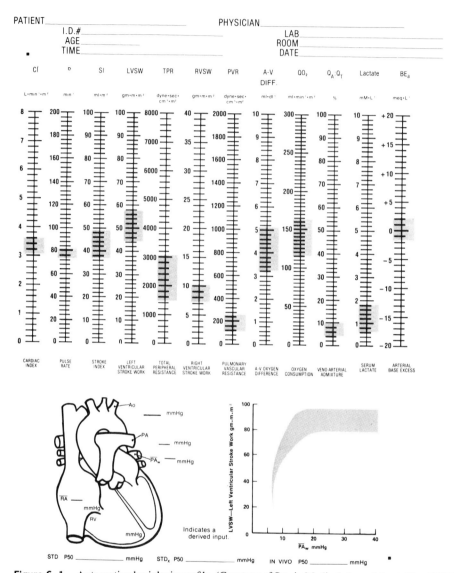

Figure 6–1. Automatic physiologic profile. (Courtesy of Stepic Medical, Long Island City, N.Y.)

sures. The systolic pressure (PAS) is obtained during the systolic phase of the cardiac cycle and reflects the pressure generated by the contraction of the right ventricle (normal 15 to 25 mm Hg). The pulmonary artery diastolic pressure (PAD) is obtained when the cardiac cycle is in the diastole and reflects diastolic filling pressure of the left ventricle (normal 8 to 10 mm Hg). The right ventricular preload is reflected by the central venous pressure (CVP) (normal 2 to 6 mm Hg or 2 to 7 cm H_2O).

The afterload is the impedance to cardiac

ejection during systole imposed by vascular resistance, blood pressure, and blood viscosity and is represented by the peripheral vascular resistance or total peripheral resistance (TPR). The pulmonary vascular resistance is a measure of the impedance applied by the pulmonary circuitry to the systolic effort of the right ventricle (PVR). The contractility refers to the state of health of the heart muscle and the ratio which the muscle fibers can shorten circumferentially around the bolus of blood within the ventricles. An intricate part of the evaluation of myocardial contractility is the ventricular performance curve, in which cardiac index is plotted against PCWP. The concept of the Frank-Starling mechanism implies that as the myocardium stretches with increased intraventricular volume, the reflected pressure (CVP or PCWP) increases respectively. When the myocardium contracts it will do so with greater force, thereby creating a greater stroke volume and cardiac output. The Sarnoff ventricular function curve is a plot of stroke work (the product of stroke volume and mean aortic blood pressure) against end diastolic pressure or end diastolic volume. It provides a good evaluation of myocardial contractility because it includes consideration of afterload and preload. The stippled area as seen in Figure 6–1 represents normal contractility.

As previously mentioned, in order to measure the amount of blood ejected from the left ventricle each minute, the thermodilution method is used. This method of calculating the output utilizes the theory of temperature change as an indicator of circulating volume. When the thermistor port of the pulmonary artery catheter is attached to a cardiac computer, it will provide the computer with an accurate reading of blood temperature. A specific amount (10 ml) of 5 per cent dextrose solution is injected through the proximal lumen, the thermistor senses the change in temperature in the pulmonary artery and the computer calculates and digitally displays the cardiac output in liters/minute.

THE HYPERDYNAMIC TRAUMA STATE

The trauma patient presents typically during the acute phase of injury with the sympatho-adrenal axis activated and a hormonal milieu characterized by increased levels of catecholamines and glucocorticoids. Hemodynamically, this is reflected by a hyperdynamic state (Fig. 6–2). Left ventricular function is markedly increased with elevated cardiac index, pulse rate, stroke index, and left ventricular stroke work. The total peripheral resistance (afterload) is diminished. Classically, these patients reflect the hypermetabolic state by increased levels of oxygen consumption. The facet of oxygen transport that manifests the adequacy of oxygen delivery is the arteriovenous oxygen content difference. In these patients this is normal; however, it should be below

normal levels due to the rapid transit and flow of blood through the arteriovenous bed. From a therapeutic standpoint strong consideration should be given to increasing volume replacement to augment the cardiac index further, thereby diminishing the oxygen extraction manifested by the high normal AVo_2 difference. The chamber pressures and pulmonary artery pressures are relatively normal. The Sarnoff curve as a reflection of ventricular function is nearly normal but tending toward hypovolemia.

The general impression from this evaluation is that the patient is slightly hypovolemic, is in a hyperdynamic state, and is compensating with slightly increased oxygen extraction. Depending on the injuries and clinical evaluation of this patient, appropriate selection of fluid replacement and continuous monitoring would be indicated. Certainly, the typical multiple trauma victim does not require invasive monitoring. Nevertheless, in cases of multiple associated injuries (especially when there is evidence of thoracic trauma with myocardiac contusion or significant pulmonary contusion as well as cerebral injuries) the data derived from the pulmonary artery catheter facilitates management.

THE HYPOVOLEMIC STATE

The problems most frequently confronting the clinician managing multiple trauma victims usually are related to causes of the hypovolemic state. Fluid losses may be either internal or external. The causal states for internal pooling with hypovolemia in spinal cord injury patients who frequently sustain associated thoracoabdominal and extremity trauma may be secondary to hemothorax, hemoperitoneum, and retroperitoneal bleeding from vertebral and other fractures. During prolonged hospitalization of these patients occult fluid losses occur secondary to ascites and intestinal obstruction, especially when patients have chronic liver disease and previous laparotomies.

The more obvious reasons for hypovolemia are most often secondary to external fluid losses following trauma (hemorrhage). However, many of these patients who sustain head trauma suffer from diabetes insipidus. Patients who initially are borderline diabetic (diabetes mellitus) actually become floridly hyperglycemic, developing significant polyuria and hyper-

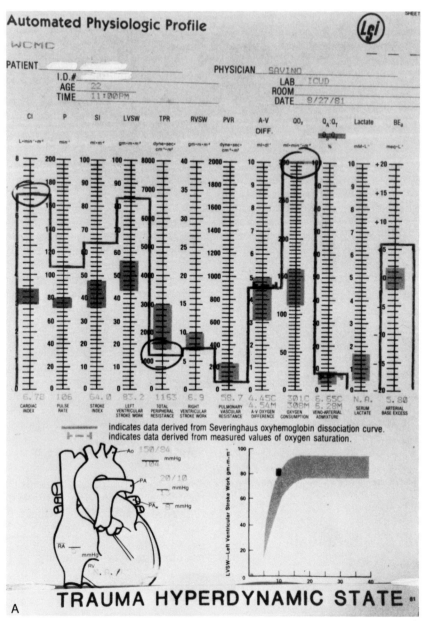

Figure 6-2. *A* and *B*, Note increased cardiac index, left ventricular stroke work, and oxygen consumption with diminished total peripheral resistance.

osmolality. Not uncommonly in patients with cord trauma or fractures of the thoracolumbar spine the gastrointestinal tract functions abnormally, with the development of paralytic ileus with associated fluid losses from vomiting. Tube feedings via the GI tract are hyperosmolar and frequently these individuals develop severe dehydration as a result of diarrhea.

In patients with associated head injury, hypothalmic malfunction is indicated by excessively high fevers and perspiration. These ven-

tilator-dependent patients usually have increased insensitive loss of water from the lung as well. Most patients with high levels of intracranial hypertension require excessive doses of mannitol and other diuretic therapy, which causes excessive loss of fluid and associated hypovolemia.

Evaluation of the profile indicates that this patient's PCWP is zero, with pulmonary artery pressures and systemic blood pressures also decreased (Fig. 6-3). Evaluation of the ventricu-

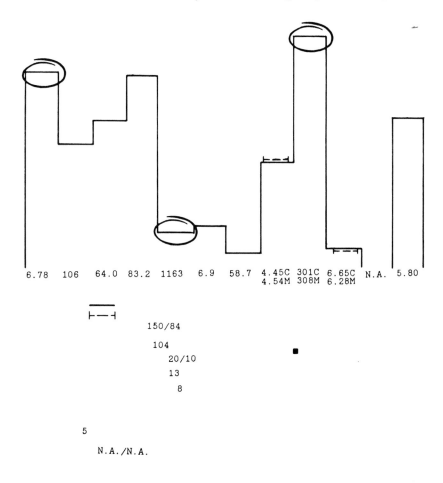

```
6.78   106   64.0  83.2  1163   6.9   58.7  4.45C  301C  6.65C  N.A.  5.80
                                            4.54M  308M  6.28M
```

```
├──┤
         150/84

         104
           20/10
            13
             8


   5
      N.A./N.A.
```

B   **TRAUMA HYPERDYNAMIC STATE**

Figure 6–2 *Continued*

lar function curve reveals the asterisk to be to the left of the stippled normal area, indicating the need for increased preload or volume. Left ventricular function is diminished secondary to the low volume; consequently the cardiac index is decreased, and a compensatory increase in pulse rate and total peripheral resistance (afterload) is seen.

The therapeutic maneuvers required in this patient are oxygen administration and increased fluid administration, especially blood, if the circumstances warrant. The need for oxygen must be emphasized because the oxygen demands of this patient are unknown. However, the prime determinants of oxygen delivery to the peripheral tissues are the cardiac output and hemoglobin level. The increased pulmonary shunting may be effectively managed with increased oxygen administration alone or, perhaps if the patient is in respiratory distress, intubation and management with me-

chanical ventilation and manipulation of respiratory parameters.

FLUID OVERLOAD IN RESUSCITATION

Not uncommonly in the management of multiply injured patients who require transfusions and fluid resuscitation (especially in cases of retroperitoneal bleeding, pelvic fractures, and long bone fractures of the lower extremities), resuscitative efforts can be excessive. Particularly in elderly patients and in patients with poor myocardial reserve who are not monitored with pulmonary artery catheters, fluid overload can precipitate congestive heart failure changes manifested on the profile (Fig. 6–4).

The PCWP is elevated beyond normal range and the systemic blood pressure remains rela-

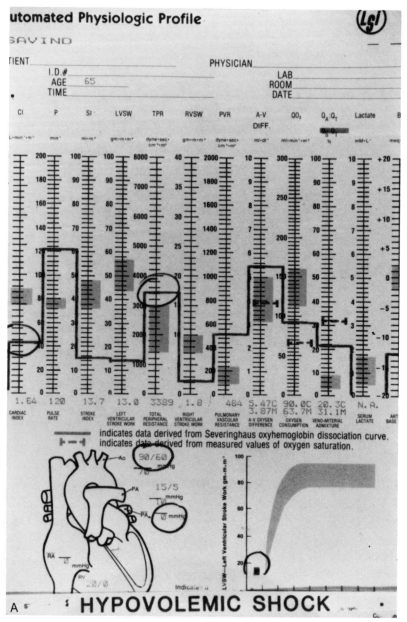

Figure 6–3. *A* and *B*, Note diminished wedge pressure, cardiac index with increased total peripheral resistance, and arterial venous contrast difference.

tively normal. The Sarnoff ventricular function curve demonstrates the asterisk displaced to the right of the stippled area, corresponding to poor myocardial performance. Left ventricular function is suppressed as evidenced by suppressed cardiac index, stroke index, and left ventricular stroke work.

Interestingly, the total peripheral resistance (afterload) and the pulse rate are augmented, indicating an increased adrenergic response. Right ventricular function in response to the elevated pulmonary artery pressures and pulmonary vascular resistance reveals relatively normal right ventricular stroke work.

To compensate for the diminished oxygen consumption relating to the suppressed cardiac output, the arterial venous oxygen content difference is increased. The shunt fraction is slightly elevated consistent with pulmonary congestion and poor oxygenation of the blood passing through the lung. Note the suppressed PVO_2 value of 32.0 mm Hg and the depressed

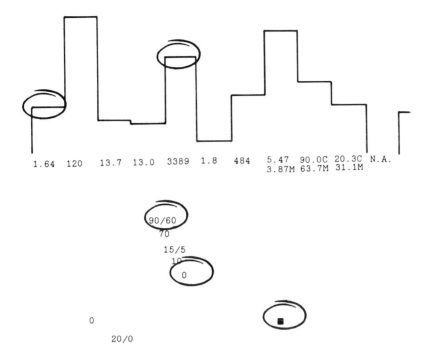

1.64 120   13.7 13.0 3389 1.8   484   5.47 90.0C 20.3C N.A.
                                             3.87M 63.7M 31.1M

90/60
70
15/5
10
0

0

20/0

B   HYPOVOLEMIC SHOCK

Figure 6–3 *Continued*

venous oxygen saturation of 59 per cent. Normal values would be approximately 40 mm Hg and 70 per cent saturation, respectively.

The poor perfusion in these patients is usually reflected by increased lactate levels and diminished base excess, both consistent with ensuing acidosis. The oxygen half-life pressure of hemoglobin (P-50) values were above normal: 35.1 mm Hg. The oxygen dissociation curve plots oxyhemoglobin saturation as a function of blood oxygen tension. The shape and position of the oxyhemoglobin dissociation curve is an expression of the affinity of hemoglobin for oxygen.[3] The P-50 defines the position of the curve when the hemoglobin molecule is half saturated at constant pH and temperature. An increase in oxygen affinity lowers the P-50 (shift to the left) from a normal value of 27 mm Hg. Factors precipitating these changes are decreases in temperature, carbon dioxide and ionized sodium, potassium, and hydrogen concentration (alkalosis, pH increase), 2,3 diphosphoglycerate (2,3-DPG), and adenosine triphosphate (ATP). A decrease in oxygen affinity raises the P-50 value (shift to the right of the curve). Factors precipitating these changes are increases in temperature, carbon dioxide and ionized sodium, potassium, and hydrogen con-

centration (acidosis, pH decreases), 2,3 DPG, and ATP. The shift to the right in this particular patient made oxygen transport more efficient. A frequent cause for a shift to the left of the curve, i.e., lower P-50 levels, is related to multiple blood transfusions, which produce low 2,3 DPG levels, thereby diminishing oxygen transport.

From a therapeutic standpoint this patient requires increased oxygen administration and possibly intubation. The increased preload (PCWP) should be treated by diminished fluid administration and possibly diuretics. If on a repeat profile the diminished cardiac output and ventricular function persist in this patient, strong consideration should be given to the use of inotropic agents such as dobutamine, dopamine, and digitalis.

THE PATIENT WITH SEVERE HEAD INJURY

Electrocardiographic abnormalities and elevated levels of the myocardial isoenzyme creatinine phosphokinase (CPK-MB) are common in young, previously healthy patients sustaining severe head injuries. Myocardial ne-

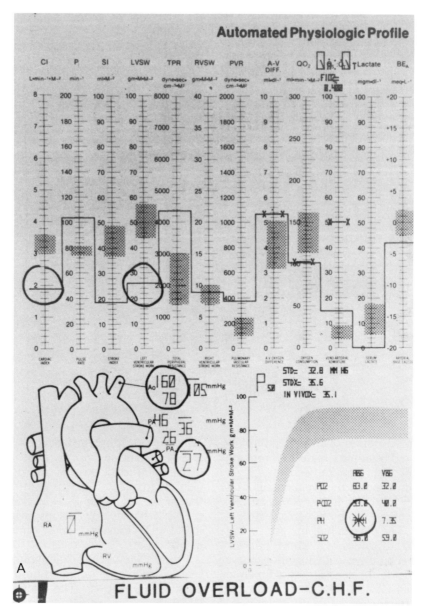

Figure 6–4. *A* and *B*, Note diminished cardiac index and left ventricular stroke work with increased blood pressure and total peripheral resistance.

crosis is often found at autopsy in patients that die of their central nervous system injuries. It is generally thought that these findings result from sympathetic hyperactivity and represent myocardial injury. Some studies of sequential cardiovascular parameters suggest that a relationship exists between cardiac function following head trauma and survival. Brown noted that a low cardiac output early in the course of a head injury characterized the patients who eventually die.[4] Popp reported that a persistently low cardiac output following head injury was associated with increased mortality.[5] The low cardiac output may be a result of myocardial damage from a more severe cerebral injury or from intravascular volume depletion from diuretic treatment (mannitol, furosemide), or the low cardiac output may contribute to the cerebral injury. Studies in animals confirm that the latter is at least possible because both hypovolemia and propranolol administration produce a decreased cardiac output and a decreased cerebral blood flow even when cerebral perfusion pressure is preserved.[6]

F1O2 = 0.400

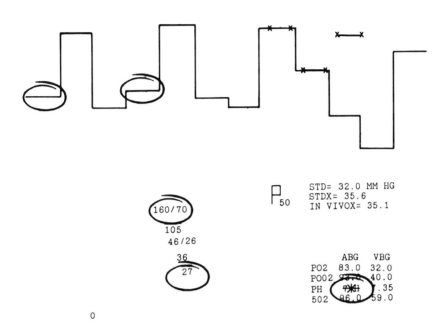

STD= 32.0 MM HG
STDX= 35.6
IN VIVOX= 35.1

160/70
105
46/26
36
27

	ABG	VBG
PO2	83.0	32.0
POO2	93.0	40.0
PH	7.41	.35
502	96.0	59.0

0

B   **FLUID OVERLOAD—C.H.F.**

Figure 6–4 *Continued*

Standard therapy dictates the use of intracranial pressure monitors (ICP) to be utilized in patients with severe head injury. Therapeutic interventions to maintain the ICP below 20 mm Hg include hyperventilation with associated alkalosis (which allegedly diminishes cerebral edema), mannitol, sedation with barbiturates, head elevation, and, more controversially, steroids. Most of these modalities (particularly sedation and diuretics) precipitate a fall in preload and cardiac output. The fall in preload may not be obvious from the measurement of PCWP. Frequently, trauma patients have normal myocardial function; however, patients with central nervous system injury have a varied left ventricular compliance or distensibility. One must remember that the PCWP provides a pressure reflection of the end diastolic volume of the left ventricle with the mitral valve open. However, if the myocardial compliance is diminished, lesser volumes will still be reflected with high wedge pressures, thereby making an excellent case for frequent monitoring of cardiac output in these patients in order to prevent diminished tissue perfusion, particularly to the brain.

For purposes of discussion, myocardial ischemia, right ventricular dilatation and overload, shock, positive and expiratory pressure (PEEP), pericardial effusion, and inotropic drugs have all been implicated in decreasing left ventricular compliance in critically ill patients. Vasodilating drugs such as nitroprusside and nitroglycerin and relief of ischemia can in-

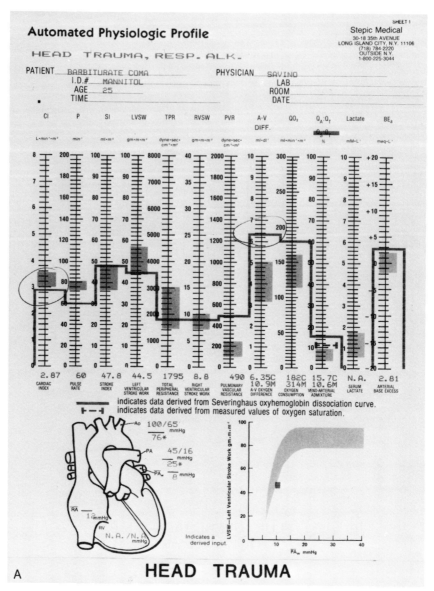

Figure 6–5. *A* and *B*, Note depressed ventricular function with increased oxygen extraction reflected by increased AVO_2 content difference.

crease left ventricular compliance by diminishing afterload, thereby relaxing the ventricle in order to accept a greater end diastolic volume.

The presented automated physiologic profile is of a typical patient with severe head injury who required treatment involving barbiturate coma, continuous mannitol infusion, respiratory alkalosis, and elevated head posture to maintain normal intracranial pressures (Fig. 6–5). Note the low normal PCWP and diminished ventricular function as depicted by the Sarnoff ventricular performance curve. Left ventricular function is diminished with diminished cardiac output. The AVO_2 content difference is increased consistent with increased extraction peripherally to compensate for the diminished output.

For purposes of managing these patients, it is not always necessary to know the precise preload. PCWP, although it does not reflect the absolute left ventricular end diastolic volume (LVEDV), is an excellent guide to the amount that the preload can be increased in an attempt to maximize cardiac output without producing pulmonary edema. If cardiac output remains inadequate with a PCWP of 16 to 18 mm Hg,

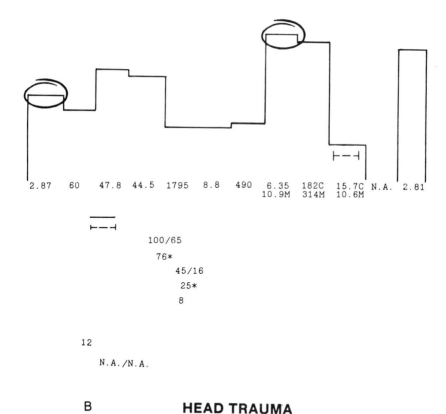

```
    2.87   60   47.8  44.5  1795   8.8   490   6.35  182C  15.7C  N.A.  2.81
                                               10.9M 314M  10.6M
```

```
                      100/65
                        76*
                           45/16
                            25*
                             8
```

```
        12
          N.A./N.A.
```

B   HEAD TRAUMA

Figure 6–5 *Continued*

other therapeutic interventions, such as administration of inotropic agents (dopamine and dobutamine) or afterload-reducing agents should be used.

SPECIFIC HEMODYNAMICS OF SPINAL CORD INJURY

In a recent review Luce described the significant cardiovascular complications in spinal cord injured patients.[7] The cardiovascular complications in spinal cord trauma are characterized by autonomic hyperactivity and hyporeactivity. Experimental studies suggest that the immediate response to acute spinal cord trauma is occasionally a transient period of hypertension.[8,9] Eidelberg[10] demonstrated that compression of the cervical, thoracic, or lumbar cord produces a brief rise in both systolic and diastolic blood pressures, usually accompanied by some degree of bradycardia. The electrocardiogram reveals a left ventricular strain pattern and ventricular ectopy during this period, followed by systemic hypotension. Transection of the cord at T1 completely elim-

inates the hypertension and ECG abnormalities. Although atropine, hexamethonium, and propranolol have no effect, the response is prevented by the alpha-adrenegic antagonist phenoxybenzamine.

Although intracranial pressure and extravascular lung water were not measured in this study, Albin and colleagues[11] report transient increases in these variables after experimental cord injury. Furthermore, pulmonary edema has been described and has been related to overly aggressive fluid therapy or chest trauma, as well as only to cord injury in other instances.[12,13] Neurogenic pulmonary edema has been attributed to a massive neural discharge that increases systemic and pulmonary vascular pressures, forces blood into the central circulation, and transiently increases capillary permeability.[14] These hemodynamic effects have been duplicated by large doses of catecholamines and prevented or suppressed by adrenergic-blocking agents.

Although hypertension may occur immediately after spinal cord trauma, most patients have hypotension due to increased venous capacitance by the time they receive medical at-

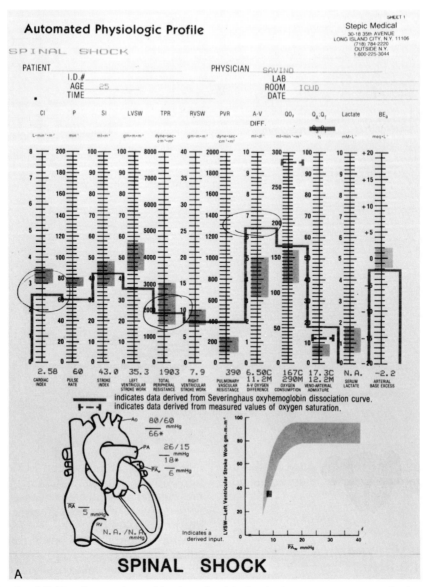

Figure 6–6. *A* and *B*, Note hypotension and bradycardia with slightly decreased TPR and cardiac index with compensatory oxygen extraction.

tention. Bradycardia progressing occasionally to heart block, and poikilothermia (in patients with complete lesions above T1) sufficient to reduce the core temperature several degrees centigrade are part of this picture, which is called *spinal shock*[8] (Fig. 6–6). Systemic vascular resistance is low in patients with spinal shock; cardiac output is normal or increased, and, depending on associated hypovolemia from associated injuries, this parameter may be decreased.[12] Because of their autonomic insufficiency, patients may become profoundly hypotensive if positioned upright. When supine,

they appear warm and well-perfused, and their systolic blood pressure rarely falls below 70 mm Hg unless bleeding from concurrent injuries is occurring.

Most chronic quadriplegics continue to manifest slightly low or normal blood pressure and pulse for weeks to months after injury (autonomic dysreflexia). Nevertheless, over 50 per cent of patients with lesions above T7 demonstrate occasional episodes of hypertension, bradycardia, muscular hypotonus, and either vasoconstrictive pallor or flushing and sweating associated with vasodilatation. These epi-

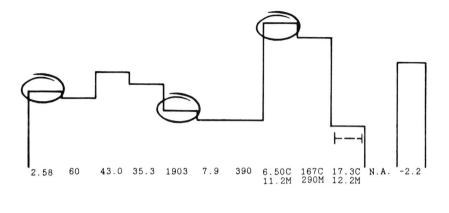

```
    2.58   60   43.0  35.3  1903  7.9   390  6.50C  167C  17.3C  N.A.  -2.2
                                              11.2M  290M  12.2M
```

```
            80/60
            66*
               26/15
               18*
               6
                                    ■
     5
        N.A./N.A.
```

B   **SPINAL SHOCK**

Figure 6–6 *Continued*

sodes most frequently are triggered by distention of hollow visceral organs, especially the urinary bladder. Apparently the trigger sensations enter the spinal cord and cause a mass sympathetic reflex that is inhibited from above in normal individuals.[15] The reflex is associated with very high levels of norepinephrine in arterial blood.

The autonomic lability of these patients dictates that vasoactive drugs and those affecting the heart be used sparingly. This provision applies equally to anesthetic agents. Rozier[15] prefers a slow, gentle induction of anesthesia and treats sympathetic deficiency or excess with the infusion of direct-acting vasoconstrictors such as Neo-synephrine, vasodilators such as nitroprusside, cardiac stimulants such as isoproterenol, and depressants such as propranolol, rather than using adrenergic agonists and antagonists that might indirectly alter catecholamine concentrations.

Albin[8] suggests induction with diazepam, fentanyl, and thiopental; intubation under pancuronium; and maintenance of anesthesia with narcotics, nitrous oxide, and pancuro-nium. Succinylcholine and other depolarizing agents should not be used during the first six months after spinal cord injury to avoid hyperkalemic crisis. Such crises apparently result from the supersensitivity of denervated muscle to acetylcholine, with subsequent sustained contractures and potassium release.[16]

Although opinions vary, most investigators agree that fluid and blood replacement should be limited in patients with spinal shock, lest pulmonary edema be potentiated.[12] On the other hand, with massive thoracic and thoracolumbar injuries, blood loss from the fracture site can be significant. The lability of these patients and their sensitivity to fluids and drugs further supports the use of hemodynamic monitoring as well as close monitoring of temperature fluctuations.

SPECIAL CONSIDERATIONS DURING THE OPERATIVE PERIOD

The patient with acute spinal cord injury who requires surgery often presents to the anesthesiologist with respiratory dysfunction, spinal shock, autonomic hyper- or hyposensitivity, hypothermia, and hyper- or hypovolemia, as previously discussed. Paraplegic patients who require repeated operative interventions may have additional problems such as autonomic hyperhyporeflexia, electrolyte imbalance, anemia, sepsis, negative nitrogen balance, adrenocortical insufficiency, and emotional instability. Thus, in addition to correcting fluid balance, the anesthesiologist must integrate the interaction of respiratory-hemodynamic-renal and fluid balance problems. Postoperative complications such as pulmonary edema, circulatory instability, renal dysfunction, and electrolyte abnormalities are usually the products of abnormalities of more than one organ or regulatory system. For instance, patients with normal lungs and cardiac function are easily able to tolerate fluid overload as opposed to those with lung contusion and increased sympathetic activity. In patients with normal cardiac and renal function, electrolyte imbalance or fluid overload rarely occurs. In patients with increased sympathetic activity, peripheral vascular resistance increases and may lead to hypovolemia and eventually reduction of cardiac output. For these reasons, monitoring of respiratory, hemodynamic, renal, and electrolyte balance is mandatory during the perioperative period for patients with spinal cord injury who may have multiple abnormalities in metabolic functions as well as the regulatory system.

Respiratory dysfunction related to spinal cord injury higher than the cervical area is well known. Ledsome and Sharp[17] reported that arterial hypoxemia frequently occurred even with normal alveolar ventilation during the first week following injury. Often unrecognized respiratory problems are reflected by progressive hypoxemia related to lung contusion. Since hypoxemia may progress during 24 to 48 hours following injury without radiologic manifestations of pulmonary edema, anesthesiologists are advised to examine arterial and mixed venous blood gases at a known inspiratory oxygen concentration and calculate pulmonary venous admixture. Particularly in these patients fluid overload should be avoided carefully.

When peripheral and pulmonary vasculature tones are altered by injury of the spinal cord and associated abnormalities of sympathetic activities,[18] CVP or PCWP ceases to reflect preload expressed as the left ventricular end diastolic volume (LVEDV). With increased sympathetic activity, CVP or PCWP can be normal even though hypovolemia or decreased preload may be present. On the contrary, most anesthetic agents increase compliance of venous capacitance vessels, especially when vasodilators are used. In this circumstance, fluid overload can occur at normal CVP or PCWP. With these considerations, induction of anesthesia should proceed slowly, while direct arterial pressure and PCWP (CVP) are observed. Hypotension can usually be avoided by using gradual induction with fentanyl while PCWP is maintained at the range of 7 to 10 mm Hg. Hypertension that may be associated with endotracheal intubation or surgical stimulation can be controlled either by deepening anesthesia or by the use of vasodilators such as sodium nitroprusside (SNP). In tetraplegic patients, severe bradycardia or asystole can occur in response to stimulation such as tracheal suctioning,[19] and these responses can be modified by the use of atropine. Circulatory instability may also occur associated with the position change in the patients with high spinal cord injury because of the lack of sympathetic control.

One of the main problems that occurs during surgery of the spine is hemorrhage. In recent years, the use of controlled hypotension with pharmacologic vasodilation such as SNP or nitroglycerin (TNG) has become popular in spinal surgery in order to reduce blood loss. However, cautions are warranted in applying such techniques in surgery of spinal cord injury. It is often stated that cardiac output is well maintained during hypotensive anesthesia because peripheral resistance is reduced pharmacologically.[20] However, most of the studies concerning hemodynamic effects of SNP and other vasodilators have been performed in normovolemic humans and animals, and rarely in humans when hemorrhage occurs concomitantly.[21] Acute blood loss and hypotension itself stimulate sympathoadrenal systems and the release of other stress hormones such as renin, angiotensin[22] and ADH.[23] These endogenous hormones may produce peripheral vascular constriction even during the infusion of SNP because the dosage of SNP that produces vasodilation varies and also tachyphylaxis occurs during the course of surgery.[24] Therefore, peripheral vascular resistance represents the balance between pharmacologic vasodilation effects and vasoconstrictor effect induced by hemorrhage and hypotension. Consequently, adequate tissue perfusion cannot be guaranteed during controlled hypotension unless blood loss is accurately replaced or cardiac output and peripheral vascular resistance are measured.

When vasodilators such as SNP or NTG are used, compliance of venous capacitance vessels increases and both CVP and PCWP decrease, even in normovolemic patients. Therefore, we recommend that PCWP be maintained at 7 to 10 mm Hg and not to exceed 12 mm Hg. We have found that CVP is usually 1 to 2 mm Hg lower than PCWP during hypotensive anesthesia with the patient in the prone position. Thus, if only CVP is monitored, relative fluid overload can be concealed.

Urine output has been a useful clinical index that reflects blood volume and/or hydration status. However, during anesthesia, all anesthetics decrease urine output, probably because of the decreased glomerular filtration rate.[25] Therefore, normal urine output should not always be expected. Again, if urine output is used only as an index to indicate adequacy of hydration or blood volume, overhydration of the patients can occur.

During recovery from anesthesia, sympathetic activity increases and the effects of stress hormones that might have been released during surgery such as renin, angiotensin and ADH may still exert their influence on both renal function and the peripheral vasculature.[26] Consequently, if relative overhydration occurs during surgery, blood that remained in venous capacitance vessels as well as fluid in the interstitial space may then return to the central circulation. Accordingly, rebound arterial hypertension and elevation of pulmonary pressure, PCWP, and CVP tend to occur during the immediate postoperative period.[12] If renal function is completely normal, these returned fluids can be readily removed as urine, but we have observed that diuresis is often delayed following spinal surgery. If the patients suffer from lung contusion or ARDS, the combined effect of both fluid overload and abnormal renal function may lead to pulmonary edema and hypoxemia during the recovery stage from anesthesia, which may be mistakenly interpreted as aspiration pneumonia.

For these reasons, monitoring of hemodynamic parameters such as PCWP, cardiac output, peripheral vascular resistance, and urine output and accurate replacement of blood loss are all necessary to manage patients with spinal cord injury during the perioperative period.

EARLY AND LATE SEPSIS AND RESPIRATORY INSUFFICIENCY

Trauma victims, especially quadriplegic patients secondary to cervical cord injuries, frequently experience septic complications. In an ICU environment factors to be considered are intravenous line sepsis, suppurative phlebitis, pulmonary infections, urinary tract infections, soft tissue infections, osseous infection, and, most importantly, intra-abdominal sepsis. These patients are frequently febrile, ventilator dependent, and mildly malnourished; they may require hyperalimentation and are monitored with bladder catheterization.

These patients usually remain normotensive and retain relatively normal hemodynamic pressures (Fig. 6–7). The myocardial performance may reveal hypovolemia to normality. Left ventricular function usually involves a hyperdynamic state with increased cardiac output and a classic finding of peripheral vasodilation (TPR). The AVO_2 difference is usually low, associated with shunting and rapid flow with somewhat diminished oxygen unloading. However, in the depicted profile, the AVO_2 difference is normal; this indicates increased extraction. The oxygen consumption value is slightly elevated. Essential to the management of early sepsis is the optimization of oxygen consumption or uptakes. To determine oxygen demands, particularly in septic patients, the cardiac output should be progressively increased with preload, afterload, and inotropic maneuvers until the oxygen consumption level reaches a plateau. When stabilization occurs, oxygen demands have been satisfied. Inability to normalize metabolic parameters reflecting acidosis usually indicates inadequate perfusion and anerobic glycolysis. In this situation further efforts toward optimization are necessary in order to accomplish the state of hemodynamic equilibrium.[27]

Unfortunately, hypotensive levels progress rapidly in many patients (Fig. 6–8). The PCWP in this profile reflects early congestive cardiac failure documented in the ventricular function curve. Left ventricular function parameters demonstrate diminished cardiac index, stroke index, and left ventricular stroke work. At this late stage of sepsis, the peripheral resistance is high normal secondary to vasconstriction. All of these findings are secondary to suppressed cardiac function. As the pulmonary artery wedge pressure rises in the evolution of the septic process, further depression in cardiac re-

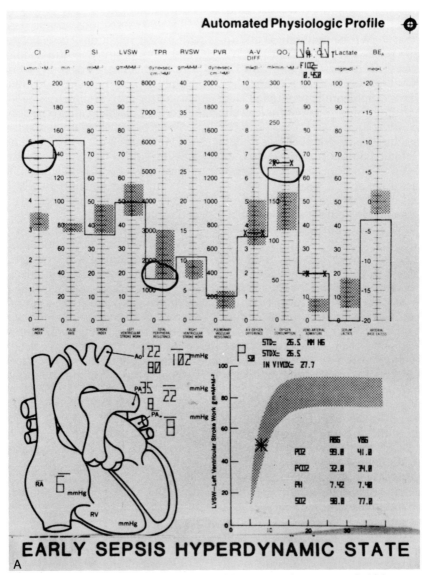

Figure 6–7. *A* and *B*, Note increased cardiac index with diminished TPR with unexpectedly high compensatory AVO_2 content difference.

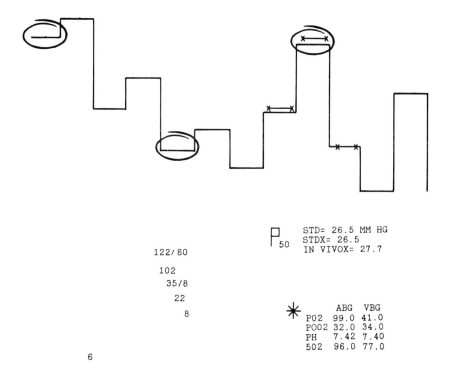

$$P_{50} \quad \begin{array}{l} \text{STD= 26.5 MM HG} \\ \text{STDX= 26.5} \\ \text{IN VIVOX= 27.7} \end{array}$$

122/80

102

35/8

22

8

6

	ABG	VBG
PO2	99.0	41.0
PCO2	32.0	34.0
PH	7.42	7.40
SO2	96.0	77.0

B EARLY SEPSIS HYPERDYNAMIC STATE

Figure 6-7 *Continued*

serve occurs and cardiac index and left ventricular stroke work fall. Oxygen transport–derived parameters in this patient reflect significant elevation of pulmonary vascular resistance and a marked increase in venoarterial admixture (pulmonary shunting). These factors are the earliest changes characteristic of the adult respiratory distress syndrome (ARDS) even before clinical evidence of respiratory distress occurs and clearly before the chest x-ray reveals diffuse infiltrates.

Therapeutic interventions should aggressively seek the source of sepsis, which should be treated. From a hemodynamic standpoint, optimizing this patient's hemodynamic status requires inotropic support (dopamine or dobutamine). Oxygen therapy is essential; often these patients are in respiratory distress with poor ventilation requiring intubation and mechanical ventilatory support. High tidal volumes and positive end expiratory pressure (PEEP) are required to maintain relatively normal oxygen and carbon dioxide gas tensions.

It has been proposed that tissues are unable to utilize oxygen effectively, perhaps as a consequence of transient hypoxemia, hypotension, or hypoperfusion, and that steroids result in improved metabolism and oxygen utilization when used in the early septic state. A similar advantage to steroids has been demonstrated with a rightward shift of the oxygen dissociation curve with high P-50 values.

Worthy of mention is the effect of PEEP on the hemodynamics of these patients. The optimal level of PEEP will produce the greatest cardiopulmonary benefits. These benefits are reflected by the primary and calculated parameters of the profile. Previous studies have demonstrated that at a PEEP greater than 10 cm H_2O, the PCWP and CVP do not accurately reflect left ventricular filling pressures. For every 5 cm H_2O increase of PEEP, the PCWP usually increases by approximately 1 mm Hg; therefore, cardiac output measurements are essential to guarantee optimal pulmonary blood flow when high PEEP is used. Due to increased intrathoracic pressure PEEP may obstruct the venous return to the heart, thereby reducing cardiac output and oxygen delivery to tissues. Therapeutic interventions

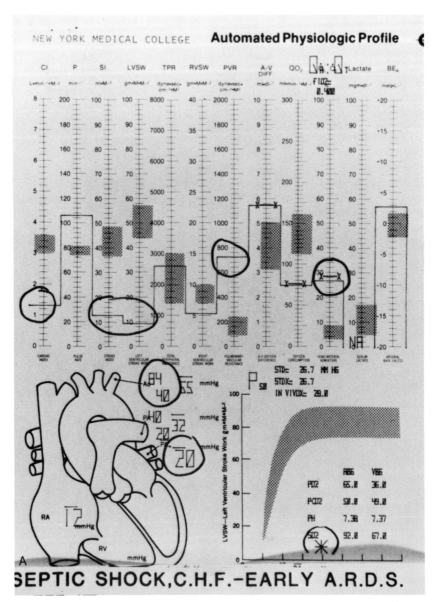

Figure 6–8. *A* and *B*, Note hypotension diminished cardiac index and LVSW with compensatory increased AVO$_2$ content difference. Note increased PVR and pulmonary shunt.

F102=0.400

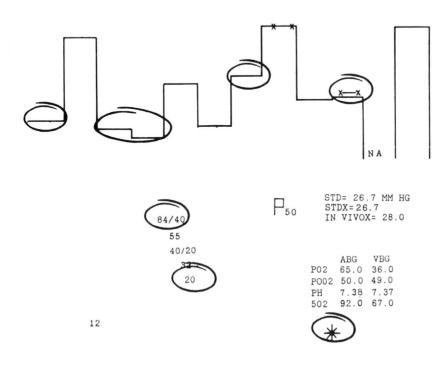

STD= 26.7 MM HG
STDX= 26.7
IN VIVOX= 28.0

	ABG	VBG
PO2	65.0	36.0
PCO2	50.0	49.0
PH	7.38	7.37
SO2	92.0	67.0

B   **SEPTIC SHOCK,C.H.F.— EARLY A.R.D.S.**

Figure 6–8 *Continued*

to combat the negative effects of PEEP frequently require preload manipulations with crystalloids, colloids, red blood cells, inotropic agents to adjust contractility, and afterload reducers to lower pulmonary and systemic vascular resistance in order to maintain an optimal cardiac index.[28]

REFERENCES

1. Cohn JD, Enger PE, Del Guercio LRM: The automated physiologic profile. Crit Care Med 3:51, 1975.
2. Shoemaker WC, Appel PL, Bhard R.: Clinical trial of an algorithm for outcome prediction in acute circulatory failure. Crit Care Med 10:390, 1982.
3. Border JR, Gallo E, Shenk WG: Alterations in cardiovascular and pulmonary physiology in the severely stressed patient. J Trauma 6:976, 1966.
4. Brown RS, Shoemaker WC: Sequential hemodynamics in patients with head injury: evidence for an early hemodynamic effect. Ann Surg 177:187, 1973.
5. Popp AJ, Gottlieb ME, Paloski WH et al: Cardiopulmonary hemodynamics in patients with serious head injury. J Surg Res 32:416, 1982.
6. Davis DH, Surdt TM, Jr.: Relationship of cerebral blood flow to cardiac output, mean arterial pressure, blood volume and alpha and beta blockade in cats. J. Neurosurg 52:745, 1980.
7. Luce JM: Medical management of spinal cord injury. Crit Care Med 13:126, 1985.
8. Albin MS: Acute spinal cord trauma. *In* Shoemaker WC, Thompson WL, Holbrook PR (eds): Textbook of Critical Care. Philadelphia, W.B. Saunders Co., 1984, pp 928–936.
9. Alexander S, Ken FWL: Blood pressure responses in

acute compression of the spinal cord. J Neurosurg 38:326, 1973.

10. Eidelberg EE: Cardiovascular response to experimental cord compression. J Neurosurg 38:326, 1973.

11. Albin MS, Bunegin L, Helsel P: Intracranial pressure and cardiovascular responses in experimental cord transection. Crit Care Med 7:127, 1979.

12. Meyer GA, Berman IR, Doty DB: Hemodynamic responses in quadriplegia with and without chest trauma. J Neurosurg 34:168, 1971.

13. Poe RH, Reisman JL, Rodenhouse TG: Pulmonary edema in cervical spinal cord injury. J Trauma 18:71, 1978.

14. Theodore J, Rubin ED: Speculations in neurogenic pulmonary edema. Am Rev Respir Dis 113:405, 1976.

15. Rozier MF: Preoperative evaluation of patients with diseases that require special preoperative evaluation and intraoperative managment. In Miller RD (ed): Anesthesia. New York, Churchill-Livingstone, 1981, pp 21–93.

16. Granert GA, Theye RA: Pathophysiology of hyperkalemia induced by succinyl choline. Anesthesiology 43:89, 1975.

17. Ledsome J, Sharp JM: Pulmonary function in acute cervical cord injury. Am Rev Respir Dis 124:41, 1981.

18. Welply NC, Mathias CJ, Frankel HL: Circulatory reflexes in tetraplegics during artificial ventilation and general anesthesia. Paraplegia 13:172, 1975.

19. Lawson NW: Sodium nitroprusside-induced hypotension for supine total hip replacement. Anesth Analg 55:564, 1976.

20. Gustafson C: Circulatory effect of hemorrhage during sodium nitroprusside induced hypotension. Acta Anesth Scand 29:502, 1985.

21. Kaneko Y, Ikeda T, Udea H: Renin release during acute reduction of arterial blood pressure in normotensive subjects and patients with renovascular hypertension. J Clin Invest 46:705, 1967.

22. Zubrow AB, Plasma renin catecholamine, and vasopressin during nitroprusside-induced hypotension in ewes. Anesthesiology 58:245, 1983.

23. Miller ED, Ackerly JA, Vaughn D, et al: The renin-angiotensin system during controlled hypotension with sodium nitroprusside. Anesthesiology 47:257, 1977.

24. Priano LL: The effect of anesthesia on renal blood flow and function. 1984 Annual Refresher Course Lectures No. 240, American Society of Anesthesiologists, Inc.

25. Khambatta HJ, Stone JG, Kahn E: Hypertension during anesthesia on discontinuation of sodium nitroprusside–induced hypotension. Anesthesiology 51:127, 1979.

26. Shibutani K, Komatsu T, Bhalodia R, et al: Rebound hemodynamic responses after the withdrawal of nitroprusside in anesthetized patients. Anesthesiology 59:A16, 1983.

27. Savino JS, Del Guercio LRM: Preoperative assessment of high-risk surgical patients. Surg Clin North Am 65:763, 1985.

28. Savino JS, Vo N, Kim KH, Gupte P: Monitoring respiratory complications in critically ill patients. Infections in Surgery 2:565, 1983.

7

Ultrasound Examination for the Evaluation of Spinal Cord Injured Patients

MATS ASZTÉLY, M.D.

The radiologist has a key role in the integrated approach to the spinal cord injured patient. He is expected to supply the necessary imaging information to the clinician directly responsible for the care of these patients. In this chapter I intend to describe the use of diagnostic ultrasound, one of several modalities of diagnostic radiology, and to point out its advantages compared with those of methods traditionally used in the care of these patients.

From a practical organizational point of view, many patients with spinal cord injuries are now being cared for in special facilities with their own radiologic services. Historically, these facilities have been oriented toward the use of general radiologic methods, and diagnostic ultrasound has not always been available. If this review of ultrasound for the evaluation of spinal cord injured patients is instrumental in leading to its increased use for this purpose, these patients will undoubtedly benefit.

In the initial emergency situation these patients often present with multisystem injuries in which accurate and fast diagnosis is necessary. Imaginative use of diagnostic ultrasound can be of great value in this situation. In an early phase of treatment of some of these patients, stabilizing surgery of the spine is considered necessary; perioperative ultrasound is increasingly used in this context. During the rehabilitation phase there is need for continuous follow-up of these patients, a need which diagnostic ultrasound can be used to fill.

IMMEDIATELY AFTER THE TRAUMA

Half of the patients with spinal cord injuries present with other major traumatic lesions. It is therefore important to screen all patients to find such injuries. Clinical and basic x-ray examinations should be done first; the findings should highlight specific problems in which specialized imaging methods will be used. Diagnostic ultrasound plays an important role in this situation because it can be used to perform examinations at the bedside without the problems of ionizing radiation. It must be emphasized that ultrasound as a supplementary diagnostic tool should be used under the supervision of the radiologist chiefly responsible for the patient. The harmlessness of the method should not lead to its uncritical utilization and unnecessary examinations.

In the initial work-up there is no value to diagnostic ultrasound for evaluation of the traumatized spine. It would be possible to evaluate paraspinal hemorrhage utilizing ultrasound, although this use has not been reported in the literature. These patients will probably be examined with computed tomography, which not only gives information about the spine and the spinal cord but also about the surrounding soft tissue. The same applies to head injuries: ultrasound is seldom used for diagnosis of cranial mid-line shift because of the availability of computed tomography.

When chest injuries are suspected, x-rays should be done at first hand. For further evaluation for pericardial or pleural hemorrhage, diagnostic ultrasound is the confirming method. If there is a direct suspicion of pericardial hemorrhage, myocardial trauma, or rupture of a valve or a tendinous cord of the heart, ultrasound examination is directly indicated.[1] The presence of blood in the pericardium will sometimes be difficult to recognize due to unexpected acoustic properties of the blood. Careful examination technique is necessary. Because post-traumatic hemopericardium or hemothorax can show up slowly,[2] the examination should be repeated at predefined intervals.

The effects of abdominal trauma can be studied successfully using ultrasound. As mentioned already, its use should be managed by the radiologist reponsible for work-up of the patient. For study of the upper abdomen for organ rupture, ultrasound scanning of liver and spleen will be accurate.[3] The findings at diaphragmatic rupture or rupture of the duodenum, however, are often atypical,[4] and supplementary abdominal flat films will be necessary. For study of the urinary tract, excretory urography should be preferred as the initial examination because it can show displacement of and leakage from kidneys, ureters, and bladder as well as the urethra. For follow-up after the status of the urinary tracts has been determined, ultrasound examination will be sufficient.[5]

One specific situation in which ultrasound is useful is the evaluation of the patient for acute abdominal complications caused by stress or cardiovascular disorders when diagnostic problems arise because of the impaired sensorium. Flat films, including films obtained using horizontal beam direction, are the main basis of diagnosis; however, the supplementary use of ultrasound can in certain situations be rewarding. In cases involving ileus, the amount and volume of entirely fluid-filled bowel loops might be more easily defined by ultrasound than by abdominal films because the chronic constipation common in these patients can obscure the impression of bowel obstruction.

A severe abdominal condition described in patients with spinal injuries, as well as in patients with other types of injuries after major trauma, is post-traumatic acalculous cholecystitis.[6,7] Deteriorating general clinical condition and elevated white count, serum bilirubin, and alkaline phosphatase should raise suspicion of this condition. At ultrasound examination a large-volume, acalculous gallbladder with thickened walls is seen.[8] If the criteria for thickened walls and large volume that are used are set for high sensitivity, the numbers of false-positive results will be significant. The diagnosis should, therefore, be confirmed using cholescintigraphy. The aforementioned diagnostic approach is also valid in diagnosis of ordinary acute cholecystitis involving calculus formation when further confirmation of the diagnosis will be obtained with the observation of calculi in the gallbladder at ultrasound examination.

The incidence of deep venous thrombosis in patients with spinal injuries is significant. The gold standard diagnostic method, phlebography, often cannot be utilized because it necessitates that the patient be placed in an upright position.[9] In order to deal with this diagnostic problem, several noninvasive methods have been used. Among these are the fibrinogen uptake test, impedance plethysmography, thermography, and ultrasound examination alone or in combination with Doppler examination (duplex Doppler). Of these methods only ultrasound will be discussed in this chapter. Several authors have presented the results of long series of studies involving ultrasound. Their results are satisfactory, with the examination having high predictive values.[10-12] The equipment necessary for this examination is cost-efficient and not complicated to use.

Several diagnostic criteria for deep venous thrombosis at ultrasound examination have been tested: The most simple way to examine the veins of the lower limb for thrombosis is to verify whether the veins collapse under pressure as applied by the transducer. A fully collapsible vein is considered free of thrombus. The ultrasound study can be made more comprehensive by studying the blood flow in the veins utilizing Doppler technique, either alone or in combination with ultrasound imaging. Detection of normal flow with normal variations synchronous with breathing and Valsalva maneuvers signifies absence of venous thrombosis.

A drawback of the ultrasound method is low accuracy of detection of deep venous thrombosis of the calf only, especially of the lower part of the calf. Practically, this seems to be of minor significance because of the low complication rate of untreated calf thrombosis.

Altogether, there is no specific problem present involving the acute phase of spinal cord injured patients when diagnostic ultrasound is the single preferred method. It should be used as one of several necessary and useful radiologic methods.

DURING SURGERY

As mentioned elsewhere in this book, stabilizing surgery of spinal fractures often is found to be necessary in patients with spinal cord injuries. In a few patients with progressive symptoms, decompressing surgery also is considered valuable. The introduction of high-resolution dynamic scanners using transducer heads with a design that permits the introduction of the ultrasound transducer into the operating field has led to clinical studies using perioperative ultrasound examination of the spinal canal.[13-18] It has been shown that the lumen of the spinal canal in the operating area can be visualized with high resolution. The width and the topography of the lumen can be shown as well as the

relationship of the cord to the lumen of the spinal canal. Compromise of the lumen by fracture fragments or displacement of the elements of the spine can also be shown. Incidentally, it is worth mentioning that this method can be used for perioperative study of tumors and other focal lesions of the cord as well. The method is established in an increasing number of institutions in which spinal surgery is performed. The value of the supplementary information obtained at operation in spinal cord injured patients is, however, not entirely settled. It seems to be of value to avoid complications in surgery of patients with spinal fractures and minor neurologic effects. In the patient with manifest neurologic transection of the cord, the presence of a compromised lumen of the spinal

Figure 7–1. *A* and *B*, Perioperative ultrasound examination of the spinal canal. *A* was obtained with a 5 MHz transducer and *B* with a 7.5 MHz transducer. Both examinations were made after laminectomy was performed; the dura, however, was not opened. The operating area was filled with saline before scanning. Both images depict a sagittal midline view, the cranial direction to the left on the image and dorsal direction upward. Short white arrows indicate the enclosure of the spinal subarachnoid space, the dura and the arachnoid dorsally and the arachnoid, the dura and the dorsal longitudinal ligament ventrally. Within this space the cord is seen surrounded by a small volume of CSF. In *A*, a small area of cystic degeneration of the cord is seen (white long arrow), otherwise the cord and the subarachnoid space appear normal in both images. Closure of the subarachnoid space ventral to the cord is the most common sign of a narrow vertebral canal.

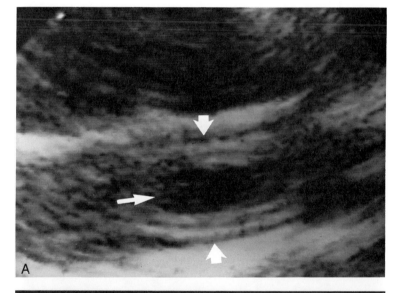

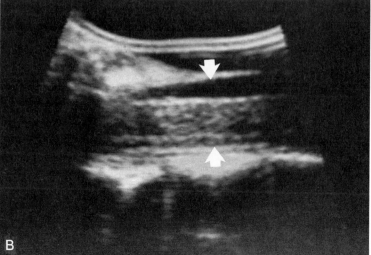

canal or bone fragments in the canal probably is of academic interest only.

In situations after initial surgery when complicating neurologic symptoms appear, ultrasound examination preoperatively using the laminectomy as an "acoustic window" or perioperatively at reoperation can help locate complicating bone fragments or degenerative cystic lesions.

DURING REHABILITATION

The necessity of close cooperation between radiologist and the physician in charge of the spinal cord injured patient during the initial emergency situation has already been emphasized. The same level of cooperation is necessary during the rehabilitation of the patient.

The most common types of complicating morbidity during rehabilitation of spinal cord injured patients are complications involving the lungs and the urinary tract. Research leading to increasing knowledge of these problems has led to significantly decreased occurrence. Favorable results are by no means guaranteed, and again the role of the radiologist is to supply the physician in charge with relevant imaging data.

The radiologist will usually be called upon to survey the urinary tract. Another area of interest is complicated pressure sores. Ultrasound

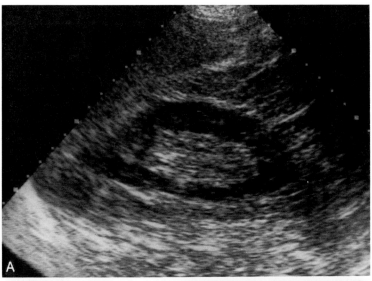

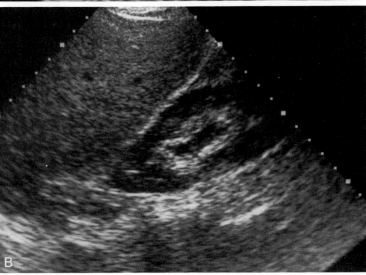

Figure 7–2. *A* and *B*, Ultrasound screening examination of the kidneys of a patient six months after multiple trauma resulting in cervical cord lesion and a right side pelvic fracture. No sign of urinary tract infection. Both kidneys are imaged from the flank in the plane giving the longest possible axis of the kidney. Cranial direction to the left on the image, ventral-lateral upward. On the image the kidneys appear as oval structures with a well-defined delineation (the capsular fat) and parenchyma giving low level echoes (dark-gray areas). The sinus (vessels, collecting system, and hilar fat) appears as a fairly homogenous area with high level echoes (a light area) in the left kidney (*A*). In the right kidney, *B*, the sinus appears as an area surrounding an area with low level echoes. This is slight hydronephrosis. The lighter gray area in the upper left part of *B* is the liver.

can of course be used as a general diagnostic tool in this population, in whom morbidity and mortality tend to be high.

THE URINARY TRACT

The main subject for diagnostic ultrasound during the rehabilitation phase of the spinal cord injured patient is the urinary tract. The main urologic problem of the spinal cord injured patient is impaired drainage of the bladder caused by the cord injury. This leads to a high risk of obstructive nephropathy and urinary tract infection. The modern management of these patients therefore has to a large extent been based on radiologic imaging of the urinary tracts. The impact of ultrasound diagnosis in this area is striking. An example is a recommendation to make repeat intravenous pyelograms every three to six months that was given in a major textbook on the subject of radiologic imaging of spinal cord injured patients.[19] In a study published only a year after the book by the same authors, a recommendation is given to perform these controls using diagnostic ultrasound.[20] The objective of radiologic imaging of the urinary tract is to verify the occurrence of hydronephrosis, ureterectasis, urinary tract calculi, renal parenchymal disease, and vesicoureteral reflux at bladder emptying. The occurrence of the first four conditions can easily be investigated using routine scanning with static or dynamic scanners. Several studies on this modality have been published giving data on accuracy as high as or even better than with intravenous pyelography.[5,20] To study the dynamic processes of reflux and bladder emptying, dynamic scanning is preferable. Using microbubbles in saline for filling the bladder for ultrasound cystography (easily accomplished by shaking the bottle just before infusion), the dynamics of urinary bladder filling and reflux if present can be observed. To study the process of bladder emptying, transrectal probes have been used successfully.[21,22] The capability of making a prolonged display of the ureter using realtime ultrasound has been utilized to give visual feedback of the micturition process to patients with dyssynergia. A high rate of improvement has been reported in a group of spinal cord injured patients with detrusor-sphincter dyssynergia through utilization of this procedure.

In this context the phenomenon of autonomic dysreflexia that can be encountered during bladder filling in some of these patients should be remembered. Awareness of this complication and preparedness for immediate action if it appears are as important during ultrasound vesicoureterography as when the x-ray counterpart is done.

Finally, when intravenous pyelography and ultrasound imaging of the kidneys are compared, the importance of the functional element in IVP often is mentioned. It is useful to note that the accuracy of intravenous pyelography as a functional study is very low, far less

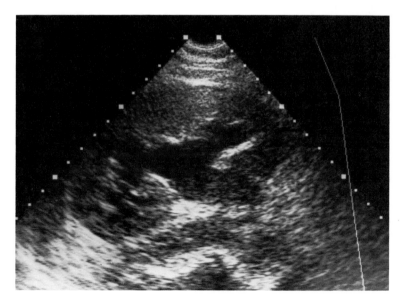

Figure 7–3. Right kidney of patient with spinal cord lesion and urinary tract infection. The kidney is depicted as described for Figure 7–2A, although the examination plane is slightly more lateral. Dilatation of the calyces, the pelvis, and the upper part of the ureter is seen. The thickness of the sinus fat is reduced as compared with Figure 7–2B, a sign of further advanced hydronephrosis.

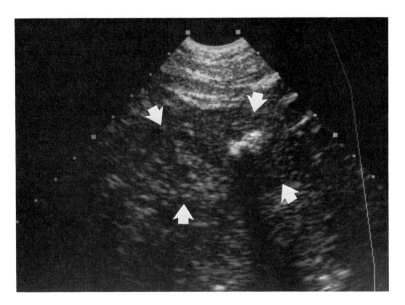

Figure 7–4. Left kidney of patient with spinal cord lesion and recurrent urinary tract infections. The kidney is not well defined toward the surrounding soft tissue (white short arrows); the same applies to the sinus area. This is a sign of postinflammatory reaction with formation of fibrous tissue in the kidney parenchyma. In the lower part of the kidney there is a high level echo with a zone with few echoes medially—a "shadow." This is a 1 cm calculus in the lower pole of the kidney. No hydronephrosis is present.

than common laboratory tests such as serum creatinine or BUN (which are not very accurate either). To obtain high accuracy data, function tests utilizing nuclear medicine are the methods of choice. These methods are easily applicable to bedridden patients.

PRESSURE SORES

The diagnosis of early changes of pressure sores is clinical. In spite of the most painstaking care, spinal cord injured patients sometimes get pressure sores complicated by deep necrosis, infection, and formation of abscesses, sometimes rather distal from the skin defect. In the diagnosis of abscesses a truly integrated approach to the imaging problem is necessary. In reports dealing directly with the study of pressure sores and their complications, ultrasound has been found inferior to computed tomography as an aid in diagnosis.[23,24] The ease with which the ultrasound examination can be performed and its high sensitivity make it an effective screening procedure. A skilled examiner will be able to discern anatomic deviations and collections of fluid or gas. If the results of this examination are considered equivocal or negative by the radiologist, computed tomography (when clinically indicated) should be done.

REFERENCES

1. Feigenbaum H: Echocardiography, 3rd ed. Philadelphia, Lea & Febiger, 1981, pp 478–496.

2. Parmley LF, Maniow WC, Mattingly TW: Nonpenetrating traumatic injury of the heart. Circulation 18:378, 1958.
3. Van Sonnenberg E, Simeone JF, Mueller PR, et al: Sonographic appearance of hematoma in liver, spleen and kidney: A clinical, pathologic and animal study. Radiology 147:507, 1983.
4. Amman AA, Brewer WH, Haull KI, et al: Traumatic rupture of the diaphragm: Real-time sonographic diagnosis. AJR 140:915, 1983.
5. Calenoff L, Neiman HL, Kaplan PE, et al: Urosonography in spinal cord injury patients. J Urology 128:1234, 1982.
6. Deitch EA, Engel JM: Acute acalculous cholecystitis. J Am Surgery 142:290, 1981.
7. Branch CL, Albertson DA, Kelly DL: Post-traumatic acalculous cholecystitis on a neurosurgical service. Neurosurgery 12:98, 1983.
8. Worthen NJ, Uszler JM, Funamura JL: Cholecystitis: Prospective evaluation of sonography and Tc-HIDA cholescintigraphy. AJR 137:973, 1981.
9. Kaufman HH, Satterwhite T, McConnell BJ, et al: Deep vein thrombosis and pulmonary embolism in head-injured patients. Angiology 34:627, 1983.
10. Sumner DS, Lambeth A: Reliability of Doppler ultrasound in the diagnosis of acute venous thrombosis both above and below the knee. Am J Surg 138:205, 1979.
11. Barnes RW: Ultrasound techniques for evaluation of lower extremity venous disease. In Zwiebel WJ (ed): Introduction to vascular ultrasonography. New York, Grune and Stratton, 1982, pp 273–288.
12. Cronan JJ, Dorfman GS, Grusmark J: Lower-extremity deep venous thrombosis: Further experiences with and refinement of ultrasound assessment. Radiology 168:101, 1988.
13. Eismont FJ, Green BA, Berkowitz BM, et al: The role of intraoperative ultrasonography in the treatment of thoracic and lumbar spine fractures. Spine 9:782, 1984.
14. Quencer RM, Morse BM, Green BA, et al: Intraoperative spinal sonography: Adjunct to metrizamide CT in the assessment and surgical decompression

of posttraumatic spinal cord cysts. AJR 142:593, 1984.

15. Jokich PM, Rubin JM, Dohrmann GJ: Intraoperative ultrasonic evaluation of spinal cord motion. J Neurosurg 60:707, 1984.

16. Rubin JM, Dohrmann GJ: The spine and spinal cord during neurosurgical operations: Real-time ultrasonography. Radiology 155:197, 1985.

17. Pasto ME, Rifkin MD, Rubenstein JB, et al: Real-time ultrasonography of the spinal cord: Intraoperative and postoperative imaging. Neuroradiology 26:183, 1984.

18. Montalvo BM, Quencer RM, Green BA, et al: Intraoperative sonography in spinal trauma. Radiology 153:125, 1984.

19. Calenoff L (ed): Radiology of spinal cord injury. St. Louis, CV Mosby, 1981.

20. Brandt TD, Neiman HL, Calenoff L, et al: Ultrasound evaluation of the urinary system in spinal cord injury patients. Radiology 141:473, 1981.

21. Shapeero LG, Friedland GW, Perkash I: Transrectal sonographic voiding cystourethrography: Studies in neuromuscular bladder dysfunction. AJR 141:83, 1983.

22. Perkash I, Friedland GW: Using transrectal sonography to teach patients with spinal cord injuries to restrain their bladders. Radiology 152:228, 1984.

23. Firooznia H, Rafil M, Golimbu C, et al: Computerized tomography in diagnosis of pelvic abscess in spinal cord injured patients. Comput Radiol 7:335, 1983.

24. Hendrix RW, Calenoff L, Lederman RB, et al: Radiology of pressure sores. Radiology 128:351, 1981.

25. Morin ME, Baker DA: The influence of hydration and bladder distension on the sonographic diagnosis of hydronephrosis. JCU 7:192, 1979.

26. Hooton TM, O'Shaughnessy EJ, Clowers D, et al: Localization of urinary tract infection in patients with spinal cord injury. J Infect Dis 150:85, 1984.

27. Rosenfield AT, Taylor KJ, Weiss RM: Ultrasound evaluation of bladder calculi. J Urol 121:119, 1978.

Efficacy of Magnetic Resonance Imaging in the Diagnosis of Spinal Cord Trauma

LINDA A. HEIER, M.D., and CARL E. JOHNSON, M.D.

It has only been with the advent of magnetic resonance (MR) imaging that direct visualization of the spinal cord has been achieved. In the past, the level of the spinal cord injury has been inferred from the presence of adjacent spinal subluxation or fracture depicted on the plain film or CT examination. Only the invasive techniques of myelography and CT myelography could provide an outline of the cord. With enlargement or compression of the cord, internal derangement of the spinal cord parenchyma was again inferred. The value of direct spinal cord imaging is apparent because neurologic deficits do not necessarily correlate with the degree of spinal canal narrowing. In a review of 75 burst fractures, the neurologic deficit corresponded to the level of the burst fracture but did not correlate with the degree of spinal canal narrowing.[1]

MR also directly visualizes the spinal column ligaments, and unlike CT, with which ligament rupture can only be inferred, ligamentous dehiscences can be identified on MR. Initial experience has found that the conspicuity of disc herniations is much greater on MR than on CT or CT myelography. The characterization of soft tissue injuries with MR imaging cannot be matched by any other modality.

While fractures are not as obvious on MR as compared with CT or plain films, they are usually visible. The multiplanar imaging capabilities of MR are extremely advantageous in a patient who cannot be moved. The direct coronal and sagittal images obtained by MR are at least equivalent and usually superior to the reformatted coronal and sagittal images obtained on CT.

MR BASICS

The basic physics of MR imaging is beyond the scope of this chapter. However, briefly, MR "visualizes" a slice of tissue by constructing an image from the returning radiofrequency pulses that are generated when the body's hydrogen protons are stimulated by a radiofrequency pulse at the *Larmor frequency* within a magnetic field. The Larmor frequency is the frequency at which magnetic protons will precess (i.e., rotate like a spinning top) around the direction of the magnetic field in which they are placed. The Larmor frequency depends upon the magnetic field strength, which is measured in teslas (T). If radiofrequency (RF) energy at the Larmor frequency is provided to protons precessing at the Larmor frequency, resonance occurs. This means that the additional energy causes the angle of precession to increase so that the nuclei tip away from the main magnetic field, or z axis. If the RF energy is sufficient to cause the precessing nuclei to tip 90 degrees into the xy or transverse plane, the associated RF pulse is said to be a 90 degree pulse. Protons precessing in the transverse plane will induce signal in a receiver coil, and this signal forms the basis of the MR image.

When the RF pulse is over, two types of relaxation mechanisms begin to change the precession patterns of the tipped nuclei. Relaxation is exponential. The T2 relaxation time refers to the time required for most (63 per cent, or e^{-1}) of the protons precessing in the transverse plane to get out of phase. T2 is also called the *spin-spin* or *transverse relaxation time*. The T1 relaxation time refers to the time required for most (63 per cent, or e^{-1}) of the tipped nuclei to once again realign with the main magnetic field. T1 is also known as the *spin-lattice* or *longitudinal relaxation time*. Essentially, T1 and T2 tell us something about the physical and chemical environments of the hydrogen protons. By imaging first with emphasis on T1 weighting and then with emphasis on T2 weighting, the superb tissue characterization of MR is obtained.

Various manipulations of the RF pulses applied to the magnetic field provide predominance of either T1 or T2 weighting. The most commonly used RF pulse sequence is a so-called spin-echo (SE) sequence in which a 90 degree pulse is followed by a 180 degree pulse. The signal intensity of tissue in a spin-echo sequence is dependent on three tissue parameters and two instrument parameters. Unique to each tissue is its hydrogen density, T1, and T2. By manipulating the two instrument parameters, the pulse repetition time (TR), and the echo delay time (TE), images can be created in which the signal intensity contributed is either predominantly dependent upon the hydrogen density, the T1, or the T2. Short TR (300 to 500 msec) and short TE (20 to 30 msec) sequences produce a predominantly T1-weighted image. Longer TR (1500 to 3000 msec) and longer TE (60 to 120 msec) sequences produce a predominantly T2-weighted sequence. A long TR and an intermediate TE (under 60 msec) produce a proton density–weighted image. Both proton density– and T2-weighted imaging can be produced by one multiecho sequence, with a long TR and the first TE being under 60 msec and the second TE being over 60 msec (e.g., TR 2000 msec/TE 40 and 80 msec).

A diagnostic examination of the spine requires both a T1-weighted pulse sequence (Fig. 8–1*A*) and a multiecho T2-weighted pulse sequence (Fig. 8–1*B* and *C*) in the sagittal plane. Axial T1-weighted images (Fig. 8–1*D*) are then angled parallel to the disc spaces through the area of interest. If the patient has underlying scoliosis, an image in the coronal plane is ex-tremely useful. It must be remembered that unlike CT, in which acquiring a single slice may only take 3 seconds, MR imaging excites an entire block of tissue in a single plane and obtains multiple slices at once. However, the times required to image these blocks of tissue are long, especially for a patient in pain. SE T1-weighted images take up to 5 minutes while SE multiecho T2-weighted images take anywhere from 8 to 20 minutes depending on the length of the TR, the number of averages, and so on. (A pulse sequence is applied several times and the signals are averaged in order to improve the signal-to-noise ratio.)

In an attempt to speed up acquisition time, gradient-echo sequences using smaller flip angles under 90 degrees without a 180 degree pulse have been utilized. Unlike spin echoes, gradient echoes achieve T1 or T2 weighting primarily by alteration of the flip angle rather than manipulation of the TR or TE. When the amount of time available for scanning is limited, they are very useful even though they have a poorer signal-to-noise ratio than do spin-echo images. A gradient-echo sequence in the coronal plane is frequently employed as a scout view in spine imaging so that subsequent sagittal images can be centered in the midline.

Gradient-echo sequences have two advantages over spin-echo sequences other than their shorter acquisition time. One is that the early stage of hemorrhage (i.e., deoxyhemoglobin) is more conspicuous than on a spin-echo sequence; the other advantage is that gradient echos are flow sensitive. While blood flow on spin-echo sequences appears as absent signal (i.e., black) (see Fig. 8–5), flow on gradient-echo sequences appears hyperintense (bright) (Fig. 8–2*C*). Areas of nonflow or thrombosis on gradient-echo sequences appear hypointense (dark).

An image of the entire spine from the foramen magnum to the sacrum can be obtained if the large-body RF coil is utilized. However, images from the body coil do not have the resolution required for diagnosis of spinal cord trauma. A secondary surface RF coil must be applied to the region of the spine that is of interest. The surface coil improves the signal-to-noise ratio over a limited distance allowing thinner slices with an improved spatial resolution. If the level of the injury is indeterminant, a screening examination can be performed with a sagittal body coil image; after review, the surface coil can be applied to the region of interest.

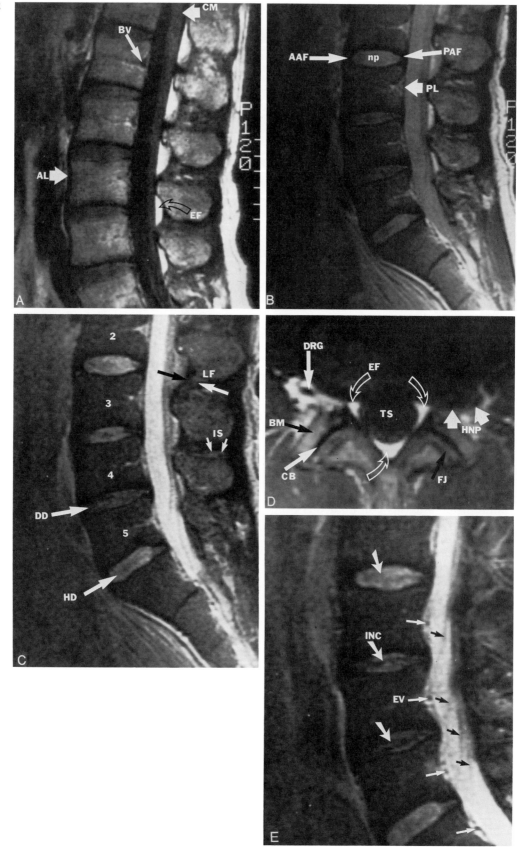

Figure 8–1 *See legend on opposite page*

Figure 8–1. This 39-year old man presented with low back pain radiating into the left leg following a parachute jump. *A*, Spin-echo TR 500/TE 20 msec T1-weighted sagittal image in the midline. CM = conus medullaris; BV = basivertebral vein; AL = anterior longitudinal ligament; EF = epidural fat. *B*, Spin-echo TR 2000/TE 40 msec multiecho proton density–sagittal image in the midline. AAF = anterior annulus fibrosis; NP = nucleus pulposis; PAF = posterior annulus fibrosis, PL = posterior longitudinal ligament. *C*, Spin-echo TR 2000/TE msec multiecho T2-weighted sagittal image in the midline. LF = ligamentum flavum; IS = intraspinous ligament; DD = desiccated disc; HD = hydrated disc. Note the loss of disc signal and disc height involving the L4/5 disc space consistent with degenerative disc disease. The signal loss is presumed to represent desiccation of the disc with loss of water as compared with the normally hydrated L5/S1 disc. *D*, Spin-echo TR 650/TE 20 msec axial image angled through the L4/5 disc space. HNP = herniated nucleus pulposis; EF = epidural fat; TS = thecal sac; DRG = dorsal root ganglion; BM = bone marrow; CB = cortical bone; FJ = facet joint. Note the large, very lateral herniated nucleus pulposis that is filling the neural formina. *E*, Spin-echo TR 2000/TE 80 msec multiecho T2-weighted image in the sagittal plane just off the midline. INC = intranuclear cleft; EV = epidural veins. The small black arrows indicate the nerve roots of the cauda equina.

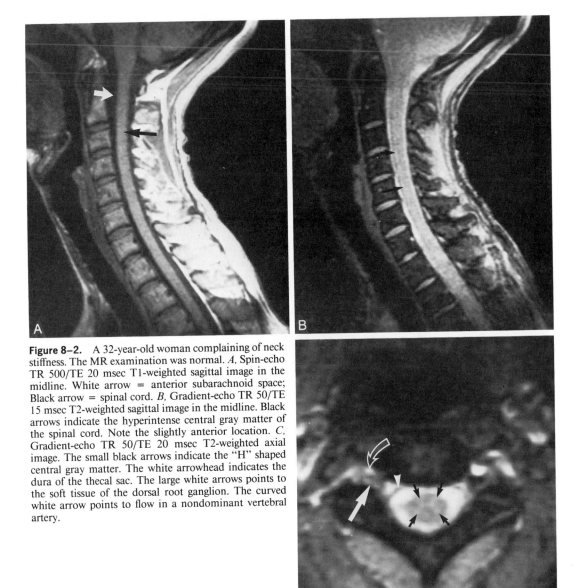

Figure 8–2. A 32-year-old woman complaining of neck stiffness. The MR examination was normal. *A*, Spin-echo TR 500/TE 20 msec T1-weighted sagittal image in the midline. White arrow = anterior subarachnoid space; Black arrow = spinal cord. *B*, Gradient-echo TR 50/TE 15 msec T2-weighted sagittal image in the midline. Black arrows indicate the hyperintense central gray matter of the spinal cord. Note the slightly anterior location. *C*, Gradient-echo TR 50/TE 20 msec T2-weighted axial image. The small black arrows indicate the "H" shaped central gray matter. The white arrowhead indicates the dura of the thecal sac. The large white arrows points to the soft tissue of the dorsal root ganglion. The curved white arrow points to flow in a nondominant vertebral artery.

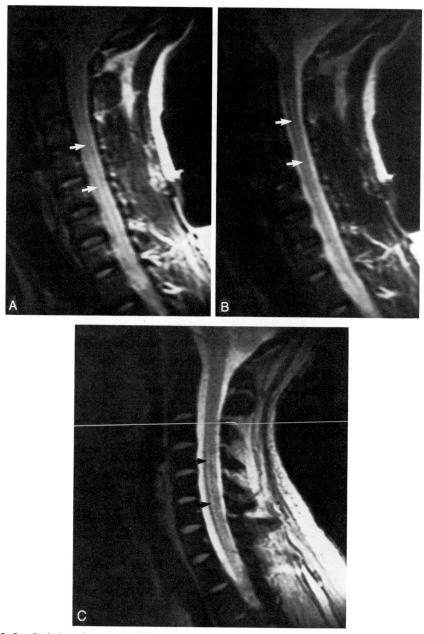

Figure 8–3. Sagital cervical spine MR images of an asymptomatic 32 year-old male. *A,* Spin-echo TR 2000/ TE 40 msec multiecho proton density–weighted image. *B,* Spin-echo TR 2000/TE 80 msec multiecho T2-weighted image. The small white arrows indicate a truncation artifact in the middle of the cervical cord. The matrix is 256 × 128. *C,* T2-weighted image with a 256 × 256 matrix. The central right truncation band has disappeared leaving a thin strip of hyperintensity in the anterior portion of the cord, which represents the central gray matter.

NORMAL ANATOMY

The anatomy of the spinal column will be discussed only with regard to unique MR appearances and the pathomechanics of spinal injury.

According to the Denis three-column concept,[2] the spine can be divided into anterior, middle, and posterior columns. The anterior column consists of the anterior vertebral body, the anterior longitudinal ligaments, and the anterior annulus fibrosis. The middle column consists of the posterior vertebral body, the posterior longitudinal ligament, and the posterior annulus fibrosis. The posterior column consists of the bony neural arch, the ligamen-

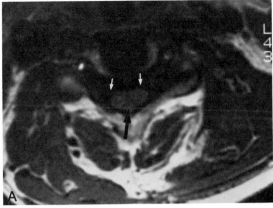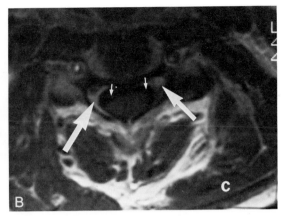

Figure 8–4. Images of an asymptomatic 32-year-old man. *A,* Axial spin-echo TR 600/TE 20 msec T1-weighted image through the C3/C4 disc space. *B,* The same image following gadolinium enhancement. The small white arrows indicate the ventral rootlets as they cross the subarachnoid space. The black arrow indicates the hypointense white matter of the dorsal columns. The large white arrows indicate the enhancement seen in the dorsal root ganglion and the meningeal sheath.

tum flavum, the intraspinous ligament, and the capsules of the apophyseal joints. All the preceding ligamentous structures are clearly identified on MR imaging (see Fig. 8–1). In stable injuries, the middle column is intact and in unstable injuries it is disrupted. Ligamentous structures, including joint capsules and the annulus fibrosis, are hypointense on both the T1- and T2-weighted images (Fig. 8–1).

The cortical bone of the vertebral body endplates and the posterior elements of the spine are also hypointense on both the T1- and T2-weighted images (Fig. 8–1*D*). Bone containing marrow found in the vertebral bodies has a slightly higher signal intensity on both T1- and T2-weighted images due to the fat containing marrow.

The intervertebral disc is only slightly lower in signal than the adjacent vertebral body on the T1-weighted images (Fig. 8–1*A*). However, on the T2-weighted images, the central portion of the disc is hyperintense. Presumably this is due to the hydration of the nucleus pulposis, in contrast to the more desiccated fibrous structure of the annulus, which exhibits dark signal (Fig. 8–1*B*). A low-intensity horizontal band is seen within normal lumbar discs in patients over the age of 30 on the sagittal T2-weighted images (Fig. 8–1*E*). This so-called *internuclear cleft* is thought to represent an invagination of the annular lamellae of the annulus into the nucleus.[3] This real anatomic finding should not be confused with truncation artifacts that occur between high-contrast interfaces such as the vertebral endplates and surface of the spinal cord.[4] The artifact is a sharp, thin band located

midway between the endplates, unlike the intranuclear cleft, which is broader and less distinct.

Fat is quite hyperintense on the T1-weighted images and fades slightly on heavily T2-weighted images. While there is essentially no fat in the cervical spine, the epidural fat that outlines the thecal sac in the thoracolumbar spine is especially helpful as it outlines the posterior elements (Fig. 8–1*D*).

Cerebrospinal fluid (CSF) is hypointense on the T1-weighted images but becomes ex-

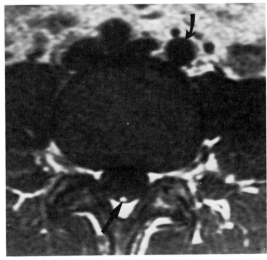

Figure 8–5. A 33-year-old man with low back pain. The spin-echo axial TR 600/TE 20 msec T1-weighted image at the level of the L4/L5 disc demonstrates hyperintense fat in the filum terminalae. This should not be mistaken for hemorrhage.

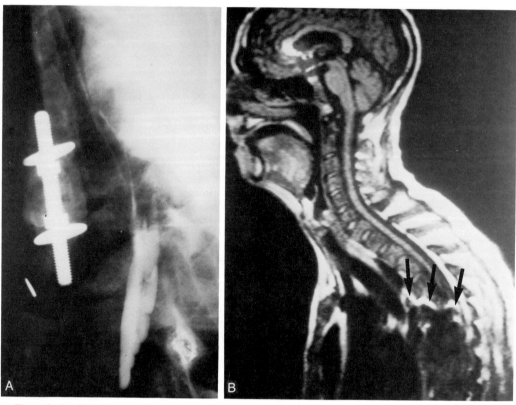

Figure 8–6. This 62-year-old man had resection of a vertebral body for renal cell carcinoma with placement of a short rod and methylmethacrylate in the defect. *A,* Lateral plain film of a pantopaque myelogram. *B,* Spin-echo sagittal T1-weighted MR. Arrows indicate the metallic artifact caused by the rod.

tremely hyperintense on the T2-weighted images, giving a "myelographic effect" in which the cord is outlined by bright CSF (Figs. 8–2B and C and 8–3B). The normal pulsations of CSF can cause flow artifact (see Fig. 8–27B and C). These can be accentuated or minimized with various sequence manipulations, which will be further discussed in the section on the chronic injury.

Both the spinal cord and nerve roots are of intermediate intensity on the T1-weighted images (Fig. 8–2A). The spinal cord is mildly hy-

TABLE 8–1. Signal Intensities of Tissue

HIGH-INTENSITY T1	HIGH-INTENSITY T2
Fat	Fluid, CSF
Marrow	Hemorrhage (subacute)
Hemorrhage (subacute)	Inflammatory/edematous tissue
	Neoplastic tissue
INTERMEDIATE-INTENSITY T1 AND T2	
Muscle/neural tissue	
Hyaline articular cartilage	
LOW-INTENSITY T1	LOW-INTENSITY T2
Fluid, CSF	Calcification
Inflammatory/edematous tissue	Hemorrhage (chronic and acute)
Neoplastic tissue	
Hemorrhage (acute and chronic)	
VERY LOW-INTENSITY T1 AND T2	
Cortical bone	
Air	
Ligaments and tendons	
Fibrocartilage/annulus	

perintense on the proton-density image but is hypointense compared with the adjacent CSF on the heavily T2-weighted image (Figs. 8–2*B* and *C*). While the internal architecture of the cord can be appreciated on spin-echo imaging, it is more obvious with gradient-echo images. For unknown reasons the T1 relaxation time of gray and white matter in the spinal cord does not correspond to that in the brain. The posterior white matter columns and corticospinal tracts are hypointense compared with the adjacent gray matter on the T1-weighted images (see Fig. 8–4*A*). On the T2-weighted images, the central gray matter, which is H- or butterfly-shaped, is hyperintense compared with the adjacent white matter tracts (Fig. 8–2*C*). On sagittal T1-weighted images, the central gray matter in the cervical cord can sometimes be appreciated as a thin hypointense stripe on the T1-weighted images and as a mildly hyperintense stripe on the T2-weighted images (Figs. 8–2*B* and 8–3*C*). Again, this normal anatomic structure should not be confused with a truncation artifact (Figs. 8–3*A* and *B*). MR is also capable of visualizing both the ventral and dorsal nerve rootlets as they cross the subarachnoid space toward the neural foramina (Fig. 8–4). The dorsal root ganglion is also routinely identified. In the cervical spine it is seen as an ovoid soft tissue structure located between the articular pillar and vertebral artery (Fig. 8–2*C*). With surface coil imaging, the fanning of the nerve roots in the conus medullaris and cauda equina is appreciated (Fig. 8–1*E*). Occasionally fat is identified in the filum terminale (Fig. 8–5).

Frequently, anterior epidural veins can be identified in the cervical and lumbar spine. These are hypointense on spin-echo images (Fig. 8–1*E*). It has not yet been possible to visualize the arterial supply of the spinal cord on MR imaging.

Following intravenous injection of the MR contrast agent gadolinium, the spinal cord and nerve roots are not enhanced as they have an intact blood-brain barrier. The foraminal veins, dorsal root ganglion, and the dural sheath surrounding the ventral and dorsal roots do enhance (Fig. 8–4).

THE ACUTE INJURY

As long as the spine is easily and mechanically reducible, the bony injury is considered acute. This stage lasts at least 3 weeks. However, in the spinal cord, the acute stage is usu-

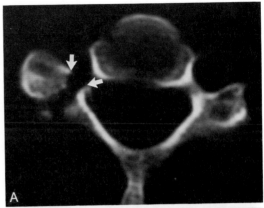

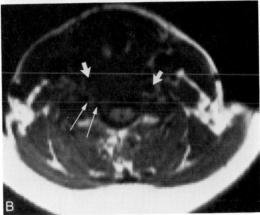

Figure 8–7. This 42-year-old woman was in a motor vehicle accident. *A*, Axial CT scan with white arrows demonstrating a fracture through the intervertebral foramen and base of the right transverse process. *B*, Spin-echo TR 500/TE 35 msec T1-weighted axial MR. The thin white arrows delineate the dehiscence in the cortical bone through the base of the transverse process. The fracture line itself is mildly hyperintense compared with the very dark cortical bone. The thick white arrow on the left demonstrates a patent left vertebral artery while the opposite arrow indicates that the right vertebral artery is thrombosed as no flow void is present.

ally considered the 5- to 7-day period following the trauma when the histologic changes in the cord are critical.

Optimal MR Technique

The patient with an acute spinal cord injury presents a unique challenge to MR imaging. This challenge results because the medical status of trauma victims frequently is unstable, and traction devices are often ferromagnetic. Consequently, these devices will either distort the image or get pulled into the magnet.

As a rule, unstable patients requiring life support systems and constant monitoring are

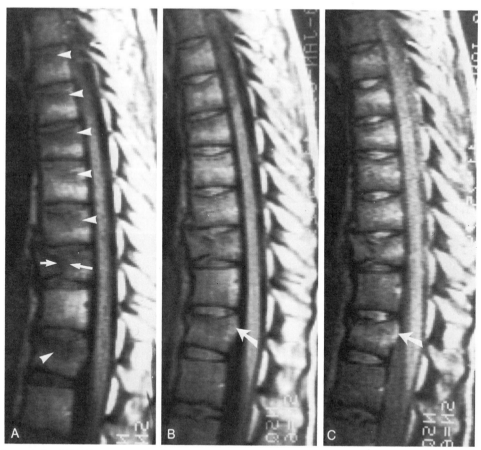

Figure 8–8. This 22-year-old woman jumped off the Verranzano Narrows Bridge nine days before this MR examination. *A,* Spin-echo TR 500/TE 35 msec T1-weighted sagittal MR in the midline. The white arrows demonstrate a hypointense vertical fracture through the vertebral body. Multiple hypointense endplate compression fractures are indicated by the white arrowheads. *B,* Spin-echo TR 2000/TE 40 msec proton density sagittal MR in the midline. *C,* TR 2000/TE 80 msec T2-weighted sagittal MR in the midline. The white arrow demonstrates a retropulsed fragment which does not cause any cord compression.

not examined with MR, as these electrical devices usually will not function within the magnetic field. Stable ventilated patients are not candidates for MR imaging for the same reasons. Recently, ventilators have been successfully modified (longer tubing) to allow their use within four feet of a self-shielded magnet.[5] MR compatible ventilators are currently under development.

Traction devices are another obstacle. Weights are usually iron and magnetic—i.e., they will be deflected in the magnetic field. If skull tongs and weights have been used to reduce a dislocation and there is no question of a retropulsed fragment, the head and neck are immobilized under the guidance of a neurosurgeon, and the weights are removed. As a rule, skull tongs are made of stainless steel and are nonmagnetic. This can be checked with a household magnet. Although the tongs will cause image distoration adjacent to their implantation in the head, they usually do not do so at the level of the cervical spine, allowing diagnostic images to be obtained. Most stainless steel alloys used for human implantation are nonmagnetic,[6] but they do exhibit some ferromagnetic properties within a strong magnetic field. This causes local magnetic field distortion and signal loss resulting in an artifact (Fig. 8–6). Once the examination is performed, the traction is reapplied outside the magnetic field.

If constant traction is required in the case of a retropulsed fragment that has been reduced, use of a pulley system tied to the patient's tongs or halo with nylon rope and weighted with water-filled plastic bags has been successful.[7]

Patients in a halo vest are another challenge. The four support rods frequently do not allow

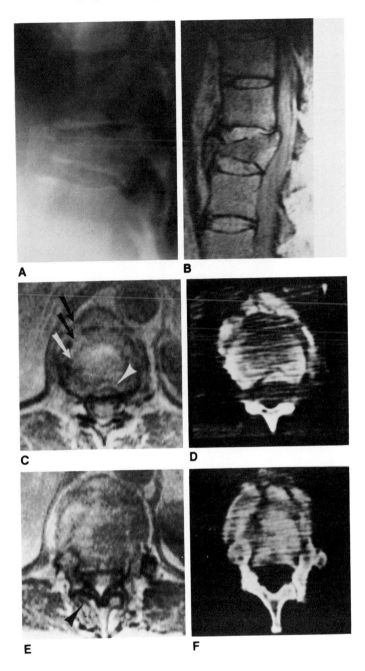

Figure 8-9. A 62-year-old woman with bowel and bladder incontinence and mild sensory loss after a T12 compression fracture from a motor vehicle accident 2 weeks before the MR study. *A,* Lateral radiograph. Both endplates of T12 are compressed and bone is displaced anteriorly and posteriorly. *B,* Spin-echo TR 1500/TE 60 msec sagittal MR. The proton density image clearly displays bulging of the anterior longitudinal ligament, bone fragments, disc, and fractured endplates. The T11/T12 disc and posterior inferior corner of T12 are bright with hemorrhage. *C,* Spin-echo TR 1500/TE 60 msec axial MR image through the superior endplate of T12. Two peripheral arching black lines circumscribe the expanded body (black arrows). A third, fainter inner dark line is evident (white arrow). Also note the curvilinear white line (arrowhead). *D,* Axial CT at approximately the same level explains the origin of the lines in C. *E,* Spin-echo TR 1500/TE 60 msec axial MR image at the mid T12 level. Faint dark and light lines in the body indicate fractures. Note the abnormal orientation of the right facet joint and misshapen right T11 inferior process (arrowhead). Retropulsed bone compresses the thecal sac and flattens the spinal cord. *F,* CT scan at the same level as E. Fractures are better seen. The spinal canal detail is poor, and there is no way to estimate from the extent of canal narrowing the degree to which the spinal cord is impinged upon. (From McArdle CB et al: Surface coil MR of spinal trauma: Preliminary experience. AJNR 7:885, 1986.)

the placement of a large surface coil directly onto the back of the patient's neck. Images may have to be obtained with the body coil, resulting in poorer resolution, or with a smaller coil that fits between the rods, limiting the area of examination. Again, most halo vests with their supporting bars and pins are made of stainless steel and can be placed within the magnetic field. Unfortunately, they result in much more distortion of the image than the smaller tongs do. Particularly, the posterior two supporting bars and the metallic buckles on the vest result in artifacts that may or may not obscure the area of interest. If on routine scanning the artifacts do overlap an area of critical interest, a 90 degree change of the phase-encoding axis may project the artifact off the spine. The ferromagnetic artifacts that occur with stainless steel halo vests can be eliminated if the halo vests are constructed of plastic reinforced with titanium, aluminum, or graphite. There may still be a small amount of

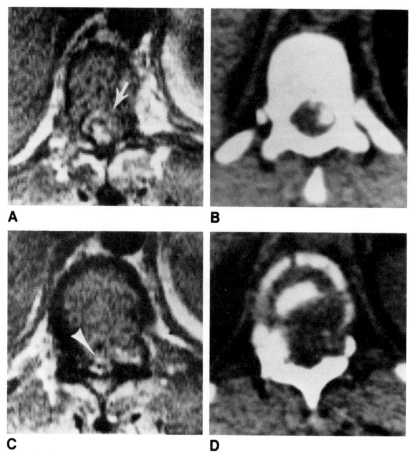

Figure 8-10. This 43-year-old woman had complete paraplegia after compression fractures of T11 and T12, imaged 3 days after trauma. *A,* Spin-echo TR 1000/TE 38 msec axial MR image at the inferior T11 level. The thecal sac is displaced to the right by an intermediate mass (arrow). The spinal cord has increased signal. *B,* Axial CT scan at the level A. Intermediate signal mass on MR is a bony fragment from the T11 body. *C,* Spin-echo TR 1000/TE 38 msec axial MR at the T11/12 disc level. The spinal canal is markedly narrowed by intermediate signal mass contiguous with the disc. The spinal cord appears as a bright slit (arrowhead). *D,* Axial CT scan at the same level. The degree of spinal cord compression is less evident. (From McArdle CB et al: Surface coil MR of spinal trauma: Preliminary experience. AJNR 7:885, 1986).

metallic artifact resulting from eddy currents rather than ferromagnetism, but the image distortion is much less.[8]

As a general rule, the surface coil is centered at the level of the patient's neurologic deficit or the bony injury as ascertained on plain films. The following anatomic landmarks have proved fairly reliable in our experience and that of others.[9] The thyroid cartilage prominence is at C4, the largest spinous process is at C7, the suprasternal notch is at T2, the sternal angle is at T4, the inferior angle of the scapula is at T7, the xyphisternal junction is at T9, and the umbilicus is at T12. Both T1- and T2-weighted spin-echo images are performed in the sagittal plane. Axial spin-echo T1-weighed images are also performed through the level of

interest and angled through the disc spaces. If the injury is very recent, i.e., within the first 24 hours, a gradient-echo sagittal image is also performed in an attempt to detect early hemorrhage. As the signal-to-noise ratio improves on gradient-echo images, some of the long spin-echo sequences may be replaced with gradient-echo sequences in the interest of time and patient comfort.

Extramedullary Abnormalities

Fractures are most easily seen on the T1-weighted and proton-density images. The signal intensity of a fracture line varies depending on the type of bone structure through which it is running. A fracture through the cortex will

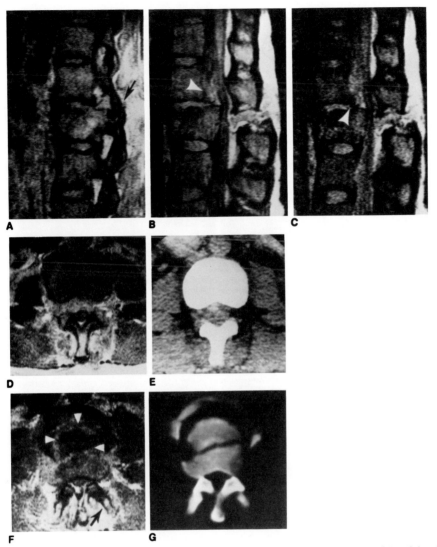

Figure 8–11. A 23-year-old man with lower extremity weakness after a motor vehicle accident 6 days before the MR. *A,* Spin-echo TR 1500/TE 38 msec left parasagittal MR scan. Note the locked facet (arrow). *B,* Spin-echo TR 1500/TE 28 midsagittal scan. Note the interruption of the supraspinous and intraspinous ligaments, ligamentum flavum, and posterior longitudinal ligament. Medium intensity material lies between L2 and the intact bulging anterior longitudinal liagment. High intensity material lies posterior to the L1 vertebral body (arrowhead). *C,* Spin-echo TR 1500/TE 76 msec sagittal MR at the same level as in *B,* On the second echo, the amorphous material anterior to L1 has the lower signal of bone while the collection posterior to L2 has the higher intensity feature of blood. A remnant of torn posterior ligament (arrowhead) is outlined by bright signal from the disrupted disc. *D,* Spin-echo TR 900/TE 38 msec axial section at the inferior level of L1. The narrowed thecal sac is posteriorly displaced by a high signal collection in the anterior epidural space. *E,* Axial CT scan at the same level shows high density in the anterior epidural space confirming a hematoma. *F,* Spin-echo TR 900/TE 38 msec axial section at the superior L2 level. The spinal canal is critically narrowed by a retropulsed L2 body. Note the locked inferior processes of L1 anterior to the superior L2 "naked facets" (arrow). Arrowheads outline the contour of the superior endplate of the L2 body; the peripheral ring of avulsed cortex is contained by the anterior ligament. *G,* Axial CT scan at the same level shows the locked facets and fractures, all seen on the MR scan. (From McArdle CB et al: Surface coil MR of spinal trauma: Preliminary experience. AJNR 7:885, 1986.)

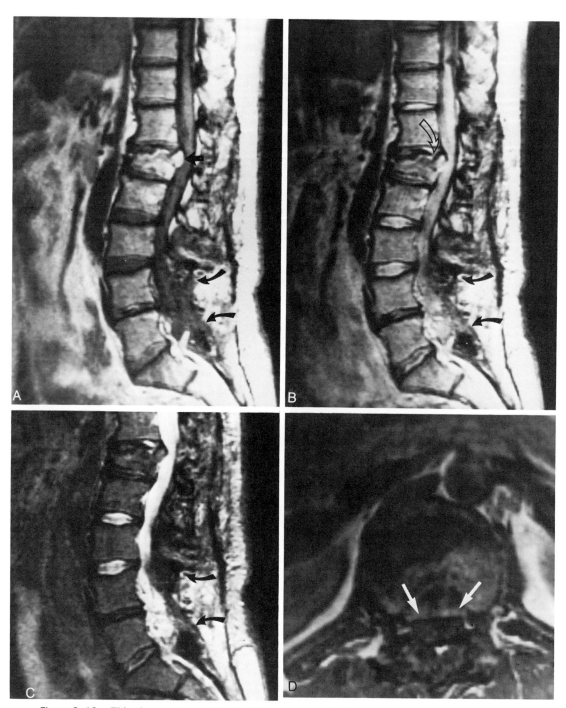

Figure 8–12. This 42-year-old man fell off a ladder two weeks before the MR examination. *A,* Spin-echo TR 600/TE 25 msec T1-weighted sagittal MR in the midline. The black arrow demonstrates the hyperintense retropulsed fragment from the compressed L1 vertebral body. The curved black arrows indicate a laminectomy defect. The laminectomy was performed for a previous disc herniation. *B,* Spin-echo TR 2000/TE 40 msec proton density–weighted sagittal MR also in the midline. The open curved black arrow indicates a fracture through the cortex of the superior endplate. *C,* Spin-echo TR 2000/TE 80 msec T2-weighted sagittal image at the same level. Note that the retropulsed fragment is hypointense. Many of the lumbar discs have lost height and signal consistent with degeneration. *D,* Spin-echo TR 1000/TE 25 msec axial image through the L1 vertebral body. The white arrows indicate the retropulsed fragment compressing the thecal sac.

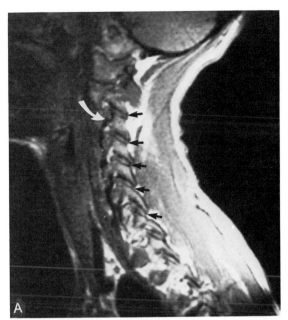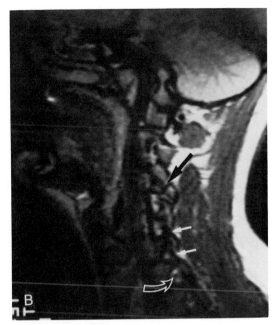

Figure 8–13. *A,* Parasagittal TR 500/TE 20 msec T1-weighted MR of a 34-year-old woman with neck stiffness secondary to a whiplash injury. The small black arrows indicate the normally aligned facet joints. The curved white arrow indicates the vertebral artery. *B,* This 39-year-old policeman was assaulted several years before the MR examination. The parasagittal TR 2000/TE 40 msec proton density–weighted image demonstrates an old fracture through a facet joint indicated by the black arrow. Note that the dehiscence is well corticated, indicating its age. The small white arrows indicate the normally aligned facet joints below. The curved white arrow indicates a nerve root within a neural foramen.

appear light or mildly hyperintense (Fig. 8–7), whereas the same fracture running through bone marrow will appear dark or hypointense (Fig. 8–8). Cortical fractures are the most clearly defined, while fractures through the marrow are less obvious. While fractures, particularly through the vertebral body, are readily diagnosed on MR, there is no question that their conspicuity is greater on CT (Fig. 8–9). This is particularly apparent with posterior element fractures, especially in the cervical spine. In the thoracolumbar spine, the posterior elements are well outlined by fat, and as a result their cortices are easily seen. However, in the cervical spine, there is little fat around the posterior elements, and as a result cortical dehiscences are difficult to see here. Retropulsed bony fragments also tend to be more conspicuous on CT. However, MR demonstrates the thecal sac compression caused by fragments much better than does CT [9–12] (Figs. 8–9 to 8–11). Acutely fractured vertebral bodies are hyperintense compared with normal intact vertebral bodies on T2-weighted images. This is also apparent to a lesser degree on the proton-density images. Initially, the T1-weighed images show no change in signal intensity, but

after a week the fractured vertebral bodies may become either hypointense (Fig. 8–8*A*) or hyperintense[9] (Fig. 8–12*A*). This delayed hyperintensity may be from hemorrhage in the bone marrow.

The alignment of the spinal column is clearly assessed with sagittal MR; the modality has proved superior to lateral plain films and sagittally reformatted CT. The information obtained is most comparable to plain film tomography, although not quite as detailed (Fig. 8–13).

Ligamentous ruptures are identified as an interruption of a hypointense band best seen in the sagittal plane. Ruptures of both the anterior and posterior longitudinal ligaments, ligamentum flavum, interspinous, and supraspinous ligaments are all identifiable (Fig. 8–11).

One of the greatest contributions of MR in the management of spinal trauma is identification of herniated discs in the cervical and thoracic spine. A fracture-dislocation with an associated disc herniation is an indication for an anterior rather than a posterior surgical decompression. While this diagnosis can be made with CT myelography, it usually requires 1.5 mm thick slices angled through the disc spaces,

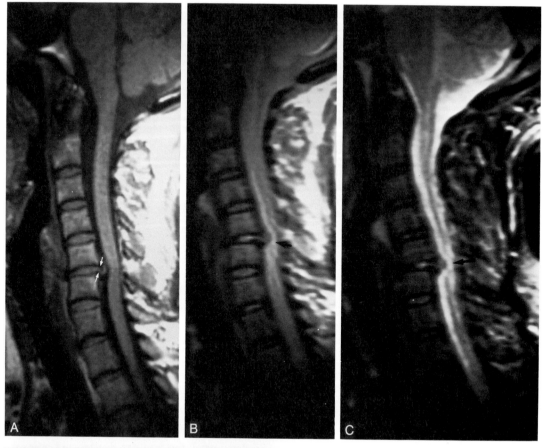

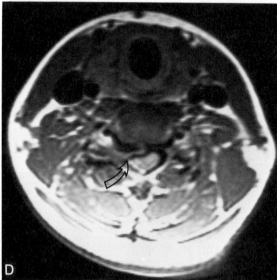

Figure 8–14. This 34-year-old woman suffered a flexion injury in a motor vehicle accident. *A,* Spin-echo TR 800/TE 20 msec T1 weighted sagittal MR in the midline. The small white arrows indicate a dehiscence in the annulus of the disc. Note the nucleus pulposis herniated into the spinal canal with the associated compression of the cervical cord. *B,* Spin-echo multi-echo TR 2000/TE 60 msec proton density sagittal MR at the same level as A. The herniated disc is again well seen (arrow). *C,* Spin-echo TR 2000/TE 120 msec T2-weighted sagittal MR, which is the second echo of the sequence in B. Note the high signal in the spinal cord adjacent to the herniated disc (arrow). This most likely represents edema from the cord compression. *D,* Spin-echo TR 800/TE 20 msec T1-weighted axial image angled through the C5/6 disc. Note that the large herniation fills the neural foramina on the right at this level (curved arrow).

which are not routinely performed. Other problems are encountered in making the CT diagnosis of cervicothoracic disc herniations. These include artifact through the level of the shoulders obscuring the spinal canal, posterior

layering of intrathecal contrast material failing to outline the ventral disc protrusion, and an anterior epidural hematoma mimicking a herniated disc. On sagittal MR sections, disc material is easily seen protruding into the spinal

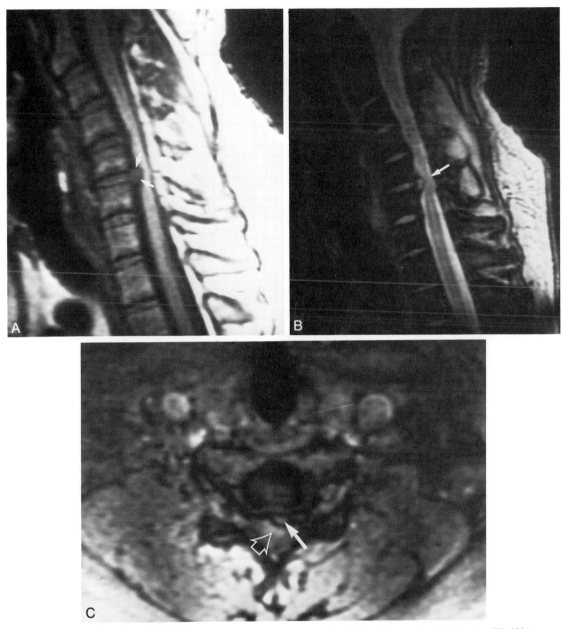

Figure 8–15. This 31-year-old man experienced neck pain after diving into a pool. *A,* Spin-echo TR 600/
TE 20 msec T1-weighted sagittal MR in the midline demonstrates a very large herniation of the C5/6 disc
(arrows). *B,* Gradient-echo TR 100/TE 17 msec T2-weighted sagittal MR also in the midline. Note the hyperintense signal in the adjacent spinal cord consistent with cord edema secondary to compression (arrow).
C, Gradient-echo TR 50/TE 17 msec T2-weighted axial image angled through the C5/6 disc space. The herniation is clearly identified (closed white arrow), as is the adjacent cord edema (open arrow).

canal (Figs. 8–14 to 8–16). Unless a dehiscence
is identified in the annulus (Fig. 8–14), it is difficult to determine whether a disc is bulging dif-
fusely or focally herniated without axial images
angled through the disc spaces, which should
be performed just as with CT scanning. In the
cervical spine it can be difficult to distinguish a

herniated disc from the bony ridges associated
with degenerative disc disease. This distinction
may be easier on gradient-echo images than on
spin-echo images, as the cortical bone of the
posterior ridges is usually very dark compared
with the disc material.

Epidural hematomas usually can be seen as

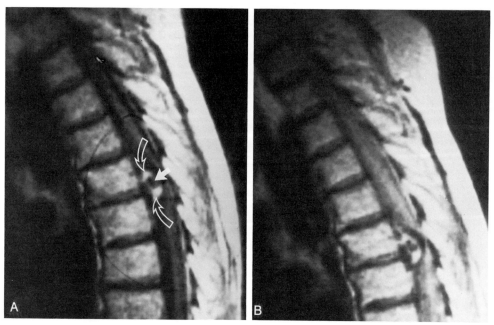

Figure 8–16. This 72-year-old woman fell out of bed and experienced mid thoracic pain. *A,* Spin-echo TR 500/TE 20 msec T1-weighted sagittal MR in the midline. There is a thoracic disc herniation. This case is unusual in that the hypointense disc fragment (white arrow) is surrounded by hyperintense hemorrhage (open arrows). *B,* Spin-echo TR 1500/TE 40 msec proton density sagittal MR also in the midline. The signal intensities of the disc fragment and hemorrhage do not appreciably change.

areas of slightly increased signal intensity on both the T1- and T2-weighted images as soon as 24 hours after the injury (Fig. 8–17).[9,12] Although acutely the signal characteristics are not much different from disc material, it is the anatomic location that allows the diagnosis to be made. Epidural hematoma does not protrude from the disc space and it runs along the top of the posterior longitudinal ligament or the ligamentum flavum.

Another major advantage of MR is its ability to aid in identification of associated soft tissue injuries outside the spinal canal. An example of this is thrombosis of the vertebral artery following a fracture through a vascular foramen (Fig. 8–7).

Intramedullary Abnormalities

Cord concussion and/or edema is visualized as a hyperintense area on both the proton density– and T2-weighted images (Figs. 8–18*B, C* and 8–19*A, B*). The T1-weighted images may be normal (Fig. 8–18*A*) or may show slight expansion of the cord at the level of the signal abnormality. This type of injury appears to be the most benign. There can be complete resolution of the neurologic symptoms (Fig. 8–18). If T2-weighted axial images are performed through

the level of the injury, it is theoretically possible to correlate a clincially determined central, anterior, or posterior cord syndrome with the MR-defined anatomic location of the lesion within the cord (Fig. 8–20). If time permits this sequence can be performed, but the sagittal T2-weighted images are sufficient to define the level of abnormality.

MR can differentiate spinal cord hemorrhage from edema because hemorrhage has the same signal characteristics in the spinal cord as it does in the brain. While this has not been pathologically proven in the human spinal cord, the findings have been experimentally confirmed in animals.[13,14] As a rule, hyperacute hemorrhage under 48 hours tends to be isointense or slightly hypointense to the brain on all pulse sequences. At this stage, the hematoma is presumed to consist of intact red blood cells containing oxyhemoglobin. Acute hemorrhage under one week old becomes increasingly hypointense on the T2-weighted images. This is thought to be due to the development of deoxyhemoglobin within the intact red blood cells. Subacute hemorrhage over a week old appears hyperintense on both the T1- and T2-weighted images due to the development of free methemoglobin. Finally, chronic hemorrhage is hypointense on all pulse sequences,

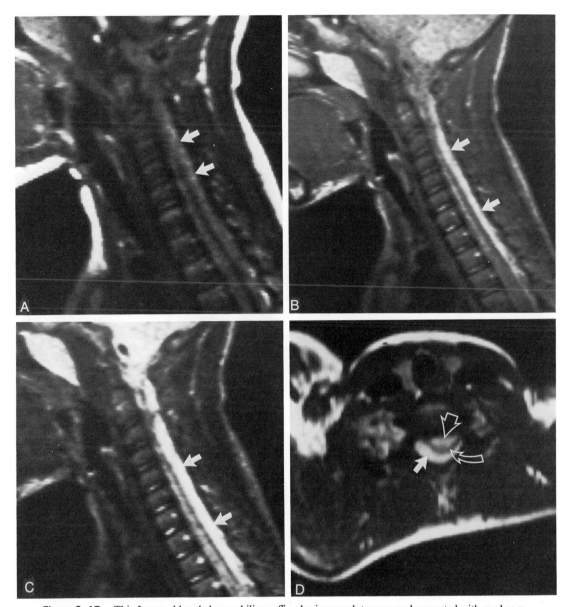

Figure 8–17. This 5-year-old male hemophiliac suffered minor neck trauma and presented with cord compression some two hours later. *A,* Spin-echo TR 1500/TE 35 msec T1 weighted midline sagittal image. *B,* Spin-echo TR 2000/TE 40 msec proton density–weighted sagittal MR also in the midline. *C,* Spin-echo TR 2000/TE 80 msec T2-weighted sagittal MR also in the midline. The white arrows indicate hyperintense hemorrhage seen in the posterior aspect of the spinal canal on all pulse sequences. Note that the hemorrhage becomes increasingly bright the more heavily T2-weighted the sequence has become. *D,* Spin-echo TR 950/TE 35 msec T1 weighted axial image. The solid white arrow indicates the hyperintense epidural hematoma which is seen to displace the spinal cord to the left as indicated by the straight open arrow. The compressed subarachnoid space and dura is indicated by the curved arrow.

presumably due to the formation of hemosiderin.[15] The MR appearance of hemorrhage, however, is somewhat unpredictable. Although hematomas tend to age in an orderly fashion, the evolutionary changes of hemorrhage are highly variable in time. It also must be remembered that hematomas evolve earlier at the pe-riphery than in the center. Thus, subacute hemorrhage will have a hyperintense outer rim on both the T2- and T1-weighted images, as a result of methemoglobin formation, before the center does.

Typically, acute spinal cord hemorrhage appears on the T2-weighted images as a central

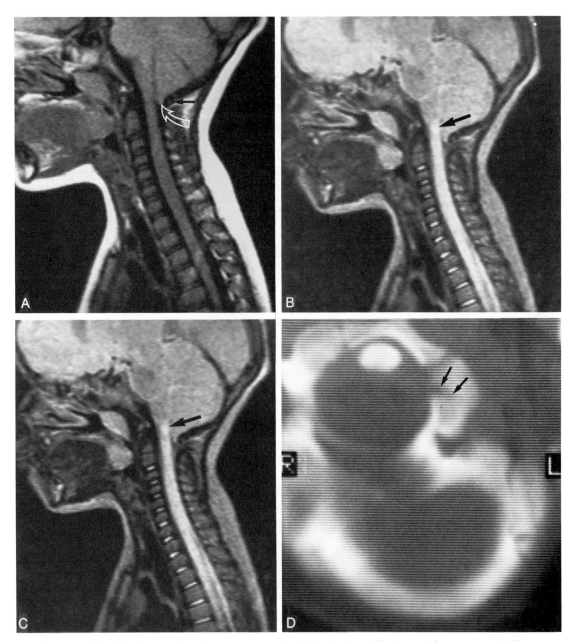

Figure 8–18. This 2½-year-old child was asleep on her father's chest while he was lying on a couch. The child fell off the couch and the father pulled her back up by lifting underneath her arms. Three hours later the baby woke complaining of neck pain and heavy arms which eventually became flaccid. Subsequently, a CT and MR of the neck were performed at our institution. *A,* Spin-echo TR 500/TE 35 msec T1-weighted sagittal MR in the midline. The examination is unremarkable on this pulse sequence except for the incidental Chiari I malformation. The white curved arrow indicates the cerebellar tonsils which protrude through the foramen magnum to the level of C1. The black arrow indicates the posterior arch of C1. *B,* Spin-echo TR 2000/TE 40 msec proton density–weighted sagittal MR also in the midline. A hyperintense lesion is identified at the cervicomedullary junction. *C,* Spin-echo TR 2000/TE 80 msec T2 weighted sagittal MR also in the midline. The hyperintense lesion is again noted. This appearance is consistent with cord edema. *D,* Axial CT examination through the arch of C1. Arrows indicate the fracture through the lateral mass of C1. The patient's neurologic function completely recovered after three weeks.

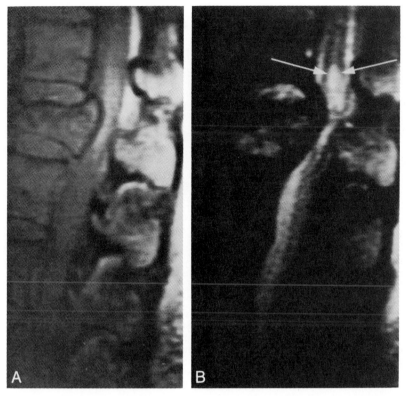

Figure 8–19. This is the MR examination of a patient 6 hours after a helicopter crash. *A,* Spin-echo TR 2000/TE 20 msec proton density–weighted image sagittal MR in the midline. *B,* Spin-echo TR 2000/TE 80 T2-weighted sagittal MR also in the midline. A comminuted fracture of L1 with retropulsion of the fracture fragment is identified. The intraspinal edema/contusion (arrows) is seen as hyperintensity within the cord. (From Kulkarni MV et al: Acute spinal cord injury: MR imaging at 1.5 T. Radiology 164:837, 1987.)

area of hypointensity with a thin rim of peripheral hyperintensity (Figs. 8–21 to 8–23). The signal on the T1-weighted images is variable.

Kulkarni et. al., in a series of 50 patients with spinal cord injury, identified those with an MR signal pattern consistent with cord hematoma as having the worse neurologic prognosis.[16] It is also indicative of spinal cord transection. This was called a type I MR pattern, while the signal characteristics of cord edema were termed type II, which had the best prognosis. They identified a third pattern, which had signal characteristics consistent with both hemorrhage and edema. This group had a variable prognosis.[16,17] Hemorrhage is much better seen on gradient-echo images than spin-echo images in the acute stages, so if the patient's injury is less than one week old, routine gradient-echo imaging should probably be performed. It appears that MR may have some predictive value in establishing the prognosis of the patient with a spinal cord injury.

Differentiating a spinal cord infarction from edema is probably not possible on the basis of

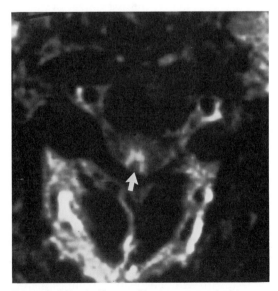

Figure 8–20. A 49-year-old man presented with posterior column symptoms only. Spin-echo TR 2000/TE 85 msec T2-weighted image in the axial plane through the cervical spine. Note that the abnormality is confined to the posterior columns alone (arrow).

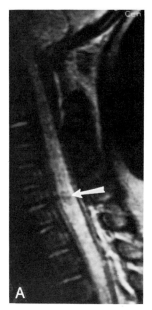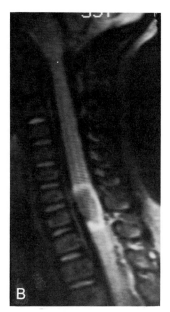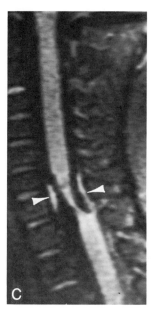

Figure 8–21. *A,* Sagittal spin-echo TR 2000/TE 80 msec T2-weighted sagittal image in the acute phase of spinal cord hemorrhage 48 hours after a motor vehicle accident demonstrates a decrease in signal (arrow) within the cord. The cord is enlarged. *B,* T2-weighted sagittal image five days after the trauma shows a central area of hypointensity surrounded by peripheral hyperintensity. *C,* Sagittal T2-weighted MR five weeks following the trauma shows that the cord hemorrhage has resolved, revealing a nearly complete transection of the cervical cord. Hemorrhage along the ligaments is seen anterior and posterior to the cord lesion (arrowheads). (From Kulkarni MV et al: Acute spinal cord injury: MR imaging at 1.5 T. Radiology 164:837, 1987.)

signal characteristics alone. Follow-up examinations are probably the only reliable method. Cord edema should resolve, while cord infarction will develop into encephalomalacia or atrophy.

If MR is available, the assessment of the spinal cord injured patient can be considered complete with the screening plain film examination, an MR, and a plain CT if further delineation of bony injuries is required. Myelography and CT myelography are nearly obsolete, although the diagnosis of nerve root avulsion and/or dural tear is made more easily on these modalities than on MR (Fig. 8–24).

THE CHRONIC INJURY

Optimal MR Technique

The role of MR in the previously injured spinal cord is even more definitive than in the acute injury. The entities that cause post-traumatic progressive myelopathy are all best visualized with MR. These abnormalities include cysts (both intramedullary and subarachnoid), myelomalacia, adhesions, and cord compression by disc (Fig. 8–25) or bone (Fig. 8–26).

Since post-traumatic sequelae, especially

cysts, can extend well above or below the original site of the trauma, a T1-weighted sagittal screening examination should be performed with the body coil to determine whether a multilevel surface coil examination will be required. Initially, spin-echo sagittal T1-weighted images are performed. If there is no evidence of any cystic structure, the usual routine examination, which utilizes motion-compensating gradients, is performed. When a cerebrospinal fluid (CSF) intensity collection is identified either within the spinal cord or subarachnoid space, two sets of spin-echo sagittal T2-weighted images are performed. The first utilizes motion suppression gradients and the second is done without any effort to suppress CSF motion. This is an attempt to determine how much fluid motion, or turbulence, is occurring. Preliminary work by Quencer suggests that pulsatile cysts may be undergoing active expansion and that a stronger case for shunting such cysts can be made.[18]

Intramedullary Abnormalities

A parenchymal cord injury results in persistent signal abnormalities on MR. Myelomalacia appears as an ill-defined region of low intensity on the T1-weighted images that be-

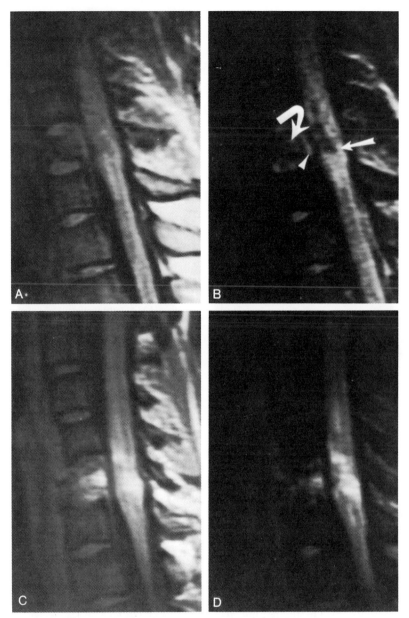

Figure 8–22. These images were obtained in a patient following a diving accident. *A*, Sagittal spin-echo TR 2000/TE 20 msec proton density–weighted image. *B*, Sagittal spin-echo TR 2000/TE 80 msec T2-weighted image in the same plane. There is a central hypointensity with a rim of peripheral hyperintensity with hemorrhage. A fracture and increased signal is identified in C6 (curved arrow). The increased signal intensity seen posterior to C6 represents hemorrhage along the posterior longitudinal ligament (arrowhead). *C*, Sagittal spin-echo TR 2000/TE 20 msec proton density–weighted image 13 days after trauma. *D*, Sagittal spin-echo TR 200/TE 80 msec also in the same plane. The initial hypointensity has disappeared and the lesion has multifocal areas of increased signal in the spinal cord. (From Kulkarni MV et al: Acute spinal cord injury: MR imaging at 1.5 T. Radiology 164:837, 1987.)

comes either isointense or slightly hyperintense to CSF on the T2-weighted images (Figs. 8–21*C* and 8–22*C*, *D*). No pulsation artifacts will be seen within the myelomalacic cord. Distinguishing an area of myelomalacia from an intramedullary cyst that may require surgical in-tervention can be difficult. Intramedullary cysts or syrinx cavities have a well-defined margin and may contain fluid pulsations (Fig. 8–27). Myelomalacia tends to involve a short segment opposite the bony injury (Fig. 8–21*C*), while a syrinx cavity is likely to extend over

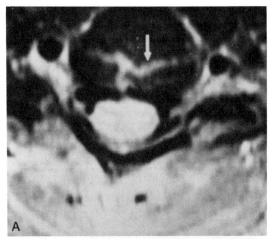

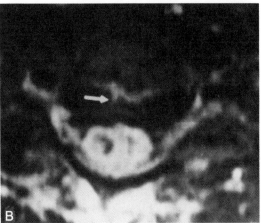

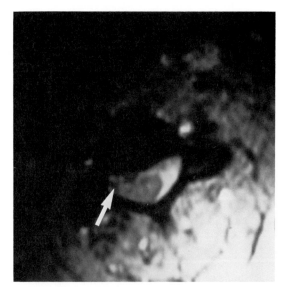

Figure 8–24. This 26-year-old man was involved in a motor vehicle accident and suffered an avulsion of the left brachial plexus. This axial gradient-echo TR 50/TE 20 msec T2-weighted image demonstrates the spinal cord to be pulled to the right by the intact nerve root (white arrow). Note the empty subarachnoid space on the opposite side where the nerve roots are avulsed.

Figure 8–23. *A*, Axial spin-echo TR 2000/TE 20 msec proton density image. *B*, Spin-echo TR 2000/TE 80 msec T2-weighted image in the same plane. The patient was imaged 12 hours after a diving injury and bilateral rounded foci of hypointensity were identified at the gray-white matter junction on the T2-weighted image. The fracture in the vertebral body is also seen (arrows). (From Kulkarni MV et al: Acute spinal cord injury: MR imaging at 1.5 T. Radiology 164:837, 1987.)

multiple levels (Fig. 8–27). Distinguishing microcysts under 1 cm in diameter from myelomalacia is of no clinical significance as these cavities are too small to shunt.[18–20]

Cord atrophy is usually an obvious diagnosis (Fig. 8–27*A*) but when a syrinx cavity attenuates most of the cord parenchyma, the appearance on the sagittal image may be confusing. An axial spin-echo image will usually clarify the intramedullary nature of the syrinx cavity.

Extramedullary Abnormalities

Loculated subarachnoid cysts may develop due to subarachnoid adhesions. These CSF collections will usually displace the spinal cord

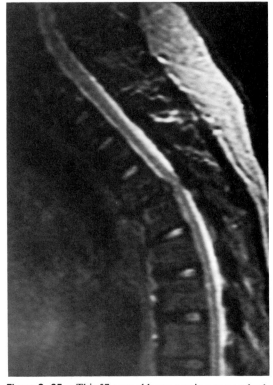

Figure 8–25. This 57-year-old man was in a rear-end collision automobile accident six months before the present MR examination. A thoracic spine series at the time of the accident was normal. He returned to his physican complaining of increasing severe upper back pain. This sagittal spin-echo TR 2000/TE 80 msec T2-weighted MR examination demonstrates a ventral subluxation of T4 on T5 accompanied by a herniated thoracic disc, which is causing cord compression.

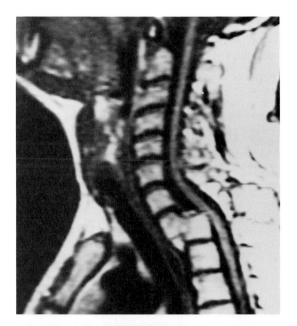

Figure 8–26. This 33-year-old man was in a motor vehicle accident a year before this examination. Initial plain films demonstrated a fracture of the T2 vertebral body but there was no evidence of subluxation. In the last 6 months, the patient has had increasing midscalpular pain and leg weakness. This spin-echo TR 600/TE 20 msec T1-weighted sagittal MR dramatically demonstrates the marked anterior subluxation of T1 forward on T2. The posterior superior corner of the T2 vertebral body impinges upon the anterior surface of the spinal cord.

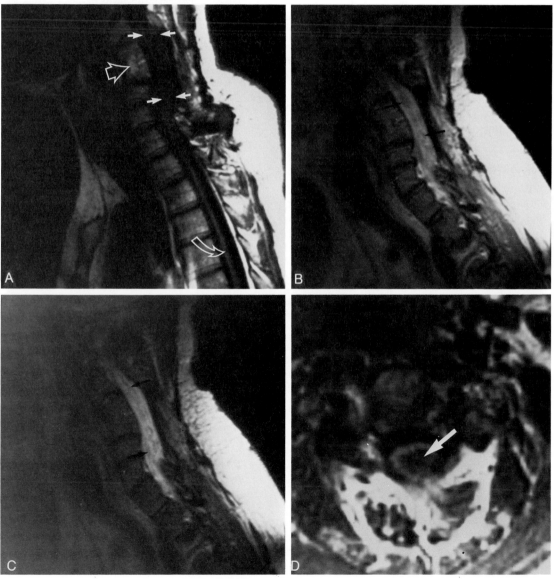

Figure 8–27 *See legend on next page*

Figure 8–27. This 44-year-old man was in a motor vehicle accident two years previously and suffered a flexion injury with a teardrop fracture of C5. Subsequently, he underwent an anterior fusion at C4. He presented with increasing neurologic deficit. *A,* Spin-echo TR 600/TE 25 msec T1-weighted sagittal MR in the midline. Note the expansion of the cervical cord (small arrows) above and below the level of the fusion (open arrow). Note the hypointensity within the center of the expanded cord consistent with a cystic cavity. Note the marked cord atrophy below the level of the injury indicated by the opened curved arrow. *B,* Spin-echo TR 2000/TE 40 msec proton density–weighted sagittal image also in the midline. *C,* Spin-echo TR 2000/TE 80 msec T2-weighted image in the same plane. The small arrows indicate the hypointense pulsation artifact seen within the syrinx cavity. *D,* Spin-echo TR 1000/TE 25 msec T1-weighted axial image demonstrating the large syrinx cavity within the cord (arrow).

and may flatten it. It is the presence of this mass effect that allows this lesion to be differentiated from spinal cord atrophy.

Although little has been written on the MR appearance of post-traumatic arachnoiditis, it is presumed that its appearance would not differ from a postoperative etiology. Arachnoiditis may appear as a soft tissue mass filling the subarachnoid space, centrally clumped nerve roots within the thecal sac, or as an "empty" thecal sac with thickened nodular dura secondary to peripherally adherent nerve roots.[21] These abnormalities are best seen on T2-weighted images, although they can be recognized on T1-weighted images. Moderate to severe arachnoiditis may show mild enhancement with gadolinium; however, the use of gadolinium adds little to the MR diagnosis of arachnoiditis.

Acknowledgment

We would like to thank Drs. J. Pagani and C. McArdle for the use of their cases and Ms. Susan Cunningham for the preparation of the manuscript.

REFERENCES

1. Atlas SW, Regenbogen V, Rogers LF, Kim KS: The radiographic characterization of burst fractures of the spine. AJNR 7:675, 1986.
2. Denis F: Spinal instability as defined by the three-column spine concept in acute spinal trauma. Clin Orthop 189:65, 1984.
3. Aguila LA, Piraino DW, Modic MT, et al: The intranuclear cleft of the intervertebral disc: magnetic resonance imaging. Radiology 155:155, 1985.
4. Czervionke LF, Czervionke JM, Daniels DL, Haughton VM: Characteristic features of magnetic resonance truncation artifacts. AJNR 9:815, 1988.
5. Mirvis SE, Joslyn JN, Young JWR, et al: Magnetic resonance imaging at 1.5 T in the evaluation of acute spine trauma. Chicago, RSNA Scientific Exhibit, Nov 29–Dec 4, 1987.
6. Shellock FG: Magnetic resonance imaging of metallic implants and materials: A compilation of the literature. AJR 151:811, 1988.
7. McArdle CB, Wright JW, Prevost WJ, et al: Magnetic resonance imaging of the acutely injured patient with cervical traction. Radiology 159:273, 1986.
8. Mirvis SE, Geisler F, Joslyn JN, Zrebeet H: Use of titanium wire in cervical spine fixation as a means to reduce magnetic resonance artifacts. AJNR 9:1229, 1988.
9. McArdle CB, Crofford MJ, Mirfakhraee M, et al: Surface coil magnetic resonance of spinal trauma: Preliminary experience. AJNR 7:885, 1986.
10. Kodoya S, Nakamura T, Kobayashi S, et al: Magnetic resonance imaging of acute spinal cord injury. Neuroradiology 29:252, 1987.
11. Mirvis SE, Geisler FH, Jelinek JJ, et al: Acute cervical spine trauma: Evaluation with 1.5-T magnetic resonance imaging. Radiology 166:807, 1988.
12. Tarr RW, Drolschager LF, Kerner TC, et al: Magnetic resonance imaging in recent spinal trauma. J Comput Assist Tomogr 11:412, 1987.
13. Chakeres DW, Flickinger F, Bresnahan JC, et al: Magnetic resonance imaging of acute spinal cord trauma. AJNR 8:5, 1987.
14. Hackney DB, Asato R, Joseph PM, et al: Hemorrhage and edema in acute spinal cord compression: Demonstration by magnetic resonance imaging. Radiology 161:387, 1986.
15. Gomori JM, Grossman RI, Goldberg HI, et al: Intracranial hematomas: Imaging by high field magnetic resonance. Radiology 157:87, 1985.
16. Kulkarni MV, McArdle CB, Kopanicky D, et al: Acute spinal cord injury: Magnetic resonance imaging at 1.5 T. Radiology 164:837, 1987.
17. Kulkarni MV, Bondurant FJ, Rose SL, Narayana PA: 1.5 Tesla magnetic resonance imaging of acute spinal trauma. Radiographic 8:1059, 1988.
18. Quencer RM, Sheldon JJ, Post MJD, et al: Magnetic resonance imaging of the chronically injured cervical spinal cord. AJNR 7:457, 1986.
19. Quencer RM: The injured spinal cord: Evaluation with magnetic resonance and intraoperative sonography. Radiol Clin North Am 26:1025, 1988.
20. Gebarski SS, Maynard FW, Gabrielsen TO, et al: Post-traumatic progressive myelopathy. Radiology 157:379, 1985.
21. Ross JS, Masaryk TJ, Modic MT, et al: Magnetic resonance (MR) imaging of lumbar arachnoiditis. AJNR 8:885, 1987.

Neurologic Evaluation and Neurologic Sequelae of the Spinal Cord Injured Patient

JACK STERN, M.D., Ph.D.

. . . an ailment not to be treated.

This description was given to spinal cord injury when Egyptian physicians first recognized such syndromes in the 17th century B.C.[1]

Even in the recent past the treatment of spinal cord injuries has been approached with a sense of futility and hopelessness. It has been difficult to shake off the overriding sense that this is the most devastating of all injuries. This is an injury that causes, in a moment, a lifelong physiologic, emotional, social, and economic alteration . . . an injury that devastates the patient as well as the family unit . . . an injury that always has the same unalterable course: paralysis, spinal instability, fear of further neurologic deterioration, sepsis, pressure sores, and a seemingly unending series of medical complications and the eventual shortening of life span.

This fatalistic attitude was changed in large part through the pioneering work of individuals such as Guttman[2] and Borrs.[3] They identified the need for an organized and categorized approach to this devastating human injury. Other significant contributions have been effected as a result of the United States Veterans' Administration and its continuous support and establishment of federally designated spinal cord injury centers.

The primary goals in the mangement of the spinal cord injured include the early identification of the degree of neurologic impairment and protection of the spinal cord from further neurologic deterioration.

STRATEGY OF CARE

Whenever spinal cord injury is suspected, the goal is to prevent further development of a worsening neurologic condition. This can be accomplished by adequate immobilization. Nothing is more tragic than the case of a patient with minimal neurologic deficit who becomes quadriplegic because neck immobilization was delayed or ineffective.

In order to more fully evaluate the degree of spinal cord injury, both in its intial stages and possible progression, it is imperative that the examiner understand the anatomy of the spinal canal and the classifications of spinal cord injury syndromes.

BASIC SPINAL ANATOMY

Spinal anatomy can be arbitrarily divided into three broad biomechanical categories. The first includes the vertebral bony column and its attendant ligaments and muscles (vertebral column unit); the second is composed of the spinal cord, its associated nerves, and its membrane investments, including the dura (spinal cord unit); and the third consists of the spinal cord vasculature (the spinal vascular unit). These categories are not strictly accurate because all tissues that compose the spinal system are intimately related. However, the categories are clinically useful in relating biomechanical distortion of vertebral and spinal vascular units to function of the cord unit.[4]

The Vertebral Column

The spinal column consists of 33 vertebra: 7 cervical, 12 thoracic, 5 lumbar, 5 fused sacral, and 1 coccygeal, which results from the fusion of four separate bodies.

The stability and mobility afforded the human body is the mechanical responsibility of this unit. All of the individual bony elements composing the spine articulate by means of the intervertebral disc and by posterolateral joints, with the exception of the first two cervical and sacral vertebrae. The very strong annulus fibrosis of the discs provides stability of the synarthroses between the vertebral bodies. The diarthrodial apophyseal joints are stabilized by their capsule as well as by the intrasupraspinous ligaments and the ligamentum flavum. Ligamentous structures, as a result of their intrinsic tensile strength and elasticity, as well as the engineering design utilized in their points of origin and termination, provide an almost ideal structural unit for stability and mobility. The articular processes are flat and small in the cervical region; those in the upper thoracic region are directed upward and backward. In the lumbar region the articular surfaces are large and point inward and outward. In all cases the upper surfaces of the lower vertebral articulate with lower facets of the superior vertebrae. Further stability is afforded to the thoracic spine through the rigidity of the thoracic cage.

THE SPINAL CORD. The spinal cord is a cylindric extension of the brain stem, suspended by means of a monotonous repeating series of nerve roots and ligaments in a fluid-filled cavity confined by relatively inelastic fibrous membrane, the dura. The true spinal dura is a continuous extension of the inner layer of the cranial dura, firmly attached circumferentially at the foramen magnum. Frequently, it is also in close approximation with the posterior surfaces of the first and second cervical vertebra and more loosely associated with a posterolongitudinal ligament in both the lumbar and cervical regions. At the second sacral level the dural investment is penetrated by the filum terminale, which is a direct extension of the pia mater in continuity with the inferior tapering spinal cord. The filum terminale and its covering of narrow dura continue as a multiple-layered structure to blend finally with the periosteum of the dorsal surface of the coccyx as the coccygeal ligament.

The interface between the spinal dura and the vertebral column is a true space, known as the *epidural space,* containing numerous venous plexuses, fat, and ligaments of the vertebral unit. Through this space the entering and existing nervous elements of the cord also pass, as do significant numbers of vascular structures supplying the cord substance.

Within the dural sac, two additional membranes surround the spinal cord. These membranes, together with the dura, are known as the *spinal meninges.* One of these membranes, the pia mater, is intimately applied to the external surface of the cord. A loosely arranged structure, referred to as the *arachnoid,* is interposed between the dura proper and the pia. This constitutes the third element of the spinal meninges. The spinal dura and the leptomeninges, by reason of their intimate relationship to the existing nerve roots, virtually cuff these structures as they terminate their association at the intervertebral foramen.

The ligamentous suspensory elements of the cord itself are known as *dentate ligaments.* Twenty-one of the these processes are attached to the inner surface of the dura and the lateral surface of the cord. The first dentate is just cephalad to the first cervical roots, and the lowest ligament is found between the last thoracic or just above the first lumbar roots. Although the significance of their supportive function to the cord remains controversial, these tough, small triangular ligaments securely anchor the cord to the dural surface.

The paired spinal roots present a constant reminder of the segmental arrangement present in the substance of the spinal cord. They are divided anatomically into the anterior (motor) and posterior (sensory) roots and are blended together in the form of spinal roots exiting through their cuff of spinal dura at the intervertebral foramina. Aside from their obvious neurophysiologic function they are also considered by some to provide mechanical fixation of the cord, especially at the cervical level in certain pathologic states.

The Spinal Vasculature

Anatomically,[5] the substance of the spinal cord is supplied by branches from a number of major vessels, including the vertebral and posterocerebellar arteries. Regional profusion is provided by branches from the thoracic and abdominal aorta as well as the deep cervical, intercostal, lumbar, and lateral sacral arteries. Lateral spinal arteries, originating from all of these parent vessels, eventually terminate in the anterior and posterior radicular arteries. The anterior radicular artery entering at each side of the cord with each anterior root (only six to eight of these vessels are of significant caliber) joins with the anterior spinal artery, which descends on the ventral surface of the cord after its formation from branches from both the vertebral arteries. Within the cranium, small branches of the vertebral or posteroinferior cerebellar arteries continue caudally over the dorsal surface of the cord, usually as two small trunks known as the *posterior spinal arteries.* Only five to eight of the posterior radicular arteries are of sufficient size to provide meaningful profusion to the cord. The largest radicular arteries, both anterior and posterior branches, usually enter the cord circulation at the upper lumbar region. Although the venous drainage of the spinal cord may be variable, its anatomic pattern is similar to those of the arteries.

The magnitude of any spinal injury also depends on the ability of the vertebra spinal cord and vascular units to attenuate the energy delivered via force vectors involving flexion, extension, compression and rotation, shear, and tension. Flexion injuries usually produce compression of the vertebral bodies with disruption of posterior longitudinal liagments as well as herniation of the intervertebral disc. In general, extension injuries can produce fractures of the posterior elements of the vertebral column and disruption of the anterior longitudinal ligaments. With compression injuries one may see explosion fractures of the vertebral bodies and ligamentous rupture. Rotational injuries usually produce disruption of the ligamentous structures, fractures, and fracture dislocation of the facets and may damage the mid section of the vertebral bodies. In the cervical region rotational-flexion and rotational-extension injuries are common, with severe damage occurring to the ligamentous and bony structures. All this of course may have a devastating effect upon the spinal cord unit itself.

NEUROLOGIC EVALUATION

Neurologic characterization of a spinal cord injury requires definition of the level of damage. Motor levels are most objectively determined using specific tests for each nerve root of the sacral, lumbar, and brachial plexuses. Thoracic motor levels are less exactly localized but can be approximated by careful evaluation of intercostal and abdominal muscles. Sensory levels tend to be the least precise but must be assessed and carefully documented.

Sensory levels are most accurately determined by beginning in the area of sensory deficit and proceeding into areas of normal sensation. The dermatomal pattern must be followed in order to obtain an accurate appraisal of the sensory level. There is an interface between the C4 and T2 dermatomes between the clavicles and the nipples because the dermatomes of the brachial plexus (C5 to T1) extend onto the upper limb. Therefore, the finding of a "sensory level" on the upper part of the chest demands that sensation also be examined on the arm and hand. Confusion can be avoided if the upper extremity is placed in the "anatomic" position (palm up) and if sensation is sequentially tested on the clavicle (C4), lateral aspect of the arm (C5), forearm and thumb (C6), middle finger (C7), little finger (C8), medial aspect of the forearm just below the elbow (T1), and medial aspect of the arm (T2).

The nipples approximate the T4 level and the umbilicus T10. The groin crease corresponds to L1, knee to L3, the medial aspect of the dorsum of the foot to L5, and the lateral aspect to S1. As already noted, testing of the sacral dermatomes is of critical importance in determining whether an injury is complete or not and is too often omitted. Lifting of the leg allows testing of posterior aspect of the calf and thigh (S2). The perineum and perianal areas are innervated by S4 and S5. Anorectal sensation can be evaluated as part of the digital rectal examination.

The sensory examination is especially important because rational management of patients with a spinal cord injury depends to a large extent upon whether the patient has a complete or incomplete physiologic transection of the spinal cord, and, if incomplete, whether the neurologic deficit is progressing or resolving with the passage of time. Early determination of the direction of the clinical course is crucial since there is evidence to suggest that the trauma to the spinal cord initiates an intrinsic tissue-destructive process that proceeds via time-related steps. It is possible that some of these steps can be prevented or even reversed by medical or surgical treatment. However, the opportunity for such therapeutic maneuvers probably exists for only a short period of time. Therefore, documentation of the neurologic examination is imperative.

CLASSIFICATION OF SPINAL CORD LESIONS[6]

Complete Lesions

Complete lesions result with immediate abolition of segmental reflex responses caudal to the lesion and demonstrate the unequivocal absence of motor or sensory function distal to the injury in the absence of spinal shock.

Complete Cervical Injury

Cervical lesions of the spinal cord involve many individual differences, variation within segments, and concomitant features such as local edema. It is convenient to consider segmental lesions at different levels starting from below, including T1 because of the hand involvement. The relationship between the cord segments and vertebral levels must be noted, especially the observation that the spinal cord levels are higher than the vertebral levels. A simple rule to determine the segmental cord levels is to add one to the spinous process level for the cervical cord and two for the upper thoracic cord. Complete transection of a T1 segment results in a partial loss of power of interossei, lumbricals, and abductor pollicus plus complete paralysis of the abductor pollicus brevis and all voluntary motion below, save for the diaphragm. Sensation is absent over the medial forearm and in all areas below it, excluding the C3 to C4 innervation extending below the clavicle. Horner's syndrome is present.

Complete transection at C8 level results in clinical findings that include the aforementioned signs plus paralysis of the lumbricals and interossei with a clawhand (main en griffe). Although partial weakness of the finger flexors and other hand muscles persists, there is usually good recovery of flexion and extension at the wrist. The sensory loss extends to the hand to include the fourth and fifth fingers.

Injury at the C7 segment follows a pattern already noted, with the addition of marked and abiding weakness of the finger and wrist flexors and the triceps muscle. The extensor carpi radialis longus receives innervation from C6; accordingly, extension of the wrist is present and usually predominates in wrist movement with deviation to radial side. The position of the hand with extended wrist and flexed fingers is often known as a preacher's hand, or main du prédicateur. This retained function is all-important for later rehabilitation. Horner's syndrome may occur at this or higher levels but is usually not as well defined as the C8, T1, and T2 lesions, presumably because of the involvement of the ciliospinal center of Budge and Waller with lower lesions.

The shift from a C7 to a C6 lesion involves changes that are particularly marked. Triceps and extensor carpi radialis groups are now weaker and may function insignificantly. Biceps, brachialis, and brachioradialis muscle power is not normal but is unopposed at the elbow to give a fairly constant flexed posture. The deltoid muscle is weakened but remains functional. The arm may be gently abducted if the patient lies in the supine position, since the adductors of the shoulder are preferentially weakened. The clavicular head of the pectoralis major muscle receives innervation from C5 and hence function may be demonstrable. This is not true for the sternal head, because its innervation comes slowly from the lower segment. The biceps reflexes are absent or diminished; the sensory level extends to include the thumb, lateral aspect of the forearm, and arm.

Complete transection of the C5 level results in added paralysis of the biceps, brachialis, brachioradialis, and deltoid muscles. Elevation of the shoulder is preserved with some external rotation. The arm is otherwise flail and is areflexic. Diaphragmatic breathing is reduced initially but recovers and stabilizes with time. Anesthesia is almost complete over the arm save for a strip extending down over the shoulder and the anterior aspect of the upper arm.

Complete transection in the upper cervical segments above C5 leads to respiratory failure because of the loss of phrenic innervation from C3 through C5. Formerly, most of these patients were lost. However, the current emphasis on early resuscitation, adequate artificial ventilation, and potent antibiotic coverage results in the survival of significant numbers of quadriplegics with high-level transection. In time some phrenic nerve function may return and may, with auxillary respiratory muscle function, provide adequate spontaneous respiration. Phrenic nerve stimulators may also be used in selected patients.

Acute and complete spinal cord lesions above the C3 segment are almost invariably fatal unless immediate respiratory support is provided. An incomplete lesion in this region may involve the lower cranial nerves and nuclei, pyramidal decussation, sensory and motor tracts and nuclei, respiratory and autonomic centers and tracts, and upper cervical nerve roots. Less commonly, compression and occlusion of the verterbral or anterior spinal artery may result in an infarction extending through the cervical medullary area simulating a concurrent upper cervical cord and brain injury.[7]

Lesions in the upper cervical spinal cord occasionally produce a peculiar pattern of sensory deficit over the face. This is described as the *Déjérine (onion peel) pattern* of sensory loss and results from the involvement of the descending tract of the trigeminal nerve, which extends down as far as the C4 segment of the spinal cord. The most caudal portion of this tract carries impulses from the outermost part of the face, whereas the central areas are represented at higher levels. Pain and temperature sensation become altered in a centripetal manner from the outermost part of the face as the lesion in the trigeminal tract extends upward—hence an onion peel pattern of sensory loss.

Serious respiratory disturbances[8,9] often follow high cervical cord lesions. Irritation of the phrenic nerve may lead to hiccups, dyspnea, and coughing. Destruction of this nerve results in paralysis of the diaphragm. Bradycardia is less common; it is attributed to interruption of the fibers ascending to cardiovascular center in the medulla oblongata. Occlusion of the vertebral arteries or thrombosis of the anterior spinal artery may cause a high cervical cord infarction, resulting in quadriplegia, impairment of various sensory modalities, bladder and bowel dysfunction, and respiratory and vasomotor disturbances.

The C1 and C2 spinal cord segments are most susceptible to injury. Direct cerebral vertex impact may be transmitted to the C2 segment of the cord—this is well documented clinically and experimentally. The atlantoaxial junction may be disrupted by sudden and excessive forces, whereas acute torsion of the cervical spine may damage the vertebral arteries as they exit over the C1 lamina.

Complete Thoracolumbar Injuries

It is important to differentiate between a cord injury and injury to the nerve roots. Roots just proximal to the cord injury will often be contused and initially may malfunction but may recover over several months. Also, because the spinal cord terminates between the first and second lumbar vertebrae, fractures and dislocations distal to this level will damage roots to the cauda equina rather than the cord. Lower motor neuron findings will be present. Some injuries of the thoracolumbar junction may involve the conus medullaris. Damage to the conus carries a poorer prognosis but rarely can early neurologic examination distinguish this from pure cauda equina injury. The level of the vertebral damage may suggest the presence or absence of conus injury.

Syndromes of Incomplete Spinal Cord Injury

Awareness of a common constellation of neurologic signs following incomplete spinal cord injury alerts the examiner through the identification of the following specific syndromes.[10]

Central Cord Syndrome

This syndrome is commonly seen with hyperextension injuries of the cervical spine. It is particularly noted in the elderly and is sometimes without radiographic evidence of vertebral injury. However, it may occur with flexion injuries. Central cord syndromes are also associated with syringomyelia and intramedullary spinal cord tumors.

The cardinal feature of the central cord syndrome is the presence of disproportionate weakness of the arms as compared with the legs. The anatomic basis may be explained as follows: The corticospinal and spinothalamic tracts are organized in such a way that sacral fibers are most peripheral and cervical fibers are most central. Therefore, in the central cord syndrome motor and sensory fibers are less severely affected in the lower extremities than in the upper extremities. It is therefore possible that the most peripheral sacral, and perhaps the adjacent lumbar, fibers escape injury, and thus "sparing" of some motor and/or some sensory function occurs in corresponding areas of the perineum, genitalia, and lower extremity. Paralysis in the upper extremity is usually profound, particularly in the hands and fingers. This is due to the fact that the medial, i.e., cervical, portion of the corticospinal tract and the alpha motor neurons in the anterior gray horn are both damaged at the level of the injury.

Incomplete lesions, with sparing of at least some of the sacral fibers, carries a relatively good prognosis. Many patients are eventually able to ambulate, at least with some mechanical support. Some regain bowel and bladder continence. Prognosis for gaining useful function of the hand is usually much less favorable for the reasons described.

As with the other incomplete lesions of the spinal cord, a "pure" syndrome is rarely encountered. This is due in part to the vagaries of the spreading tissue edema but more specifically, in the cases of central cord syndrome, to the presence of the potentially variegated structure of the hematomyelic cavity. In fact, the classic central cord syndrome is that found with syringomyelia. The cavity lies in the midline or in the paracentral position and interrupts the decussating pain and temperature fibers to give a dissociated sensory loss. The arms, shoulder, and upper thorax are often involved in a capelike distribution. Weakness and atrophy of the small muscles of the hand are early symptoms and are caused by anterior horn cell involvement. Later, muscle power in the forearm, arm, and shoulders is lost as the syrinx enlarges and fibrillations and fasciculations become widespread. The lesions progress to include the corticospinal tracts with spastic paralysis, hyperreflexia, ascending plantar responses, and a neurogenic bladder, and the dorsal columns with loss of proprioception, vibration sensation, and hypoesthesia. Also commonly seen with a classic syrinx but uncommonly seen with acute central cord syndromes are trophic changes in the hands and Horner's syndrome with involvement of the ciliospinal centers at C8 and T1.

Anterior Cord Syndrome

This syndrome is usually seen with flexion injuries and may be associated with acute traumatic herniation of an intervertebral disc. Pure anterior cord syndromes are rare. The syndrome involves injury to the anterior part of the spinal cord that is supplied by the anterior spinal artery: the anterior gray horn including alpha motor neurons and the tracts including the corticospinal and spinothalamic tracts of the anterior and lateral white matter. Only the posterior gray horn and both posterior columns are spared. Thus, below the level of the injury, variable degrees of paralysis coincide with diminution of pain and temperature sensation, but not with light touch, joint position sense, or vibratory sensation. Pure anterior horn cell syndrome is characterized by lower motor neuron signs of flaccid weakness, atrophy, and areflexia.

Lateral Cord Syndrome, the Syndrome of Brown-Séquard

The Brown-Séquard or hemisection syndrome is seen with unilateral lesions of the cord and consists of ipsilateral motor neuron weakness, posterior column sensory loss, and vasomotor and pseudomotor changes, plus contralateral loss of pain and temperature sensibilities. These findings are present at a level one of more segments distal to a lesion. Ipsilateral lower motor neuron weakness and analgesia or hypalgesia are found over a narrow band at the sight of injury as a result of local damage to incoming or outgoing fibers or their cells of origin. In practice, the classic Brown-Séquard syndrome is rarely seen. Instead, a partial Brown-Séquard syndrome is commonly found with cervical cord involvement of many kinds and consists of simple combinations of the two most prominent features of the syndrome: ipsilateral spastic weakness and contralateral analgesia and thermoanesthesia.

In contrast is the type of sensory loss produced by peripheral nerve transection, in which all modalities of somatic sensation are lost together, demonstrating anesthesia in the involved area. In the Brown-Séquard syndrome each half of the body exhibits a dissociated sensory loss, in which there is a loss of some of the sensory modalities without loss of the other.

Posterior Column Syndrome

This rare syndrome is associated with hyperextension injuries. In its purest form only posterior column sensation is lost. In general, prognosis for recovery is good.

Root Syndromes

Above the cauda equina, one or perhaps two nerve roots are frequently compressed as a result of vertebral subluxation or even acute disc herniation. Local cervical pain radiating into the shoulder or down the arm is characteristic of cervical root compression. Although the patient may complain of tingling or numbness, objective sensory changes referable to a single nerve root are unusual due to overlap of adjacent dermatomes. However, isolated weakness of a muscle or loss of a reflex referable to an involved root is often demonstrable. Traumatic lesions of the cauda equina due to thoricolumbar or lumbar spinal injuries usually involve multiple roots with highly variable, often asymmetric patterns of motor and sensory loss.

Some or all deep tendon reflexes are usually absent. Involvement of midsacral roots may denervate the bladder even if the motor and sensory function of lumbar roots is found to be intact. It is important to test sacral root function as well because injuries of the lumbosacral spine usually involve nerve roots rather than the spinal cord itself; the occurrence of isolated sacral root involvement producing saddle hypalgesia is just as possible as sacral root sparing. Since spinal roots and nerves are part of the peripheral nervous system, regeneration can occur provided that anatomic continuity of the root or nerve is preserved. Thus, spontaneous motor and sensory recovery is often seen, sometimes even after prolonged intervals. Whenever a nerve root remains compressed the chances of recovery are usually enhanced by closed or open (operative) decompression.

It should be pointed out that digital rectal examination is a key part in the determination of whether a spinal cord injury is complete or not. If the patient can feel the palpating finger or voluntarily contract perineal muscles around it, the lesion is incomplete. Rectal sensation is seldom absent in the presence of true voluntary perianal muscle contraction, but sensation is often preserved in the absence of voluntary motor activity. In either case the prognosis for further motor and sensory recovery is favorable. Demonstrable rectal tone by itself, without rectal sensation or voluntary contraction, does not constitute evidence of an incomplete lesion, since some tone may be preserved by local reflexes alone. The bulbocavernosus reflex is used to demonstrate that reflex perianal muscle contraction is present. If this spinal reflex arc is intact and rectal sensation and voluntary perianal muscle contraction are absent, the examiner has good evidence of complete isolation of at least the sacral cord segments. This implies that there is no physiologic continuity between the lower spinal cord and the supraspinal centers. Acute interruption of the supraspinal innervation of autonomic bladder centers in the spinal cord usually renders the bladder at least temporarily inactive and hypotonic.

SPINAL SHOCK

The term *spinal shock* was introduced by Hall, who described the neurogenic form, with its characteristic early areflexia and flaccidity.[11] Hall also conducted animal studies, carried on in frogs, in which reflex activity was lost with spinal cord injury and then increased within a few minutes. In humans this latency extends to a few weeks. In the interval, marked hypertonia is present and virtually all reflex action is absent, with the exception of the anal reflex. The presence of spinal shock indicates that, in the primate and especially in the human, cord function is highly dependent on influence from above, and that the capacity for independent action is much less than in lower animals. Spasticity appears after the period of spinal shock. The latter may be defined as exaggerated activity of the extensor posture mechanisms.[12]

The probable anatomic basis for this phenomenon is the interruption of descending inhibitory fibers of the corticobulboreticular and the caudatospinal and the cerebelloreticular and the reticulospinal pathways. Hypertonicity is found, together with hyperreflexia and clonus. The latter is, in effect, an expression of repeated stretch reflexes that travel through simple monosynaptic pathways.

SPASTICITY

Reflex activity other than that found with deep tendon responses appears as well and precedes the appearance of spasticity. This is of two types: one involves the sacral parasympathetics with reappearance and strengthening of the anal and bulbocavernous reflexes; the other is the primitive withdrawal response, which is quite variable but which consists primarily of flexion at the knee and flexion and abduction at the hip. These movements are often combined with extension of the great toe and fanning of the toes as in the Babinski response. The extension movement is actually a primitive flexion withdrawal; *dorsiflexion* may be a better term.[13] Another manifestation of the withdrawal response is the fact that the afferent discharges from the plantar responses can be elicited from wide areas on the leg and thigh. This mass reflex, or mass response, may develop later; it involves violent bilateral flexion and adduction action of the legs and abdominal contractions that are coupled with evacuations of the bladder and rectum, plus reflex sweating. Its presence points to a wide extension of activity through much of the isolated cord. The stimulus is usually excessive and is associated with an infected full bladder or a large pressure sore or sepsis. Fortunately, modern care of the paraplegic or quadriplegic is such that these problems can largely be eliminated and consequently the mass reflex is uncommonly seen now. Paraplegia-in-flexion was a frequent finding in the past. Its presence was thought to point to a complete lesion as opposed to an incomplete one with paraplegia-in-extension. Paraplegia-in-flexion has largely disappeared, again because of better care. The *flexor spasm* constitutes the third phenomenon in this group. These spasms are frequently violent. They may be initiated by stimulation of intact skin or by stimulation from a pressure sore. These are less common than in the past but have not disappeared. Other indications of the mass reflex, such as reflex sweating, may be seen in isolation. There is a complete loss of all sensory modalities with complete lesions. This is often associated with a zone of hyperpathia at the level of the injury. These patients are later aware of what would normally be appreciated as visceral pain. Sensations may be transmitted by way of the phrenic nerves, which contain sensory fibers although they are primarily motor. These enter the cord at C3 to C4 and C5 levels and hence are at least partially above most cervical lesions. Impulses may also travel along the autonomic nervous system. A third mechanism associated with autonomic hyperreflexia is a reflex vasoconstriction in the paralyzed area that occurs in response to visceral overdistention, which usually involves the bladder. A hypertensive crisis ensues and the patient notes severe headache, flushing of the face, stuffiness in the nose, and a pounding heartbeat.

Patients are sometimes aware of unpleasant phantom sensations in the acute phase; these often involve localized areas such as the genitals. They may be severe intially but tend to disappear during rehabilitation.

AUTONOMIC CHANGES

Changes in vasomotor control are very important in considering autonomic changes.[14] Spinal shock has already been discussed. The second type of shock is *vascular*. This occurs in the acute period and is due to a sudden loss of sympathetic control. Experimental and clinical studies place the vasomotor pathways in the ventrolateral white matter. Blood pressures may remain low for a brief period of one to two days. This hypotension is different from that found with the usual traumatic shock in that it is accompanied by a slow rather than a fast pulse. The second phase is that of postural hypotension. This persists for many weeks after the injury and can be detected by placing the patient on a tilt table. The presence of postural hypotension reflects the slow return of vasomotor tone. Careful monitoring of the blood pressure is required during tilting in this phase. Because the pressure may fall precipitously, it may pass the lower level of autoregulation of blood flow for the brain as well as for the spinal cord above the lesion. Bladder involvement is also prominent in the state of spinal shock.[15,16] There is absence of active or reflex contraction of the detrusor muscle; therefore, the bladder distends beyond the passive obstruction at the neck. If this is unchecked, urinary retention occurs with overdistention and eventually overflowing continence. The period of bladder shock usually parallels the period of spinal shock, i.e., one to six weeks. Reflex detrusor contractions then appear under ideal circumstances. Age and quality of bladder care are important factors. These contractions may be noted prior to the reappearance of deep tendon reflexes. The mechanism is that of simple reflex action without afferent and efferent arcs through S1, S3, and S4, paralleling the monosynaptic reflex for skeletal muscle. The end result is a full automatic bladder, which is now common.

Sexual malfunction[17,18] is another prominent manifestation of interruption of the control of the autonomic nervous system. In the male priapism or passive engorgement is common in the acute phase. Reflex erections return later at about the same time as reflex detrusor action. Ejaculations are usually not possible with complete cervical cord transections. These require more complicated, integrated reflex action through the lumbar sympathetic system. Orgastic sensations are absent with complete lesions, but alternative sites for similar feelings may develop above the level of transection. Ovulation may be suppressed in the female for one or two months but is unaffected thereafter. Pregnancy and normal delivery are possible.

Gastrointestinal function is also seriously impaired. Ileus and fecal retention are routine in the acute phase. Ulcerations in the upper gastrointestinal tract are uncommon but are well known. These may be the result from unbalanced actions of the vagus nerve. Bowel function returns after the period of initial spinal shock and proceeds until the establishment of autonomic rectum with reflex defecation. This parallels reflex bladder and reflex erection activities.

The loss of sweating is another feature of autonomic involvement. Complete cervical transection leads to a loss of sweating throughout the body, since the entire sympathetic outflow is interrupted. Reflex action returns later as noted. Pilomotor function is also affected. Heat control is a major problem and the one that is particularly difficult to manage in patients with high lesions. Late adaptations occur with the return of local vasomotor responses.

REFERENCES

1. Elsberg, CA: The Edwin Smith surgical papyrus and diagnosis and treatment of injuries to the skull and spine 5,000 years ago. Ann. Med. Hist. 3:271, 1931.
2. Guttman L: Spinal Cord Injuries: Comprehensive Management and Research. London, Blackwell Scientific Publications, 1973.
3. Borrs, E, Comarr, AE: Neurological Urology. Baltimore, University Park Press, 1971.
4. Albin, MS: Acute cervical spinal injury. Crit Care Clin 1:267, 1985.
5. Dommise, GF: The arteries and veins of the human spinal cord from birth. Edinburgh, Churchill Livingstone, 1975.
6. Schneider, RC, Crosby, EC, Russo, RH, Gosh, HH: Traumatic spinal cord syndromes and their management. Clin Neurosurg 20:424, 1973.
7. Schneider, RC, Crosby, EC: Vascular insufficiency of brain stem and spinal cord in spinal trauma. Neurology 1:643, 1969.
8. Bellamy R, Pitts, FW, Stauffer, ES: Respiratory complications in traumatic quadriplegia: Analysis of 20 years' experience. J Neurosurg 39:596, 1973.
9. Frost, ER: The physiopathology of respiration in neurosurgical patients. J. Neurosurg 50:669, 1979.
10. McQueen JD, Khan, MI: Evaluation of patients with cervical spine lesions. In The Cervical Spine. Philadelphia, JB Lippincott, 1983.
11. Hall, M: Four Memories of the Nervous System. London, 1840.
12. Lindsley, DF, Schriner, LH, Magoun, WH: Electromyographic study of spasticity. J Neurophysiol 12:197, 1949.
13. Landau, WM, Clare, MW: The plantar reflex in man with special references to some conditions where the extensor response is unexpectedly absent. Brain 82:321, 1959.
14. Kurnick, NB: Autonomic hyperreflexia and its control in patients with spinal cord lesions. Ann Intern Med. 44:678, 1956.
15. O'Flynn, JD: Neurogenic bladder in spinal cord injury. Urol Clin North Am 1:155, 1974.
16. Thomas DG, Smallwood, R, Graham, D: Urodynamic observations following spinal trauma. J Urol 47:161, 1975.
17. Comarr, AE: Sexual function among patients with spinal cord injury. Urol Int 25:134, 1970.
18. Weiss, HD: Physiology of penile erection. Ann Intern Med. 76:793, 1972.

Urologic Evaluation and Management of the Spinal Cord Injured Patient

10

GEORGE F. OWENS, M.D., F.A.C.S., and
JOSEPH C. ADDONIZIO, M.D., F.A.C.S.

The incidence of traumatic spinal cord injury is approximately 3 per 100,000 population. Motor vehicle accidents and falls account for a majority of the cases. Recreational (especially diving) accidents and gunshot and stab wounds also account for a significant number of spinal cord injuries. A majority of those injured are between 15 and 34 years of age. Associated injuries are the rule in patients sustaining spinal cord injury. Consequently, immediate management of these patients should be approached in a team fashion.

Because of the high incidence of genitourinary tract injury in association with multiple trauma, a complete evaluation of the GU tract is warranted at the time of presentation regardless of the presence or absence of hematuria. This should include computerized tomography (CT) of the abdomen and pelvis or an intravenous urogram (IVU). Magnetic resonance imaging (MRI) may also prove helpful. If bladder or urethral injury is suspected, a cystogram and retrograde urethrogram should also be performed.

Initially, a catheter is placed in the bladder and left indwelling to monitor urine output. The patient is stabilized and, if required, immediate surgical repair of associated injuries is accomplished without delay.

GOALS OF UROLOGIC CARE

The primary concern of the urologist in caring for the spinal cord injured patient is to maintain renal function. Renal failure ranks as one of the most common late causes of death in male patients. The three primary causes of renal failure are (1) bladder and sphincter dysfunction resulting in high-pressure voiding and impaired renal tubular drainage, (2) urinary tract infection, and (3) amyloid disease as a result of chronic pressure sores.

Secondly, the urologist is concerned with affording the patient an acceptable means of bladder emptying. After a thorough assessment of the dynamics of micturition in each patient, the mechanism of voiding dysfunction can be defined and appropriate therapy instituted.

A third concern is the sexual rehabilitation of the spinal cord injured patient. In the male this entails providing him with the means to maintain an erection adequate for sexual activity, and for those patients desiring children, an acceptable method of retrieving or producing viable sperm.

ANATOMY AND PHYSIOLOGY

In order to formulate a complete urologic care plan and to understand and properly interpret the radiologic and urodynamic procedures performed on the spinal cord injured patient one needs at least a basic understanding of the anatomy and neurophysiology of the GU tract.

Anatomic Considerations

The kidneys lie in the retroperitoneum protected by the lower ribs and perirenal fatty tissue. The kidneys are supplied by renal arteries arising directly from the aorta just below the superior mesenteric artery. Anterior to the artery lies the renal vein, which drains directly into the inferior vena cava. The renal pedicles are relatively fixed and therefore renal vascular injury must be considered in severe trauma. The renal pelvis lies posterior to the artery. The ureters are fixed at the ureteropelvic junction and, consequently, are susceptible to avulsion at this point in deceleration injury. The remainder of the ureter courses to the bladder freely in the retroperitoneum. Blood supply is from the aorta and iliac arteries. The ureters course below the internal iliac artery and enter the bladder posteriorly and inferiorly through an oblique intramural tunnel. It is this tunnel that provides the antireflux mechanism during voiding. Each ureter is surroudned by an incomplete collar of detrusor smooth muscle. The bladder wall consists of an outer adventitial layer, a smooth muscle layer, and an inner urothelium. The muscle layer is formed by interlacing large-diameter smooth muscle cells. The trigone of the bladder is composed of a deep detrusor layer and a more superficial muscle layer constituted of small diameter smooth muscle cells. This layer extends down into the posterior urethra. The posterior urethra is attached to the pubis by the puboprostatic ligament. The membranous urethra is that portion surrounded by the urogenital diaphragm. The bulbous urethra lies free within the perineum and scrotum. The remainder of the anterior urethra, the pendulous urethra, courses through the penis.

Neuroanatomic and Physiologic Considerations

The spinal cord ends at the level of the first lumbar vertebra. Below this level lies the conus medularis and the cauda equina. The respective nerve roots exit from the corresponding intervertebral space. Injury below the first lumbar vertebra (L1) results in so-called *lower motor neuron lesions* and injury above L1 results in *upper motor neuron lesions.* On the basis of evolving knowledge of the innervation of the lower urinary tract, this classification is somewhat antiquated. It is, however, still in common use and is therefore mentioned.

Innervation to the lower urinary tract is via parasympathetic, sympathetic, and somatic nerves. The anterior segments of the pelvic plexus serve as the final common pathway for the autonomic innervation of the bladder and urethral sphincter. Preganglionic parasympathetic nerves arise from the intermediolateral gray columns of the third and fourth sacral segments of the spinal cord (S3 and S4) and run in the pelvic nerve to ganglia lying in or on the bladder wall. Postganglionic fibers then course directly to the detrusor muscle bundles. The neurotransmitter for these nerves is acetylcholine (Ach).

Sympathetic preganglionic nerves arise in the intermediolateral gray matter of the thoracolumbar cord from the tenth thoracic to the second lumbar (T10 to L2). These fibers enter the sympathetic ganglia and the postganglionic fibers, then course to the pelvic plexus and the hypogastric nerve. The neurotransmitter for the postganglionic nerves in this case is norepinephrine. The somatic nerves to the external urethral sphincter are derived from the pudendal nerve. Recent studies suggest that these nerves run with the pelvic nerve. They arise from the anterior horn of S2 to S4. They are classified as alpha motor neurons but do not exhibit the behavior typical of alpha motor neurons elsewhere in the body. The pelvic floor muscles are innervated by typical alpha motor neurons arising from S2, S3, and S4. The perineal portion of the pelvic floor is innervated mainly by fibers from S2, S3, and S4, and the upper pelvic floor muscles from S3 and S4.

Neuroanatomy of Sexual Excitation

The parasympathetic innervation to the penis responsible for reflex erection is derived from the pelvic nerves (S2 to S4) via the nervi erigentes. The sympathetic nerves arise from the thoracolumbar segments T11 to L2 and innervate the seminal vesicles, vas deferens, and posterior urethra. These nerves are responsible for psychogenic erections. Somatic innervation derived from sacral segments S2 to S4 via the pudendal nerve supply the bulbocavernosus, ischiocavernosus, striated urethral sphincter, and perineal muscles and is responsible for ejaculation. Seminal emission is derived from sympathetic fibers from the thoracolumbar segments T11 to L2 coursing via the hypogastric nerve.

INITIAL MANAGEMENT

Immediate Care—Paraplegic and Quadriplegic

Of paramount importance in the evaluation of the spinal cord injured patient is a systems approach in the assessment of associated injuries. Once the patient has been stabilized and other injuries requiring immediate attention have been cared for, the patient can be transferred to a neurosurgical intensive care unit. A small bore catheter, No. 12 French or No. 14 French, is left indwelling in the bladder for the first 48 hours. This allows close monitoring of the urine output during the immediate postinjury period.

Spinal Shock Phase—Paraplegic and Quadriplegic

Once the patient is hemodynamically stable, the indwelling catheter is removed and intermittent catheterization is started. Both sterile and clean techniques are employed in different spinal injury centers. An acceptable approach is to employ sterile technique when catheterization is performed by the nursing staff in quadriplegics and initially in the paraplegic. When the paraplegic patient has been instructed in self-catheterization, a method of clean self-catheterization (CSIC) is utilized.

Prolonged initial management with an indwelling urethral catheter is to be discouraged. Calcifications can form around the catheter, resulting in refractory urinary tract infections and bladder stones. In males the incidence of urethritis and epididymitis is greater with indwelling urethral catheters. Fistulas and stricture formation are also more likely after prolonged urethral catheterization.

Bacteriuria occurs in virtually all patients on intermittent catheterization regardless of which technique, clean or sterile, is used. Culture to identify the species of bacteria as well as urinalysis to assess the degree of pyuria should be performed routinely, i.e., once monthly, to determine if medical therapy is indicated. Routine antibiotic prophylaxis has not been demonstrated to decrease the incidence of clinically important urinary tract infections and therefore is not recommended. The bacteriuria is, in general, tolerated without adverse effects in the majority of patients. Certainly if the patient appears clinically ill without any other obvious source of infection, treatment with an appropriate antibiotic on the basis of previous culture results should be instituted to sterilize the urine.

Prompt initiation of intermittent catheterization during the acute phase facilitates the overall long-term urologic management of all patients with injury to the spinal cord. The achievement of a "balanced bladder" is the ultimate goal in management. A balanced bladder can be defined as a bladder with sufficient capacity to store urine reliably and empty sufficiently without undue high pressure or vesicoureteral reflux, so that residual urine is not more than 30 per cent of bladder capacity nor greater than 125 cc.

Catheterization can be started at intervals of every six hours. A small-caliber, straight catheter, i.e., No. 12F or No. 14F, straight catheter should be used. The interval of catheterization should be adjusted in order to obtain between 300 and 350 cc of urine with each catheterization. Paraplegic patients can be taught self-catheterization during this phase of treatment. Typically, within two to six weeks the bladder will begin to function in an upper motor neuron (suprasacral) type of injury.

INTERMEDIATE MANAGEMENT

Work-up and Evaluation—Urodynamic Studies

During this phase of managment the achievement of a balanced bladder is the goal of therapy. A complete evaluation of the patient should be performed in all cases. It is during this period that urodynamic monitoring of the lower urinary tract should be initiated. Carbon dioxide or water can be used as the medium. Water is usually preferable because its properties make it a more reliable and reproducible medium for assessment of bladder capacity and intravesical pressures. Its use, especially in the initial evaluation, is recommended.

Intravesical pressures are monitored by a small (4F or 5F) tube within the bladder. The bladder is filled via a separate larger catheter. Alternatively, a multiple-lumen catheter can be used, but such a catheter usually precludes measuring pressure and flow simultaneously due to the large size required. If accurate recording of flow is not required, however, it is a perfectly acceptable monitoring device. Intraabdominal pressures are monitored by placing a catheter in the rectum; in the female the vagina can also be used. The electrical activity of the external urethral sphincter or pelvic floor musculature is recorded by placing wire electrodes or needles percutaneously into the muscle. The proper position can be confirmed by observing action potentials on an oscilloscope or other suitable monitoring device. Patch electrodes can be used but are less specific in reflecting activity of the muscle group in question.

In all patients who are voiding, a simultaneous uroflow and EMG should be performed. The finding of detrusor-sphincter dyssynergia is apparent when a decrease is present in flow associated with an increase in muscle activity. Monitoring both intravesicle and intra-abdominal pressures permits calculation of the pressure generated by the bladder (detrusor) by subtracting the abdominal pressure from the total intravesical pressure: $(P_{detrusor} = P_{vesical} - P_{abdominal})$. If available, videourodynamics should be performed. This allows for visualization of the dynamics of voiding while the pressures are recorded simultaneously. It aids in differentiating internal from external sphincter detrusor dyssynergia and identifying low and high pressure reflux and aids in confirming the proper location of the pressure monitors within the urinary tract. The response of the bladder to filling and during voiding can thus be visualized and recorded. Cystoscopy can also be performed at this time.

In general, patients can be classified into two broad categories: those having suprasacral lesions and those with cauda equina or conus lesions. Suprasacral lesions are associated with bladder hyperreflexia and detrusor-sphincter dyssynergia. Cauda equina and conus lesions are associated with bladder areflexia. When a management program is planned, preserving renal function and helping the patient to achieve an acceptable life style are the two major considerations. Lesions may be complete or incomplete and the degree of dyssynergia will vary accordingly. In all cases the treatment should be tailored to the individual rather than fitting the individual into a preconceived treatment protocol.

Quadriplegics with Suprasacral Lesions

In the majority of cases, these patients will develop spontaneous voiding after a period of spinal shock. Detrusor contractions can be initiated by suprapubic tapping or some other stimulus. Dyssynergia will be present to varying degrees. Urodynamic studies help identify filling and voiding vesicular pressures and

allow measurement of residual urine. If bladder pressure is not significantly elevated (less than 60 to 70 cm H_2O) the amount of residual urine acceptable (less than 75 cc and uninfected), spontaneous or stimulated voiding is an acceptable method of management.

External urine collection devices, now available for men and women, can be used to protect against incontinence. There are a variety of types of condom catheters on the market. In most cases one can be found that is acceptable and reliably remains in place. Women can wear any of the high-absorbancy pads now marketed by several companies.

When dyssynergia causes significant obstruction, high voiding pressures are generated that will accelerate the development of renal failure. In those patients with external sphincter-detrusor dyssynergia the external sphincter can sometimes be successfully ablated with pharmacologic therapy. Alpha sympatholytics such as phentolamine, phenoxybenzamine, and prazosin have been used successfully. Skeletal muscle relaxants (dantrolene and baclofen) have also been employed successfully. Transurethral external sphincterotomy to ablate the sphincter can also be performed and is without the side effects of long-term medication. Occasionally, transurethral resection of the prostate and bladder neck is required to resect the internal urethral sphincter. In older patients with prostate hyperplasia, transurethral resection may be necessary to relieve the obstructive prostate.

If hyperreflexia results in too-frequent detrusor contractions, anticholinergics such as propantheline or smooth muscle relaxants such as oxybutynin (which also has anticholinergic type of activity) or musculotropics such as flavoxate can be used to control the bladder. Spontaneous voiding is still an option. In selected patients with some use of their upper extremities or with patients able to have 24-hour care, the bladder can be paralyzed with anticholinergics and intermittently catheterized. Alternatively, a suprapubic cystostomy in the male or an indwelling bladder catheter in the female can be used to collect urine. However, because of the long-term complications of indwelling catheters (urinary tract infection, calculi, contracted bladder, hematuria, catheter blockage) they should be considered a second-line therapeutic choice. The use of transurethral catheters in the male is especially discouraged because of the additional complications of urethritis, epididymitis, urethral stricture, and urethrocutaneous fistulous formation.

Quadriplegics with Areflexic Bladders

In certain patients with multiple levels of injury, the quadriplegic patient will not have any detrusor activity. Oral cholinomimetic therapy with bethanechol has not been demonstrated to be effective in any well-controlled studies. These patients generally require catheter drainage. Currently, clinical trials of sacral nerve stimulation are being conducted. Initial results are promising, and bladder stimulation will probably become a clinically feasible choice in the near future.

Paraplegics with Suprasacral Lesions

In these patients as in others, the achievement of a balanced bladder is the goal of therapy. Patients with an acceptably low vesical voiding pressure can be allowed to void into an external collection device. As mentioned, these are now available for men and women. For those patients with a high vesicular voiding pressure, and for those few men unable to wear a condom catheter (or similar device), and for those women unable to remain satisfactorily dry with a collection device or pad, an alternative management protocol must be devised.

For those patients with hyperreflexia and high intravesicular pressure, the first line of therapy should be medication to paralyze the bladder and intermittent catheterization to empty it. Occasionally, the patient may be able to void with abdominal straining without causing harmful high pressure voiding (> 60 to 70 H_2O). The Credé maneuver should be avoided, as it is associated with high "voiding pressures." The use of oxybutynin, propantheline or flavoxate will in most cases successfully control the hyperreflexic bladder. Oxybutynin (Ditropan) is the author's drug of choice. The dose must be titrated to obtain the desired response. Typically a patient is started on 5 mg b.i.d. and the dose is increased as needed up to 5 mg t.i.d. or q.i.d. Complete bladder paralysis is the end point of therapy in order to maintain a low pressure system. The patients catheterize themselves, utilizing a clean technique starting with six-hour intervals and adjusting the time between catheterizations so as to obtain approximately 350 to 400 cc with each catheterization. Men can apply a condom catheter in between catheterizations and women can wear an appliance or incontinence pad to protect against breakthrough bladder contractions.

Those patients with hyperreflexic bladder that is unresponsive to anticholinergic medication and who exhibit detrusor-sphincter dyssynergia pose a difficult management problem with respect to obtaining a balanced bladder. Medical ablation of the sphincter can be attempted with alpha blockers and/or antispasmodics such as dibenzyline or baclofen, respectively; however, the success rate is low. Traditionally, male patients have undergone transurethral sphincterotomy, rendering them incontinent, and worn condom catheters to collect the urine. For those patients with the less common detrusor-internal sphincter dyssynergia, a transurethral resection of the bladder neck and prostate can be attempted. The justification for these procedures is that through ablation of the source of obstruction the patient will be able to void successfully and not experience dangerous high intravesicular pressures. Unfortunately, the success rate of transurethral sphincterotomy is not always high. An alternative treatment is partial cystectomy with bladder augmentation using a segment of detubularized bowel. Ileum or colon can be employed. Detubularization is required to obliterate bowel contractions and avoid creation of a high-pressure system.

Paraplegics with Areflexic Bladders

For those patients unable to empty the bladder by abdominal straining, the treatment of choice is intermittent catheterization. A regimen of clean intermittent self-catheterization offers significant advantages over the use of indwelling bladder catheters. Urethrocutaneous fistulas, urethritis, bladder calculi, bladder contracture, urinary tract infection, and urosepsis are more common with indwelling catheters. The incidence of hospitalization to treat these complications is also higher with indwelling catheters increasing the cost of care for these patients.

Patients should be instructed in the method of clean intermittent self-catheterization as well as a program of urinary acidification. Intake should be adjusted to produce a steady urinary output and permit the patients to catheterize themselves on an acceptable schedule.

A certain number of patients will be unable or will refuse to perform self-catheterization. Tapping the suprapubic region or manually stimulating the anal spincter or pulling on the pubic hair will in some cases induce a detrusor contraction. This can be combined with abdominal straining or the Credé maneuver to empty the bladder.

LONG-TERM MANAGEMENT

Patients should remain in spinal care programs during their rehabilitation and recovery. As time passes the nature of the bladder dysfunction may change or complications may develop. There is no universally accepted best method of management. In general, especially in males, indwelling urethral catheters should be avoided. Women tolerate catheterization better than men do, and acceptable external collection devices are still not widely available. Therefore, catheterization is more often the management option employed in women. The decision to perform any surgical procedure, e.g., external sphincterotomy, transurethral resection of the prostate, or bladder augmentation, should be postponed until the treating physician is sure that the results of the spinal cord injury are not transient. This usually means waiting several months to a year before performing any definitive surgical procedures.

One must keep in mind the basic tenets of urologic care: to preserve renal function and to aid in providing an acceptable functional lifestyle. Overall, most patients are managed by condom drainage. Indwelling catheters, mostly in women, and intermittent catheterization are the next most common methods of long-term management. Throughout the intermediate phase of management, patients should be observed for spontaneous voiding.

Once the long term-management strategy has been decided on, the patient should continue to be evaluated periodically. To date, there are no reliable early predictors of future complications. In long-term management, therefore, problems must be identified as early as possible. Patient awareness and teaching are integral to the successful long-term management. They should be instructed to report any changes in their routine or in bladder function. Urinalysis should be monitored on a regular basis. Leukocyte esterase, nitrite, and protein content and pH balance can all be easily monitored at home by dipstick analysis of the urine.

Periodic microscopic examination and culture should also be performed at least every three months and at times monthly, depending on the clinical situation. Assessment of renal function is also necessary. Serum electrolytes, creatinine, and blood urea nitrogen should be checked at least yearly if not biannually. Creatinine clearance should be checked annually, since serum creatinine can be misleading as an indicator of renal insufficiency in spinal cord injury patients with muscle atrophy. The intravenous urogram (IVU) has traditionally been used to assess renal function. Its use is, however, not without complications, and other techniques with less potential harmful complications are now available. Evaluation of renal function with radionuclides offers a useful alternative. ^{131}I or ^{123}I hippuran scans or ^{99}Tc DTPA or DMSA are simple effective tests to assess renal function. A plain film of the kidney, ureter, and bladder (KUB) should be done to check for calculi. When indicated, a renal sonogram, IVU, cystogram, or voiding cystourethrogram can be ordered to further delineate any abnormal finding. A nuclear scan and KUB should be done yearly. Urodynamics are not done routinely. Instead, they are performed if any changes are noted on the routine studies and urodynamic information is necessary to determine proper therapy. Whatever procedures are used and whatever schedule is employed, it is important to continue followup because complications can occur many years postinjury. With more patients surviving longer, continued screening is essential.

SEXUAL REHABILITATION

Erection and ejaculation are both parasympathetic and sympathetic nervous responses. Parasympathetic nerves from S2 to S4 innervate the corpora cavernosa and sympathetic nerves from the thoracolumbar erection center (T11 to L2) contribute to erections. Emission and ejaculation occur through stimulation of the sympathetic nerves from T12 to L2 and pudendal nerves originating from the somatic sacral roots (S2 to S4). Sexual function will depend on the level and completeness of the injury. Suprasacral lesions tend to result in reflex erections but no psychologically induced erections. Conus or cauda equina lesions generally are associated with no erections at all. Emission and ejaculation depend on the intactness of the sympathetic outflow from T11 to L2 and the somatic nerves from S2 to S4, the hypogastric and pudendal nerves, respectively.

Approximately 67 per cent of spinal cord injury patients will have erections, while only about 10 per cent will ejaculate. In most patients it will take up to 6 months for recovery of sexual function. For those patients with satisfactory erections but with retrograde ejaculation who desire children, the semen can be obtained from the bladder. The urine is sterilized and alkalinized and the bladder emptied. After ejaculation the bladder is catheterized and irrigated with buffered medium such as Ham's F-10, and the semen collected and washed for insemination. For those patients unable to have erections or who have a lack of seminal emission, transrectal electroejaculation and glandular vibratory stimulation can be utilized to induce erections and ejaculation. Intrathecal neostigmine injection is no longer used to stimulate erections. Patients with lesions above T6 are at risk of autonomic dysreflexia as a result of the stimulation. Therefore close monitoring of vital signs is especially important in these patients. In patients with retrograde ejaculation desiring children, the semen is collected as described previously. Semen quality is generally impaired, with poor motility being the most common abnormality. There is also a higher percentage of abnormal morphology. This is a relatively new technology and one would expect higher success rates as the methods are refined.

Not all patients are candidates for stimulation. Penile prosthesis, either semirigid or inflatable, offers an alternative therapy for these patients. The procedure is relatively simple and the success rate high and complication rate low.

SPECIAL CONSIDERATIONS

Urinary Tract Infection and Urolithiasis

A general consensus does not exist concerning the use of antimicrobial therapy in the spinal cord injured patient. Most investigators would agree that prophylactic antimicrobials are not necessary in those patients who are catheter free. Some authors do suggest prophylaxis in those patients with indwelling catheters or on intermittent catheterization. However, several excellent large studies have failed to demonstrate an advantage to long-term antimicrobial prophylaxis; therefore, this author does not utilize it. Significant pyuria (> 50 leukocytes per high-power field) and symptomatic bacteriuria—that is, bacteriuria associated with fever or significant symptoms—should be treated with an appropriate antibiotic. Empiric therapy can be started on the basis of the results of the most recent routine urine culture and then adjusted on the basis of culture and sensitivities of specimens sent off before therapy was started.

Bladder calculi cause significant irritative signs and are often infected. In general, they should be removed when detected. For calcification around indwelling catheters, a solution of 10 per cent hemiacidrin in water can be used to irrigate the bladder. One should take care to monitor the serum magnesium in patients undergoing this therapy because hypermagnesemia is a potential complication. For those patients with larger bladder calculi which cannot be irrigated free, transurethral electrohydraulic lithotripsy is usually effective in fragmenting the stone, thus allowing its aspiration to rid the bladder of the fragments. For very large stones or stones not amenable to lithotripsy, open cystolithotomy is required.

Approximately 8 per cent of spinal cord injured patients will develop renal calculi. Recurrence rates are high. The incidence of renal calculi is highest in the first year after injury and higher in patients with bladder calculi. The occurrence of struvite stones is greatly increased in the spinal cord injury patient. Up to 98 per cent of stones in these patients have some degree of struvite as opposed to 15 per cent of stones in the general population that are struvite in composition. The presence of struvite is associated with deterioration in renal function in up to 50 per cent of patients. They are typically infected, usually by urease-producing bacteria, and are associated with chronic urinary tract infection. Because of impaired mobility and calcium resorption the spinal cord injury patient is also more likely to develop calcium stones.

The presence of an asymptomatic stone does not require intervention. However, urinary obstruction, recurrent infection, and renal impairment are all indications for intervention. For those patients able to tolerate the procedure, extracorporeal shock wave lithotripsy (ESWL) offers a nonsurgical approach to elimination of the stone. Alternatively, percutaneous endourologic nephrolithotomy or nephrolithotripsy for renal stones and transureteral endoscopic lithotripsy or removal of ureteral stones are now widely available and are the "surgical" procedures of choice in treatment of urolithiasis. Although the initial treatment of an asymptomatic stone remains conservative, rarely is it justified with the availability of ESWL and endourology to leave a symptomatic stone untreated.

Autonomic Dysreflexia (Hyperreflexia)

More than 80 per cent of patients with lesions above T6 will exhibit signs and symptoms of this disorder. Urinary retention with bladder distention is one of the most common causes of this syndrome. Its occurrence is a medical emergency. Signs and symptoms include hypertension, sweating above the level of the lesion, piloerection, restlessness, anxiety, bradycardia, pounding headache, and flushed face. It is secondary to massive sympathetic outflow. Other urologic causes include catheterization, urinary tract infection, testicular torsion, electroejaculation, distention of the renal pelvis, and urologic procedures. The immediate treatment is removal of the stimulus. In cases of bladder distention, either catheterization to relieve retention or replacement or irrigation of an obstructed indwelling catheter is indicated. The patient should be placed with the head elevated; other potential causes such as fecal impaction should be ruled out. If the patient does not respond to removal of the offending stimulus, pharmacologic therapy is indicated. Rapid decrease in blood pressure can be achieved by continuous intravenous administration of nitroprusside. Alternatively, one can also use hydralazine, ganglionic blockers such as pentolinium and trimethaphan, diazoxide, phentolamine, amyl nitrate inhalation, and occasionally spinal anesthesia. Nitroprusside in 100 mg/cc concentration in 5 per cent dextrose and water offers the quickest response and the best control. Initial therapy with 1 mg/kg/min is started, and the dose titrated to achieve normal pressure. An arterial line or some other method is required for continuous monitoring of the blood pressure.

Phenoxybenzamine, an alpha blocker, has been used in treatment of recurrent autonomic dysreflexia. Pentolinium and mecamylamine (ganglionic blockers) have also been suggested as has guanethidine.

New Treatment Modalities

The artificial urinary sphincter has been successfully placed in patients with spinal cord lesions. In those patients with areflexic bladders and incompetent bladder outlets it has been successfully implanted and used in conjunction with intermittent catheterization. It also has potential as a substitute sphincter for those patients requiring sphincterotomy. Initial problems with erosion at the site of cuff placement have been rectified by design changes. Careful choice of the proper cuff pressure and size is required to prevent complications.

Bladder contraction by selective stimulation of the anterior nerve roots via implantable electrodes is now being performed at several medical centers and offers great promise in the control of bladder function. Inhibition of bladder contractions by nerve stimulation is also in clinical trials and if successful will offer another alternative to pharmacologic manipulation. These methods of extradural nerve root stimulation to control detrusor and sphincter activity are perhaps the most exciting advances since the concept of intermittent catheterization was first introduced.

CONCLUSION

As length of survival increases in patients with spinal cord injury, proper urologic management becomes even more important. As our knowledge of the physiology of micturition extends, we can expect significant advances in treatment methods for the spinal cord injury patient. Further study is needed to identify early predictors of potential complications and bladder function. These, together with the rapid technologic advances being made, will allow these patients to live a longer, more normal life. In the foreseeable future we may be able to override the neural dysfunction by externally stimulating selected nerves, thereby reproducing a normal micturition reflex. We have for the most part advanced beyond the need for urinary diversion, and soon patients may be managed catheter free and without the need for pharmacologic intervention or surgical procedures.

RECOMMENDED READINGS

1. Anderson RU, Hsieh-Ma ST: Association of bacteriuria and pyuria during intermittent catheterization after spinal cord injury. J Urol 130:299, 1983.
2. Barrett DM, Goldwasser B: The artifical urinary sphincter: Current management philosophy. AUA Update Series 5:2, 1986.
3. Barton CH, Khonsari F, Vaziri ND, et al: Effect of modified transurethral sphincterotomy on autonomic dysreflexia. J Urol 135:83, 1986.
4. Bedbrook GM: The development and care of spinal cord paralysis. Paraplegia 25:172, 1987.
5. Bennett CJ, Seager SW, Vasher EA, McGuire EJ: Sexual dysfunction and electroejaculation in men with spinal cord injury: Review. J Urol 139:453, 1988.
6. Berard E, Depassio J, Pangau N, Landi J: Self-catheterization: Urinary complications and the social resettlement of spinal cord injured patients. Paraplegia 23:386, 1985.
7. Chagnon S, Leroy F, Vallee Ch, Blery M: Cinefluoroscopic study of the micturition and cystomanometry in patients with spinal cord injuries. A

comparative study in 50 cases. J Radiologie 66:26, 1985.

8. Chagnon S, Vallee Ch, Laissy JP, Blery M: Comparison of ultrasound and intravenous urography imaging of the urinary tract for investigation of 50 patients with spinal cord injuries. J Radiologie 66:801, 1985.

9. Culkin DJ, Wheeler JS, Nemchausky BA, et al: Percutaneous nephrolithotomy in spinal cord injury population. J Urol 136:1181, 1986.

10. DeVivo MJ, Fine PR: Predicting renal calculus occurrence in spinal cord injury patients. Arch Phys Med Rehabil 67:722, 1986.

11. Dimitrijevic MM, Dimitrijevic MR, Illis LS, et al: Spinal cord stimulation for the control of spasticity in patients with chronic spinal cord injury: I. Clinical Observations. Cent Nerv Syst Trauma 3:129, 1986.

12. Dimitrijevic MR, Illis LS, Nakajima K, et al: Spinal cord stimulation for the control of spasticity in patients with chronic spinal cord injury: II Neurophysiologic Observations. Cent Nerv Syst Trauma 3:145, 1986.

13. Dimitrijevic MR: Neurophysiology in spinal cord injury. Paraplegia 25:205, 1987.

14. Dudognon P, Labrousse C, Lubeau M, et al: Early vesico-ureteral reflux following conus medullaris injury: Case report. Paraplegia 24:194, 1986.

15. Ergas Z: Spinal cord injury in the United States: A statistical update. Cent Nerv Syst Trauma 2:19, 1985.

16. Erickson RP: Autonomic hyperreflexia: Pathophysiology and medical management. Arch Phys Med Rehabil 61:431, 1980.

17. Falls WF, Stacy WK: A prospective analysis of renal function in patients with spinal cord injuries and persistent bacilluria. Milit Med 151:116, 1986.

18. Fellstrom B, Butz M, Danielson BG, Ljunghall S: The effects of methenamine-hippurate upon urinary risk factors for renal stone formation. Scand J Urol Nephrol 19:125, 1985.

19. Gardner BP, Parsons KF, Soni BM, Krishnan KR: The management of upper urinary tract calculi in spinal cord damaged patients. Paraplegia 23:371, 1985.

20. Gardner BP, Parsons KF, Machin DG, et al: The urological management of spinal cord damaged patients: A clinical algorithm. Paraplegia 24:138, 1986.

21. Gocking K, Gebhardt K: Indikation und ergebnisse der transurethralen 12-uhr-sphinkterotimie in der therapie der neurogenen blasenentleerungsstorungen bei querschnittslakmung. Z Urol Nephrol 79:207, 1986.

22. Gosling JA, Dixon JS, Lendon RG: The autonomic innervation of the human male and female bladder neck and proximal urethra: J Urol 118(2):302ff, 1977.

23. Green BA, Eismont FJ: Acute spinal cord injury: A systems approach. Cent Nerv Syst Trauma 1:173, 1984.

24. Green BG, Sloan SL: Penile prosthesis in spinal cord injured patients: Combined psychosexual counselling and surgical regimen. Paraplegia 24:167, 1986.

25. Grundy D, Russell J: ABC of spinal cord injury: Urological management. Br Med J 292:249, 1986.

26. Grundy D, Swain A, Russell J: ABC of spinal cord injury. Early management and complications—I. Br Med J 292:44, 1986.

27. Grundy D, Swain A, Russell J: ABC of spinal cord injury: Early management and complications—II. Br Med J 292:123, 1986.

28. Grundy D, Russell J: ABC of spinal cord injury: Later management and complications—I. Br Med J 292:677, 1986.

29. Halstead LS, VerVoort S, Seager SWJ: Rectal probe electrostimulation in the treatment of anejaculatory spinal cord injured men. Paraplegia 25:120, 1987.

30. Hoffberg HJ, Cardenas DD: Bladder trabeculation in spinal cord injury. Arch Phys Med Rehabil 67:750, 1986.

31. Hughes JT: Historical review of paraplegia before 1918. Paraplegia 25:168, 1987.

32. Kakulas BA: The clinical neuropathology of spinal cord injury: A guide to the future. Paraplegia 25:212, 1987.

33. Lockhart JL, Vorstman B, Weinstein D, Politano VA: Sphincterotomy failure in neurogenic bladder disease: J Urol 135:86, 1986.

34. Lloyd LK: New trends in urologic management of spinal cord injured patients. Cent Nerv Syst Trauma 3:3, 1986.

35. Lloyd LK, Kuhlemier KV, Fine PR, Stover SL: Initial bladder management in spinal cord injury: Does it make a difference? J Urol 135:523, 1986.

36. McGuire TJ, Kumar VN: Autonomic dysflexia in the spinal cord-injured. Postgrad Med 80:81, 1986.

37. Mathe JF, Labat JJ, Lanoiselee JM, Buzelin JM: Detrusor inhibition in suprasacral spinal cord injuries: Is it due to sympathetic overactivity? Paraplegia 23:201, 1985.

38. Maynard FM, Glass J: Management of the neuropathic bladder by clean intermittent catheterization: 5 year outcome. Paraplegia 25:106, 1987.

39. Mohler JL, Barton SD, Blouin RA, et al: Evaluation of creatinine clearance in spinal cord injury patients. J Urol 136:366, 1986.

40. Nance PW, Shears AH, Givner ML, Nance DM: Gonadal regulation in men with flaccid paraplegia. Arch Phys Med Rehabil 66:757, 1985.

41. Perkash I, Martin DE, Warner H: Reproductive problems of paraplegics and the present status of electroejaculation. Cent Nerv Syst Trauma 3:13, 1986.

42. Pietronigro DD, DeCrescito V, Tomasula JJ, et al: Ascorbic acid: A putative biochemical marker of irreversible neurologic functional loss following spinal cord injury. Cent Nerv Syst Trauma 2:85, 1985.

43. Raeder JC, Gisvold SE: Perioperative autonomic hyperreflexia in high spinal cord lesions: A case report. Acta Anaesthesiol Scand 30:672, 1986.

44. Rao KG, Hackler RH, Woodlief RM, et al: Real-time renal sonography in spinal cord injury patients: Prospective comparison with excretory urography. J Urol 135:72, 1986.

45. Rossier AB, Fam BA: From intermittent catheterization to catheter freedom via urodynamics: A tribute to Sir Ludwig Guttman. Paraplegia 17:73, 1979.

46. Ruuter ML: Cystometrographic patterns in predicting bladder function after spinal cord injury. Paraplegia 23:243, 1985.

47. Ruuter ML, Lehtonen TA: Bladder outlet surgery in men with spinal cord injury. Scand J Urol Nephrol 19:241, 1985.

48. Stover SL, Lloyd LK, Nepomuceno CS, Gale LL: Intermittent catheterization: Follow-up studies. Paraplegia 15:38, 1977–78.

49. Talalla A, Bloom JW, Nguyen Q: Successful intraspinal extradural sacral nerve stimulation for bladder emptying in a victim of traumatic spinal cord transection. Neurosurgery 19:955, 1986.

50. Thomas DG: Spinal cord injury. In Murphy AR, Stephenson TP, Wein AJ (eds): Urodynamics, Principles, Practices and Applications. New York, Churchill Livingstone, 1984.

51. Viera A, Merritt JL, Erickson RP: Renal function in spinal cord injury: A preliminary report. Arch Phys Med Rehabil 67:257, 1986.

52. Warner H, Martin DE, Perkash I, et al: Electrostimulation of erection and ejaculation and collection of semen in spinal cord injured humans. J Rehabil Res Dev 23:21, 1986.

53. Wein AJ: Drug treatment of voiding dysfunction. Part I: Evaluation of drugs: treatment of emptying failure. AUA Update Series 7:106, 1988.

54. Wein AJ: Drug treatment of voiding dysfunction. Part II: Drug treatment of storage failure. AUA Update Series 7:114, 1988.

55. Wu Y, Nanninga JB, Hamilton BB: Inhibition of the external urethral sphincter and sacral reflex by anal stretch in spinal cord injured patients. Arch Phys Med Rehabil 67:135, 1986.

56. Wyndale JJ: Urology in spinal cord injured patients. Paraplegia 25:267, 1987.

57. Wyndale JJ: Urethral sphincter dyssynergia in spinal cord injured patients. Paraplegia 25:10, 1987.

58. Yalla SV: Spinal cord injury. In Krane RJ and Siroky MB (eds): Clinical Neurology. Boston, Little, Brown and Co, 1979.

Renal Insufficiency in Patients with Spinal Cord Injury

11

N. D. VAZIRI, M.D. ——————————————————————————————

ACUTE RENAL INSUFFICIENCY IN SPINAL CORD INJURED PATIENTS

Spinal cord injured patients are at increased risk for acute renal insufficiency. A variety of factors can result in acute renal failure in this population. Rhabdomyolysis and shock associated with the trauma leading to spinal cord injury can cause acute renal failure. Hemodynamic impairment associated with sepsis originating from the urinary tract and other sites can lead to ischemic renal injury and acute tubular necrosis. Likewise, use of aminoglycoside antibiotics for the treatment of urinary tract and other infections can produce toxic acute tubular necrosis. In addition, intravascular administration of radiocontrast material used for intravenous urography and other diagnostic procedures can cause acute renal insufficiency. Acute interstitial nephritis associated with the use of a wide variety of antibiotics including penicillin derivatives, methicillin, cephalosporins, sulfa derivatives, as well as many other drugs, can lead to acute renal failure. Similarly, use of various nonsteroidal anti-inflammatory drugs such as salicylates, indomethacin, ibuprophen, and newer agents can impair renal hemodynamics and cause azotemia.

Acute azotemia can occur under three different pathophysiologic conditions: (1) renal hypoperfusion leading to a reduction of glomerular filtration rate and increased tubular reabsorption of filtrate (prerenal azotemia), (2) urinary obstruction (postrenal azotemia), and (3) acute renal insufficiency caused by potentially reversible renal parenchymal injury (intrinsic renal failure), several examples of which were mentioned earlier.

Prerenal Azotemia

Prerenal azotemia is a common form of acute renal insufficiency that occurs in a variety of conditions characterized by renal hypoperfusion. The latter may be due either to a fall in perfusion pressure or to an intense rise in renal vascular resistance (Table 11–1). The associated renal hypoperfusion leads to a fall in glomerular filtration rate and increased tubular reabsorption of filtrate. This results in the retention of nitrogenous waste products (azotemia) and a reduction in urine output. It should be noted, however, that urine output may be inappropriately high in patients with tubulo-interstitial diseases (common in spinal cord injured patients) and various other conditions listed in Table 11–1. Therefore, the absence of oliguria should not be construed as evidence against the diagnosis of prerenal azotemia in such cases. Another frequent feature of prerenal azotemia is reduced urinary sodium concentration (less than 20 mEq/L) and fractional excretion of sodium (less than 1 per cent). This is due to enhanced tubular reabsorption of this cation. Fractional excretion of Na (FENa) can be simply calculated from simultaneous measurements of Na and creatinine concentrations in the serum and spot urine using the following formula:

$$FENa = UNa/SNa \div U\ Creat/S\ Creat \times 100$$

where UNa and SNa represent urinary and serum sodium concentrations and U Creat and S Creat stand for urinary and serum creatinine concentrations, respectively. Once again, the expected low urinary sodium concentration

134

TABLE 11–1. Causes of Prerenal Azotemia

A. Reduction of intravascular volume
  1. Abnormal gastrointestinal losses: diarrhea, emesis, fistulas, drainage
  2. Hemorrhage
  3. Excessive diuresis: diuretics, partial or postobstruction, chronic tubulointerstitial nephropathies, potassium depletion, lithium administration, osmotic diuresis, central or nephrogenic diabetes insipidus, hypercalcemia
  4. Sequestration in third space: ileus, burns, peritonitis, pancreatitis, traumatized tissue
B. Cardiovascular disorders: cardiac failure, pericardial tamponade, massive pulmonary embolism, renal arterial occlusion
C. Decreased peripheral vascular resistance: gram-negative sepsis, vasodilatory drugs, and so on
D. Renal vasoconstriction: prostaglandin inhibitors, severe liver disease, surgery, and anesthesia

and FENa may not be attained in patients with sodium-losing states (e.g., diuretic administration, tubulointerstitial nephropathies, and mineralocorticoid deficiency) despite renal hypoperfusion. This may be particularly true in some patients with long-standing spinal cord injury suffering from neuropathic bladder dysfunction, chronic pyelonephritis, and urolithiasis. Other urinary indices useful in the diagnosis of prerenal azotemia include increased urinary osmolality (> 500 mOsm) as well as urine to serum concentration ratios of urea (> 8) and creatinine (> 40). These indices reflect the rate of water reabsorption by the tubules; this is expectedly increased in the face of renal hypoperfusion. It should be noted that patients with impaired urinary concentrating ability may fail to meet these criteria despite severe renal hypoperfusion. This may be the case in certain patients with chronic spinal cord injury complicated by chronic pyelonephritis and amyloidosis exhibiting urinary concentration defect. Patients with prerenal azotemia often exhibit a disproportional rise in serum urea nitrogen concentration compared with that of creatinine (serum BUN to creatinine > 20). This is due to enhanced tubular reabsorption of fluids associated with renal hypoperfusion in which urea is carried passively from the tubular lumen to the peritubular circulation. Normally, serum BUN to creatinine ratio ranges from 10 to 20 in normal individuals. However, the ratio may be greater in spinal cord injured patients due to lower serum creatinine concentration. The latter is due to decreased muscle mass and the resulting creatinine production associated with muscle atrophy in patients with chronic paraplegia or quadriplegia. This should be considered in the interpretation of BUN to creatinine ratio in such patients. The ratio can be quite helpful, however, when compared with patient's previous values. In contrast to the chronic phase, subnormal serum creatinine concentrations are not observed in the acute phase of spinal cord injury when the muscle mass reduction has not yet occurred. In fact, increased release of creatinine may raise its concentration in patients with rhabdomyolysis associated with the initial trauma or uncontrolled muscle contractions.

Relative increases in hemoglobin, hematocrit, and serum protein values may be indicative of hemoconcentration due to dehydration, while a rapid fall in hemoglobin and hematocrit values may signify internal or external hemorrhage. An increase in serum bicarbonate concentration may suggest contraction alkalosis and points to the prerenal nature of azotemia, since azotemia of other types tends to cause acidosis. However, several exceptions exist, including prerenal azotemia caused by diarrhea that is associated with acidosis resulting from bicarbonate losses. Likewise, prerenal azotemia is associated wtih reduced serum bicarbonate concentration in patients with renal tubular acidosis; this may be relatively common in patients with long-standing spinal cord injury. In contrast, gastric fluid losses by nasogastric suctioning or protracted vomiting as well as excessive alkali intake can lead to alkalosis in patients with established renal failure.

Careful attention to the history and physical findings remains an essential part of the assessment of patients with azotemia. Elucidation of the sequence of events leading to the problem is of utmost value. The presence of thirst, dry mouth, lightheadedness, orthostatic symptoms and palpitation, reduced skin turgor, supine and orthostatic tachycardia and hypotension or blood pressure values less than the patient's usual values, and poor jugular venous filling or pulsations suggest intravascular volume depletion. Likewise, a rapid weight loss may reflect dehydration. In some cases it may be difficult to determine hemodynamic status with certainty using bedside evaluation. More invasive procedures such as measurement of central venous pressure or pulmonary wedge pressure may be required to establish the diagnosis and to guide the therapy in such cases. Prompt recognition and correction of prerenal azotemia is of vital importance, because failure to recognize and correct this situation can lead to ischemic parenchymal injury and acute tubular necrosis, which is a serious condition. Moreover, renal hypoperfusion markedly increases the risk of renal damage associated with nephrotoxic antibiotics, radiocontrast material, septicemia, rhabdomyolysis, and intravascular hemolysis.

Treatment

Treatment of prerenal azotemia depends on the nature of the underlying condition responsible for renal hypoperfusion. For instance, patients with pure volume depletion respond to appropriate fluid replacement and correction of the fluid and electrolyte deficits. Volume depletion associated with hemorrhage can be corrected by packed red blood cell transfusion and normal saline. Intravascular volume contraction due to the sequestration of plasma in the devitalized tissue following extensive burns or crush injury may be compensated for with normal saline. Due to the marked differences in the composition of fluids from various segments of the gastrointestinal tract, proper replacement therapy for dehydration from such losses requires measurement and close monitoring of electrolytes in the serum and sometimes in the fluid that is being lost. As a rule, dehydration associated with normal serum sodium concentration or mild hyponatremia should be initially replaced with normal saline, whereas dehydration associated with marked hyponatremia or hypernatremia may require hypertonic saline or 5 per cent dextrose in water, respectively, as the initial therapy. Subsequently, maintenance fluid therapy should be determined by the nature and content of fluids being lost. For instance, proper fluid replacement for diarrhea is 5 per cent dextrose in water supplemented with sodium bicarbonate 45 mEq (one ampule of 7.5 per cent) and potassium chloride (KCl) 20 to 30 mEq per liter. In contrast, gastric fluid losses are replaced with one fourth to one half normal saline supplemented with 10 to 20 mEq/L of KCl, whereas small intestinal, biliary, and pancreatic losses require normal saline solution. Replacement for losses associated with excessive diuresis should be determined by regular monitoring of the urinary electrolytes. For instance, excessive losses in central or nephrogenic diabetes insipidus require free water with no or little sodium and potassium, whereas postobstructive diuresis or the polyuric phase of acute tubular necrosis often requires replacement with one half normal saline and potassium supplementation. Prerenal azotemia associated with use of prostaglandin inhibitors responds

to drug withdrawal, while that associated with sepsis requires proper antibiotic administration as well as intravenous fluids to support hemodynamic status. Patients with severe heart failure may benefit from afterload reduction and digitalis preparations. However, occasionally cardiac function is so poor that considerable prerenal azotemia may persist despite all available measures. In such cases mild to moderate prerenal azotemia should be accepted as a compromise. Rarely, prerenal azotemia leads to clinical uremia requiring chronic peritoneal dialysis to control azotemia and fluid balance in diuretic-unresponsive patients with advanced stages of heart disease.

The amount of fluids required to correct the deficits in hospitalized patients with prerenal azotemia can be estimated from the intake and output data. In addition, survey of daily weight provides a valuable clue as to the magnitude of fluid deficits. Becasue hasty correction of fluid and electrolyte abnormalities may lead to substantial morbidity and even mortality, caution should be used in determining the rate of fluid administration. As a rule, no more than 50 to 75 per cent of the estimated deficits should be replaced during the first 24 hours. This is particularly true in elderly patients and others with an impaired cardiovascular system. The response to fluid administration should be regularly assessed employing simple clinical parameters including pulse rate, blood pressure, jugular venous pulsation, and heart and lung examinations. The appearance of bibasilar rales and S3 gallop suggests cardiopulmonary congestion and requires prompt cessation or marked reduction in the rate of fluid administration. When vigorous correction of fluid deficits is desired and the status of the patient's cardiovascular tolerance is undefined, fluid replacement should be guided by direct monitoring of central venous pressure (CVP) or pulmonary artery wedge pressure.

Monitoring of CVP is often adequate when rapid fluid administration is indicated in patients without significant cardiopulmonary disease. Central venous pressure ranges between 2 to 12 cm water in euvolemic normal persons and could fall to zero or negative values in volume depletion. A fluid challenge with 200 to 300 ml of normal saline should be administered during the 10 to 20 minute interval before vigorous fluid administration is begun. Ordinarily this causes very little change in the CVP of a volume-depleted subject with an intact cardiopulmonary system. A rise in CVP greater than 5 cm water in response to the fluid challenge is indicative of cardiac insufficiency and calls for prompt cessation of fluid delivery.

In patients with chronic or acute pulmonary disorders, tricuspid stenosis, constrictive pericarditis, pericardial tamponade, and an unstable cardiovascular system, pulmonary artery wedge pressure provides a reliable index as to the left ventricular function and should be used instead of CVP when rapid fluid administration is desired.

Postrenal Azotemia

Partial or complete urinary tract obstruction should be seriously considered in the differential diagnosis of azotemia in patients with acute or chronic spinal cord injury. Various causes of urinary tract obstruction are listed in Table 11–2. Spinal cord injured patients are particularly prone to several types of urinary tract obstruction, the most prominent of which is neuropathic bladder dysfunction. In patients with indwelling catheters, obstruction of the catheter by calcific deposits, purulent debris, and blood clot can cause postrenal azotemia. Bilateral ureteral obstruction by purulent debris and sloughed papillary tissue can cause azotemia in spinal cord injured patients, who are extremely prone to acute and chronic pyelonephritis.[1] Another potential cause of obstruction is urolithiasis, which is quite prevalent in this population.[2-4] Several factors appear to be responsible for stone formation in this setting. These include hypercalciuria during the early phase of spinal cord injury, hyperuricosuria, hyper-oxaluria, supersaturation with magnesium ammonium phosphate associated with urinary tract infection with urease-producing organisms, abnormal urine flow, and reduced urinary excretion of citrate, pyrophosphate, and orthophosphate (major inhibitors of stone formation).[2,5-9] In addition, disruption of the ureters or their occlusion by retroperitoneal hematoma associated with the initial trauma can cause azotemia during the acute phase of spinal cord injury.

In order for obstruction to cause significant azotemia, it must affect both kidneys or a solitary functioning kidney. Consequently, obstruction at the level of urethra or bladder neck or involvement of both ureters or the ureter to the single functioning kidney should be considered. The associated obstruction may be either complete or incomplete. Complete obstruction is manifested by anuria, whereas incomplete obstruction may present with polyuria or fluctuating urinary volume. It should be noted that due to the associated sensory deficits acute bladder distention is usually asymptomatic in such patients.

Patients with urinary tract obstruction may exhibit hypertension. In addition, acute bladder distention may lead to autonomic dysreflexia in patients with spinal cord injury above T7. Acute autonomic dysreflexia can present with severe hypertension, flushing, diaphoresis, pounding headache, cardiac dysrhythmias, and various CNS abnormalities including subarachnoid bleeding, convulsions, coma, and even death.[10-12]

In patients with incomplete obstruction, BUN rises out of proportion to serum creatinine. Consequently, BUN to serum creatinine concentration ratio usually increases above the patient's usual values. This is due to increased tubular reabsorption of urea associated with the obstruction-induced slowing of fluid flow rate in the tubules. It should be re-emphasized that BUN to creatinine ratio is usually higher in patients with long-standing spinal cord injury when compared with able-bodied individuals due to lower than usual serum creatinine concentrations in the former population. Once again, concurrent rhabdomyolysis (which raises serum creatinine) and protein malnutrition or severe liver disease (which reduce BUN) can mask the effect of partial obstruction on BUN to creatinine ratio. In contrast to partial obstruction, complete obstruction with anuria leads to proportional elevations of BUN and serum creatinine concentrations.

Urinary sodium concentration and frac-

TABLE 11–2. Causes of Urinary Tract Obstruction

A. Intrarenal obstruction: uric acid, sulfa drugs, myeloma casts
B. Extrarenal
  1. Intraluminal: Calculi, purulent debris, sloughed papillae, fungal ball, blood clot, tumors and polyps, strictures, trauma, ureteroceles, anterior and posterior urethral valves
  2. Extraluminal
    a. Reproductive system abnormalities: malignant and benign tumors, cysts, pregnancy, endometriosis, ureteral ligation during gynecologic surgery, ovarian and pelvic infections and abscesses
    b. Retroperitoneal: retroperitoneal fibrosis (primary, secondary) tumors, hematoma, urinoma, infection, and surgical disruption
    c. Gastrointestinal pathology: malignancies, chronic inflammatory bowel diseases, pancreatic pseudocyst, appendiceal abscess
    d. Vascular abnormalities: aneurysms, aberrant vessels, retrocaval ureters

tional excretion of sodium (FENa) are generally increased (greater than 20 mEq/L and more than 1 per cent, respectively) in obstructive uropathy. This is due to the resulting impairment of sodium transport in the tubules. However, this is not true during the early phase of acute obstruction when sodium reabsorption is enhanced and the aforementioned urinary indices are reduced. Consequently, acute obstruction may transiently mimic prerenal azotemia from a biochemical standpoint.

In some cases obstructive uropathy leads to hyperkalemic distal renal tubular acidosis. This is due to the impairment of potassium and hydrogen ion secretion associated with defective distal sodium reabsorption. Its indications are hyperchloremic metabolic acidosis and hyperkalemia. Another common consequence of obstructive uropathy is vasopressin-resistant urinary concentration defect. This abnormality is responsible for polyuria associated with partial obstruction as well as postobstruction diuresis.

Diagnosis and Management

The patient should be carefully examined for the presence of bladder distention, which can be further evaluated by straight catheterization. In patients with indwelling catheters the catheter should be tested to rule out luminal obstruction.[13] When there is doubt, ultrasonography can be safely used to detect and localize possible urinary tract obstruction. In addition, radionuclide scanning modalities may be employed to study renal blood flow and to compare renal function on each side as well as to assess the extent of renal parenchymal damage. In most cases the diagnosis is readily made from clinical findings with or without ultrasonography. However, on rare occasions it is necessary to resort to other diagnostic modalities such as retrograde or antegrade pyelography, computed tomography, or magnetic resonance imaging.

Once the diagnosis of obstruction is established, the necessary measures should be taken to restore urine flow as soon as possible to minimize irreversible parenchymal damage. In addition, vigorous antibiotic therapy should be instituted if urinary tract infection is also present. Supportive measures including hemodialysis or peritoneal dialysis should be employed as indicated to control severe azotemia and the associated fluid, electrolyte, and acid-base disorders.

Controversy exists concerning the rate of emptying of the overly distended bladder. Some authors believe that rapid drainage in such cases may lead to a marked fall in the luminal hydrostatic pressure with resultant hemorrhagic cystitis, hypotension, and even shock. However, other investigators note that hydraulic pressure in the distended bladder falls to the normal range with the removal of the first one or two deciliters of urine. Therefore, continued emptying has little effect on the luminal pressure and as such it may not be necessary to employ slow, gradual bladder emptying as previously recommended.

A brisk diuresis often follows the relief of obstruction in patients with postrenal azotemia. This is due to a combination of factors including volume expansion, increased osmotic load (elevated urea concentration), defective tubular transport of salt and water, and vasopressin resistance. In the majority of cases postobstructive diuresis is self-limited (lasting one or two days) and appropriate for the state of volume expansion. Consequently, it does not lead to volume and electrolyte depletion in most patients. However, it is quite severe, persistent, and inappropriate in a minority of patients who exhibit volume and electrolyte depletion if not given proper replacement therapy. This is associated with impaired tubular reabsorption of water, sodium, magnesium, and phosphorus as well as potassium and bicarbonate wasting. In such cases urinary losses need to be replaced with appropriately formulated intravenous fluids. It is often necessary to measure urinary and serum electrolytes every six hours as a guide for the fluid replacement. In addition, body weight and orthostatic pulse rate and blood pressure should be closely monitored to assess intravascular volume and hemodynamic status. As a rule, urine output may be replaced with one half normal saline solution to which sodium bicarbonate and potassium chloride can be added as needed. Magnesium sulfate (2 ml ampules containing 4 mEq of Mg) can be added to the NaCl solution. If preferred, magnesium sulfate may be administered intramuscularly instead. When phosphorus supplementation is indicated, it can be provided using either 42 per cent sodium phosphate or 45 per cent potassium phosphate solutions available in 15 ml ampules containing 45 mmol of phosphate and 66 mEq of sodium or 60 mEq of potassium, respectively. These phosphate preparations may be mixed with either 5 per cent dextrose or one half normal saline solutions and administered intravenously.

At times it is difficult to differentiate continued postobstructive diuresis from that driven by volume expansion associated with fluid administration. In such cases it may be appropriate to lower the rate of fluid administration while closely monitoring pulse rate, blood pressure, urine output, body weight, BUN concentration, and (if available) central venous pressure or pulmonary artery wedge pressure. Continued polyuria despite occurrence of hypotension, tachycardia, reversal of the declining BUN values, and an abnormal fall in CVP or wedge pressure suggest continued postobstructive diuresis. Appropriate fluid replacement should be continued in such instances. In contrast, appropriate reduction in urine output with maintenance of stable hemodynamic status suggests iatrogenic polyuria driven by fluid administration. In these patients further parenteral fluid replacement should be reduced or discontinued.

Acute Intrinsic Renal Failure

Unlike prerenal and postrenal azotemia acute intrinsic renal failure is usually associated with renal parenchymal injury and is not immediately reversible upon withdrawal of the offending factor. However, complete or partial recovery often occurs after variable periods with the reversal of the underlying pathophysiologic process and repair of the associated tissue damage. Acute intrinsic renal failure may result from ischemic insults, nephrotoxic injury, or hypersensitivity reaction (Table 11–3).

TABLE 11–3. Classification of Acute Intrinsic Renal Failure

A. Ischemic acute tubular necrosis (ATN)
  1. Severe volume depletion: hemorrhage, dehydration, cardiovascular collapse
  2. Surgical complications
  3. Trauma, rhabdomyolysis
  4. Septic shock
  5. Severe pancreatitis
B. Nephrotoxic insults
  1. Nephrotoxic antibiotics: aminoglycosides, cephaloridine, amphotericin B, colistin, vancomycin
  2. Iodinated radiographic contrast media
  3. Anesthetic agents: methoxyfluorane, enflurane
  4. Ethylene glycol poisoning (antifreeze)
  5. Cyclosporine administration
  6. Heavy metal poisoning, organic solvents
  7. Anticancer agents: methyl-CCNU, mithramycin, Adriamycin, cis-platinum
C. Acute interstitial nephritis
  1. Drug-induced
  2. Infections
  3. Autoimmunity
  4. Idiopathic

Not infrequently a combination of toxic and ischemic insults is operative in the genesis of acute intrinsic renal failure in a given patient. A common example of such dual insult is aminoglycoside administration in septic patients. Established acute renal failure due to ischemic and nephrotoxic insults is usually, but not always, associated with histologically demonstrable tubular epithelial cell necrosis. Hence, the term *acute tubular necrosis* (ATN) is commonly used to define these conditions. However, other terms including *acute vasomotor nephropathy* (AVN) and *lower nephron nephrosis* have been also used. In the next section those forms of acute renal failure that are more likely to occur in spinal cord injured patients are briefly discussed.

Ischemic Acute Tubular Necrosis

As noted earlier, mild to moderate renal hypoperfusion leads to prerenal azotemia that is associated with no renal parenchymal damage and is immediately reversible upon restoration of adequate renal perfusion. More severe and more prolonged renal hypoperfusion can lead to incipient ATN, in which urine osmolality is lower (300 to 500 mOsm) and urine output is somewhat higher than in the prerenal phase. While incipient ATN is not immediately reversible, it is rapidly reversed (in two to three days) with the restoration of adequate renal perfusion. Further reduction in renal blood flow results in established acute renal failure with histologic changes of acute tubular necrosis. Recovery of renal function in this case takes considerably longer and is related to the severity of ischemic insult and the patient's age and nutritional and metabolic state. Finally, extreme states of renal hypoperfusion can cause partial or complete cortical necrosis. The latter is usually associated with complicated pregnancies (e.g., placenta previa, septic abortion, abruptio placentae), profound shock, overwhelming sepsis, and disseminated intravascular coagulation. The condition leads to partial or complete loss of renal function on a permanent basis. Thus, renal ischemia can result in a continuum of renal disorders ranging from no parenchymal damage to severe irreversible destruction of the kidney.

Because of the high incidence of urinary tract infection, urinary tract instrumentations, infected pressure sores, osteomyelitis, and other infections, spinal cord injured patients are at increased risk of sepsis and associated hemodynamic disorders. In addition, the initial trauma responsible for spinal cord injury can cause hemorrhagic shock and loss of fluids into the traumatized tissue. Moreover, the associated rhabdomyolysis and myoglobinuria can cause intense renal vasoconstriction. These and other events can lead to ischemic acute renal failure in such patients.

Toxic Acute Tubular Necrosis

Despite its small size, the kidney receives a large portion (20 per cent) of the cardiac output and is often capable of generating very high concentrations of toxic drugs and their metabolites. Therefore, the kidney is highly susceptible to injury with various drugs and toxic agents. Nephrotoxic insults can result in acute renal failure, chronic renal failure (e.g., analgesic nephropathy), or glomerular damage with proteinuria (e.g., gold, penicillamine, and so on).

Various drugs or poisons can cause acute renal failure by three different mechanisms: (1) production of a prerenal state by depleting volume (e.g., diuretics, cathartics), increasing renal vascular resistance (e.g., prostaglandin inhibitors), or reducing peripheral vascular resistance (e.g., potent vasodilators); (2) production of intrarenal tubular obstruction directly (e.g., sulfa drugs) or indirectly (e.g., massive uric acid release with chemotherapy in cancer patients); and (3) intrarenal cell injury (e.g., aminoglycosides, radiocontrast media, heavy metals, carbon tetrachloride). A brief mention was made earlier in this chapter of drug-induced prerenal and postrenal azotemia. The following discussion is intended to provide an overview of drug-induced acute renal failure due to intrarenal cell injury. This is of particular relevance in spinal cord injured patients, who frequently require various medications including antibiotics and radiographic studies with radiocontrast material.

MECHANISMS OF CELL INJURY IN TOXIC ACUTE TUBULAR NECROSIS. Nephrotoxic agents may produce cell injury by affecting the plasma membrane, mitochondria, endoplasmic reticulum, lysosomes, or the cell nuclei. Plasma membrane can be affected by different mechanisms, including (1) direct interaction with membrane constituents leading to altered membrane permeability (e.g., amphotericin that reacts with cholesterol present in the membrane to produce aqueous channels, thereby impairing ion transport) or those interacting with pump functions (e.g., heavy met-

als), (2) interference with the enzymatic reactions and loss of enzymatic activity within the plasma membrane as evidenced by histochemical studies and marked enzymuria, and (3) alteration of tubular epithelial cell surface area due to destruction or loss of surface membrane (e.g., brush border), impaired membrane formation, or internalization of membrane.

Mitochondria are among the major targets of toxic insults and are affected by practically all nephrotoxic agents studied. Interference with mitochondrial function may mediate cell injury by limiting the energy supplies (ATP production), generation of free radicals, or impaired heme metabolism.

Lysosomes are the main intracellular site of accumulation of toxic compounds including heavy metals and aminoglycoside antibiotics. It is conceivable, but not proven, that nephrotoxic cellular injury may be in part mediated by either the resultant impairment of normal lysosomal function or release of potent hydrolytic enzymes from the affected lysosomes. The lysosomal changes are particularly striking in proximal tubules of aminoglycoside-treated man and animals who show enlarged lysosomes with formation of myeloid bodies. The myeloid bodies represent enlarged phospholipid-laden lysosomes caused by inhibition of phospholipases by aminoglycosides.

Endoplasmic reticulum is the locus of protein synthesis and mixed function oxidases and is one of the major sites of intracellular calcium sequestration. Therefore, toxic agents affecting endoplasmic reticulum can cause cell injury by either inhibition of protein synthesis or activation of phospholipases (by calcium freed from damaged endoplasmic reticulum) and generation of free radicals. For instance, halogenated hydrocarbons are metabolized by the endoplasmic reticulum to produce free radicals, which are thought to be involved in the genesis of hepatic and possibly renal injury. With regard to the cell nucleus, certain toxic agents may produce cell damage by inhibiting nucleoprotein synthesis.

Drugs Causing Acute Tubular Necrosis

With rapid proliferation and introduction of new pharmacologic agents the number of drugs capable of causing acute tubular necrosis continues to grow. These include nephrotoxic antibiotics, iodinated radiographic contrast media, heavy metals, certain antineoplastic agents, and a group of other drugs and chemicals (see Table 11–3). ATN associated with a number of drugs likely to be used in spinal cord injured patients is presented in this chapter.

AMINOGLYCOSIDE-INDUCED ACUTE TUBULAR NECROSIS. Aminoglycoside antibiotics are widely used in the treatment of infections with various gram-negative organisms. A mild to moderate deterioration of renal function occurs with parenteral use of these drugs in 10 per cent of the treated patients. It should be noted that the incidence of severe acute renal failure requiring dialytic therapy is considerably lower.

A number of factors can increase the risk of clinically significant acute renal failure with aminoglycosides. Long duration and high doses of the drug clearly increase the likelihood of ATN. Likewise, sequential courses of aminoglycoside therapy within days or weeks of each other can cause acute renal failure. Pre-existing renal disease and advanced age are thought to increase the risk of renal failure. Concomitant use of other potentially nephrotoxic agents such as radiographic contrast media, loop diuretics, cephalosporins, amphotericin, methoxyflurane, and clindamycin is also considered to potentiate aminoglycoside nephrotoxicity. Dehydration, circulatory impairment, and potassium depletion are definite risk factors. It is important to note that use of the popular formulas employing serum creatinine level for calculation of aminoglycoside dosage may have grave consequences in chronic spinal cord injured patients and elderly individuals. As noted earlier, because of the reduction in muscle mass and creatinine production, serum creatinine is often substantially lower than expected for the given level of renal function in these patients. Consequently, with use of such formulas, higher than necessary doses may be given, increasing the risk of nephrotoxicity as well as ototoxicity.

The earliest laboratory manifestation of aminoglycoside-induced renal injury is appearance of enzymuria (brush border, lysosomal, and cytosolic enzymes) that may be detected within a day or two following the institution of therapy in nearly all patients or normal volunteers. In addition, aminoglycosides damage proximal nephron and can thereby produce renal glucosuria, tubular proteinuria (increased urinary excretion of beta$_2$-microglobulin), aminoaciduria, and potassium and magnesium wasting. The last may cause profound hypokalemia and hypomagnesemia with the expected biochemical and physiologic consequences. The promi-

nent effect of aminoglycoside-induced injury in distal nephron is impaired urinary concentrating ability with ADH resistance, which appears early in the course of therapy and may persist for prolonged periods.

Considerable controversy exists as to the relative nephrotoxicity of various aminoglycosides. It appears that tobramycin may be somewhat less nephrotoxic than amikacin and netilmicin, which are thought to be as nephrotoxic as gentamicin. However, according to some reports, amikacin and netilmicin may be less nephrotoxic than gentamicin. Due to the severe nephrotoxicity of neomycin, this drug is not used systemically, and caution should be exercised with its enteral use because of its partial absorption through the gastrointestinal tract. With regard to other aminoglycosides, the choice of the agent should be based on the result of antibiotic sensitivity testing.

Clinical Considerations. Demonstrable increases in serum creatinine concentration and decreases in glomerular filtration rate usually do not appear before 7 to 10 days of therapy with aminoglycosides. However, this can occur more rapidly when risk factors are present. It is important to emphasize that patients with aminoglycoside-induced ATN are usually nonoliguric, with daily urine output ranging between 500 to 2000 ml. Consequently, the presence of normal urine output should not be regarded as evidence of adequate renal function. Instead, serial measurement of serum creatinine should be obtained to monitor renal function.

Every effort should be made to prevent this complication. Maintenance of adequate hydration and normal potassium level during therapy is helpful in reducing the risk of ATN. When possible, concomitant use of cephalosporins, loop diuretics, and radiocontrast media should be avoided. The risk of ATN is considerably increased when serum gentamicin or tobramycin peak and trough levels exceed 10 μg/ml and 2 μg/ml, respectively. Therefore, it is important to avoid such concentrations by regularly monitoring serum drug levels and making the necessary dosage adjustments. When antibiotic sensitivity testing indicates that a less nephrotoxic antibiotic may be effective, the aminoglycoside should be replaced by this agent. However, if necessary, the drug should be continued at lower doses or preferably longer intervals. It should be noted that because of aminoglycoside accumulation in the kidney, renal insufficiency may progress despite discontinuation of therapy.

AMPHOTERICIN NEPHROTOXICITY. Amphotericin, a polyene antibiotic, is a widely used antifungal agent with well-known nephrotoxicity. Both the antifungal and nephrotoxic actions of amphotericin are caused by its interaction with cholesterol content of the cell membrane. The cholesterol-amphotericin complexes formed in the cell membrane serve as aqueous channels that allow easy passage of small particles of solutes such as water, potassium, hydrogen ion, and various other solutes.

Amphotericin nephrotoxicity can be manifested by distal renal tubular acidosis, potassium wasting, renal magnesium wasting, nephrogenic ADH-resistant diabetes insipidus, and ultimately renal insufficiency with acute tubular necrosis.

The severity of the associated renal abnormalities depends on the dose and duration of therapy. Cumulative doses of less than 600 mg rarely cause appreciable renal dysfunction, whereas as many as 80 per cent of patients exhibit nephrotoxicity with cumulative doses between 2 and 3 gm. Nearly all patients receiving more than 5 gm of amphotericin show significant renal insufficiency. Although use of mannitol and sodium bicarbonate has been shown to afford some protection against amphotericin nephrotoxicity in experimental animals, their protective value in a clinical setting remains unproven. While irreversible renal failure may occur with amphotericin, complete or at least partial recovery is usually achieved with discontinuation of therapy. Magnesium and potassium wasting readily improve with cessation of amphotericin administration, while distal renal tubular acidosis may persist for many months. Patients receiving amphotericin should be regularly monitored for the occurrence of nephrotoxicity by serial determinations of serum electrolytes and BUN, creatinine, and magnesium levels. Hypokalemia and distal renal tubular acidosis are managed with alkali and potassium supplementation. Likewise, magnesium depletion should be treated with oral or parenteral magnesium compounds. When BUN values exceed 50 mg/dl, amphotericin administration should be stopped if possible and resumed later with improvement of renal function. When therapy is deemed necessary despite occurrence of significant azotemia, alternate-day dosing should be attempted.

Acute Tubular Necrosis Associated with Radiographic Contrast Agents. Deterioration of renal function as a result of the administration of radiographic contrast agents is recognized with increasing frequency. This is, in part, due to increased physician awareness of this complication, to the advent of new imaging techniques (computed tomography and digital angiography), to increased use of the conventional modalities (intravenous urography and angiography), to administration of multiple tests in a short period to reduce the length of hospitalization, and to the aggressive approach used in the management of critically ill patients with multiple risk factors, as well as to the use of high doses to maximize the resolution of the study. The majority of the contrast agents currently available for intravascular administration consist of various salts of the triiodinated benzoic acid. As a result of their low PK values, these salts maintain their anionic form in the circulation and as such are not lipophilic, are not reabsorbable, and are exclusively distributed within the extracellular compartment. They are primarily excreted by the kidney and carry a substantial osmolar load. This is thought to be involved in the genesis of the associated nephrotoxicity. A number of agents have been recently introduced with half the osmolality of the existing compounds and are currently under investigation in this country and abroad. The incidence of nephrotoxicity is thought to be considerably lower with these compounds. Iopanoic acid is a lipid-soluble compound used for oral cholecystography. Although renal insufficiency can occur following oral cholecystography, it is a rare occurrence and is usually associated with the administration of several doses of iopanoic acid.

The degree of radiocontrast-induced renal impairment varies from a mild transient renal failure with normal urine output to a severe oliguric variety requiring dialytic intervention. In the mild and transient variety, serum creatinine rises to its peak value within three to four days following the exposure and returns to the baseline level within one to two weeks. Patients with severe ATN develop oliguria, which appears during the first day following contrast administration and lasts for two to six days. This results in a progressive azotemia which increases in severity within five to ten days and reverses within two to three weeks. In contrast to oliguric ATN of other origins, urinary sodium concentration and fractional excretion of sodium may be extremely low in oliguric ATN caused by radiocontrast material. Another important clinical consideration is the apparent dissociation between urinary specific gravity and urine osmolality. While the osmolality of the urine often approximates that of serum, its specific gravity may be exceedingly high (due to the large atomic weight of iodine). Urinary excretion of various markers of proximal tubular injury, including enzymes and ligandin, increases in patients with radiocontrast-induced ATN. However, these markers are too sensitive and nonspecific and usually appear even in the absence of clinically significant renal impairment.

The reported incidence of clinically significant renal failure following administration of radiocontrast material is less than 2 per cent in patients with no discernible risk factors. However, a number of conditions have been found to greatly increase the risk of radiocontrast-induced ATN. The most prominent risk factor is pre-existing renal disease, the severity of which clearly correlates with the occurrence of superimposed acute functional impairment.

Diabetes mellitus is another important risk factor especially when associated with diabetic nephropathy. It fact, recent evidence suggests that the role of diabetes mellitus as a risk factor is primarily related to the associated renal disease rather than to the presence of diabetes per se. Likewise, old age with the accompanying nephrosclerosis and diminished nephron mass may be a distinct risk factor. Multiple myeloma has been also reported to predispose to radiocontrast-induced acute and sometimes irreversible renal failure. However, the risk is considerably reduced with the use of modern contrast agents and proper hydration before, during, and after procedure. Dehydration is another important predisposing condition, particularly in those with other risk factors such as diabetes, pre-existing renal disease, and multiple myeloma. Administration of large doses of the contrast agents and use of multiple studies in a short period (one to two days) increases the probability of nephrotoxicity especially in the presence of other risk factors. The risk of ATN is substantially increased in patients with prior history of radiocontrast nephrotoxicity.

The pathogenesis of acute renal failure associated with radiocontrast agents is not clearly known and several mechanisms may be involved. These include (1) direct tubular epithelial damage as evidenced by vacuolization, degeneration and necrosis of the tubular cells on histologic examination, and appearance of enzymes and other markers of tubular injury in the urine; (2) intrarenal obstruction by sloughed tubular cells, proteinaceous casts (i.e. Tamm-Horsfall glycoprotein or Bence Jones protein), or uric acid (due to the known uricosuric effect of these agents); and (3) renal vasoconstriction which follows the initial vasodilation and is normally transient (lasting a few minutes) but can last considerably longer in the presence of activated renin-angiotensin system.

Every effort should be made to prevent this iatrogenic complication by observing the following points: (1) All the possible risk factors should be identified and alternative diagnostic procedures used in those at increased risk when possible (e.g., ultrasonography, MRI, and radionuclide scanning). (2) Dehydrating preparatory measures such as routine use of cathartics and overnight fasting should be avoided in high-risk patients. (3) Adequate hydration should be considered using intravenous fluids before, during, and after the procedure when needed. (4) The dose of the contrast agent should be kept to a minimum and multiple sequential studies within one to two days should be avoided. (5) Administration of mannitol (12.5 to 25 gm given intravenously) shortly before or after radiocontrast exposure may afford some degree of protection against severe renal failure in certain high risk patients.

Acute Renal Failure with Topical Iodine Preparations. Excessive use of topical iodine preparations has been reported to lead to acute deterioration of renal function in some patients. In addition to azotemia, the patients may exhibit metabolic acidosis, pseudohyperchloremia, hypernatremia, and hyperosmolality. Hyperthyroidism or hypothyroidism, hypoxemia, and leukopenia may also occur in this condition. Elevation of serum iodine level and history of topical iodine administration confirm the diagnosis. This syndrome may occur in spinal cord injured patients with extensive pressure sores in whom topical iodine preparations are used in cleaning the open wounds.

ACUTE TUBULAR NECROSIS ASSOCIATED WITH RHABDOMYOLYSIS. Rhabdomyolysis and hemoglobinuria can occur as a result of the initial trauma leading to spinal cord injury. In addition, a variety of other conditions including metabolic disorders, toxic insults, various infections as well as pressure necrosis, seizures, and hyperpyrexia may cause rhabdomyolysis in patients with established spinal cord injury. Approximately 33 per cent of able-bodied persons with rhabdomyolysis develop ATN. Although incidence of ATN in spinal cord injury patients with rhabdomyolysis is not known, it is expected to be equal to or greater than that seen in individuals without spinal cord injury.

Clinically, the patient may present with dark-brown urine that tests positive for occult blood with no or disproportionally few red blood cells. In addition, the affected muscles may exhibit pain, tenderness, or swelling. Biochemically, ATN associated with myoglobinuria may differ from that caused by other factors by more pronounced hyperkalemia, hyperuricemia, and hyperphosphatemia. These features are attributed to the flux of potassium, phosphorus, and nucleoproteins from the damaged muscle fibers. Marked initial hypocalcemia and subsequent hypercalcemia have been also reported. The former is thought to be due to the rise of calcium $\times$ phosphate product, which leads to precipitation of calcium in the soft tissues, while the latter is due to the mobilization of calcium deposits during the recovery phase of ATN. According to some authors, the rise in serum creatinine may be greater than usual in ATN associated with rhabdomyolysis because of the release of both creatinine and creatine from the damaged muscles. However, it is not a constant feature of myoglobinuric ATN. Serum levels of creatine phosphokinase (CPK), aldolase, aspartate aminotransferase (AST or SGOT), and lactate dehydrogenase (LDH) rise dramatically in patients with rhabdomyolysis as a result of release of these enzymes from the damaged muscles. Therefore, measurement of CPK or other intracellular enzymes is essential in the diagnosis of rhabdomyolysis. Also useful is analysis of serum or urine or both for the presence of myoglobin. The precise mechanism by which myoglobinuria causes ATN is not known. However, ischemia associated with renal vasoconstriction combined with normal or increased oxygen requirement to maintain inefficient transport function demonstrated in this condition may be involved.

Adequate hydration along with urinary alkalinization using bicarbonate and use of mannitol or furosemide can be effective in preventing ATN in patients undergoing rhabdomyolysis.

PATHOGENESIS OF RENAL FAILURE AND PATHOLOGIC CHANGES IN ACUTE TUBULAR NECROSIS. Several mechanisms have been implicated in the genesis of acute renal failure associated with ischemic and toxic insults. These include (1) tubular obstruction by swollen epithelial cells, necrotic epithelial debris, or myoglobin casts in rhabdomyolysis; (2) back leak of the filtrate through damaged tubular epithelium, thereby negating glomerular filtration; (3) persistent afferent arteriolar constriction and/or efferent arteriolar dilatation leading to a fall in glomerular capillary pressure and net filtration forces (hence the term acute vasomotor nephropathy); and (4) decreased glomerular capillary wall permeability coefficient (Kf). In most cases no single mechanism can fully account for profound reduction of renal function in ATN; instead, several mechanisms appear to be operative simultaneously.

Pathologic changes include tubular cell necrosis and regeneration, loss of brush border, dilatation of Bowman's space, tubular casts, vasa recta hematopoiesis, interstitial edema, and inflammation. These changes are generally mild and scattered.

DIAGNOSIS. Diagnosis of ischemic and or toxic acute intrinsic renal failure requires exclusion of other causes such as prerenal azotemia, postrenal failure, acute interstitial nephritis, renal vascular disorders, and rapidly progressive glomerulonephritis. Close attention should be given to the sequence of events leading to renal failure. Careful assessment of fluid balance and hemodynamic status (as noted under prerenal azotemia) is of utmost value in the diagnosis of ischemic ATN. The pharmacologic regimen used before and after the onset of renal failure should be carefully reviewed for determination of possible nephrotoxicity as well as any need for dosage adjustment of renally excreted or metabolized drugs. Obstruction should be ruled out as previously noted under postrenal azotemia. In addition, chronic renal failure should be excluded as the cause of azotemia in patients whose cases are previously unknown to the managing physician. Several clues may suggest chronic renal insufficiency as a cause of azotemia. These include previous history of hypertension, history of chronic edema, hematuria, polyuria, nocturia and pruritus, presence of renal osteodystrophy, bilateral contracted kidneys, band keratopathy, and carbomylated hemoglobin. The presence of anemia, hypocalcemia, and hyperphosphatemia is of less value in making the diagnosis because these conditions can rapidly occur in acute renal failure.

The finding of tubular epithelial cells and debris, renal tubular cell casts or granular casts—particularly muddy brown casts—is indicative of ATN. However, a relatively inactive urinary sediment may be seen in some cases. Mild proteinuria and occasional erythrocytes may also be present. In contrast, heavy proteinuria and hematuria suggest glomerulonephritis while concurrent nephrotic syndrome and acute renal failure may be related to the use of certain nonsteroidal anti-inflammatory agents. Acute interstitial nephropathy is often associated with leukocyturia with or without eosinophiluria or eosinophilia. A positive urine test for occult blood in the absence of proportional hematuria suggests acute renal failure caused by myoglobinuria, hemoglobinuria, or methemoglobinuria. The presence of large quantities of urate crystals or amorphous uric acid may indicate acute uric acid nephropathy, while the finding of oxalate crystals may suggest renal insufficiency caused by ethylene glycol poisoning or methoxyflurane anesthesia. It thus appears that a meticulous urinalysis can be helpful in the differential diagnosis of acute renal failure.

Loss of urinary concentrating ability is one of the earliest, most consistent, and longest-lasting manifestations of ischemic or toxic acute tubular necrosis. This is evidenced by a low urine to serum creatinine concentration ratio (less than 20), the presence of isosthenuria (urine to plasma osmolality ratio less than 1.1), and urine osmolality less than 350 mOsm.

Impaired tubular reabsorption of sodium and its increased urinary concentration (> 20 mEq/L) and fractional excretion (FENa >1 per cent) remain useful in distinguishing oliguric ATN from prerenal azotemia, in which these indices are reduced. However, they are not of value in the diagnosis of acute renal failure caused by nonoliguric ATN and that caused by acute interstitial nephritis, radiographic contrast agents, severe liver disease, nephrotic syndrome, or advanced heart failure, in which urinary sodium concentration and FENa may be reduced due to relative preservation of tubular transport of this cation.

Urinary excretions of beta$_2$-microglobulin and various enzymes released from the damaged tubular epithelial cells (e.g., ligandin, *N*-acetyl-betaglucosaminidase, lysozyme, and LDH) increase in patients with acute tubular necrosis.[13] In fact, the rise in urinary excretion of some of these markers may precede the onset of renal failure. However, the reported changes are quite nonspecific and can occur under a variety of other conditions. Moreover, the tests are costly and are not readily available for routine clinical use.

Occasionally, the diagnosis of the underlying cause of acute deterioration of renal function remains unclear despite extensive evaluations. Renal biopsy may be necessary to make the definitive diagnosis in such cases.

ACUTE INTERSTITIAL NEPHRITIS (AIN). AIN is a relatively common cause of acute renal insufficiency. Exposure to a growing

TABLE 11–4. Causes of Acute Interstitial Nephritis

A. Drugs (partial list)
 1. Antimicrobial agents: penicillin, synthetic penicillin analogs, cephalosporins, tetracyclines, sulfanamides, rifampin, trimethoprim-sulfa preparations
 2. Nonsteroidal anti-inflammatory drugs: zomepirac, tolmetin, fenoprofen, indomethacin, naproxen, phenylbutazone, diflunisal, mefenamic acid
 3. Miscellaneous: phenindione, warfarin, thiazides, furosemide, allopurinol, azathioprine, phenytoin, cimetidine
B. Infections: diphtheria, leptospirosis, staphylococcal, streptococcal, brucellosis, Legionnaires' disease, toxoplasmosis, mononucleosis, CMV, syphilis, falciparum malaria, and so on
C. Immunologic disorders: systemic lupus erythematosus, Goodpasture's syndrome
D. Idiopathic

number of drugs, a variety of infections, and certain immunologic disorders such as systemic lupus erythematosus, cryoglobulinemia, and Goodpasture's syndrome can cause AIN. In addition, idiopathic AIN has been reported in which no discernible cause can be identified (Table 11–4).

Pathologic features of AIN include the presence of edema and cellular infiltrate consisting of mononuclear cells, plasma cells, eosinophils, and neutrophils. In addition, patchy tubular changes are usually present and include epithelial cell degeneration, necrosis, or tubular atrophy. Occasionally tubular invasion by the inflammatory cells can be seen on histologic examination of the tissue. In addition, granulomatous lesions are rarely found in the interstitial region.

CHRONIC RENAL INSUFFICIENCY

Chronic renal insufficiency is a serious and common complication of long-standing spinal cord injury. In a large necropsy series reported by Tribe and Silver in 1969, renal insufficiency was the primary cause of death in the great majority (75 per cent) of cases studied.[14] In a subsequent report published in 1977 by Hackler[15] chronic renal failure was found to be the principal cause of death in 45 per cent of a group of World War II and Korean War veterans with traumatic spinal cord injury. A preliminary report by Borges and Hackler on a group of Vietnam War veterans appears to indicate further reduction in the percentage of deaths from renal causes (20 per cent).[16] The reported improvement was attributed to the use of external sphincterotomy in the majority of patients in the latter study.[16] Long-term follow-up of a large group of civilian spinal cord injured patients recently reported by Price shows an even greater reduction in renal mortality (14 per cent) as compared with the previous studies.[17] The impressive success in preservation of renal function and prevention of renal insufficiency in this series has been attributed to intensive patient education, prevention and control of infection, prevention of reflux, and most importantly special attention to maintenance of urine flow and bladder drainage.

Pathogenesis

Several processes are usually involved in the genesis of chronic renal insufficiency in patients with long-standing spinal cord injury including chronic pyelonephritis, nephrolithiasis, reflux nephropathy, amyloidosis, and hypertensive nephrosclerosis.[18] *Chronic pyelonephritis* with chronic active urinary tract infection was present and contributed to end-stage renal disease in 100 per cent of 43 spinal cord injured patients reported by our group.[19] A similar observation had been previously reported by other investigators.[14] Infection ascends by way of catheters, fecal contamination, and cross infection with infected pressure sores. The infection is perpetuated by the presence of indwelling catheters, urinary calculi, and impaired urinary drainage. A hematogenous route is also possible considering the associated bowel dysfunction and occasional need for manual control of fecal impactions. The combination of active infection and functional obstruction often leads to vesicoureteral reflux, which further contributes to the destruction of renal parenchyma.

In addition to causing tubulointerstitial injury, *reflux nephropathy* may lead to focal glomerulosclerosis. This presents with proteinuria and contributes to progressive renal insufficiency and hypertension. Although the precise mechanism responsible for focal glomerulosclerosis is not known, glomerular capillary hypertension and hyperfiltration necessitated by progressive nephron loss may be the culprit.

Nephrolithiasis is another frequent finding among patients with long-standing spinal cord injury, particularly those with persistent urinary tract infection. A number of factors are involved in the genesis of this abnormality. Although hypercalciuria due to immobilization is common during the early phase of spinal cord injury, it is usually absent or less pronounced during the chronic phase of the disease. In fact, urinary calcium excretion may be reduced in those with chronic renal impairment probably due to the associated impairment of vitamin D metabolism and secondary hyperparathyroidism. However, we have found substantial hyperoxaluria in a group of spinal cord injured patients with varying degrees of renal insufficiency.[9] The observed hyperoxaluria may be due to increased intestinal absorption of oxalate occasioned by the associated impairment of bowel motility. We have also found a decrease in urinary citrate level in our patients.[9] These observations were subsequently confirmed by other investigators.[5] Reduction in the urinary content of citrate, which is a potent inhibitor of stone formation, may be of significance in the genesis of urolithiasis in this population. However, urinary tract infection—particularly that caused by urease-producing organisms—is the most important factor. Such infections can facilitate formation of struvite stones by providing an abundance of ammonium while greatly increasing the urinary pH. Stasis associated with functional obstruction as well as inflammatory debris associated with active infection further facilitate stone formation. Development of urolithiasis contributes to renal deterioration by producing further obstruction and, more importantly, by complicating the treatment of urinary tract infection. Moreover, sequential studies have revealed a significant fall in renal plasma flow in spinal cord injured patients developing nephrolithiasis.[20]

Amyloidosis is another major factor contributing to development of renal insufficiency in patients with long-standing spinal cord injury. In addition, amyloidosis is the major cause of heavy proteinuria frequently seen in this population. According to the results of autopsy studies reported by Tribe and Silver,[14] 50 per cent of the patients studied showed renal amyloidosis. In a more recent study of 43 spinal cord injured patients with end-stage renal disease, we found an even greater prevalence (81 per cent) of renal amyloidosis.[18] The greater incidence of renal amyloidosis in our patients was thought to be caused by their longer survival occasioned by maintenance hemodialysis enabling the disease to progress beyond that seen in patients who died of renal insufficiency. Infected pressure sores and osteomyelitis, commonly present in this population, appear to be responsible for secondary amyloidosis in spinal cord injured patients. The possible role of persistent active urinary tract infection in the genesis of amyloidosis has been also suspected but has not been proven.

Finally, *hypertensive nephrosclerosis* appears to contribute to progression of renal insufficiency in spinal cord injured patients with renal involvement.[18] This observation underscores the importance of hypertension control in this condition.

Prevention

Chronic renal insufficiency is an entirely preventable complication of spinal cord injury. This is evidenced by the steady decline in mortality from renal causes, which parallels the technical and therapeutic improvements reflected in the data published during the last two decades.[15-17] Measures designed to prevent and control urinary tract infection and provide satisfactory urinary flow constitute the principal approach to preservation of renal function in spinal cord injured patients. When possible, bladder drainage should be achieved by spontaneous voiding without the use of catheters or other appliances. Intermittent catheterization employing meticulous aseptic techniques is the second method of choice when the former option is not feasible. If this is not practical, triggered voiding and condom catheter should be considered for male patients with incontinence. Less desirable measures, including indwelling catheterization, suprapubic catheters, and diversions, should be used if other options are not applicable. External sphincterotomy may be quite useful in lowering the intravesicular pressure and vesicoureteral reflux as well as allowing a catheter-free status in patients with detrussor-sphincter dyssynergia.[16] The procedure has been shown to lead to a balanced bladder in the majority of patients and to reverse vesicoureteral reflux in 40 to 75 per cent of patients with this condition.[16]

Also important is prevention and treatment of urolithiasis. Measures directed at prevention and treatment of urinary tract infection, as well as provision of satisfactory urine flow, are essential in preventing the occurrence of struvite stone, which is the most common type of calculi in spinal cord injured patients. Those with calcium oxalate stones may benefit from reduction in dietary oxalate content, improved bowel care, and pyridoxin supplementation to reduce endogenous oxalate production. In addition, adequate calcium intake can reduce oxalate absorption by chelation of dietary oxalate within the intestine. The patients should be also advised against consuming large quantities of vitamin C, which may serve as a precursor for endogenous oxalate, as well as foods with high oxalate content. The role of citrate supplementation in the management of stone diathesis in spinal cord injured patients has not been evaluated. However, sodium or potassium citrate may be useful in those patients with renal tubular acidosis. Use of a urease inhibitor may be of considerable value in the management of patients with struvite stones. Recently, one such preparation has been marketed in the United States. Careful evaluation of safety and efficacy of this preparation is required in those patients with staghorn struvite calculi.

With regard to amyloidosis, prevention and proper management of chronic pressure sores and the underlying osteomyelitis appears to be essential for prevention of this serious complication. In addition, a number of other major complications including sepsis and cross-contamination of urinary tract and other organs can be avoided with successful prevention and management of pressure sores and osteomyelitis.

Clinical and Laboratory Features

Progression of renal disease results in a gradual decline in excretory and endocrine functions of the kidney with eventual development of end-stage renal disease (ESRD). Impairment of excretory function is manifested by a gradual fall in glomerular filtration rate and the associated progressive azotemia. As noted earlier, the magnitude of elevation of serum creatinine concentration in spinal cord injured patients is considerably lower than the familiar values seen in the able-bodied individuals with comparable degrees of renal insufficiency. This is due to the reduction of muscle mass, which results in endogenous production of creatinine in this population. For this reason the urinary excretion of creatinine is also reduced in spinal cord injured patients. Moreover, serum concentration and urinary excretion of creatinine are lower in quadriplegics as compared with paraplegic individuals with comparable levels of renal function.[21] It should be noted that creatinine clearance (when determined from urinary and plasma values) is not affected by the differences in creatinine production and as such is equally useful in the assessment of glomerular filtration rate in spinal cord injured and in normal persons. However, extreme caution should be used when creatinine clearance is calculated from serum creatinine concentration using either nomograms or mathematic equations developed and widely used in able-bodied populations. We compared creatinine clearance measurements obtained from urine and serum collections with those calculated from serum creatinine concentration using an equation popularized by Cockroft and Gault:[22]

$$Ccr = \frac{(140 - age) \times wt\ (kg)}{72 \times Scr\ (mg/dl)}$$

for men and

$$Ccr = \frac{(140 - age) \times 0.85\ wt\ (kg)}{72 \times Scr\ (mg/dl)}$$

for women where Ccr represents creatinine clearance (ml/min), wt stands for body weight, and Scr represents serum creatinine concentration (mg/dl). In this study, we found that while the measured and calculated values closely approximated one another in the able-bodied group, the latter substantially overestimated the true creatinine clearance in spinal cord injured patients. Specifically, the calculated creatinine clearance overestimated the true value by 20 per cent in paraplegics and 40 per cent in quadriplegics, necessitating the use of correction factors of 0.8 and 0.6 in the respective populations.[21] In contrast to serum creatinine concentration, which is reduced in spinal cord injured patients, urea nitrogen concentration in these patients is comparable with that found in able-bodied persons with the same level of renal function, dietary protein intake, and metabolic states.[23]

URINARY, FLUID, ELECTROLYTE, AND ACID-BASE DISORDERS. Advanced renal disease in spinal cord injured patients often manifests a combination of glomerular and tubulointerstitial disorders.[23] For instance, we have found a high incidence of nephrotic-range proteinuria in those patients with severe renal disease, indicating altered glomerular capillary wall permeability.[23] This was usually associated with secondary amyloidosis and sometimes focal glomerulosclerosis. In addition, some features of tubulointerstitial disease were nearly always present, including polyuria, impaired concentrating ability, impaired sodium conserving capacity, renal tubular acidosis, and sometimes hyporeninemic hypoaldosteronism. The latter is manifested by persistent or episodic hyperkalemia and hyperchloremic metabolic acidosis. With the progression of renal disease toward end-stage renal failure, uremic acidosis with widened anion gap ensues, reflecting in-

sufficient tubular hydrogen ion secretion combined with inadequate glomerular clearance of neutral salts of inorganic and organic metabolic acids. Chronic acidosis, in turn, leads to the consumption of bone buffers and thereby contributes to the uremic osteodystrophy.

Although ability to conserve sodium and water is usually impaired in most spinal cord injured patients with mild to marked renal disease, fluid and sodium overload can occur when glomerular filtration rate is greatly reduced. This can lead to hypertension, cardiac failure, and pulmonary edema.

Normally, urine is the principal route of potassium excretion. In response to the progressive nephron loss, tubular secretion of potassium rises and colonic mucosa begins to secrete potassium into the feces in an attempt to maintain potassium homeostasis. However, in the presence of severe renal insufficiency, these adaptive mechanisms fail to maintain potassium homeostasis, and hyperkalemia ensues. Severe hyperkalemia can occur with less severe renal insufficiency when large amounts of potassium enter the extracellular fluid compartment through parenteral routes (e.g., inadvertent intravascular administration of potassium-containing fluids), or ingestion of large amounts of potassium-containing material (e.g., salt substitutes, potassium-rich foods). Likewise, excessive release of potassium from the intracellular compartment (e.g., severe hemolysis, rhabdomyolysis, ischemic tissue necrosis, hypercatabolic state) can lead to severe hyperkalemia in patients with impaired renal function. Alternatively, conditions capable of adversely affecting renal tubular transport of potassium, such as reduced distal sodium delivery, oliguria, hyporeninemia, hypoaldosteronism, use of potassium-sparing diuretics (e.g., amiloride, triamterene, spironolactone) and prostaglandin synthetase inhibitors (e.g., nonsteroidal anti-inflammatory agents) can lead to hyperkalemia, even in patients with mild to moderate renal insufficiency. Likewise, constipation can contribute to hyperkalemia by limiting colonic excretion of potassium. This is of particular significance in spinal cord injured patients, who frequently suffer from impaired colonic motility and anal sphincter dysfunction, leading to fecal impactions.

Hyperkalemia can lead to severe electrophysiologic disorders resulting in life-threatening arrhythmias, cardiac conduction defects, and cardiac arrest as well as skeletal and respiratory muscle weakness and paralysis. Accordingly, hyperkalemia represents one of the most critical complications of renal insufficiency in spinal cord injured and able-bodied patients alike.

Patients with severe renal insufficiency are unable to fully excrete a dietary load of magnesium. Consequently, hypermagnesemia can readily occur in such patients, particularly when magnesium-containing antacid or laxative preparations are used. Hypermagnesemia is manifested by loss of deep tendon reflexes, skeletal muscle weakness and paralysis, cardiac conduction defect, and depressed mental status.

ENDOCRINOLOGIC DISORDERS. Although the kidney is best known for its excretory function, it has a major role in the endocrine system. The endocrine functions of the kidney are multifaceted and involve production of certain hormones (e.g., erythropoietin, $1,25(OH)_2D_3$, prostaglandins), regulation of hormone production by other glands (e.g., renin-aldosterone system), metabolism and excretion of hormones (e.g., polypeptide and steroid hormones), and serving as a target organ for several hormones (e.g., aldosterone, parathormone, atrial natriuretic peptide, and antidiuretic hormone). Destruction of the renal parenchyma leads to parallel losses of both excretory and endocrine functions of the kidney. In addition, the profound biochemical abnormalities induced by renal insufficiency adversely affect the function of various endocrine glands and alter hormone metabolism. Accordingly, severe renal insufficiency leads to a multitude of endocrinopathies, discussion of which is beyond the scope of this chapter. In addition, spinal cord injured patients with end-stage renal disease show a variety of other abnormalities, including a high incidence of amyloidosis involving various endocrine organs which can further complicate the problem.[24]

HEMATOLOGIC COMPLICATIONS. One of the most constant and disabling consequences of end-stage renal disease is anemia, which is primarily due to erythropoietin deficiency. In addition to erythropoietin deficiency, impaired iron utilization, shortened erythrocyte life span, nutritional deficiencies, and blood loss are also involved in the genesis of anemia in patients with chronic renal failure.[25] In a study of the hematopoietic system conducted by our group, we found more severe anemia and greater transfusion requirement in spinal cord injured patients treated with hemodialysis than those found in their able-bodied counterparts.[26] In addition, we found high incidence of amyloid deposition in the bone marrow of spinal cord injured patients, which undoubtedly contributed to severity of anemia in this population.

The other hematologic complication of severe renal insufficiency is uremic platelet dysfunction, which can lead to a bleeding diathesis. Studies of coagulation and fibrinolytic pathways conducted by our group in patients with long-standing spinal cord injury and end-stage renal disease have revealed numerous abnormalities of intrinsic and extrinsic pathways, antithrombin III deficiency, and decreased protein C anticoagulant activity in the presence of increased protein C antigen concentration.[27–30] In addition, marked alterations were noted in the fibrinolytic system, with greatly reduced tissue plasminogen activator activity.[31] The coagulation and fibrinolytic abnormalities observed in this population point to a possible thrombophilic diathesis. These laboratory abnormalities are of considerable interest in view of reduced physical activity often present in these patients, a factor predisposing to venous thrombosis.

DISORDERS OF BONE AND MINERAL METABOLISM. Kidney is the principal producer of $1,25(OH)_2D$, which is the biologically active metabolite of vitamin D. This hormone is essential for calcium absorption and bone metabolism. Advanced renal insufficiency leads to deficiency of $1,25(OH)_2D$; this in turn results in osteomalacia and negative calcium balance. The latter causes secondary hyperparathyroidism and osteitis fibrosa cystica. Concurrently, impaired renal phosphorus excretion and the resultant hyperphosphatemia lead to soft tissue and vascular calcification. The bone disease is further compounded by demineralization associated with chronic acidosis and reduced physical activity often present in spinal cord injured patients with advanced renal disease. In addition, aluminum-related bone disease can occur in dialysis patients receiving large quantities of aluminum compounds used as phosphate binders to control hyperphosphatemia. Aluminum overload has been also reported in patients dialyzed against dialysates prepared with aluminum-containing water supplies. The latter problem has been solved by the widespread use of deionized water in nearly all dialysis centers in this country. Patients with markedly increased aluminum burden usually have bone and joint pain, pathologic fracture, and severe anemia. In addition, they show an inability to mineralize newly formed osteoid tissue, resulting in hypercalcemia and normal or suppressed parathormone levels. Recently, a peculiar type of amyloidosis involving bone and other tissues has been described in dialysis patients. This is thought to be due to precipitation of beta$_2$-microglobulin in the affected tissue. The disease appears as radiolucent lesions within the bone and can lead to pathologic fractures.

NEUROLOGIC CONSEQUENCES. Both central nervous system (CNS) and peripheral nerves are affected by uremia. Some of the major CNS manifestations of uremia include reversal of sleep pattern, reduction in mental status, astrixis, confusion, and coma. Uremic peripheral neuropathy can involve both sensory and motor modalities. CNS manifestations readily respond to the institution of adequate dialysis therapy. However, once significant uremic neuropathy develops, the response (if any) to dialysis therapy is slow and often incomplete. For this reason, dialytic therapy should be instituted before the occurrence of clinically significant peripheral neuropathy. The combination of uremic neuropathy with the neurologic deficits associated with the spinal cord injury can greatly magnify the patient's disabilities and should be vigorously guarded against.

CARDIOVASCULAR AND PULMONARY COMPLICATIONS. Severe renal insufficiency can lead to fluid overload, congestive heart failure, pulmonary congestion, or edema and hypertension. These abnormalities can be controlled by fluid and sodium restriction, ultrafiltration with dialysis, and use of antihypertensive agents when necessary. Pericarditis is a common complication of uncontrolled renal insufficiency and is usually associated with mild to severe bloody effusion, which can occasionally lead to tamponade. Occurrence of uremic pericarditis signifies the need for prompt institution of dialytic therapy. It should be noted that uremic pericarditis usually responds to the use of adequate dialysis. Not uncommonly, patients receiving adequate dialysis exhibit pericarditis or pericardial effusion that does not respond to further intensification of dialytic therapy. The precise mechanism responsible for dialysis-associated pericarditis is not known. In addition to pericarditis, hypertrophy and/or dilatation of cardiac chambers (particularly left ventricle) and ischemic heart disease are common occurrences in patients with advanced renal failure. In a study conducted by our group,[32] we found some cardiac abnormality in all spinal cord injured patients with end-stage renal disease. These abnormalities included fibrinous pericarditis (50 per cent), left and right ventricular hypertrophy (45 and 20 per cent), left and right ventricular dilation (40 and 30 per cent), cardiac amyloidosis (25 percent), myocardial fibrosis (45 per cent), coronary arteriosclerosis (45 per cent), and a few cases of valvular abnormalities.[32] In addition to pulmonary congestion and edema, which can occur in this population as a result of uncontrolled hypervolemia, a variety of other pulmonary abnormalities have been found in these patients with considerable frequency. These include respiratory infections such as pneumonia, pulmonary interstitial and pleural fibrosis, pulmonary arteriosclerosis, amyloid involvement, and calcification and hemosiderin deposition in the lung tissue.[33]

INFECTIONS. Bacterial infections are extremely prevalent in spinal cord injured patients with advanced renal failure. In fact, chronic infections involving urinary tract, pressure wounds, and osteomyelitis are instrumental in the development and progression of renal disease in this population. In a survey of 43 spinal cord injured patients with end-stage renal failure, practically all patients exhibited chronic active urinary tract infections, many showed infected pressure ulcers, and some had underlying osteomyelitis.[19] In addition, vascular access infection, respiratory infection, peritonitis (especially in those treated with peritoneal dialysis), and sepsis were encountered with considerable frequency. Cross-infection between pressure sores, urinary tract, and blood access or peritoneal access were common. Fever and significant leukocytosis were either absent or disproportionally mild for the severity of the associated infections, and septicemia was the immediate cause of death in greater than 50 per cent of the patients.

In addition to the bacterial infections, various viral infections such as hepatitis B, non-A non-B hepatitis, cytomegalovirus infection, and possibly HIV infection can occur in those requiring frequent blood transfusions for the treatment of symptomatic anemia.

GASTROINTESTINAL COMPLICATIONS. Anorexia, nausea, vomiting, stomatitis, gastritis, and colitis can occur with uncontrolled uremia. These manifestations usually respond to the use of adequate dialysis therapy. Elevation of gastrin level and impaired gastric HCl production are also common in patients with advanced renal insufficiency. We have found a high incidence of amyloidosis involving the liver and alimentary tract in spinal cord injured patients with chronic renal insufficiency maintained on hemodialysis.[34] In addition, iron overload and liver disease associated with hepatitis B and non-A non-B hepatitis were common due to frequent blood transfusions used to control symptomatic anemia. Likewise, the incidence of peptic ulcer disease and cholelithiasis was increased in this population.[34] Other frequent problems include fecal impaction, precocious diverticulosis, hiatal hernia, and reflux esophagitis.[35]

NUTRITIONAL DISORDERS. Many patients with end-stage renal disease exhibit evidence of protein-calorie malnutrition as assessed by various biochemical and anthropometric parameters. The degree and prevalence of protein-calorie malnutrition are even greater in spinal cord injured patients with advanced renal failure than in their able-bodied counterparts.[36] This was clearly demonstrated in a study of dialysis patients with and without spinal cord injury in which the spinal injury group exhibited a greater incidence of suboptimal dry body weight, reduced values of mid-arm circumference, triceps skin fold thickness, serum albumin concentration, serum transferrin level, and total lymphocyte count than did the able-bodied dialysis patients, who generally had suboptimal values themselves.[36] A variety of factors are thought to be operative in the genesis of protein-calorie malnutrition in this population. These include chronic disabling disease state, chronic infections, amyloidosis, anorexia, protein losses in the urine, and prescribed or self-imposed protein restriction. The presence of protein-calories malnutrition in this population may contribute to impaired wound healing and increased susceptibility to various infections. Consequently, every effort should be made to improve nutritional status in this condition.

Management

The approach to spinal cord injured patients with chronic renal disease should begin with identification and correction of any potentially reversible components of renal insufficiency. Such reversible components include urinary obstruction (functional or mechanical), active infection, renal hypoperfusion, severe hypertension and use of various endogenous or exogenous substances possessing nephrotoxic properties (e.g., those causing hyperuricemia and hypercalcemia and such drugs as aminoglycosides and nonsteroidal anti-inflammatory agents). In patients with a significant residual renal function (glomerular filtration rates greater than 10 ml/min), every effort should be made to retard progression to end-stage renal insufficiency. This can be achieved by providing satisfactory urine flow, treatment of urolithiasis, control of infections (including those of urinary tract, pressure wounds, and osteomyelitis), and ensuring maintenance of normal blood pressure and avoidance of nephrotoxic substances when possible. In addition, use of low-protein diet, angiotensin-converting enzyme inhibitors, and certain calcium channel blockers has been advocated to prevent glomerular capillary hypertension and hyperfiltration, which appear to contribute to progressive nephron loss in patients with chronic renal disease.

As noted earlier, the ability of the kidney to conserve sodium and water is usually impaired in spinal cord injured patients with chronic renal disease. Consequently, failure to maintain adequate intake can lead to hypovolemia and increased azotemia as may occur in patients placed on dietary restriction or those with nausea and vomiting, as well as patients with impaired sensorium receiving inferior care or those receiving insufficient nutrition. Likewise, conditions leading to unusual losses of sodium and water can produce severe volume depletion and deterioration of renal function. These include gastrointestinal losses (e.g., diarrhea, vomiting, and fistulas) increased insensible losses (e.g., fever and a hot environment), bleeding or fluid losses from the wounds and enhanced renal losses (e.g., diuretic therapy, osmotic diuresis such as that seen with hyperglycemia or following use of radiocontrast agents and post-obstructive diuresis). Under such circumstances, the intercurrent process should be promptly identified and corrected, hemodynamic indices should be monitored, and careful fluid and electrolyte replacements should be instituted as soon as possible. It is important to note that in spite of the inability to conserve salt and water, patients with advanced renal insufficiency often show reduced capacity to excrete large sodium and water loads. Accordingly, various clinical and hemodynamic parameters should be closely watched during fluid replacement to avoid iatrogenic hypervolemia and pulmonary edema.

When glomerular filtration falls irreversibly below 8 to 10 ml/min, one of the renal replacement modalities should be considered. These include hemodialysis, peritoneal dialysis, and renal transplantation. Published data on the use of dialytic modalities in spinal cord injured patients are limited, and information concerning renal transplantation in this population is practically nonexistent.

HEMODIALYSIS. With the use of dialytic modalities, mortality from acute renal failure can be considerably reduced and death as a direct consequence of end-stage renal disease can be prevented in the general population. For the most part these observations hold true in spinal cord injury patients with renal insufficiency. It should be noted that due to the presence of chronic active infections, amyloidosis, malnutrition and poor general condition, survival time of spinal cord injured patients (particularly quadriplegics) on maintenance dialysis is significantly shorter than that observed in able-bodied patients.[37,38] However, the author believes that spinal cord injured patients can do reasonably well on maintenance dialysis and should not be denied the use of this life-saving therapeutic modality.[39]

Blood Access. Like all extracorporeal systems, hemodialysis requires a ready access to the patient's bloodstream. Access to the bloodstream can be achieved in a variety of ways, selection of which depends on several considerations. For instance, a short-term or temporary access is appropriate for patients with acute renal failure expected to regain kidney function within a short period. Alternatively, temporary access can be used in patients with end-stage renal failure needing dialysis while awaiting placement or maturation of a long-term blood access or peritoneal dialysis access.

A variety of single- or double-lumen catheters are currently available for placement in femoral, subclavian, or jugular veins to provide temporary access to the bloodstream. Newly developed subclavian catheters equipped with a Dacron cuff placed in a subcutaneous tunnel can be kept in place for several weeks. Major complications of transcutaneous catheters include hemorrhage, thrombosis, and infection. In addition, hemothorax, mediastinal hematoma, pneumothorax, pneumomediastinum, and subclavian vein stricture can occur with subclavian catheters.

External arteriovenous shunts, which were commonly used as a blood access for acute and chronic hemodialysis during the early years after the introduction of hemodialysis, are seldom used at the present time. This is because of the high risk of infection, thrombosis, and severe blood loss associated with accidental or suicidal separation of the arterial and venous cannulas with the external shunts. Instead, a variety of surgically created internal arteriovenous communications are presently used in patients with chronic renal insufficiency. These include arteriovenous fistulas, saphenous vein grafts, bovine carotid artery grafts, and those made of polytetrafluoroethylene (PTFE). The internal blood access devices are placed subcutaneously in either upper or lower extremities and occasionally in the thoracic area. The access is cannulated with each dialysis using large needles. Infection and thrombosis, although less common than external shunts, constitute the main complications of the internal access sites as well. Likewise, hematoma, aneurysm, and pseudoaneurysm formation as well as rupture at the weakened or infected sites can occasionally occur in patients with the internal blood access. Strict aseptic measures should be taken to avoid infection, which can lead to sepsis, endocarditis, and/or loss of the access site. We have seen cross-infection of blood accesses by organisms infecting pressure sores in spinal cord injured patients with some frequency.[19,40] These observations underscore the importance of meticulous care of the blood access in this population.

Dialysates and Delivery Systems. Practically all dialysates used for hemodialysis are prepared in the dialysis facilities using one of several commercially available electrolyte concentrates and deionized water to produce a physiologic solution with the desired composition and osmolality. This is accomplished by either central delivery system, which supplies all dialysis stations with the same dialysate, or individual proportioning machines, which provide freedom to make adjustments in dialysate composition on the basis of individual patient needs.

With either of these delivery systems, large volumes (about 140 L) of dialysate are delivered during the course of a single dialysis treatment. In contrast, only a small volume of dialysate (about 5 L) is needed with dialysate-regenerating systems, in which dialysate is regenerated by certain columns that adsorb or otherwise eliminate the waste products removed from the patient.

Nearly all hemodialysis solutions used employ either acetate or bicarbonate as their principal buffer. Although it is generally well-tolerated, use of acetate-buffered dialysate is associated with a mild reduction in arterial oxygen tension (Pao_2) as well as occasional instances of hypotension and hemodynamic instability. In contrast, bicarbonate-buffered dialysate minimizes the dialysis-induced hypoxemia and affords greater hemodynamic stability. However, bicarbonate-buffered dialysates are costly and require additional machinery and maintenance work (because of deposition of calcium carbonate within the delivery system). Owing to these economic and technical drawbacks, replacement of acetate dialysates by bicarbonate dialysates has not been widely implemented.

Potassium concentration in the dialysate can be adjusted between zero to 4 mEq/L on the basis of the patient's serum level, dietary intake, and fecal and urinary excretion of potassium. As a rule, dialysates with low-potassium concentration are used in patients exhibiting marked hyperkalemia in predialysis samples. Extreme caution should be used in patients receiving digitalis preparation to avoid life-threatening cardiac dysrhythmias resulting from dialysis-induced hypokalemia.

Calcium concentration in dialysates used by most centers is about 3.5 mEq/L, which considerably exceeds plasma concentration of diffusible calcium. This results in a net transfer of calcium to the blood compartment, which helps to combat negative calcium balance commonly present in uremia. It should be noted that a lower calcium dialysate should be used in hypercalcemic patients. In addition, a lower dialysate calcium concentration should be used in patients treated with $1,25(OH)D_2$, who should receive an increased oral calcium supplement instead.

Hemodialysis Membranes. A variety of materials are used in production of hemodialysis membranes. Many of the currently available dialyzers are made of cellulose derivative such as cuprammonium cellulose (cuprophane), cellulose acetate, and regenerated cellulose membranes. Other dialyzers are made of different synthetic polymers such as polyacrylonitril (PAN) and polysulfon membranes, which possess greater permeability characteristics.

Dialyzers are classified on the basis of the chemical nature of their membrane as well as the physical configuration of the membrane (e.g., parallel plate, hollow fiber, and coil dialyzers). Various dialysis membranes differ from one another with respect to their permeability characteristics and hydraulic conductivity as well as their biocompatibility. For instance, cellulosic membranes, particularly those made of cuprophane, show greater evidence of complement activation with resultant pulmonary leukostasis and transient leukopenia than do those made of PAN, which do not produce leukopenia. It appears that while PAN membranes also activate complement system they avidly adsorb the active components. Consequently, pulmonary leukostasis, leukopenia, and other systemic consequences of complement activation do not occur during dialysis with PAN dialyzers. For this reason, polyacrylonitril dialyzers are considered the most desirable products currently available from both the permeability and biocompatibility standpoints. However, widespread use of these dialyzers has been limited by their prohibitive cost.

PERITONEAL DIALYSIS. Before the advent of indwelling peritoneal catheters, peritoneal dialysis was used only as a temporary modality in the treatment of acute renal failure. However, during the past decade peritoneal dialysis has emerged as one of the major therapeutic modalities for the treatment of end-stage renal disease.

Several different types of peritoneal dialysis have been introduced for long-term management of advanced renal failure. These include intermittent peritoneal dialysis (IPD) using automated delivery systems, continuous ambulatory peritoneal dialysis (CAPD), and continuous cycling peritoneal dialysis (CCPD). Published data on the use of peritoneal dialysis in spinal cord injured patients are limited. We have reported the experience with intermittent peritoneal dialysis in a group of spinal cord injured patients with end-stage renal disease.[41] On the basis of our experience, long-term use of IPD resulted in comparable control of azotemia and fluid, electrolyte, and acid-base disturbances when compared with hemodialysis. Moreover, patients exhibited a greater hemodynamic stability than that observed during hemodialysis. However, serum albumin concentration was considerably lower (due to protein losses with peritoneal dialysis) than that observed during treatment with hemodialysis. This is a well-recognized consequence of peritoneal dialysis and can potentially compound the underlying protein-calorie malnutrition that is frequently present in spinal cord injured patients with advanced renal insufficiency.

The other major complication of peritoneal dialysis is peritonitis. The incidence of peritonitis in patients treated by our group using IPD averaged 0.9 episodes per 100 patient/days of treatment, which was comparable with the results obtained by others in able-bodied individuals at that time. The majority of the peritonitis episodes responded to the use of appropriate antibiotics administered intraperitoneally and/or systemically. Interestingly, peritoneal infection appeared to have been caused by organisms found in the pressure sore or urinary tract, in some cases indicating cross-contamination.[19,41] In recent years use of IPD has been almost completely abandoned and has been replaced by newer, more desirable modalities (i.e., CAPD and CCPD).

With the steady improvement in the design, placement, and care of the peritoneal catheters, use of more effective aseptic procedures, and improved connection technology, the incidence of peritonitis has markedly decreased in patients maintained on CAPD and CCPD. Unfortunately, no data are presently available on the use of CAPD and CCPD in spinal cord injury patients. However, the author believes that CCPD may prove highly effective in selected spinal cord injured patients since peritoneal irrigation is carried out at night during sleeping hours automatically as programmed by the cycler system, thereby minimizing the risk of contamination associated with multiple connection/disconnection steps required for CAPD.

In general, several issues are of interest with regard to the use of peritoneal dialysis in spinal cord injured patients:

1. As noted earlier, protein loss associated with peritoneal dialysis compounds the pre-existing protein-calorie malnutrition which is prevalent in this population. Consequently, close attention should be paid to patients' dietary intakes to correct nutritional deficiencies.

2. The observation that organisms infecting pressure sores and the urinary tract can contaminate the peritoneal cavity via PD catheter underscores the importance of meticulous use of aseptic measures, prevention of pressure sores, proper management of urinary tract infections, and appropriate handling of suprapubic or indwelling urethral catheters, if present.

3. Many able-bodied individuals treated with CAPD exhibit basilar rales and atelectasis resulting from the upward pressure on the diaphragm by the instillation of dialysate in the abdominal cavity.[42] Moreover, in a study of respiratory system by our group, we found a high incidence of acute and chronic pulmonary disorders in a group of spinal cord injured patients with advanced renal disease.[33] Therefore, instillation of large volumes of peritoneal dialysate may compromise respiratory function in this population with already diminished respiratory reserve. In such circumstances, the cycler system can be programmed to reduce the volume and increase the frequency of exchanges with shorter dwell times.

4. High concentrations of glucose are used to provide the osmotic force for ultrafiltration in peritoneal dialysis. Partial absorption of glucose from the peritoneal cavity can lead to hyperglycemia during the procedure and occasionally reactive hypoglycemia within a few hours thereafter. This issue is of some interest in view of the reported high incidence of glucose intolerance among spinal cord injured patients.[43]

5. Fecal impaction, impaired intestinal motility, and abdominal muscle weakness, often present in spinal cord injured patients, can occasionally interfere with peritoneal dialysis, which itself can produce gastrointestinal disorders.[44] For instance, incomplete drainage of dialysate and/or suboptimal solute clearances may occur in such cases. This requires proper bowel care and positional changes.

DIETARY CONSIDERATIONS. The primary objective of the dietary regimen in spinal cord injured patients receiving long-term dialysis is to provide adequate nutrition while preventing fluid overload hypertension, hyperkalemia, and hyperphosphatemia.

With the use of adequate dialysis therapy, no protein restriction is usually needed. Hemodialysis patients can attain positive nitrogen balance with a protein intake of 1 gm/kg/day containing 80 per cent high-quality proteins. Many patients fail to consume sufficient protein in their diet and as such sustain a negative nitrogen balance. This can be readily ascertained by the finding of unusually low predialysis BUN values. Such patients should be encouraged to increase their protein intake or should be given one of the commercially available protein supplements specially formulated for use in dialysis patients. This is particularly relevant in spinal cord injured patients with end-stage renal disease, who often exhibit protein-calorie malnutrition.

A sodium intake of 2 gm per day is usually enough to control excessive thirst, hypervolemia, and hypertension in most dialysis patients while maintaining reasonable palatability. However, it should be noted that, because of the predominance of tubular injury, certain dialysis-dependent patients with end-stage renal disease excrete substantial quantities of sodium, water, and potassium in the urine despite negligible residual renal function. We have observed many such cases among the spinal cord injury patients and only a few among their able-bodied counterparts. These patients usually show little if any increase in body weight between dialysis treatments and as such should not be placed on strict sodium and fluid restriction.

Fluid intake in dialysis patients with little or no urine output should be restricted to about 1000 ml per 24 hours. Since the insensible losses (500 to 600 ml/day) are canceled by the metabolic production of water and water content of various foods, a fluid restriction of 1000 ml/24 hours limits the interdialytic weight gain to about 1 kg/day in anuric patients. This is generally well-tolerated in patients receiving hemodialysis three times weekly. Patients consuming large amounts of salt experience difficulty in restraining their thirst and complying with the prescribed fluid restriction. This underscores the importance of compliance with sodium restriction in dialysis patients. In patients with daily urine output exceeding 100 ml/24 hours, daily fluid intake can be increased by an amount equal to the daily urine output.

In most dialysis patients a potassium restriction of 60 to 80 mEq per day is sufficient to prevent significant hyperkalemia without rendering the diet too unpalatable. The rate of potassium removal by hemodialysis can be enhanced by reducing its concentration in the dialysate. However, this may be hazardous in patients receiving digitalis preparations because dialysis-induced hypokalemia can lead to life-threatening arrhythmias in such patients. Accordingly, dialysate concentration of potassium should not be less than 2 mEq/L and strict compliance with dietary potassium should be enforced in patients receiving digitalis preparations. As noted earlier, proper bowel function is highly important for potassium homeostasis in patients with renal failure in whom fecal potassium excretion by colon is greatly magnified.

Phosphate retention and hyperphosphatemia play a major role in the disturbance of calcium, vitamin D, and parathormone metabolism, renal osteodystrophy, and soft-tissue calcification in patients with chronic renal failure. Dietary phosphate intake should be restricted to about 0.8 gm per day. Foods with very high phosphorus content such as chocolate, dairy products, nuts, legumes, and whole grains should be avoided when possible. Generally, removal by regular dialysis and dietary restriction are insufficient to prevent phosphate retention and use of a phosphate binder is invariably required.

A number of other considerations should be given in patients treated with CAPD:

1. Due to the continuous nature of dialysis, with this procedure marked fluctuations in the volume and chemical composition of body fluids occurring with intermittent dialysis are not seen. Consequently, a more liberal dietary intake can be allowed in such patients.

2. Peritoneal dialysis results in significant protein losses averaging 9 gm per day. These losses can increase by several times in the presence of peritonitis. Consequently, a higher protein intake may be required to maintain neutral or positive nitrogen balance in CAPD patients. A daily protein intake of 1.2 gm/kg or use of protein supplements in those who cannot attain that type of intake appears to be adequate in most patients.

3. Approximately 60 to 70 per cent of glucose present in the peritoneal dialysate is usually absorbed in patients undergoing peritoneal dialysis supplying an average of 200 gm of glucose per day. Besides the unintended oversupply of calories that can lead to obesity, the flux of a huge glucose load contributes to a marked increase in serum level of triglyceride-rich very low-density lipoproteins (VLDL). For these reasons it is appropriate to reduce dietary intake of carbohydrates, cholesterol, and saturated fats in CAPD patietns.

ROUTINE MEDICATIONS. All patients undergoing long-term dialysis should receive a daily *multivitamin* preparation and *folic acid* supplement (1 mg/day) to prevent deficiency states associated with dietary restrictions and removal by dialysis. In addition, a phosphate-binding preparation almost invariably must be taken with meals to minimize phosphate absorption and hyperphosphatemia. Aluminum carbonate and aluminum hydroxide are among the most commonly used phosphate binders. However, with increasing awareness of the devastating consequences of aluminum toxicity in chronic dialysis patients, considerable interest has been given to the use of other phosphate binders. Calcium carbonate has been suggested as a possible alternative. However, when used in quantities required to control hyperphosphatemia, calcium carbonate may produce hypercalcemia, which combined with hyperphosphatemia can promote soft tissue and vascular calcification. In an attempt to minimize both risks, many nephrologists prescribe calcium carbonate and aluminum carbonate together, allowing considerable reduction in the amount of each preparation compared with that needed when only one of the two is utilized.

Other medications frequently used in chronic dialysis patients include iron preparations and various antihypertensive drugs. With the recent release of recombinant erythropoietin, regular administration of this hormone has become a routine procedure in this population.

PHARMACOLOGIC CONSIDERATIONS. Spinal cord injured patients with advanced renal disease often exhibit a variety of concurrent acute and chronic illnesses that require use of various medications. A multitude of pathophysiologic conditions present in this population, individually or in combination, can greatly alter the metabolism of many pharmacologic agents. For instance, bioavailability of drugs can be affected by altered motility and absorptive capacity of the gastrointestinal tract caused by spinal cord injury, uremia, and amyloidosis, which is prevalent in this population. Likewise, the apparent volume distribution of drugs can be influenced by the presence of edema, volume contraction, and changes of plasma protein concentration. Hypoalbuminemia, often present in this setting, can markedly affect the pharmacologic activity and degradation rate of protein-bound agents. The presence of renal disease can profoundly alter the duration of action and concentration half-life (t 1/2) of drugs that depend on the kidney for their elimination.

Moreover, uremia per se can alter protein-binding characteristics, apparent volume of distribution, and pharmacologic or biological activities of certain medications. For instance, the metabolic biotransformation of drugs that are metabolized by reduction, hydrolysis (esters or peptides), or acetylation is retarded by renal insufficiency. In contrast, the half-life of drugs that depend on hepatic microsomal oxidation for their metabolism is unaltered in uremia.

Another variable of potential importance in drug metabolism and activity is the amount of adipose tissue, lean tissue, and bone mass relative to total body weight which can be affected by the associated paralysis. In addition, concurrent use of several drugs, quite common in this population, can produce drug interactions and metabolic interferences. For instance, heparin used as the anticoagulant during hemodialysis can alter protein binding characteristics of several drugs. Dialysis itself can remove substantial amounts of drugs with relatively small molecular size (< 500 daltons), and limited or no protein-binding capacity. In contrast, large molecular sized drugs, those with high protein or tissue binding capacity, and water-insoluble agents are not appreciably removed by conventional dialysis. It should be noted that, in addition to these factors, the rate of drug removal during dialysis can vary on the basis of blood drug concentration, blood and dialysate flow rates, and the porosity of the membrane used. Accordingly, different artificial membranes and peritoneal membranes have different permeability characteristics.

Therefore, it is clear that because of the multitude of variables involved each spinal cord injury patient with advanced renal disease treated with one of the dialytic modalities represents a unique model from the pharmacologic-pharmacodynamic standpoint. Accordingly, not only is such a patient distinct from his able-bodied counterpart with or without renal failure but also from other spinal cord injury patients depending on the level of injury and its duration, nutritional status, presence or absence of renal disease or amyloidosis, concurrent medication, and type and frequency of dialysis if any. Substantial information is available on the effect of renal insufficiency and various dialysis modalities on metabolism of many drugs in the able-bodied population.[45,46] Unfortunately, pharmacodynamic studies in this population are limited and, not surprisingly, the available studies have revealed considerable heterogeneity among those studied. The matter is even more complicated in cases of spinal cord injured patients with end-stage renal disease on whom practically no pharmacodynamic studies have been performed. Practitioners have employed various formulas, including guidelines established for drug use in able-bodied persons with renal disease off and on dialysis, to estimate the initial drug dosage. The proper frequency and dosage is subsequently determined by close monitoring of the drug level or its pharmacologic effects or both. The lack of vital information in this area clearly points to the need for systematic investigation of pharmacology and pharmacodynamics in this population.

REFERENCES

1. Grundy DJ, Rainford DJ, Silver JR: The occurrence of acute renal failure in patients with neuropathic bladders. Paraplegia 20:35, 1982.
2. Burr RG: Calculosis in paraplegia. Intl Rehab Med 3:162, 1981.
3. DeVivo MJ, Fine PR, Cutter GR, Maetz HM: The risk of renal calculi in spinal cord injury patients. J Urol 131:857, 1984.
4. Nikakhtar B, Vaziri ND, Khonsari F, et al: Urolith-

iasis in patients with spinal cord injury. Paraplegia 19:363, 1981.

5. Burr RG, Nuseibeh I, Abiaka CD: Biochemical studies in paraplegic renal stone patients. 2. Urinary excretion of citrate, inorganic pyrophosphate, silicate and urate. Br J Urol 57:275, 1985.

6. Burr RG, Nuseibeh I: Biochemical studies in paraplegic renal stone patients. 1. Plasma biochemistry and urinary calcium and saturation. Br J Urol 57:269, 1985.

7. Freeman LW: The metabolism of calcium in patients with spinal cord injury. Ann Surg 129:177, 1949.

8. Minaire P, Pilonchery G, Leriche A: Hyperuricosuria and urinary lithiasis in paraplegics. Semaine des Hôpitaux de Paris 57:1409, 1981.

9. Vaziri ND, Nikakhtar B, Gordon S: Hyperoxaluria in chronic renal disease associated with spinal cord injury. Paraplegia 20:48, 1982.

10. Comarr AE: Autonomic dysreflexia (hyperreflexia). J Am Paraplegia Soc 7:53, 1984.

11. Linden R, Joiner E, Freehafer AA, et al: Incidence and clinical features of autonomic dysreflexia in patients with spinal cord injury. Paraplegia 18:285, 1980.

12. Perkash I: Problems of decatheterization. J Urol 124:249, 1980.

13. Vaziri ND, Kaupke J: Biochemical investigations of urine. In Masry S, Glassock R (eds): Textbook of Nephrology. Baltimore, Williams & Wilkins Co., 1988.

14. Tribe CR, Silver JR: Renal failure in paraplegia. London, Pitman Medical, 1969, pp 13–89.

15. Hackler RH: A 25-year prospective mortality study in the spinal cord injured patient: Comparison with the long-term living paraplegic. J Urol 117:486, 1977.

16. Borges PM, Hackler RH: The urologic status of the Vietnam war paraplegic: A 15-year prospective follow-up. J Urol 127:710, 1982.

17. Price M: Some results of a fifteen year vertical study of urinary tract function in spinal cord injured patients: A preliminary report. J Am Paraplegia Soc 5:31, 1982.

18. Barton CH, Vaziri ND, Gordon S, Tilles S: Renal pathology in end-stage renal disease associated with paraplegia. Paraplegia 22:31, 1984.

19. Vaziri ND, Cesario T, Mootoo K, et al: Bacterial infections in patients with chronic renal failure: Occurrence with spinal cord injury. Arch Intern Med 42:1273, 1982.

20. Kuhlemeier KV, Huang LLK, Fine PR, Stover SL: Effective renal plasma flow: Clinical significance after spinal cord injury. J Urol 133:158, 1985.

21. Mirahmadi MK, Byrne C, Barton CH, et al: Prediction of creatinine clearance from serum creatinine in spinal cord injury patients. Paraplegia 21:23, 1983.

22. Cockroft DW, Gault MH: Prediction of creatinine clearance from serum creatinine. Nephron 16:31, 1976.

23. Vaziri ND, Bruno A, Mirahmadi MK, et al: Features of residual renal function in end-stage renal failure associated with spinal cord injury. Int J Artif Organs 7:319, 1984.

24. Barton CH, Vaziri ND, Gordon S, Eltorai I: Endocrine pathology in spinal cord injured patients on maintenance dialysis. Paraplegia 22:7, 1984.

25. Vaziri ND: Anemia in ESRD patients. In Nissenson AR, Fine RN (eds): Current Dialysis Therapy. Philadelphia, Hanley and Belfus, 1986, pp 158–161.

26. Vaziri ND, Byrn C, Mirahmadi MK, et al: Hematologic features of chronic renal failure associated with spinal cord injury. Artif Organs 6:69, 1982.

27. Vaziri ND, Winer RL, Alikhani S, et al: Antithrombin deficiency in end-stage renal disease associated with paraplegia: Effect of hemodialysis. Arch Phys Med Rehabil 66:307, 1985.

28. Vaziri ND, Winer RL, Alikhani S, et al: Extrinsic and common coagulation pathways in end-stage renal disease associated with spinal cord injury. Paraplegia 24:154, 1986.

29. Vaziri ND, Winer RL, Patel BS, et al: Protein C abnormalities in spinal cord injured patients with end-stage renal disease. Arch Phys Med Rehabil 68:791, 1987.

30. Vaziri ND, Winer RL, Toohey J, et al: Intrinsic coagulation pathway in end-stage renal disease associated with spinal cord injury treated with hemodialysis. Artif Organs 9:155, 1985.

31. Vaziri ND: Unpublished information.

32. Pahl MV, Vaziri ND, Gordon S, Tuero S: Cardiovascular pathology in dialysis patients with spinal cord injury. Artif Organs 7:416, 1983.

33. Fairshter RD, Vaziri ND, Gordon S: Frequency and spectrum of pulmonary diseases in patients with chronic renal failure associated with spinal cord injury. Respiration 44:58, 1983.

34. Meshkinpour H, Vaziri ND, Gordon S: Gastrointestinal pathology in patients with chronic renal failure associated with spinal cord injury. Am J Gastroenterol 77:562, 1982.

35. Gore RM, Mintzer RA, Calenoff L: Gastrointestinal complications of spinal cord injury. Spine 6:538, 1981.

36. Mirahmadi MK, Vaziri ND, Gordon S: Nutritional evaluation of hemodialysis patients with and without spinal cord injury. J Am Paraplegia Soc 6:36, 1983.

37. Mirahmadi MK, Vaziri ND, Ghobadi M, et al: Survival on maintenance dialysis in patients with chronic renal failure associated with paraplegia and quadriplegia. Paraplegia 20:43, 1982.

38. Stacy WK, Falls WF, Hussey RW: Chronic hemodialysis of spinal cord injury patients. J Am Paraplegia Soc 6:7, 1983.

39. Vaziri ND, Bruno A, Byrn C, et al: Maintenance hemodialysis in end-stage renal disease associated with spinal cord injury. Artif Organs 6:13, 1982.

40. Vaziri ND: Long-term haemodialysis in spinal cord injured patients. Paraplegia 22:110, 1984.

41. Vaziri ND, Lopez G, Nikakhtar B, et al: Peritoneal dialysis in renal failure associated with spinal cord injury. J Am Paraplegia Soc 7:63, 1984.

42. Berlyne GM, Lee HA, Ralston AJ, Woolcock JA: Pulmonary complications of peritoneal dialysis. Lancet 2:75, 1966.

43. Duckworth WC, Jallepalli P, Solomon SS: Glucose intolerance in spinal cord injury. Arch Physical Med Rehab 64:107, 1983.

44. Khanna R, Oreopoulos DG: Complications of peritoneal dialysis other than peritonitis. In Nolph K (ed): Peritoneal Dialysis. Boston, Martinus Nijhoff, pp 459–460, 1985.

45. Bennett WM: Drugs and Renal Disease, 2nd ed. New York, Churchill Livingstone, 1986.

46. Gopler TA: Principles of drug usage in dialysis patients. In Nissenson AR, Fine RN (eds): Philadelphia, Hanley and Belfus, 1986, p 214.

Advantages and Disadvantages of Roentgenograms in the Diagnosis of Odontoid Fractures

12

ALAIN B. ROSSIER, M.D., IL Y. LEE, M.D., and AY-MING WANG, M.D. _____

Because undiagnosed fracture-dislocation at the C1 to C2 level may be catastrophic, early correct diagnosis is of the essence. Open-mouth views may be difficult to interpret and misleading. In many instances only tomograms will allow a correct assessment of the situation.

We report our findings in a patient who was referred to us within two hours of injury with the diagnosis of odontoid fracture without neurologic deficit. Subsequent neurologic and roentgenographic work-up negated both of these findings and disclosed other pathologic features of the cervical spine which would have not been discovered if the roentgenograms had been confined to the area suspected of having sustained major trauma. The sequence of events in this particular case seemed of sufficient interest to justify their reporting.

CASE REPORT

While walking in an airport area, a 20-year-old man hit the top of his head against the back flap of a plane wing. He fell to the ground and was unconscious for about 5 minutes. The patient was transported in the supine position to the local clinic by emergency paramedics. The sensory and motor neurologic evaluation was reported as normal. However, the roentgenograms of the cervical spine were interpreted as showing posterior displacement of C1 on C2

158

with questionable fracture of the odontoid. Past history revealed that the patient had sustained a go-cart injury as a child during which he was knocked into the air and somersaulted, landing on his right side and injuring his right elbow and knee. The patient was unconscious for 5 to 10 minutes and experienced some decrease of grip strength of the right hand, which eventually fully recovered. Cervical spine roentgenograms were reported as normal.

At the time of admission to our spinal cord injury service two hours after injury, the patient did not have any subjective complaints. He was awake and oriented and had tenderness in the upper cervical spine by palpation. Cranial nerves were all normal. Reflexes in the upper and lower extremities were 1+ and 2+, respectively. Horner's syndrome was not present, and there was no sensory deficit. However, the motor examination did reveal weakness of hand grip and wrist flexors and extensors bilaterally (3+ out of 5). Paresis was more marked on the right. Supine lateral roentgenograms of the cervical spine that had been done in the referring clinic showed what was diagnosed as posterior displacement of C1 on C2 (Fig. 12–1). The open-mouth view that was carried out in our service was inconclusive. In view of these findings, it was decided to fit the patient with a halo vest. At the time the patient was positioned for its application, another lateral roentgenogram of the cervical spine showed

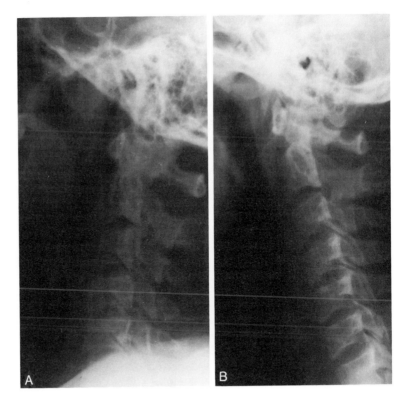

Figure 12-1. Initial roentgenograms. *A*, In the referring clinic. Apparent step off C1 to C2 secondary to rotation of the cervical spine below C2. The head is in a nearly true lateral position (superimposition of posterior border of mandibles). *B*, In the Spinal Cord Injury Service. Same misleading step off C1 to C2 secondary to rotation of the head. The cervical spine below C2 is in a nearly true lateral position (superimposition of the articular facets).

"reduction" of the retrolisthesis C1 on C2 (Fig. 12-2). The halo vest was then fitted. Lateral and anteroposterior tomograms of the suspected area were performed to better define the location of the suspected odontoid fracture (Fig. 12-3). Unexpectedly, they did not show any dens fracture or displacement. In view of the apparent discrepancy in these findings, bone scans with 99^mTc-labeled methylene diphosphonate were carried out two and eight days after injury with the hope that this would aid in making the diagnosis.[1,2] No increased uptake of the radiopharmaceutical agent could be observed in the suspected cervical area.

In view of these negative findings, the halo vest was removed. However, it was believed to be justified to carry out a metrizamide tomomyelogram to exclude any intraspinal pathology that could account for the motor deficit in the hands. No abnormality could be seen at the C1 to C3 levels. Although the cuts in the head neutral and flexion positions did not show any impingement of bone or soft tissue within the spinal canal, the cuts to the right at C6 to C7 in the head extension position were strongly suggestive of spondylotic changes impinging within the spinal canal (Fig. 12-4).

Mid and left sided cuts were normal. These

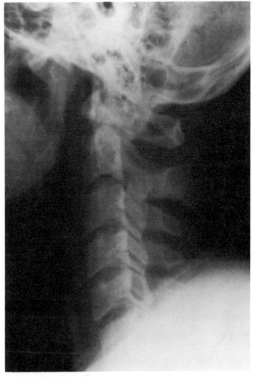

Figure 12-2. Radiograph taken at the time the halo vest was fitted. "Correction" of the step off C1 to C2. Head and cervical spine are in a nearly true lateral position.

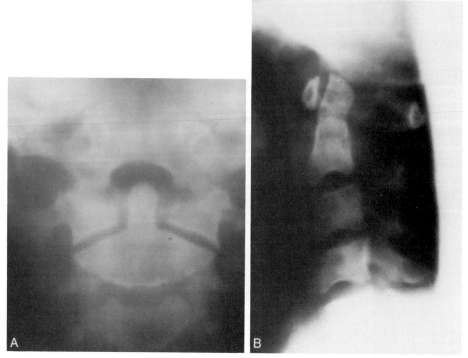

Figure 12–3. Tomograms of C1 to C2. *A*, Anteroposterior view. *B*, Lateral view. Both show no visible fracture or misalignment.

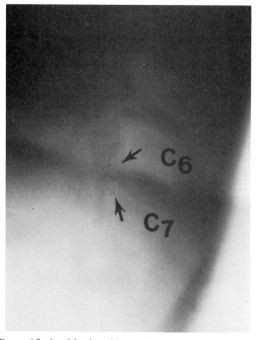

Figure 12–4. Metrizamide myelogram through the lumbar route. Tomographic cut to the right: spondylotic changes (arrows) at the posterior border of C6 to C7 vertebral bodies with some impingement within the spinal canal.

findings appeared to correlate well with the motor deficit, which was more pronounced in the right hand and wrist. The patient was fitted with a protective soft collar. At the time of discharge two weeks later the patient had fully recovered and did not show any motor deficit.

DISCUSSION

The sequence of events that took place in the case indicates the fact that roentgenograms may be misleading in the diagnosis of dens fracture dislocation. It appears that the positioning of the patient in an exact lateral projection not only of the head but also of the cervical spine segments below C2 is of the utmost importance in achieving an accurate diagnosis in traumatic odontoid pathology. The diagnosis error based upon the initial radiograms can be attributed to two factors, the importance of which appear to have been somewhat underestimated in past publications dealing with cervical spine trauma.[3-8] In the first instance one roentgenogram was not taken in a true lateral position of the cervical spine from C2 downward, although the head position was close to a true lateral (superimposition of the posterior border of the mandibles) (see Fig. 12–1*A*). In the second instance, although the roentgenogram was taken in a nearly true lateral position of the cervical spine from C2 downward, the head position was rotated to a major extent (see Fig. 12–1*B*). In order to corroborate this postulate, we have tried to duplicate the mistakes previously described by placing a patient without spine pathology in different positions of the head and neck in relation to each other. The results of these experiments have demonstrated that the aforementioned hypothesis concerning the role of the patient's head and neck positioning was correct (Fig. 12–5).

When the neck is rotated and the head is perfectly lateral, the lateral aspect of the vertebral body of C2 rotates anteriorly and causes a double contour on the film which may be mistakenly interpreted as a fracture. The time relationship between the anterior arch of C1 and the odontoid process of C2 should use a continuous straight line as a landmark.

The post-traumatic transitory neurologic deficit in the patient's hands and wrists, which did not correlate with the suggestive roentgenographic dens pathology, could have been related to the degenerative spondylotic changes at the C6 to C7 levels. The patient's previous history of weakness in the right hand following

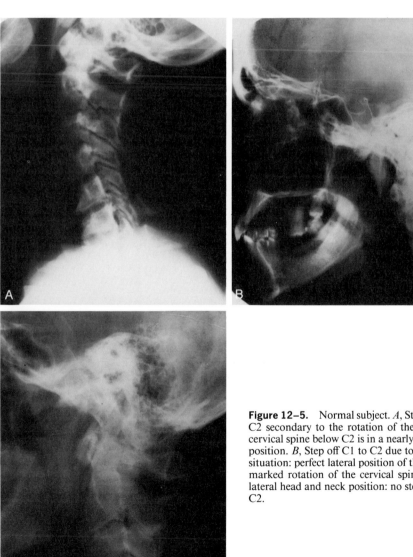

Figure 12–5. Normal subject. *A*, Step off C1 to C2 secondary to the rotation of the head. The cervical spine below C2 is in a nearly true lateral position. *B*, Step off C1 to C2 due to the reverse situation: perfect lateral position of the head but marked rotation of the cervical spine. *C*, True lateral head and neck position: no step off C1 to C2.

head and neck injury points to a similar cause-and-effect relationship.

Apart from the interesting misleading roentgenographic findings in the patient, this case presentation also illustrates another important point: investigations should not be limited to the supposedly pathologic area but should cover further possible abnormalities in other locations that could also be involved in the pathologic process as suggested by a careful neurologic evaluation. Philosophically, it must be acknowledged that our natural tendency as physicians is to focus more on previous abnormal findings rather than to look for further new pathologic features. In traumatic injuries of the spine we should not limit our investigations to what first appears to be evident on roentgenograms. It should be remembered that a careful neurologic evaluation takes precedence over radiograms, which should be guided by abnormal neurologic deficits and not vice versa.

This case seems to represent a good example of how errors may contribute positively to extend our knowledge.

SUMMARY

Missed pathology at the C1 to C2 level following an injury may have tragic consequences. Open-mouth views and lateral roentgenograms may be obscured by technical features that make their interpretation dubious. These difficulties are illustrated in a patient whose post-traumatic condition was diagnosed as odontoid fracture without neurologic deficit. However, further work-up indicated the absence of C1 to C2 pathology but disclosed neurologic deficits related to bone pathology in another region of the cervical spine. Some of the fallacies which are linked to the roentgenographic imaging of the C1 to C2 region are discussed. First, the need is emphasized for x-ray views with both the head and cervical spine in the true lateral position. Second, when one has radiographic evidence of pathology in one part of the spine, one should also study the rest of the spine.

REFERENCES

1. Bell EG, Subramanian G: The skeleton. *In* Gonçalves Rocha AF, Harbert JC (eds): Textbook of Nuclear Medicine: Clinical Applications. Philadelphia, Lea and Febiger, 1979, pp 109–128.
2. Matin P: Bone scanning of trauma and benign conditions. *In* Freeman LM, Weissmann HS (eds): Nuclear Medicine Annual 1982. New York, Raven Press, 1982, pp 81–118.
3. Braakman R, Penning L: Injuries of the Cervical Spine. Amsterdam, Excerpta Medica, 1971.
4. Gerlock AJ, Kirchner SG, Heller RM, Kaye JJ: Advanced Exercises in Diagnostic Radiology. Philadelphia, WB Saunders, 1978.
5. Harris JH: The Radiology of Acute Cervical Spine Trauma. Baltimore, Williams & Wilkins, 1978.
6. Howorth MB, Petrie JG: Injuries of the Spine. Baltimore, Williams and Wilkins, 1964.
7. Lob A: Die Wirbelsäulenverletzungen und ihre Ausheilung (ed 2). Stuttgart, Thieme, 1954.
8. McRae DL: How to look at cervical radiographs. *In* Tator CH (ed): Early Management of Acute Spinal Cord Injury. New York, Raven Press, 1982, pp 77–92.

13 Body Composition and Endocrine Profile in Spinal Cord Injured Patients

ALAIN B. ROSSIER, M.D., HERVÉ FAVRE, M.D., and
MICHEL B. VALLOTON, M.D.

Various metabolic alterations have been described in spinal cord injury patients, notably in protein metabolism, electrolyte balance, calcium-phosphorus equilibrium, and hepatic and endocrine functions.[1] We have studied the body composition of such patients, using the compartmental analysis as proposed by Moore et al.[2] Because results have demonstrated a body composition similar to that observed in patients with hyperaldosteronism, plasma aldosterone, plasma renin activity, and cortisol were measured later on in a second group of patients presenting an identical clinical setting.

Global evaluation of these patients showed a persistent increase in plasma aldosterone and plasma renin activity levels with a normal cortisol level that may account for the observed changes in body composition.

MATERIAL AND METHODS

This work is based on the study of 11 paraplegic and 6 tetraplegic male patients with spinal cord injuries. Patients' ages ranged from 17 to 55 years, with a mean age of 27 years. Each patient was carefully evaluated to exclude co-existing disturbances of cardiac, hepatic, or renal function. Control group consisted of 24 healthy subjects matched for sex and age.

Serial measurements of total body composition were made at different points in the patient's course, between the 10th and 30th days and during the second, the fourth, and the 12th months after spinal cord injury. In the control group, body composition was studied on one occasion.

Total body composition was determined by simultaneous tracer dilution method developed in our laboratory and described in detail by Busset et al.[3] In brief, on the first day of the experiment, [42]potassium (K) 150 μCi, [24]sodium (Na) 100 μCi, and [82]bromide (Br) 30 μCi was injected intravenously between 7 and 8 A.M. Twenty-four hour urine was collected. On day 2, a sample of blood was drawn 24 hours after injection of the isotopes and urine was again collected. On day 3, a second sample of blood was drawn 48 hours after injection and tritiated water 1 μCi was injected. Isotopes were counted in each of the urine and blood specimens using a beta counter (B 12 H, 20th Century Electronics LTD) for the potassium and a gamma counter (Auto gamma, Packard 410 A) for the [24]Na and [82]Br. On day 3, blood was taken two and three hours after injection of tritiated water. Two-hour urine collection was made after injection of this isotope. Tritium was measured by a beta counter (Tri-Cab, Packard). All these isotopes were purchased from Radiochemical Center Amersham (England). Details concerning the type of column used to separate isotopes and the calculation made are given elsewhere.[3] This method permits the simultaneous determination of:

- Total body water (TBW) equivalent to the tritiated water space.

- Extracellular water (ECW) equivalent to the diffusion space of ^{82}Br, corrected for both the diffusion of Br into the RBCs and for the true serum H_2O concentration.[4]
- Total exchangeable sodium (Na_e) equivalent to 70 per cent of the total Na obtained by measuring serum isotopic Na dilution in a sample taken 24 hours after injection of ^{24}Na.
- Total exchangeable potassium (K_e) equivalent to 90 per cent of the total K obtained by measurement of urine isotopic activity 48 hours after injection of ^{42}K.

The error of these determinations, for the simultaneous method, was in our hands of the order of $\pm$ 3 per cent, and the reproducibility had been shown to be of the order of $\pm$ 5 per cent.[3]

Among the values that may be derived from these direct measurements, we considered the following[2]:

- Intracellular water (ICW): the difference between TBW and ECW may be acknowledged as an index of the active cellular mass.
- The Na_e/K_e ratio: it reflects the proportion of the extracellular milieu to the cellular mass.
- The $(Na_e + K_e)/TBW$ ratio: the "mean body osmolality." Edelman et al[5] have demonstrated the close relationship existing between TBW and the total body supply of these two exchangeable cations.

In some particular situations, however, this correlation is no longer valid for unknown reasons, as demonstrated by Bartter[6] and confirmed by de Sousa et al.[7]

Average intracellular potassium concentration (AvICK) is calculated as follows:

AvICK = intracellular potassium (ICK)/ICW (mmol/L) where ICK = K − ECK and ECK = ECW × Kplasma × correction factor.[2]

According to Nagant de Deuxchaisnes et al,[8] a decrease in AvICK may be considered as the hallmark of true potassium depletion, a consequence of a cellular metabolic alteration (anoxia, acidosis, and hypercorticism). The primary metabolic defect must be corrected before potassium depletion may be remedied. This treatment is the opposite of that for potassium deficit from excessive losses, which is easily corrected by the administration of potas-

sium, and pseudodepletion, which corresponds to a reduction in cell mass without change in AvICK and is found in patients suffering from chronic debilitating disease.

Total body fat (TBF) is calculated according to the Pace-Rathbun formula[9] based on the assumption that fat contains no water and lean tissue contains 73.2 per cent water. This derivation is subject to significant error.[10]

The K_e/FFS ratio expresses the part of the lean body mass made up of cellular tissue, where FFS = body weight − (TBW + TBF).

Expression of the Results

Each form of presentation of the results of a compositional study has its drawbacks; the choice of the form of presentation must be made with regard to the ultimate goal of the study. We wished to follow the case developments of our relatively homogeneous group of patients and compare this group with a group of normal subjects. Since we could not a priori discern whether a variation in body weight was due to variations in TBF or TBW or both, we chose to express our results in absolute terms rather than relating them to body weight or TBW.

This form of expression may obscure variations from the normal but will increase the salience of the differences found and facilitate the longitudinal study of the subjects.

Endocrine Study

In view of the results obtained by the study of the body composition in the first group of patients, endocrine studies have been undertaken in a second series of patients in order to substantiate the mechanism responsible for the alterations found in the body composition of paraplegic and tetraplegic patients. Plasma aldosterone (PA), plasma renin activity (PRA), and cortisol were measured on day 1 after the injury and one and two months later, in two paraplegic and five tetraplegic male patients. The clinical features and the treatment of these patients, whose ages ranged from 20 to 55 years (mean age 30 years), were similar to those of the patients in the first series.

PRA was estimated according to Poulsen and Jorgensen,[11] and Vallotton,[12] plasma aldosterone and cortisol were measured according to Underwood and Williams.[13] Normal values have been previously established by the laboratory for normal subjects ingesting a 150 mmol sodium per day diet in supine position. Blood was drawn at 8 A.M. in supine patients. During the first three days, the patients were perfused with an isotonic saline solution containing 20 mmol of potassium per liter at a rate between 1500 and 2500 ml/24 hours. In addition, they received 6 mg of dexamethasone the first day tapered to 1 mg a day by day 6. On this treatment, extracellular fluid volume was maintained constant as judged by the blood pressure. Systolic mean blood pressure ± SD was 116 + 21 mm Hg the first day and 118 + 14 and 114 + 15 by the end of the first and second months, respectively.

Diastolic blood pressure averaged 68 ± 16 mm Hg the first day and 76 ± 9 and 73 ± 11 by the end of the first and second months, respectively. There were no statistical differences between these values. There were also no significant differences during the three periods of observation in serum sodium, potassium, and total carbon dioxide concentration. Mean serum sodium concentrations averaged 137 ± 2.8 mmol/L on day 1, 140 ± 4.0 mmol/L during the first month, and 142 ± 3.3 mmol/L during the second month. The corresponding values for potassium were 4.1 ± 0.23, 4.0 ± 0.21, 4.1 ± 0.31, and for total CO_2 26.6 ± 1.9, 26 ± 3.32, and 25 ± 2.9, respectively. These values did not differ from those recorded in the patients of the first series.

Statistics

All the values are expressed as mean ± SD. Statistical comparisons were made with the Student's t-test and double variance analysis whenever applicable.

RESULTS

Body Composition

Results and normal values are displayed in this chapter Tables 13–1 to 13–3.

Data Comparison Between Patients and Controls

The average weight of our patients is lower than that of control subjects, with an average corpulence index[14] of 12 per cent below ideal body weight (Table 13–1). Total body fat is within normal limits.

Average total body weight for the group approaches the lower limits of the normal; the distribution between the intracellular and extracellular compartments is slightly altered as evidenced by a nonsignificant elevation of the Na_e/K_e ratio. Na_e is within normal limits.

K_e is significantly decreased ($p < 0.001$), with an average absolute value of 2287 mmol. This decrease will be reflected in all the values derived from or dependent on K_e.

The Na_e/K_e ratio is raised (although not significantly) by a reduction of the denominator with a normal numerator. The $(Na_e + K_e)$/ TBW ratio is reduced significantly ($p < 0.05$). However, serum sodium concentration remains in the normal range from 135 to 143 mmol/L (average 140 mmol/L) (see Table 13–1). This implies an apparent contradiction— that is, a "low mean body osmolality" in the face of normal serum sodium and potassium

TABLE 13–1. Comparison of Mean Values Observed in Spinal Cord Injury Patients With Those of Control Subjects

	NORMAL CONTROLS N = 24	PARAPLEGICS OR TETRAPLEGICS N = 17		
		Mean ± SD	Difference	Significance
Weight (kg)	67.3 ± 7.4	59.5 ± 7.88	− 7.8	NS
TBW (Liter)	40.7 ± 5.66	36.40 ± 4.37	− 4.3	NS
ECW (Liter)	16.3 ± 1.70	17.65 ± 1.96	+ 1.35	NS
Na_e (mEq)	2830 ± 339	2751 ± 351	− 79	NS
K_e (mEq)	3096 ± 332	2287 ± 431	− 809	$p < 0.01$
TBF (kg)	9.6 ± 2.4	10.25 ± 5.08	+ 0.65	NS
ICW (Liter)	21 ± 3	18.53 ± 3.52	− 2.47	NS
Na_e/K_e	0.85 ± 1.0	1.23 ± 0.26	+ 0.23	NS
AvICK (mEq/L)	150 ± 10	118.06 ± 13.74	− 31.94	$p < 0.01$
$Na_e + K_e$/TBW (mEq/L)	155 ± 5	138.70 ± 11.67	− 16.30	$p < 0.05$
K_e/FFS (mEq/kg)	225 ± 25	174.01 ± 19.31	− 50.99	$p < 0.01$

There is a significant decrease in K_e, AvICK, $(Na_e + K_e)$/TBW and K_e/FFS. The other values do not show significant deviation from the normal (NS = not significant).

TABLE 13–2. Comparison of Measurements Made During and After One Month Following Spinal Cord Injury in 17 Patients

	DURING 1ST MONTH	2ND TO 12TH MONTHS		
	Mean ± SD	Mean ± SD	Difference	Significant
Weight (kg)	59.52 ± 6.02	59.46 ± 8.74	− 0.06	NS
TBW (Liter)	37.80 ± 3.97	35.70 ± 4.48	− 2.10	NS
ECW (Liter)	17.64 ± 1.89	17.65 ± 2.03	+ 0.01	NS
Na_e (mEq)	2643 ± 342	2805 ± 380	+ 162	NS
K_e (mEq)	2400 ± 380	2231 ± 452	− 169	NS
TBF (kg)	9.53 ± 4.23	10.57 ± 5.50	+ 1.04	NS
ICW (Liter)	20.40 ± 2.75	18.05 ± 3.92	− 2.35	NS
Na_e/K_e	1.11 ± 0.13	1.30 ± 0.29	+ 0.19	$p < 0.05$
AvICK (mEq/Liter)	114.47 ± 16.76	119.86 ± 11.99	+ 5.39	NS
$Na_e + K_e$/TBW (mEq/Liter)	133.68 ± 14.02	141.21 ± 9.70	+ 7.35	NS
K_eFFS (mEq/kg)	176.66 ± 22.69	172.84 ± 18.20	− 3.82	NS

The *t*-test shows that only the modest elevation of Na_e/K_e reaches significance, as a result of the opposite (and in themselves nonsignificant) variations in both Na_e and K_e.

TABLE 13–3. Comparison of Measurements Made Before and After Wheelchair Ambulation in 17 Patients

	BEFORE WHEELCHAIR AMBULATION	AFTER WHEELCHAIR AMBULATION		
	Mean ± SD	Mean ± SD	Difference	Significance
Weight (kg)	63.13 ± 7.34	55.83 ± 6.82	− 7.30	$p < 0.02$
TBW (Liter)	37.18 ± 4.57	35.34 ± 4.01	− 1.84	NS
ECW (Liter)	17.93 ± 2.03	17.27 ± 1.85	− 0.66	NS
Na_e (mEq)	2700 ± 391	2819 ± 343	+ 199	NS
K_e (mEq)	2300 ± 447	2270 ± 423	− 0.30	NS
TBF (kg)	12.02 ± 5.17	8.48 ± 4.49	− 3.59	NS
ICW (Liter)	19.40 ± 3.54	18.07 ± 3.91	− 1.33	NS
Na_e/K_e	1.20 ± 0.24	1.28 ± 0.28	+ 0.04	NS
AvICK (mEq/L)	114.82 ± 13.67	122.47 ± 13.02	+ 7.65	NS
$Na_e + K_e$/TBW (mEq/L)	134.61 ± 12.40	144.25 ± 8.04	+ 9.64	$p < 0.02$
K_eFFS (mEq/kg)	174.63 ± 19.75	173.40 ± 19.64	− 1.23	NS

The *t*-test shows that the only significant variations are a fall in body weight and an elevation of the $(Na_e + K_e)$/TBW ratio.

values. Such a situation has been reported earlier by Bartter et al[6] and de Sousa et al[7] without any definite explanation. In certain circumstances, the Edelman formula may not represent the true mean body osmolality, which could be the consequence of a situation of cationic inactivation.

The K_e/FFS ratio is significantly reduced ($p < 0.01$). This is logical if the weight loss is at the expense of the lean tissue (with a normal TBF) and, in particular, at the expense of the muscle mass (decrease of K_e proportionally greater than the decrease in fat-free solids (FFS) which includes organs less affected by paraplegia, such as the skeleton). Therefore, the decreased K_e/FFS ratio expresses a relatively greater loss of lean body mass (Table 13–1).

AvICK is significantly reduced ($p < 0.01$), permitting the classification of this potassium deficiency as potassium depletion.

Finally, in our patients the serum potassium was found to be within normal limits during the entire course of the study (range 3.8 to 5.2, average 4.5 mmol/L).

The body of data accumulated from the present series of measurements allows the conclusion that as a group the paraplegics and tetraplegics we treated had potassium depletion, low mean body osmolality, and weight loss at the expense of lean body mass.

Evolution of the Measurements of Parameters in the Paraplegic and Tetraplegic Group

We first tried to differentiate early from late changes. We adopted a period of one month after trauma as an arbitrary limit between the early and late stages, since the catabolic posttraumatic phase is estimated to be of about one month's duration. Measurements were made from the 10th day to one month after trauma for the early period and from two months to 12 months after injury for the late period. Table 13–2 summarizes the trend of variations occurring during these two periods.

As can be seen in Table 13–2, compared with those in normal persons, the alterations in body composition of paraplegic and tetraplegic patients exist in varying degrees from the first month after injury and remain unchanged later. Within the limits of observation of the selected parameters, with the exception of an increase in the Na_e/K_e ratio, statistical analysis does not reveal any difference between the early and the late periods. Thus, the potassium depletion, the low mean body osmolality ratio, and the weight loss are present from the first month after injury and persist thereafter.

In a second phase of investigation it was deemed necessary to look at the modifications that might take place under the influence of the patient's resumption of activity. To do so, we compared the measurements carried out before and after wheelchair ambulation, a very important step in the course of rehabilitation, during which the motor activity of the patient increases considerably. Wheelchair ambulation occurs with most of our patients at about two to three months after injury. Table 13–3 shows the direction and the statistical significance of variations observed during the periods under consideration, before and after wheelchair ambulation.

From the foregoing it would appear that the resumption of physical activity results in a weight loss at the expense of both TBF and TBW and coincides with a partial correction of the mean body osmolality. The potassium depletion persists after wheelchair ambulation and no argument can be found in favor of an increase in muscle mass.

Endocrine Results

As illustrated in Figure 13–1, plasma aldosterone and plasma renin activity levels are both above the normal values for people who receive a normal salt diet and remain supine. Elevation of both parameters appears immediately after the injury and persists for months. In contrast, the cortisol values found in the serum of these patients remain normal during the period of observation with the exception of suppressed levels observed on the first day after injury, which could be easily explained by the corticoid treatment these patients received at

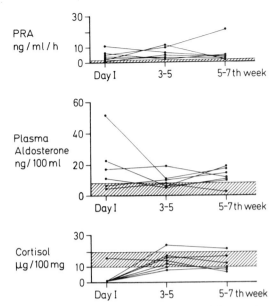

Figure 13–1. This figure illustrates the individual values of plasma renin activity (PRA), plasma aldosterone (PA), and cortisol observed during the two first months after injury in five tetraplegic and two paraplegic patients. The dashed bars represent the normal value ± 2 SD. PRA and PA values are above 2 SD in most patients, while cortisol levels fall within normal range with the exception of the first values, which are suppressed by the initial corticoid treatment.

that time. In these patients, no correlation could be found between PA and PRA.

DISCUSSION

In spite of individual variations in patients' courses, three elements were demonstrated to be common to the group: potassium depletion, low mean body osmolality, and loss of weight. The method used shows that the weight loss is a result of combined loss of TBF and TBW, especially at the expense of the intracellular water fraction, which is in agreement with the observations of Cardús et al.[15,16] Because the TBW loss amounts to more than the water contained in adipose tissue, a loss in lean body mass must be present, most probably from the muscle mass.

The persistent fall in total exchangeable potassium is the most important finding in these patients. This fall is probably composed of two elements:

- Loss of muscle mass (pseudodepletion)
- Potassium depletion syndrome, clearly demonstrated in this study by a de-

creased AvICK. This potassium depletion reveals the existence of a permanent metabolic change in the paraplegic patients.

Decreased AvICK is pronounced in the early course of our patients and persists practically unchanged throughout the period of observation. Such a perturbation is usually secondary to alterations of either metabolic (anoxia and/or acidosis) or endocrine origin.[8] The spinal cord injured person is a patient beset by numerous metabolic difficulties which may create and maintain a potassium depletion: there is an initial post-traumatic shock with vasoplegia, hypotension, anemia secondary to capillary stasis, hemolysis and decreased hematopoiesis, disorders of hemostasis and depression of cellular metabolism reflected in a decreased BMR, resulting from the combined effects of anemia, hypoxia, pain, and increased body temperature loss secondary to vasoplegia.[1] Then comes the post-traumatic catabolic phase (two weeks to six months) with a negative nitrogen balance.[17,18] From the third day, the urinary potassium losses reach a maximum and a concomitant sodium retention is found.[17] In addition, transitory BSP retention,[1] disturbances of glucose tolerance,[17] occasional feminization syndrome with gynecomastia and testicular atrophy,[19] adrenal functional disturbances, and increased urinary aldosterone excretion have been reported.[19,20]

Such changes per se are sufficient to explain a true potassium depletion. This potassium depletion is similar to that one observed in non-edematous cardiac and cirrhotic patients and differs from that which can be seen in patients with muscular wasting disease, in which AvICK remains normal.[8] This fact suggests the presence of some mineralocorticoid hormone disturbance such as secondary hyperaldosteronism or excess of cortisol. The repercussions of hypercorticism on the total body composition are an increase in Na_e/kg and a decrease in K_e. Expressed in absolute terms, we found the Na_e to be normal in our patients. Therefore, in view of the loss of body weight observed, the ratio of Na_e to body weight must be increased, which is in fact the case: the Na_e/kg in our patients averaged 50.4 mmol/kg (normal 43.3 mmol/kg), a value which is close to that one found in patients with cirrhosis or cardiac insufficiency without edema.[8]

The AvICK remains markedly decreased. Since the $Na_e + K_e/TBW$ ratio becomes partially corrected, a finding that is in agreement with Cardús and McTaggart[16] at this stage for the disease, and the serum sodium concentration remains normal, we must postulate a degree of intracellular substitution of sodium for potassium, as in secondary hyperaldosteronism.[8] Increased aldosterone excretion in spinal cord injury patients has already been reported by Claus-Walker et al.[21] Because hyperaldosteronism is the most likely mechanism for the persistent potassium depletion, we have measured plasma aldosterone, plasma renin activity, and cortisol in a second series of patients over a period of two months. Compared with results in normal persons, the results have confirmed that the paraplegics have a high aldosterone level throughout the period of observation (see Fig. 13–1).

Increased aldosterone secretion may be stimulated by different elements, some of which could be relevant to paraplegics. The most classic stimulus is hypovolemia.[22] This stimulus could be excluded in our group of patients because their blood pressure remained constant. In addition, hypovolemia implies a low exchangeable sodium and a low Na_e/kg ratio, which is in opposition to our finding of a normal exchangeable sodium and elevated Na_e/kg ratio. Hyperkalemia is another stimulus which is irrelevant to our patients because the serum potassium was found to be within normal limits all during the study.[6]

Finally, the most potent stimulus for the aldosterone secretion remains angiotensin II generated by renin. We have found elevated plasma renin activity from the immediate post-traumatic phase throughout the period of observation of two months. The initiation of the stimulation of renin secretion as well as its persistence could be explained by the vasoplegia accompanying the paraplegic condition. This vasoplegia occurs immediately after the injury and persists for the rest of the paraplegic patient's life. In view of recent "in vitro" experiments, stimulation of the PGE_2 biosynthesis by the potassium depletion may offer another explanation for the maintenance of elevated PRA and PA in paraplegic patients.[23] It should be noted that, although both PRA and PA are elevated, there is no statistical correlation between the two parameters as would normally be expected. However, this situation is not unique and has been described in other pathologic conditions such as uremia.[24]

In fact, the most remarkable finding in these patients is the persistence of a high plasma aldosterone level best explained by a permanent vasoplegia. This endocrine abnormality can induce the changes in the body composition; that is, a permanent potassium depletion with a progressive correction of the $Na_e + K_e/TBW$ ratio.

Correction of this ratio depends on the sodium retention resulting from the hyperaldosteronism, which creates a relative increase in the exchangeable sodium despite the continuing potassium depletion. At the end, as it appears from our data, the intracellular volume is reduced and the extracellular volume is slightly increased.

SUMMARY

Various metabolic alterations have been ascribed to spinal cord injury patients; 11 paraplegic and six tetraplegic male patients with spinal cord injuries were studied in regard to body composition as assessed by compartmental analysis. As body composition was shown to be similar to that observed in hyperaldosteronism, five more tetraplegics and two paraplegics were investigated with regard to plasma aldosterone, renin, and cortisol levels. The most striking finding was the persistence of elevation of both aldosterone and renin activity. This might best be explained by the chronic condition of vasoplegia in these patients. It is suggested that endocrine modifications are responsible for the changes in body composition, i.e., permanent potassium depletion with progressive correction of the total exchangeable sodium + potassium/total body water ratio. From these longitudinal metabolic studies it is concluded that potassium depletion, low mean body osmolality, weight loss at the expense of the lean body mass, and elevated plasma aldosterone level and plasma renin activity are some of the metabolic changes that take place in spinal cord injury patients.

REFERENCES

1. O'Connell FB, Gardner WJ: Metabolism in paraplegia. J Am Med Assoc 153:706, 1953.
2. Moore FD, Olesen KH, McMurrey JD, et al: The Body Cell Mass and its Supporting Environment (ed 1). Philadelphia, WB Saunders, 1963, p 535.
3. Busset R, de Sousa RC, Mach RS: Etude de la composition corporelle à l'aide de radio-isotopes chez l'homme normal et au cours de différents états pathologiques. Méthode Sem Hôp Paris 43:1312, 1967.
4. Lacroix M, Busset R, Mach RS: Utilisation comparative du soufre 35 et du brome 82 pour la détermination du volume de l'eau extracellulaire. Helv Med Acta 32:87, 1965.
5. Edelman IS, Leibmann J, O'Meara MP, Birkenfeld LW: Interrelations between serum sodium concentration, serum osmolality and total exchangeable sodium, total exchangeable potassium and total body water. J Clin Invest 37:1236, 1958.
6. Bartter FC, Barbour BH, Carr AA, Delea CS: On the role of potassium and of the central nervous system in the regulation of aldosterone secretion. In Baulieu EE, Robel P (eds): Aldosterone: A Symposium. Oxford, Blackwell Scientific Publications, 1964, pp 221–242.
7. de Sousa R, Busset R, Moser C et al: Corrélation entre sodium échangeable, potassium échangeable, eau totale et espace brome (Applications cliniques de la formule d'Edelman). Helv Med Acta 31:623, 1964.
8. Nagant de Deuxchaisnes C, Collet RA, Busset R, Mach RS: Exchangeable potassium in wasting, amyotrophy, heart disease and cirrhosis of the liver. Lancet 1:681, 1961.
9. Pace N, Rathbun EN: Studies on body composition. III. The body water and chemically combined nitrogen content in relation to fat content. J Biol Chem 158:685, 1945.
10. Quoidbach A, Busset R, Dayer AA, Mach RS: Evaluation of body composition in obesity using isotopic dilution techniques. In Vague J (ed): Physiopathology of adipose tissue, 3rd ed. Amsterdam, Excerpta Medica Foundation, 1969, pp 302–317.
11. Poulsen K, Jorgensen J: An easy radioimmunological microassay of renin activity, concentration and substrate in human and animal plasma and tissues based on angiotensin I trapping by antibody. J Clin Endocrinol Metab 39:816, 1974.
12. Vallotton MB: Parallel radioimmunoassay of angiotensin I and of angiotensin II for measurement of renin activity and of circulating active hormone in human plasma. In Federlin K, Hales CN, Kracht J (eds): Immunological Methods in Endocrinology. Stuttgart, Thieme, 1971, pp 94–100.
13. Underwood RH, Williams GH: The simultaneous measurement of aldosterone, cortisol and corticosterone in human peripheral plasma by displacement analysis. J Lab Clin Med 79:848, 1972.
14. Monnerot-Dumaine M: L'indice de corpulence et son calcul chez l'adulte. Presse Méd 63:1037, 1955.
15. Cardús D, McTaggart WG: Total body water and its distribution in men with spinal cord injury. Arch Phys Med Rehabil 65:509, 1984.
16. Cardús D, McTaggart WG: Body sodium and potassium in men with spinal cord injury. Arch Phys Med Rehabil 66:156, 1985.
17. Knowlton K, Spence WT, Rioch DMcK, et al: Metabolic changes following transsection of the spinal cord in dogs. Acta Neurovegetativa 15:374, 1957.
18. Wyse DM, Pattee CJ: The metabolic alterations of immobilization, injury and paraplegia. Part I: Protein metabolism. DVA Treat Serv Bull 8:63, 1953.
19. Wyse DM, Pattee CJ: The metabolic alterations of immobilization, injury and paraplegia. Part V: Endocrine and physiological alterations. DVA Treat Serv Bull 8:351, 1953.
20. McDaniel JW, Sexton AW: Psychoendocrine function in relation to level of spinal cord transection. Horm Behav 2:59, 1971.
21. Claus-Walker JL, Carter RE, Lipscomb HS, Vallbona C: Daily rhythms of electrolytes and aldosterone

excretion in men with cervical spinal cord section. J Clin Endocrinol Metab 29:300, 1969.

22. Laragh JH, Cannon PJ, Ames RP: Aldosterone in man. Its secretion, its interaction with sodium balance and angiotensin activity. *In* Baulieu EE, Robel P (eds): Aldosterone: A Symposium. Oxford, Blackwell Scientific Publications, 1964, pp 427–448.

23. Zusman RM, Keiser HR: Regulation of prostaglandin E_2 synthesis by angiotensin II, potassium, osmolality, and dexamethasone. Kidney Int 17:277, 1980.

24. Louis F, Zwahlen A, Favre H, Vallotton MB: Contrôle de l'aldostérone plasmatique chez les patients en hémodialyse. Schweiz Med Wschr 110:1882, 1980.

14 Nonoperative Management of Cervical Instability

DANIEL A. CAPEN, M.D., and RUSSELL W. NELSON, M.D.

Recent advances in surgical techniques have made operative management of cervical spine instability a much more popular treatment. However, there are definite indications for the utilization of nonoperative techniques to manage cervical spine instability both with and without neurologic injury. Immobilization of the spine and protection of the spinal cord from further injury remain the primary goals of both emergency treatment and long-term care.[1] The physician must be aware that excessive motion of an unstable cervical spine can facilitate further neurologic damage.

Field medical management has improved with recent improvement of emergency care systems. Initial immobilization by trained technicians frequently helps to preserve neurologic function. This is done with tongs and traction, halter immobilization, and sometimes direct application of the halo vest stabilization device either in the field or in the emergency department. Halo or tong traction provides sufficient stabilization to permit neurologic assessment and study of the spinal canal. Plans for either surgical management or long-term external immobilization can be made.

Since Nickel et al[2] popularized the utilization of halo external skeletal traction with attachment to a custom-molded vest, there have been some definitive advances in the materials utilized. These improvements permit patient tolerance of the device, easier application of the device, and long-term management with

reduction of significant complications. Also, the newer graphite posts do not interfere with cervical spine imaging.

The treating physician and surgeon must be aware that there are some selected cases in which the halo vest is essential for long-term immobilization. Definitive cervical spine injuries exist in which the halo vest has an unacceptable incidence of long-term failure of treatment on the basis of the fact that primarily ligamentous instability is involved. There are also selected upper cervical spine fractures and cervical hyperextension injuries with neurologic deficit in which appropriate management can be carried out with other types of semirigid immobilization such as the Somi brace, the Guilford brace, or the extended Philadelphia collar. All of these options are available to the treating surgeon. They help provide for selection on the basis of patient preference when this is feasible as well as according to the needs of the multiply injured patient.

External skeletal fixation has the benefit of involving no surgical risk and the capability for application and management of the device on an outpatient basis. This type of treatment is especially applicable in the patient with cervical spine instability but absolutely no neurologic deficit. It also is useful in the multiply injured patient or the systemically ill patient in whom early cervical spinal surgery is precluded.

INDICATIONS FOR NONSURGICAL MANAGEMENT

The surgeon must be aware of fracture classification and be able to identify fracture types.

Supported in part by the National Institute for Disability and Rehabilitation Research Grant No. G008535134.

The method most useful is the Allen classification of cervical spine injuries.[3] This source provides definitive information on location and extent of instability based on the radiographic picture on AP and lateral radiographs. Identification of the fracture type provides an outline for the surgeon to differentiate cases in which surgery is essential and cases in which halo vest immobilization would be useful.

The other factor critical in identifying appropriate cases for nonsurgical management is the neurologic picture. The identification of spinal cord injury and spinal shock and the patient's subsequent emergence from spinal shock are necessary in planning appropriate treatment. The usual extent of spinal shock after cord injury is 24 to 48 hours. A diagnosis of complete spinal cord injury can be made on the basis of neurologic examination only after the patient has emerged from spinal shock. In patients with completed spinal cord injury from any trauma type, the instability can be managed appropriately in a halo vest (Fig. 14–1). Facet dislocations of primary ligamentous origin and compression flexion lesions with insufficient bony comminution have a high incidence of failure with the halo. However, with a halo vest it is rare to observe late instability in fractures with significant bony comminution.

With incomplete neurologic injury, serial neurologic examinations and appropriate study of the cervical spinal canal by computed tomography (CT) or magnetic resonance imaging are required. Emergency surgical decompression is necessary in patients with documented neurologic deterioration on serial neurologic examinations. However, a patient with improving function can continue to be treated in traction or a halo vest. In a study at Rancho Los Amigos, Nelson et al[4] documented the incidence of failure and success with treatment by a halo vest immobilization (Table 14–1).

In the multiply injured patient in whom systemic illness or multiple areas of systemic trauma make surgery untenable, the halo vest may be the only option until surgery can be tolerated. It may be successful at three months in providing cervical stabilization.

Rehabilitation can take place in the halo vest,[2] although its use does provide some obstacles to dressing training, and to mobilization that are not present after surgical stabilization and use of a Philadelphia collar. These patients often require interim discharge to avoid long stays in rehabilitation hospitals.

Before the advent of utilization of a halo, prolonged bedrest in skull traction was the accepted standard treatment. Numerous medical complications occurred as a result of this treat-

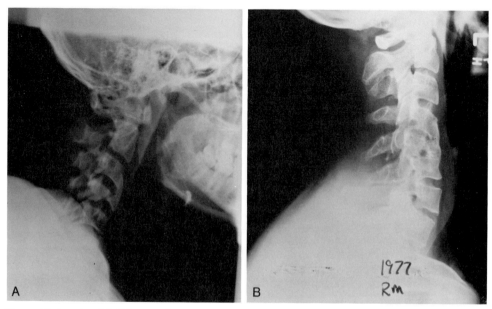

Figure 14–1. *A* and *B*, When cervical trauma produces anterior bony comminution, there is sufficient calcification and bone formation in the intradiscal spaces and along the anterior longitudinal ligament to produce stability.

TABLE 14–1. Long-Term Follow-Up of 179 Patients Treated with Halo Vest Immobilization

	TOTAL	UNSTABLE	X-RAY STABILITY
Vertical compression (all)	31	1	22
Distractive flexion			
DF$_1$*	15	7	2
DF$_2$	14	3	5
DF$_3$*	17	9	4
DF$_4$	3	0	3
TOTAL	49	19	14
Compressive flexion			
CF$_1$	10	0	1
CF$_2$	16	1	4
CF$_3$*	13	7	5
CF$_4$	13	0	12
CF$_5$	11	1	10
TOTAL	63	9	32
Compressive extension	6	1	
Distractive extension	1	0	
Lateral flexion	1	0	

*The study revealed that DF$_1$, DF$_3$, and CF$_3$ type fractures were "at risk" for late instability. Patients with all other fracture types had 90 per cent or greater incidence of bony ankylosis at three months.

ment, and this is now considered to be a much less desirable course. Although skull traction is utilized initially, the emphasis (whether by surgery or halo vest immobilization) is to help the patient achieve mobility as soon as possible. The alternative semirigid immobilization devices also provide help in achieving patient mobility.

HALO VEST APPLICATION

Garfin[5] has outlined the importance of correct halo vest application. The standard pin placement for the skull fixation is the critical point of halo application. Pin intolerance pain and pin tract infections can result from inappropriate initial application of the device.

Placement of the halo ring caudad to the biparietal diameter of the skull is critical. Avoidance of the temporalis muscle is also necessary. The cosmetic deficit from halo pins into the forehead above the eyebrows is minimal after the scar formation has matured. After the halo is applied, an appropriate well-molded and padded vest with attachments can provide for semirigid immobilization sufficient to allow for bony healing. As documented in numerous studies, there is some motion at all cervical segments in the halo vest because of the difficulty in obtaining complete rigid immobilization.[4] In most cases this motion is tolerated.

COMPLICATIONS OF HALO VEST IMMOBILIZATION

In 179 patients treated by halo vest immobilization, there were definitive complications reported. Pin loosening and pin infection were the most frequently seen complications in the highest percentage. Some scarring was noted in long-term follow-up after pin loosening and pin infection. Skin pressure sores in multiple areas were noted as a frequently seen complication as well.

The presence of severe complications such as nerve injury and dural puncture was minimal (Table 14–2). No deaths occurred. In the series

TABLE 14–2. Complications in 179 Patients Treated with Halo Vest Immobilization

	NO. OF PATIENTS	PERCENTAGE OF PATIENTS
Pin loosening	64	36
Pin sepsis	35	20
Pressure sores	20	11
Pin bleeding	2	1
Nerve injury	3	2
Dural puncture	1	1
Dysphagia	3	2
Severe scars	18 of 59 pts seen	

Many patients experienced more than one complication. Complications requiring discontinuation of the halo numbered 15 of 179. Successful treatment of loosening sepsis and pressure sores occurred in the majority of cases.

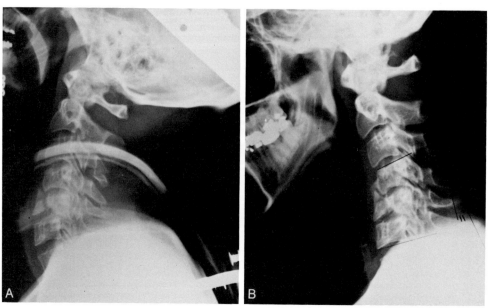

Figure 14–2. *A* and *B*, Flexion and extension radiographs showing sufficient anterior bony union to immobilize a compressive flexion type IV injury that was successfully treated with a halo vest.

of Garfin et al[5] and Nelson et al,[4] the overall complication rates approached 20 per cent.

INDICATIONS FOR HALO VEST USAGE

In a patient with an intact neurologic system the option of surgical versus nonsurgical treatment must be presented. Avoidance of potential neurologic complications is always an important factor in decision-making. In our series, at least 50 per cent success rate with halo treatment is noted. In the majority of cases a 90 per cent or greater success rate is recorded. The choice of avoidance of surgery is not irrational in this patient group.

We recommend, on the basis of our experience, that surgery can be avoided if the fracture classification fits the profile of patients successfully treated in a halo vest and if the neurologic system is totally intact (Fig. 14–2).

The other obvious candidate for halo vest usage is the systemically unstable patient. In many cases, the initial period after cervical spinal cord trauma and spinal cord injury is accompanied by a high incidence of systemic illness and complications such as pneumonia, urinary tract infection, and cardiovascular instability. Because of the nature and origin of most spinal cord trauma, there are frequently associated injuries that also prevent early surgery. In many instances surgery for spinal sta-

bilization cannot be performed and the halo vest treatment must be utilized. If after three months of immobilization there is still documented instability or excessive motion in the cervical spine, surgery can then be considered. Halo vest immobilization may be selected after anterior cervical spine decompression and fusion when there is documented accompanying posterior ligamentous instability (most often compression flexion lesions).

In some patients, immediate surgery will be required for spinal cord decompression. In these patients a second procedure in which posterior wiring and fusion or utilization of the halo vest for three months to allow for graft incorporation will be necessary to provide complete stabilization. For these patients the halo vest is protection against graft dislodgement and development of kyphotic deformity secondary to the posterior ligamentous instability.[6]

CONTRAINDICATIONS TO THE UTILIZATION OF THE HALO VEST

In some purely ligamentous injuries such as distraction flexion 1 and distraction flexion 2 injuries (formerly known as facet dislocations, unilateral and bilateral), there is total ligamentous instability and insufficient bony injury to permit healing. Utilization of the halo for three months in cases such as this often results in failure of achievement of bony union. Ligamentous injuries do best with posterior wiring and fusion, and surgical stabilization. If identification of a primary ligamentous injury can be made, early surgical stabilization is the treatment of choice.

In some combined head trauma and spinal cord injury patients when an unstable skull fracture is present, a contraindication exists to the utilization of a halo vest. This cannot provide the appropriate skeletal fixation without compromise of the fracture healing of the skull, and in many cases with massive head trauma there is no bony base that is stable enough to allow for fixation. These cases obviously require alternative forms of treatment, including surgery.

The most obvious situation in which prolonged halo vest immobilization is contraindicated is when there is a documented instance of bone and disc compressing the cervical spinal cord combined with documented worsening of neurologic function. These patients will not have improvement of neurologic function created or produced by halo immobilization. If initial traction has been applied and documented bone and disc are still present in the canal, surgical decompression is indicated. When neurologic function deteriorates, this treatment is indicated immediately.

CONCLUSIONS

The halo vest is a primary treatment of choice in nonoperative management of the cervical spine instability. It is a viable treatment alternative for many cases and in some instances it is the only treatment available for the patient. When appropriate identification of fracture classification is made, the surgeon can utilize the halo based upon results of recent research. Except for distractive flexion and compressive flexion type 3 injuries (in which the success rate is 50 per cent), the halo vest immobilization is successful in over 90 per cent of other fracture types. It is acknowledged that primary anterior bone comminution is required to effectively create a stimulus for callous formation and thereby create a significant healing environment. This is present in most fracture types other than those that only involve ligamentous injuries. If care is taken in initial application of the halo and if nursing and rehabilitation management includes detailed attention to potential skin problems, patients can usually tolerate three months of halo vest immobilization while participating in active rehabilitation. Newer materials that are radiopaque also do not interfere with appropriate study of the cervical spinal canal.

Although surgical management is emphasized in most training programs and remains the primary form of treatment of cervical spine instability, the treating surgeon must be familiar with utilization of the halo vest because it is extremely successful when appropriately applied.

REFERENCES

1. Beatson TR: Fractures and dislocations of the cervical spine. J Bone Joint Surg 45B:21, 1963.
2. Nickel VL, Perry J, Garrett A, Heppenstall M: The halo a spinal skeletal traction fixation device. J Bone Joint Surg 50-A 1400, 1968.
3. Allen BL Jr, Ferguson RL, Lehmann TR, O'Brien RP: A mechanistic classification of closed indirect fractures and dislocations of the lower cervical spine. Spine 7:1, 1982.
4. Nelson RW, Capen DA, Garland D, Waters RL: Halo vest stabilization of cervical spine fractures and dislocations. A series review and long term follow-up. AAOS Presentation, Annual Meeting, Atlanta, 1984.
5. Garfin SR, Botte MJ, Waters RL, Nickel VL: Complications in the use of the halo fixation device. J Bone Joint Surg 68A:320, 1986.
6. White AA, Johnson RM, Panjabi MM, Southwick WO: Biomechanical analysis of cervical stability in the cervical spine. Congress of Rehabilitation Research, 109:85, 1975.

Surgical Stabilization in Cervical Spine Trauma

15

DANIEL A. CAPEN, M.D.

Traumatic fracture or fracture dislocation of the cervical spine remains the most common cause for cervical spinal cord injury. Vehicular trauma, water sports, and low-velocity gunshot wounds account for 8000 to 10,000 traumatic spinal cord injuries in the United States each year. It is a disease of young people, with most series showing a preponderance of patients in their late teens and early twenties.[1-3] Spine stabilization remains a challenging problem for the surgeon.

Emergency techniques have continually improved to allow for a higher rate of survival from the initial injury. Also, advances in medical treatment have made life expectancy much longer among quadriplegics. The average life expectancy of a quadriplegic now approaches 80 per cent of normal.[4] Early treatment of cervical instability with minimal complications and maximum recovery potential is the objective. Rehabilitation to maximize functional recovery is of paramount importance. Appropriate early treatment of cervical injury facilitates the achievement of this goal. This treatment frequently includes surgery.

While it is clear that neurologic damage to the cervical spinal cord is often irreversible, some areas of the spinal cord may be only partially injured. Appropriate early treatment may protect the spinal cord from further injury and permit return of neurologic function.

Appropriate diagnosis and treatment of the patient with a damaged cervical spinal cord and unstable cervical spine is crucial to maximize the potential for recovery. With emergency treatment, attention to the total patient is essential. Frequently, with high-speed injuries, there is associated head trauma or visceral injury or both as well as cervical spine damage. It is also important to realize that multisystem complications may accompany a cervical spinal cord injury, including pulmonary, renal, gastrointestinal, and cardiovascular problems. Appropriate management of these injuries must be instituted before the decision is made to use any surgical procedure to stabilize the spine. Realignment of the skeletal elements and stabilization in a nonoperative manner may be indicated to allow for the appropriate treatment of these injuries. It is also essential to have an appropriate understanding of the diagnostic implications of the neurologic injury.

The goals of treatment of the unstable cervical spine are to realign the spine, to protect partially damaged neural tissue, and to facilitate early mobilization for rehabilitation. Restoration of near-normal canal dimensions can serve to maximize recovery. However, direct surgical removal of bone and soft tissue fragments may also be required. The achievement of decompression must be planned with consideration for patient condition, extent of instability, and timing.

While perioperative complications can be expected to occur with all surgical procedures on spinal cord injury patients (Table 15–1) the selection of the appropriate surgical approach and method of fixation is crucial. While use of both anterior and posterior stabilization techniques is warranted, inappropriate use of these procedures can result in significant complications. Before a decision concerning the surgical procedure is made, an understanding of indications for each procedure is essential.

176

TABLE 15–1. Distribution of Complications in Each Patient Group with Average Blood Loss for Surgical Procedure

COMPLICATION (NO. PATIENTS AFFECTED)	ANTERIOR FUSION	POSTERIOR FUSION	COMBINED FUSION
Wound	5	10	0
Pulmonary	4	10	0
DVT (PE)	6(2)	6(2)	1
GI	3	0	0
ENT	8	0	1
Other	0	3	1
TOTAL COMPLICATIONS	28 in 18 pts	31 in 22 pts	3 in 3 pts
Blood Loss (in ml's)	639	651	725

IDENTIFICATION OF INSTABILITY

Recognition of the location and extent of cervical spine instability is crucial in formulation of a plan for surgical stabilization as well as in selection of appropriate methods of nonoperative stabilization. A treatment plan can be made only after an accurate assessment of the type of injury is done. Repeated failure of anterior stabilization alone has led to the realization that the posterior ligaments are more frequently damaged than previously thought.[2,5–7]

We recommend utilization of the Allen classification of cervical injuries[8] to best diagnose the location and extent of instability. The use of sophisticated diagnostic equipment, including CT scanning, magnetic resonance imaging, and contrast myelography, also helps in localizing compressive lesions and helps in determining whether decompressive surgery would be beneficial. With this information the surgical procedure can be chosen to treat either posterior or anterior lesions.

POSTERIOR STABILIZATION OF THE CERVICAL SPINE

The achievement of stability from a posterior surgical approach has long been utilized. Since Hadra passed the first wire for a case of instability secondary to tuberculosis,[9] the use of internal fixation wire and bone graft on the posterior elements has been an effective method for stabilizing the spine. Rogers[10,11] first reported a large series of cases describing the efficacy of this procedure.

With many modifications, a simple interspinous process wiring technique has evolved. A drill hole through the upper spinous process with an 18-gauge wire passed around the inferior margin of the spinous process below the level of the lesion provides for an internal splint to allow for a modest amount of bone graft to be incorporated when placed along the posterior lamina and facet joints (Fig. 15–1). This procedure affords enough stability to permit halo removal and use of a Philadelphia collar for three months. It provides a low risk, low blood loss type of procedure that, in most cases, has been performed under local anesthesia in patients in whom neurologic monitoring is crucial.[12]

Posterior wiring and fusion are clearly superior in cases in which the trauma is primarily ligamentous as in distractive flexion injuries, indicating unilateral and bilateral facet dislocations. These injuries involve a significant amount of ligamentous damage both in the posterior and anterior columns, and these types of injuries are characterized by a high

Figure 15–1. *A* and *B*, The standard technique of posterior wiring and fusion with corticocancellous onlay graft is shown. Note in *B* the appropriate wire placement.

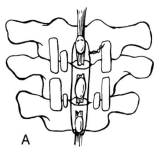
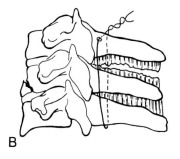

A

B

probability of late instability if treated nonsurgically.[3] The posterior wire and fusion secures the ligamentous area and allows for bone graft incorporation. Clearly, the aim is to immobilize as few segments as possible; however, in some cases, lamina fractures make a longer fusion procedure necessary.

In the compressive flexion type of injury (Fig. 15–2), there is a definite incidence of posterior ligamentous instability that can be unrecognized. This compressive flexion injury was frequently associated with complications of late instability when treated by means of a halo vest or with anterior stabilization. In a review of the Rancho Los Amigos experience and the literature, this type of fracture was frequently mistaken for a burst type of vertical compression injury. Efforts were directed at anterior stabilization because it was thought that the bony lesion was of primary importance. We now recognize that this type of injury involves both anterior and posterior instability. Surgical treatment must address the ligamentous lesion, and if decompression is needed it can be performed without risk of graft dislodgement or late kyphotic deformity.

We recommend posterior wiring and fusion for patients with complete spinal cord injury after traction reduction to the best possible lateral x-ray position. This restores stability. Later, anterior decompression may play a role. Clearly, in the patients whose lesions are complete, the anterior decompressive technique provides little hope for recovery, with the possible exception of enhanced nerve root recovery. It has been shown, however, that root escape will occur in fully one third of the patients, regardless of treatment.[12] Surgical manipulation can impair the root escape; therefore, adequate precautions must be taken even when dealing with complete neurologic injury.

One subgroup of compressive-flexion injuries requires anterior decompression because of fragments of disc and/or vertebral body protruding posteriorly into the canal. If incomplete neurologic injury is present with these compressive-flexion injuries, there may be an opportunity for recovery if the area is appropriately decompressed. Once again, however, it is important to realize that, if the goal is halo-free immobilization in this group of patients, a posterior wiring and fusion procedure would be indicated before the anterior procedure to treat the posterior ligamentous instability. At our facility we perform the posterior procedure first under local anesthesia,[13] followed in one to two weeks by the anterior decompression.

ANTERIOR CERVICAL DECOMPRESSION AND FUSION

Anterior stabilization of the cervical spine has a definite place in treatment of cervical spine injury. It is rarely indicated as a primary stabilizing procedure. When used for this purpose, it is fraught with complications of graft dislodgement and progressive kyphotic deformity in the face of posterior ligamentous instability (Table 15–2).[2,3,5,6] If unaccompanied by posterior stabilization, it should be augmented by use of a halo vest for a period of three months to allow for graft incorporation.

The technique of anterior decompression and fusion has been described by many au-

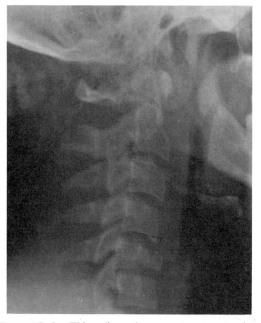

Figure 15–2. This radiograph represents a compressive-flexion lesion with occult but definite posterior ligamentous instability. The radiographs after anterior stabilization are in Figure 15–4, where the posterior ligamentous injury can be seen as kyphosis develops.

TABLE 15–2. A Comparison of Postsurgical Complications of Anterior and Posterior Stabilization Procedures

	ANTERIOR	POSTERIOR
Follow-up/total	59/88	98/114
Fusion extension	0/59	73/98
Graft/wire loss	6/59	4/98
Loss of reduction	32/59	0/98
Degenerative changes	36/59	2/98

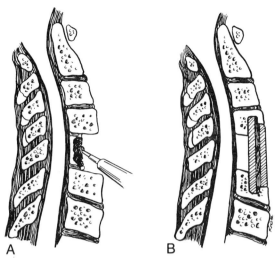

Figure 15-3. *A* and *B*, This is an artistic representation of the standard anterior decompression and fusion technique performed at Rancho. The use of fibular strut has now been substituted in favor of key-shaped tricortical iliac crest.

thors.[6,8] We utilize an anterior approach to the cervical spinal column and perform vertebrectomy and discectomy as needed (Fig. 15-3). After adequate decompression, tricortical iliac crest is keyed into the vertebra above and below the lesion (Fig. 15-4). This graft can be tailored to the appropriate length of fusion.

We would emphasize that the combination of anterior decompression and fusion is not the primary stabilization procedure of choice. It should be reserved for patients with incomplete neurologic lesions in whom recovery has reached a plateau and who have demonstrable anterior compressive lesions. In these patients, the decompressive procedure can be very beneficial. It can also be used in a patient with loss of neurologic function with anterior compressive elements.

The anterior decompressive approach is of definitive benefit in one subgroup of patients with cervical spinal cord injury who have no real demonstrable instability. These patients with traumatic spondylitic myelopathy frequently have sustained their central cord injury by a fall or hyperextension injury to the neck. In these cases, multiple levels of compression and/or spinal stenosis frequently are found. The anterior approach affords an excellent exposure to allow decompression and allows for stabilization of the unstable segments. A secondary benefit is achieved by immobilizing the segments of the cervical spine to allow for osteophyte resorption.

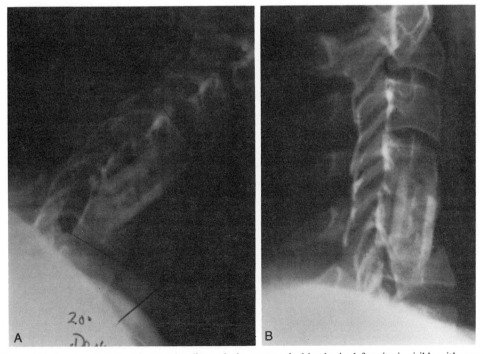

Figure 15-4. *A* and *B*, In this lateral radiograph the postsurgical kyphotic deformity is visible with more noticeable posterior interspinous process widening. Tilt and settling of the fibular strut graft are also noted. This is the postsurgical result when unrecognized ligament injury is present posteriorly (Fig. 15-2).

DECOMPRESSIVE LAMINECTOMY

No discussion of surgical treatment of the cervical spine would be complete without addressing the issue of laminectomy. Neurosurgical colleagues rely on removal of the posterior elements to allow for spinal cord recovery by revascularization and relief of pressure. It is important to note that the literature has no evidence that would statistically substantiate that removal of bony elements leads to neurologic recovery.[14,15] Although decreasing in frequency, the cervical decompressive laminectomy for trauma is still too frequently performed (20 per cent incidence). Several series of patients with complications after laminectomy including neurologic injury failure of stabilization and late deformity provide evidence for avoiding this procedure. Our series[14] presented a neurologic complication rate of 8.8 per cent and a surgical complication rate of 26 per cent directly related to early laminectomy. Decompressive laminectomy makes treatment of instability quite difficult. It makes limited posterior cervical fusion extremely difficult and causes anterior stabilization to be hazardous. A Southwick type of posterior lateral fusion is more technically demanding, requires more extensive surgery with greater blood loss, and immobilizes a longer segment of the cervical spine. In patients whose lesions are not surgically stabilized, there is a high incidence of late kyphotic deformity (42 per cent), especially in those with complete quadriplegia (Fig. 15–5).

From a statistical standpoint, the performance of post-traumatic decompressive cervical laminectomy is contraindicated. No justification can be made to support the use of this procedure. In cases of recovery with laminectomy, there are an equal number of cases with recovery without the laminectomy; no reason exists to subject the patient to a high-risk surgical procedure early on in the treatment of the lesion.

SURGICAL COMPLICATIONS

When performing posterior cervical fusion under local anesthesia, the potential for significant neurologic complications associated with application of internal wire fixation is minimal.

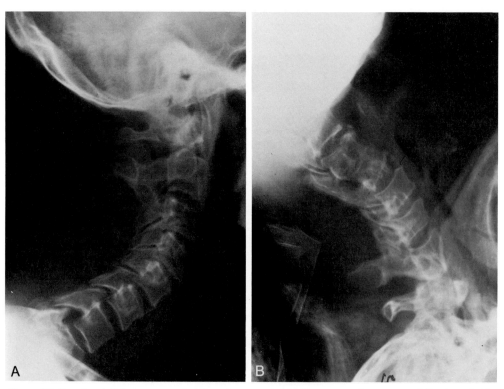

Figure 15–5. *A* and *B,* Late swan neck deformity was noted in 42 per cent of cases not stabilized surgically after decompressive laminectomy. Impaired root escape was noted and long-term loss of neck function is a concern. Clearly, stabilization of the cervical spine in this patient is made more difficult by extensive laminectomy.

The procedure can be performed without significant discomfort and is well tolerated. No major neurologic complication has occurred in 51 consecutive posterior cervical fusions using local anesthesia.

The technique of midline and lateral injection of a solution of 1 per cent xylocaine at 2 to 3 mg per pound of patient body weight is easily accomplished. To inhibit blood loss, the solution contains 1:500,000 epinephrine. In most cases 80 to 100 cc is required for the cervical surgery and 40 to 60 cc for the iliac crest graft. Because this technique is done under local anesthesia, there has been more attention given to limited exposure of posterior elements and limited application of bone grafting. Although long-term follow-up is not available, it is believed that this will reduce the 75 per cent incidence of fusion extension noted in the study of 114 cases of posterior spine fusions performed under general anesthesia.

Surgical complications associated with the anterior approach are greater than those with posterior surgery because of the potential for local tracheal and esophageal problems. However, in experienced hands, these complications are extremely rare. A 10 per cent incidence of transient reversible dysphagia or dysphonia can be anticipated. The primary late complications are associated with the error in diagnosis of location and extent of posterior ligamentous instability. Inappropriate use of the anterior surgical procedure resulted in progressive kyphosis and graft dislodgement in over 60 per cent of the cases in which anterior surgery was utilized as the primary stabilizing procedure.

achieve surgical stability. This procedure can be done safely—frequently under local anesthesia—with a minimum risk of neurologic complications. It is recommended that primary anterior stabilization of the cervical spine be reserved for the few cases in which a posterior procedure is impossible or the sole instability is located anteriorly and a halo vest apparatus is not applicable.

The anterior approach has a primary function in decompressing the cervical spine from bony fragments, disc fragments, osteophytic spurs, or spinal stenosis. In traumatic cases, the patient requires either an initial posterior fusion or a halo vest until the anterior graft incorporates, thus preventing graft dislodgement or late kyphotic deformity. It is the anterior decompression rather than cervical laminectomy that is the procedure of choice to effect relief of compressing elements on the cervical spinal cord and nerve roots.

Despite the fact that quadriparesis and quadriplegia may present concomitant health compromises, it should be noted that the posterior stabilizing procedure is relatively safe. It serves to realign the spine, to protect the existing neurologic function, and to facilitate early recovery and participation in rehabilitation. Patients suffering from this devastating injury can then learn to maximize their functional potential.

The choice of surgical treatment remains one of many primary steps that lead to the goal of total rehabilitation. The choices of surgery should be made with a view to minimizing the potential for complication, to eliminating possible neurologic damage, and to maximizing the rehabilitation potential in the shortest possible time.

CONCLUSIONS

When halo vest immobilization is not tolerated and if halo-free rehabilitation is desired, posterior surgical stabilization is a safe and effective treatment of cervical instability. Surgical decompression can be performed without significant added risk. Each surgical approach has appropriate indications that have been outlined, and when proper indications are observed, excellent long-term results can be anticipated.

From a review of an extremely large series of patients and a review of the literature, our conclusion is that a vast majority of destabilizing injuries to the cervical spine respond well to early posterior wiring and fusion. Most frequently it is the primary procedure of choice to

REFERENCES

1. Bailey RW, Badgley CE: Stabilization of the cervical spine by anterior fusion. J Bone Joint Surg 42A:565, 1960.
2. Bohlman H: Acute fractures and dislocations of the cervical spine. J Bone Joint Surg 61A:1119, 1979.
3. Capen D, Waters R, Garland D: A comparative analysis of anterior and posterior fusions. Clin Orthop Rel Res 186:229, 1985.
4. Geisler WO, Jousse AT, Wynne-Jones M, and Breithaupt D: Survival in traumatic spinal cord injury. Paraplegia 21:364, 1983.
5. Cloward RB: Treatment of acute fractures and fracture dislocations of the cervical spine by vertebral body fusion. A report of 11 cases. J Neurosurg 18:201, 1961.
6. Stauffer ES, and Rhoades ME: Surgical stabilization of the cervical spine after trauma. Arch Surg 111:652, 1976.

7. Van Peteghem PK, and Schweigel JF: The fractured cervical spine rendered unstable by anterior cervical fusion. J Trauma 19:110, 1979.

8. Allen BL, Ferguson RL, Lehman TR, O'Brien RP: A mechanistic classification of closed indirect fractures and dislocations of the lower cervical spine. Spine 7:1, 1982.

9. Hadra BE: Wiring of the spinous process in injury and Pott's disease. Trans Am Orthop Assn. 4:206, 1891.

10. Rogers WA: Treatment of fracture dislocation of the cervical spine. J Bone Joint Surg 24:295, 1942.

11. Rogers WA: Fractures and dislocations of the cervical spine, an end-result study. J Bone Joint Surg 39A:2, 1957.

12. Venos K: Rancho Los Amigos Hospital experience with root escape after spinal cord injury. Rancho Proceedings, July 1982.

13. Zigler J, Rockowitz N, Capen D, Nelson R, Waters R: Posterior Cervical Fusion Using Local Anesthesia. AAOS Meeting, 1986.

14. Capen DA, Nelson RW, Zigler JE, Sadler CR, Waters RL: Decompressive laminectomy in cervical spine trauma. A review of early and late complications. AAOS meeting, 1985.

15. Heiden JS, Weiss MH, Rosenberg AW, Apuzzo ML and Kurze T: Management of cervical spinal cord trauma in Southern California. J Neurosurg 43:732, 1975

16 Spinal Cord Injury Treatment and the Anesthesiologist

JOSEPH P. GIFFIN, M.D., and KENNETH GRUSH, M.D.

Currently on an annual basis 10,000 patients with spinal cord trauma survive the initial injury to arrive at our nation's hospitals,[1] presenting anesthesiologists and other intensive care specialists with a unique responsibility and challenge. The fact that 70 per cent of these patients are 19 to 34 years of age[2] makes this an especially poignant problem in terms of lost human potential as well as the urgency to preserve whatever function remains and restore as much lost function as possible.

While the mortality for these patients remains high, approximately 50 per cent reported in 1980,[3] recent advances in resuscitation and rehabilitation have resulted in an expanding population of long-term survivors.[2] In spite of continuing disagreement on the advisability of surgical intervention, 78 per cent of patients admitted to one spinal injury center with acute spinal cord injury underwent some type of surgical procedure.[4] Clearly, there is a need for the anesthesiologist to be familiar with the nature of spinal cord injury and its management.

Consequently, our attention in this discussion will be directed toward the acute management of spinal cord injury and the medical sequelae of spinal cord injury which may influence the anesthetic management for diagnostic and surgical procedures. Finally, current concepts of the pathophysiology of spinal cord injury will be discussed with regard to experimental as well as clinical modalities of spinal cord resuscitation which bear some hope for the restoration of useful function.

ACUTE MANAGEMENT OF SPINAL CORD INJURY

Since anesthesiologists are frequently consulted to assist in the management of patients in unstable condition arriving with severe spinal cord injury in the emergency department, a brief review of the necessary steps in stabilizing such patients follows. As in most life-threatening medical emergencies, first attention must be directed to the ABCs (airway, breathing, and circulation). Any comatose and/or multiple trauma patient must be considered to have a cord injury until proven otherwise. First, an airway is established using the jaw thrust technique while the head and neck are maintained in the neutral position. Absent ventilation after this mandates the initiation of artificial ventilation, either mouth-to-mouth or bag-valve-mask. Inability to ventilate the patient in spite of jaw thrust usually means that a foreign body is occluding the airway; this should be assessed and remedied. Although movement of the neck is contraindicated, asphyxia certainly carries a worse prognosis than cervical cord injury. It is the most common early cause of death.

Laryngoscopy and intubation should be carried out as expediently as possible with immobilization of the spine maintained. Ventilation should be given to produce a normal minute ventilation (75 to 80 ml/kg). In the breathing patient, supplemental oxygen and intensive observation are indicated.

Once these goals are satisfied, the systemic

blood pressure should be supported at normal levels with the judicious administration of intravenous fluids if hypotension is present. Ventilatory and circulatory management of these patients are discussed in greater detail below.

Between 25 to 65 per cent of spinal cord injury patients have associated problems, the most common being head, chest, abdominal and skeletal injuries.[5] These may complicate ventilatory and circulatory problems resulting from the cord injury, and a high index of suspicion is necessary in evaluating these patients. As soon as feasible, appropriate roentgenographic studies should be completed (including magnetic resonance imaging and computed tomographic scans). Initial laboratory determinations should include CBC, arterial blood gases, serum electrolytes, serum creatinine, and any other study dictated by the individual patient's intrinsic illnesses or associated injuries.

Once the ABCs have been addressed and life-threatening deficits managed, the next priority becomes rapid transport of the patient with the spine immobilized to a major trauma center or, when feasible, to an acute cord injury center.[5] Upon arrival at the hospital, diagnostic studies to determine the extent of injury and whether surgery is indicated are initiated, followed by appropriate medical therapy.

MEDICAL COMPLICATIONS OF SPINAL CORD INJURY AND THEIR MANAGEMENT

Respiratory Complications

Depending on the level and degree of spinal cord injury, respiration may be impaired by paralysis of abdominal, intercostal, diaphragmatic, and accessory muscles of respiration progressively as the site of trauma moves from low thoracic to high cervical or even brainstem levels. Loss of motor function originating at C3 to C5, giving rise to the phrenic nerves, results in diaphragmatic paralysis (major contribution from C4) as well as the loss of intercostal and abdominal motor function. High quadriplegia (C4 or above) results in a severe, life-threatening decrease in all standard measures of respiratory mechanics and dynamics—forced vital capacity (FVC), forced expiratory volume in one second (FEV_1), peak inspiratory and expiratory force and flow, and total pulmonary compliance. Only the accessory muscles of inspiration (sternocleidomastoid, scalenes, and trapezius) function during inspiration. Lower

rib cage and abdominal paradox is seen as the hemidiaphragms passively respond to the changes in intrathoracic pressure caused by accessory muscle activity. As the upper rib cage expands (less than with intact intercostal muscles), upward diaphragm motion decreases intra-abdominal pressure, resulting in inward movement of it and the lower rib cage. The reverse occurs during expiration. The paradoxical diaphragm motion and its cephalad displacement decrease the efficiency of already diminished muscle activity in effecting gas exchange.[6] Tidal volume, inspiratory and expiratory reserve volumes (IRV and ERV), and functional residual capacity (FRC) are critically reduced, while residual volume (RV) is increased.[7]

Alveolar hypoventilation results in hypercarbia. Hypoventilation, atelectasis, and airspace collapse associated with the decrease in FRC relative to closing volume produce ventilation-perfusion ($\dot{V}/\dot{Q}$) mismatching and cause hypoxemia. Respiratory function in this case is worst in the supine or Trendelenburg positions, as abdominal contents displace the diaphragm further cephalad, and it improves if other variables (e.g., blood pressure) permit some degree of head and thorax elevation. Global hypoventilation often worsens further during sleep, occasionally progressing to sleep apnea, which has been attributed to diminished carbon dioxide responsiveness.[8,9]

Sighing and coughing are essential to maintain alveolar patency and pulmonary toilet. A near-normal inspiratory reserve is required in the former case, while the generation of pressure against a closed glottis and maintenance of flow following glottic opening is essential in the latter. Decreases in IRV, ERV, FVC, peak inspiratory and expiratory force and flow, as well as inability to splint the diaphragm accompanying diaphragmatic, intercostal, and abdominal paralysis cause inability to cough and clear airway secretions or to sigh and diminish atelectasis.[10]

Low quadriplegic patients with partial or complete integrity of diaphragmatic innervation will have variable diaphragmatic strength. Also, the diaphragms are prevented from achieving their optimal, steeply domed fiber length-tension position at end-expiration because of intercostal and abdominal muscle paralysis; hence, their inspiratory efficiency is impaired. Adding to this effect is the upper rib cage paradoxical *inward* motion during inspiration (lower rib cage and abdominal paradox in high quadriplegics).[10] The resulting decrease in respiratory capacity may produce $\dot{V}/\dot{Q}$ mismatching and hypoxemia.

Five months after injury, a group of these patients was found to have a 50 per cent decrease in FVC, peak expiratory and inspiratory flow, and inspiratory and expiratory reserve volumes. Decreases in expiratory flow were much less at low lung volumes (at 25 per cent of total lung volume, flow was 72 per cent of the predicted value) than at higher lung volumes (55 per cent of predicted value). This was taken to implicate muscle weakness rather than intrinsic airway disease, airway compression, or decreased lung compliance as the primary cause of the decreased flow rates: normally, initial expiratory flow rate is effort dependent, whereas late expiratory flow rates are effort independent and are limited by airway compression, which increases resistance proportionately to thoracic pressure. Muscle weakness, therefore, would decrease early expiratory flow as well as end-expiratory resistance. Assuming the Trendelenburg position, by shifting the diaphragms cephalad to a more mechanically advantageous starting fiber length, actually increased IRV and FVC an average of 300 ml.[11]

The importance of the extent of diaphragmatic involvement is emphasized by a study comparing quadriplegics having complete cord lesions at the C5 to C6 level, with an average FVC of 1.5 L (24 per cent of predicted), to those having complete lesions at C4 with an average FVC of 1.3 L (21 per cent of predicted). Four of 11 patients with C5 to C6 lesions required oxygen, but only two required mechanical ventilation. All five patients with C4 lesions received oxygen and were ventilated. Although both groups approximately doubled their vital capacities over the next three months and were breathing unassisted, two patients having C4 level lesions displayed postural hypoxemia and hypercarbia.[12]

The significance of at least some presence of intercostal muscle activity on EMG was demonstrated by measured decreases in FRC, transpulmonary pressure at FRC, and static expiratory compliance in patients lacking parasternal intercostal EMG activity. These three values remained normal in those who displayed such EMG activity—a finding attributed to a postulated role for tonic inspiratory intercostal activity in helping to determine FRC, which has usually been attributed to passive chest wall recoil balanced against lung compressibility. This would increase transpulmonary pressure, increase FRC, maintain alveolar inflation, and improve lung compli-

ance.[13] The same investigators have found previously unsuspected participation of the pectoralis major and possibly other muscles during expiration, accounting for the persistence of a small ERV in patients with paralysis of all commonly accepted expiratory muscles.[7] Training directed at both expiratory and inspiratory accessory muscles and diaphragms combined with any functional intercostal recovery can result in improved strength and endurance as well as decreased likelihood of fatigue.[14]

Although respiration is less compromised in low quadriplegics and paraplegics than in high quadriplegics, those with low lesions are still at risk for hypoventilation, $\dot{V}/\dot{Q}$ mismatching, and retention of secretions paralleling the changes in respiratory parameters already outlined. Aside from diaphragmatic and intercostal muscle strength, a key factor in overall respiratory function is the contribution of the abdominal muscles in increasing expiratory pressure directly as well as improving the efficiency of the intercostals in forced expiration or coughing by preventing paradoxical movement of the diaphragm into the abdomen. The importance of abdominal muscle tone in optimizing diaphragmatic position for inspiration has already been discussed. The abdominal weakness or paralysis accounts for the persistence of respiratory complications, especially retained secretions and pulmonary infections seen in some paraplegics with intact diaphragms and intercostal muscles.

Evaluation of the respiratory status of a spinal cord injury patient should be directed toward any obvious signs of hypoxemia or dyspnea, tidal volume, FVC, FEV_1 respiratory rate, and minute volume, as well as observation of abdominal and thoracic movement, which should indicate the level of respiratory muscle impairment. Accessory muscle activity can be detected by inspection and careful palpation of the muscles involved or electromyography as needed. Arterial blood gas analysis should be done as soon as feasible.

Any comatose, apparently apneic or cyanotic patient or those unable to manage their secretions should be endotracheally intubated as soon as possible, as has usually already been done before arrival at the hospital in severely compromised patients. Immobilization of the spine is essential in preventing extension or completion of an incomplete lesion. In cervical injuries, the head should be maintained in the neutral position (neither flexed nor extended) by *gentle* traction (the aim is *not* reduction) so as to avoid neck movement during intubation.

Blind nasotracheal intubation, as well as laryngoscopic or flexible fiberoptic oral or nasal intubation, are all possible and should be chosen on the basis of the ability to accomplish the task both as quickly as possible and without disturbing the existing cervical alignment.

A wide selection of laryngoscope blades, endotracheal tube sizes, a fiberoptic laryngoscope, cricothyroidotomy apparatus, supplemental oxygen, manual and mechanical ventilation equipment, suction apparatus, and other resuscitation equipment and drugs should be available and ready for use. Surgical tracheostomy back-up should also be available. Sedation and/or neuromuscular blockade is not advisable in view of the further respiratory compromise and loss of muscular cervical splinting that they cause. Superior laryngeal nerve block and meticulous topical anesthesia will improve patient tolerance when time and airway status permit their use. The distinct possibility of sinus arrest or complete heart block resulting from unopposed vagovagal reflexes following pharyngeal and tracheal stimulation in lesions above T4 should be borne in mind and can be prevented by 0.6 mg of atropine administered intravenously.[15] Some investigators question this practice as rarely needed and prefer treatment with atropine on an occurrence basis. Although tracheostomy is rarely needed acutely, once the indications for anterior cervical fusion have been excluded, early tracheostomy provides greater patient comfort and makes eating, talking, and pulmonary toilet easier in those patients who will require prolonged mechanical support.

Once intubation has been accomplished, ventilatory assistance is indicated in patients displaying an elevated $PaCO_2$ or a borderline PaO_2 in the face of maximal sustainable ventilatory efforts. Spontaneously breathing intubated patients with adequate ventilation should be given supplemental oxygen, and continuous positive airway pressure (CPAP) may be added incrementally to normalize FRC, thus reducing atelectasis and $\dot{V}/\dot{Q}$ mismatching while improving compliance and lessening the work of breathing. Frequent respiratory assessment is mandatory, especially in view of the frequent cephalad extension of injuries which can occur in the acute period.

No mode of ventilation is inherently superior,[10] although synchronized intermittent mandatory ventilation (SIMV) has the theoretical advantages of greater hemodynamic stability and continuing exercise of functional muscles. Positive end expiratory pressure (PEEP) may be added for considerations already mentioned. The recent introduction of variable pressure support ventilation, in which all spontaneous breaths can be supported at any desired pressure level and synchronized with variable frequency mandatory machine breaths, combines many of the advantages of SIMV with the security of controlled or assist-control ventilation in terms of compensating for potential muscle fatigue. In the exclusively pressure-support mode, fine tuning of muscle work load is possible for training and weaning purposes.

In cases of complete lesions above C3, alternatives to chronic positive pressure ventilation include radiofrequency electrophrenic stimulation in patients with damaged phrenic nuclei but intact phrenic nerves,[16] or intermittent negative pressure ventilation in an iron lung when the phrenic nerves are interrupted. Chronic subtotal diaphragmatic dysfunction can be managed by means of a rocking bed, chest cuirass, or pneumobelt.[6]

Respiratory complications are the most common cause of death in acute spinal cord injury, with pneumonia being the most important after anoxic death at the time of injury.[17] In patients with chronic, stabilized conditions, respiratory infections decrease and cause less than 10 per cent of the febrile episodes. The importance of aggressive pulmonary toilet in addressing this problem was evidenced by a 33 per cent decrease in prolonged ventilation as a result of such measures as careful monitoring of pulmonary function, vigorous chest physical therapy, and early bronchoscopy and lavage if lobar collapse develops as shown by chest roentgenographs.[18] Any fever accompanied by leukocytosis or physical and/or radiographic evidence of pneumonitis should be aggressively treated.

Cardiovascular Complications

The hemodynamic sequelae of spinal cord injury follow a sequential pattern beginning at the moment of injury. First, it has been well documented experimentally[19] that for 3 to 4 minutes following spinal cord compression, a sudden drastic increase in systolic blood pressure, between 200 and 250 mm Hg, occurs. This has been attributed both to an early thoracic sympathetic outflow and to a later, adrenally mediated secretion of catecholamines.[20] The possible role of this abrupt pressor response in augmenting the extent of hemorrhagic necrosis and releasing possible mediators of secondary injury is discussed in the section on pathophysiology.

Experimental cord injury has also been shown to result in transient but significant increases in intracranial pressure, blood-brain barrier permeability, brain water, and extravascular lung water with a marked decrease in cerebral blood flow.[21] This investigation verified the extreme increase in blood pressure (to a mean of 225 mm Hg), which lasted for 6 minutes, and also showed increases in pulmonary artery pressure, pulmonary capillary occlusion pressure, central venous pressure, and cardiac output. However, the intracerebral and pulmonary changes occurred before the cardiovascular changes were fully developed. This, along with the fact that phentolamine pretreatment sufficient to prevent the cardiovascular changes did not prevent the brain and lung events, seems to support independent but causally linked mechanisms producing both processes. At any rate, this work is compatible with the clinically observed susceptibility to pulmonary[22] and cerebral edema seen during resuscitation of spinal cord injured patients and reinforces the advisability of early hemodynamic monitoring to guide fluid management in these patients.

Since spinal cord injury patients rarely reach medical attention within minutes of their injury, acute hypertension is rarely, if ever, observed. Most patients manifest varying degrees of hypotension. This phase, commonly called *spinal shock,* features hypotension, bradycardia, decreased total peripheral resistance, low or normal central venous pressure, and normal or elevated cardiac output.[22] Orthostatic and other pressor reflexes are diminished or absent, and thermoregulation is lost. At the same time, somatic and visceral motor and sensory loss below the level of the lesion is observed. The extent of these changes is a result of the level of the cord injury. Injuries at or above T1 may result in mean blood pressures as low as 40 mm Hg. The observed bradycardia may be due to unopposed vagal tone secondary to loss of the cardiac accelerator fibers (T1 to T4), but many believe that the Bainbridge reflex caused by a fall in right atrial and central venous pressures is a more important contributing factor, as bradycardia is seen with lesions below T4. The critical level above which significant hypotension will be manifested is T6 to T7.

This phase of spinal shock may last days to weeks but is more abbreviated than the period of skeletal muscle–flaccid paralysis. Unfortunately, no one has delineated the point at which the sympathetic neurons regain their functional ability, now autonomous from higher control; but it is clear that they do regain some tonic activity as well as the ability for reflex reaction as evidenced by the unpredictable onset of potentially catastrophic sympathetic reflex spasticity.

Alterations in cardiovascular function during the subacute and chronic phases of spinal cord injury feature the persistence of a slightly low to normal blood pressure and pulse rate in most patients punctuated by episodes of severe hypertension in up to 85 per cent of patients with lesions at or above T6. These hypertensive spasms are triggered by day-to-day stimuli—most often distention of a hollow viscus, such as bladder or rectum. Other stimuli—including temperature, contractions of labor, and surgery—may be particularly potent.[23] The tendency toward reflex hypertension is called autonomic hyperreflexia. Its symptoms include facial paresthesias, nasal congestion, severe headache, dyspnea, nausea and blurred vision. Typical diagnostic signs are vasoconstrictive pallor, sweating, and piloerection below the level of the lesion,[24] vasodilation and flushing above the lesion site, accompanied by bradycardia and severe hypertension.[25] Subarachnoid and retinal hemorrhages have been observed, which eventuate in syncope, convulsions, and finally death if the hypertension continues unabated.[23]

The neuroanatomical correlates of this syndrome include stimuli arising from somatic or visceral receptors causing afferent impulses that follow their normal course via the posterior columns and spinothalamic tracts. Spinal cord section prevents these impulses from reaching the brain, but they do synapse with cells of the intermediolateral gray, giving rise to efferent sympathetic discharges. Normally these reflexes are localized in nature, but after spinal cord injury they tend to involve most of the sympathetic system below the level of the lesion. The usual homeostatic inhibitory impulses from higher centers following the initial arrival of the afferent impulses are never triggered. Intense, unabated somatic and visceral muscle contractions, arteriolar spasm, sweating, and piloerection are caused by the unchecked sympathetic reflexes below the cord lesion. Above the cord lesion, the hypertension caused by the arterioloar spasm and adrenal secretion activates carotid sinus and aortic arch baroreceptors as well as other CNS reflexes to cause vagally induced bradycardia as well as generalized vasodilation. These measures, however, are insufficient to prevent the hypertension when the lesion is above the origin of the splanchnic sympathetic outflow (T4 to T6). The time at which spastic autonomic or somatic reflex activity supersedes spinal shock and flaccid paralysis is difficult to predict and may occur one to three weeks or more after injury.[25]

Cardiac arrhythmias and electrocardiographic abnormalities may also contribute to cardiovascular risk in these patients. Acute, midthoracic spinal cord compression, besides producing hypertension, also usually resulted in sinus or nodal bradycardia in monkeys. Moreover, this initial response often preceded the pressor response. The initial bradyarrhythmias were followed by premature atrial and ventricular contractions, A-V dissociation, or ventricular tachycardias. Atropine prevented the bradycardia, whereas propranolol prevented the delayed ventricular tachyarrhythmias.[26] The electrocardiogram frequently shows ST-T wave changes variously interpreted as left ventricular strain pattern or consistent with subendocardial ischemia.[10,27] Similar arrhythmias have been reported in 75 per cent of autonomic hyperreflexia episodes.[24] The potential for severe bradycardia, heart block, and even cardiac arrest pursuant to tracheal stimulation in these patients has already been noted.[15]

Management of these cardiovascular problems is dictated by the physiological alterations that produce them. In the case of hypotension, a conservative approach is usually indicated, the urgency of treatment being proportional to the degree of hypotension and the symptomatology (CNS, cardiac, renal, and the like) produced. The etiology of the hypotension is usually a decreased venous return following sympathetic denervation, which causes increased venous capacitance as well as some degree of decreased arteriolar tone. However, cautious addition of volume is indicated in view of decreased cardiac reserve. This deficit in ability to accommodate excess volume is a natural consequence of the inability to further increase venous capacitance as the venous reservoir becomes full. Central venous pressure increases relatively little until the point when volume equals capacity and then rises abruptly. On the other hand, left ventricular and left atrial pressures increase proportionately with filling volume, and such indices as pulmonary capillary occlusion pressure (PCOP) will provide an early measure of volume status before CVP finally rises equivalently. Furthermore, sympathetically mediated reflex increases in heart rate and contractility are not possible in the event of lesions above T1.[28] Finally, the possibility of altered pulmonary capillary permeability to water during the acute phase of spinal cord injury, as already discussed, may play a role in the observed susceptibility to pulmonary edema during resuscitation of these patients, as occurred in 44 per cent of patients in one series.[22]

In view of these findings, early use of pulmonary artery catheters in monitoring fluid resuscitation during spinal shock would seem prudent. Not only are filling pressures and volume status readily assessable, but cardiac output and total peripheral resistance (TPR) can also be measured and manipulated if they are found to contribute to the hypotension. One clinical investigator[29] has used pulmonary arterial hemodynamic monitoring to categorize three groups of spinal cord injury patients. Rapid fluid infusion (50 ml/min in 250 ml increments), leg raising, or military anti-shock trousers (MAST) were used to increase central volume. One group of patients displayed a 3 to 4 mm Hg rise in PCOP, which settled to a level 2 mm Hg above control, with concomitant increases in cardiac output. A second group showed similar increases in PCOP, which then returned to baseline, with no net change in cardiac output. The third group showed progressive increases in PCOP and no change or a fall in cardiac output. He interpreted these findings as indicating adequate volume loading in the first instance, the need for more volume in the second group, and excessive volume and/or an indication for inotropic support in the last group. These guidelines seem appropriate in optimizing filling pressures at the lowest value yielding adequate cardiac output and perfusion pressures.

If, in spite of volume loading, cardiac output and mean arterial pressure are such that spinal cord and other organ hypoperfusion seems likely, inotropic support is indicated. One study compared the efficacy of either dopamine or transfusion in raising mean arterial pressure and augmenting SCBF in rats. Although both yielded improvements in these two variables, transfusion alone was better than dopamine alone.[30] The demonstration that naloxone-mediated increases in systemic blood pressure and spinal cord blood flow may be mediated by augmented endogenous plasma dopamine levels in the systemic circulation also suggests that this inotrope may be used when indicated without adversely affecting the potential for spinal cord recovery.[31]

The management of autonomic hyperreflexia is problematic in conscious patients, since the offending stimulus is not perceived, and headache or other symptoms of an already severely elevated blood pressure is usually the first clue that an episode is in progress. The aim in chronic spinal cord injury patients is, therefore, to avoid known stimuli through such measures as regular self-catheterization. Persistent attacks may require surgical or chemical ablation of the afferent pathways initiating the reflex through such measures as sacral neurotomy, dorsal rhizotomy, and use of subarachnoid phenol or alcohol. Pharmacological regimens investigated for preventing or treating autonomic hyperreflexia have included ganglionic blockers (trimethaphan, hexamethonium, pentolinium), catecholamine depleters (guanethidine), alpha-adrenergic blockers (phentolamine, phenoxybenzamine) and direct-acting vasodilators (nitroprusside). Unfortunately, many of the studies were small, lacked controls, or featured concomitant use of anesthetics. Consequently, comparison of the various drugs is difficult. Unpleasant side effects have also limited their usefulness. Finally, the ability to control visceral and somatic muscle spasm is not achieved when blood pressure is controlled only by adenergic blockers or direct-acting vasodilators. Basically, any treatment regimen for an acute episode that controls the arteriolar spasm and arrhythmias while maintaining cardiac output is acceptable.

Attempts at the prevention of autonomic hyperreflexia during surgery and anesthesia have met with more success. Schonwald et al.[32] reported a series of 219 patients with spinal cord injuries. Of the patients with lesions at or above T5, 33 per cent underwent general anesthesia with halothane (37 cases) or enflurane (12 cases), and none of these developed autonomic hyperreflexia or arrhythmias. Of nine patients in this group receiving nitrous oxide–narcotic anesthesia, two developed intraoperative hyperreflexia. In 97 cases of spinal anesthesia with tetracaine, no attacks occurred, but one lidocaine spinal anesthetic apparently wore off before the end of urological surgery, resulting in autonomic hyperreflexia. The author noted the level of injury as a major factor influencing the technical ease and feasibility of lumbar subarachnoid block, with low levels of injury resulting in failure in 3 of 19 patients, most likely

as a result of previous spinal surgery or traumatic distortion of the anatomy.

It should be borne in mind that successes in preventing hyperreflexia intraoperatively are not infrequently reversed by episodes occurring in the recovery room as the patient recovers from anesthesia; therefore, continued intensive monitoring and such measures as temperature regulation and bladder or bowel evacuation should be the routine.

Significant arrhythmias, such as ventricular tachycardia, are usually attendant to episodes of autonomic hyperreflexia and can likewise be prevented by adequate anesthetic depth or neural blockade in the surgical patient, or the other modalities discussed previously for day-to-day prophylaxis. Any life-threatening tachyarrhythmia that does occur in spite of prophylactic measures should be treated with beta-adrenergic blockers (concurrent alpha-adrenergic blockade is mandatory if significant hypertension is present) or other indicated antiarrhythmics. The baseline high vagal tone of these patients should be kept in mind, and atropine and pacemaking capability should be available if the combination of vagal tone and antiarrhythmic therapy results in sinus arrest, heart block, or too slow a rate to support adequate cardiac output. The potential need for atropine to treat the vagal reflexes attending tracheal stimulation should be anticipated.

Genitourinary Complications

Acute renal failure, although uncommon, may occur in spinal cord injury patients as a result of hypotension, dehydration, sepsis, use of nephrotoxic drugs, acute obstruction, associated kidney trauma, and other influences. During the chronic phase of spinal cord injury, renal failure becomes a progressively more important cause of death, accounting for 20 to 75 per cent of mortality.[17] In one series, renal failure caused only 4.5 per cent of all deaths in patients surviving only two years but caused 60 per cent or more of deaths among those surviving more than 10 years. Overall, renal failure is the factor producing death in 36 per cent of all spinal cord injury patients.[25] Pyelonephritis, amyloidosis, and hypertension were the most commonly identified proximate causes of death.[17]

Urinary retention, more often a problem in the flaccid lower motor neuron bladder than in the spastic upper motor neuron type, predisposes the patient to autonomic reflexes and cystitis. Vesicoureteral reflux may result from this cause as well as neurogenic causes, and repetitive ascending pyelonephritis occurs, leading eventually to secondary renal and adrenal amyloidosis and insufficiency. Neuropathic bladder outflow obstruction often contributes to the problem. Renal calculi tend to be recurrent in these patients. They are most often of the triple phosphate variety associated with urease-producing bacteria (e.g., Proteus spp.); however, some investigators believe that hypercalciuria may play a limited role.[17] A large proportion of surgery in chronic spinal cord injury patients is devoted to cystoscopy, urological invasive diagnostic studies, stone removal, lithotripsy, and urinary drainage or diversion procedures.

Urinary tract infections are a persistent problem. One autopsy series found a 90 per cent incidence of genitourinary disease including acute and chronic pyelonephritis (65 per cent), cystitis (74.5 per cent), nephrolithiasis (11.8 per cent), and other genitourinary infections (39.2 per cent). Another pathological study reported secondary amyloidosis in almost all specimens with an average postinjury survival of 12 years.[25] Prophylactic drug regimens have not been successful in substantially decreasing bacteriuria and bacteremia. Intermittent bladder catheterization seems to result in fewer infections and fewer instances of urolithiasis and renal dysfunction when compared with indwelling catheterization, at the expense of considerable time and equipment, but conclusive prospective studies are lacking.[17]

Renal insufficiency causes disturbances of the fluid and electrolyte, cardiovascular, and other systems. Hyponatremia, hypoproteinemia, hypocalcemia, increased extracellular and total body water, hypertension, and congestive heart failure may all be caused or exacerbated. These, as well as altered drug clearance, are clearly of concern to the anesthesiologist, and careful evaluation of renal function is a must. The avoidance of potentially nephrotoxic drugs is obviously advisable.

Proteinuria is usually the earliest sign of renal dysfunction, although it is qualitative rather than quantitative.[25] Serum creatinine studies may be misleading in view of the decrease in muscle mass seen in chronic quadriplegics. Although intravenous pyelography allows excellent visualization of the upper urinary tract, it is limited by potential allergic reactions, discomfort of the procedure and preparation, potential nephrotoxicity of the contrast material, cumulative radiation, and

the fact that significant functional impairment may precede detectable anatomical alterations. Renal scintigraphic determination of effective renal plasma flow seems to be a sensitive indicator of renal dysfunction and also correlates with the presence of calculi and altered renal architecture and may be used for serial follow-up of these patients and in determining the need for an intravenous pyelogram.[33,34]

Sexual dysfunction is the usual finding in these patients. Male patients suffer from impotence and decreased or absent ability to achieve orgasm and ejaculation. Infertility is frequent; abnormal spermatocytes are seen. The effects are more pronounced the higher the lesion, and no underlying endocrinological cause has been found. Female patients have altered sexual function on the basis of sensory and motor deficits, although normal menses usually resume within one to three months of the injury.[17] Female fertility seems to be unimpaired, although premature labor and delivery are more common. Sensory loss may make labor unknown to the mother, predisposing to delivery under unfavorable conditions. Weekly examination after 32 weeks of gestation is advised, and bedrest is indicated if any effacement is detected. Autonomic hyperreflexia is a major threat. It may be triggered by bowel or bladder stimuli as well as labor itself. Induction of labor has also been associated with a high risk of hyperreflexia and is relatively contraindicated. Spinal and epidural analgesia and anesthesia seem to decrease hyperreflexive episodes effectively.[35]

Abnormal Response to Depolarizing Muscle Relaxants

Of great importance to the anesthesiologist is the massive translocation of intracellular potassium from skeletal muscle to the extracellular space following the administration of a depolarizing muscle relaxant such as succinylcholine. This phenomenon may occur as early as three days after injury and is thought to result from the denervation process of overgrowth and spread of cholinergic nicotinic receptors to include extrajunctional sarcolemma. This results in supersensitivity to depolarizing agents whereby the entire affected muscle mass depolarizes synchronously and releases large amounts of potassium into the circulation.[36]

A number of important points should be emphasized. First, the magnitude of potassium release is more a function of the amount of muscle mass affected than of the amount of drug given: 20 milligrams of succinylcholine have been noted to result in a serum potassium concentration of 13.6 meg/L.[37] Also, the causative overgrowth of receptors may well occur before spasticity replaces flaccid muscle paralysis. Finally, pretreatment with a "defasciculating" dose of nondepolarizing relaxants does not reliably block the occurrence of significant hyperkalemia. Since the precise onset of supersensitivity is unpredictable, depolarizing agents should be avoided in all spinal cord injury patients.

Should the inadvertent administration of succinylcholine occur, electrocardiographic changes progress from atrial conduction disturbances to prolonged PR interval ($>$ 7 mEq/L), tall peaked T waves (7 to 9 mEq/L), progressive widening and aberration of the QRS complex ($>$ 6 to 7 mEq/L), and finally to sinusoidal ventricular complexes and ventricular fibrillation when serum potassium concentration exceeds 12 to 14 mEq/L.

Pharmacological treatment includes sodium bicarbonate (44 to 88 mEq) and glucose-insulin (1 to 2 units per 5 gm of dextrose) administration to shift potassium intracellularly, as well as calcium (0.5 to 1 gm) to antagonize the membrane effects of potassium. Hyperventilation may also be employed acutely. If circulation fails, CPR is, of course, mandatory to support cellular metabolism (which will resequester the potassium in 10 to 15 minutes) as well as to circulate resuscitative drugs.

Altered Thermoregulation

Temperature regulation is impaired for a number of reasons. Afferent information to the hypothalamic thermoregulatory center is interrupted. Sympathetic denervation causes cutaneous vasodilation, which increases heat loss. Also, inability to shiver limits the ability to increase body temperature. Spinal cord injured patients, therefore, become relatively poikilothermic. Efforts to avoid both hypothermia and hyperthermia are necessary. The use of a heating-cooling mattress, variable operating room temperatures, the adjustment of ventilator circuit temperature and humidity, and intravenous fluid temperatures tailored to the situation will allow either raising or lowering of body temperature as indicated.

Other Systemic Alterations

Spinal cord injury produces alterations in a number of other systems, the more salient of which will be summarized here. Several recent reviews detail and discuss these and other sequelae in more detail.[10,17] Besides the changes in fluid and electrolyte status caused by the occurrence of renal insufficiency, hypercalcemia and hypercalciuria have been observed in the early stages of spinal cord injury. This phenomenon occurs most often in young male patients, seems to result from calcium release from denervated (flaccid) muscle and possibly from bone stores, and occurs in the first year with a peak around 10 weeks after injury. It is more common in higher level injuries, and serum sodium and parathyroid hormone levels are normal.[38] When hypercalcemia is severe, symptoms include anorexia, nausea and vomiting, abdominal pain, polyuria, constipation, dehydration, psychosis, depressed mental status, and eventually coma. Shortening of the QT interval is seen on the electrocardiogram. Hypertension and ventricular arrhythmias may occur. Treatment includes rehydration with saline, potent diuretics, glucocorticoids, and if necessary, calcitonin. In contrast, long-term spinal cord injury patients develop osteoporosis as a result of increased calcium loss and, especially in the case of supervening renal failure, become hypocalcemic.

The skin of denervated areas becomes atrophic and susceptible to pressure sores. Underlying bone is at risk of osteomyelitis. In addition, pathologic fractures often result from the osteoporosis. Skeletal muscle spasticity or contractures complicate skin and general patient care, and make surgical positioning difficult.

Heterotopic calcification occurs below the level of injury in 50 per cent of patients, primarily involving the proximal two joints of the upper and lower extremities. Alkaline phosphatase is elevated, and acute inflammation may be apparent at the involved site. Commencing weeks to months after injury, the process usually stabilizes within one and a half years and may vary from asymptomatic to a debilitating condition that decreases range of motion.[17]

Average metabolic rates are usually depressed after injury, but catabolism and hypoproteinemia can occur acutely, especially when infection occurs. Increased protein and caloric intake can overcome this tendency.

Endocrine function has usually been normal when assessed, with two possible exceptions. A number of investigators have documented moderate glucose intolerance, often with hyperinsulinemia, suggesting relative resistance to endogenous insulin (glucagon levels were normal).[39] Secondly, the potential for adrenal insufficiency after steroid therapy should be considered.

Hematological studies show anemia in 52 per cent of patients with normal kidney function, which may be either normocytic hypochromic in nature (56 per cent) or normochromic (32 per cent). Possible causes for these anemias include increased plasma water in response to augmented venous capacity, significant pressure sores, as well as chronic or severe urinary tract infections.

The digestive system is affected as well. Gastrointestinal bleeding may occur acutely in up to 20 per cent of patients. Gastric distention, ileus, and nonspecific liver dysfunction with a normal serum bilirubin are common complications—usually occurring during the first week after injury and resolving over several weeks, although occasionally persisting longer. Pancreatitis also occurs, but it is unknown if this is related to the cord injury per se. Diagnosis of these and other intra-abdominal emergencies may be difficult as a result of altered sensation. Vomiting may occur *without* pain or nausea. The newly described syndrome of gastroduodenal motor dysfunction, possibly secondary to loss of adrenergic inhibitory control, features altered motility, pain, and vomiting. It is seen in certain spinal cord injury cases and responds to low doses of adrenergic agonists such as ephedrine.[40] Gastric and bowel distention and the tendency toward vomiting in most of these disorders warrants a high index of suspicion and preparation for airway protection on the part of the anesthesiologist. The distention itself may hinder ventilatory ability.

Last but not least, chronic pain is a problem in many of these patients. It can cause and reinforce the tendency toward depression that is often present. Proper management of pain and psychosocial support have proved essential for adaptation and rehabilitation of the patient.

ANESTHETIC MANAGEMENT OF PATIENTS WITH SPINAL CORD INJURY

In view of the high percentage of spinal cord injury patients with associated injuries, the anesthesiologist may be required to care for these patients during initial diagnostic procedures, during emergency operations aimed at managing life-threatening trauma elsewhere in the body (e.g., closed head injury, hemorrhage), for emergency spinal decompression, or for other procedures (e.g., urological, plastic) during the more chronic phase of injury. The forgoing discussion of acute and chronic derangements in systemic function provides the basis for rational and safe anesthetic management as well as daily care of these patients.

Acutely, maintenance of normal acid-base and blood gas parameters, as well as adequate spinal cord perfusion pressures, is paramount in importance. Experimental work in cats has suggested that there is no therapeutic advantage of either hypercarbia or hypocarbia over normocarbia in terms of both neurologic recovery and histological tissue preservation. Although not statistically significant, mortality and tissue preservation results suggested that hypocarbia may be less harmful than hypercarbia in the acute postinjury period.[41] Consequently, it seems prudent to maintain $PaCo_2$ in the 35 to 40 mm Hg range. Management of closed head injury with increased intracranial pressure would take precedence in this area ($PaCo_2$ maintained between 25 and 30 mm Hg).

Hypoxemia must be prevented by careful attention to minimizing significant physiologic shunting, which is suggested by the inability to maintain a Pao_2 greater than 60 mm Hg with an FIo_2 of 50 per cent. Possible contributing causes such as hemothorax or pneumothorax, pulmonary embolization of fat or thrombi, foreign body or gastric content aspiration, and noncardiogenic pulmonary edema should be searched for and either excluded or treated appropriately. PEEP may be required to decrease shunting and increase oxygenation once pneumothorax or other reversible causes of hypoxemia have been excluded. However, the possible negative effect of PEEP on cardiac output and intracranial pressure must be considered. In case the patient is not already intubated and this is necessary, it should be carried out as during acute resuscitation, with caution used in avoiding neck displacement, managing airway reflexes, avoiding aspiration, and with the capability of treating severe vagal bradycardia or arrest.

Cardiovascular management, as discussed already, most frequently requires judicious repletion of intravascular volume to restore normal venous return and filling pressures. However, it should be recalled that 3 of 19 patients in the study cited on volume loading in the acute postinjury period actually showed decreased cardiac output and progressive increase in PAOP. This required decreasing or eliminating halothane or other myocardial depressants or even the use of an inotrope.[29] During the phase of spinal shock, lasting anywhere from three days to six weeks (average of three weeks), the advantages of pulmonary artery catheter monitoring are obvious in maintaining hemodynamics and avoiding pulmonary edema. Also, when it is employed, it allows quantitation of shunt and monitoring of the respiratory and hemodynamic effects of PEEP.

In choosing fluids for perioperative resuscitation and maintenance, the use of glucose containing solutions is questionable. Recent investigations have documented deleterious effects of the hyperglycemia resulting from dextrose infusion on the neurological outcome after cerebral[41a] and spinal cord[41b] ischemia. In the latter study, Drummond and Moore showed that mild to moderate increases of plasma glucose averaging only 40 mg/dl tripled the incidence of paraplegia in rabbits subjected to transient spinal cord ischemia following aortic occlusion (9 of 10 dextrose-treated animals as compared with 3 of 10 control animals). The authors considered end products of hypoxic glucose metabolism, such as lactate (which has experimentally verified adverse effects on physiological and histological outcome after cerebral ischemia), to be the most likely mechanism by which enhanced glucose availability could worsen tolerance to ischemia. However, this was not elucidated by the study design. Of note was the lack of correlation between the magnitude of plasma glucose elevation and the extent of neurological injury. This result was thought to be possibly attributable to differences in intracellular glucose availability not reflected by extracellular concentration, perhaps as a result of varying insulin effect. In light of these findings, routine use of dextrose containing fluids, as part of initial resuscitation or perioperatively in cases in which the development or worsening of spinal cord ischemia is possible, should be confined to those instances in which a definite medical indication exists and close monitoring and control of plasma glucose is possible. The data were not sufficient to recommend that an already-elevated plasma glucose be lowered emergently when encountered intraoperatively. Keeping in mind electrolyte, neuromuscular, and other potential systemic alterations is also necessary, with management as already outlined.

Of relevance for surgery during the acute phase of spinal cord injury or for any procedure that might feasibly result in new or worsened injury, Cole and coworkers[41c] recently investigated the effect of various anesthetic regimens on the susceptibility to ischemic SCI on anesthetized rats in a controlled, blinded fashion. Of the three agents investigated—halothane, fentanyl/nitrous oxide, and subarachnoid lidocaine—all increased the duration of ischemia required to produce spinal cord injury. No one agent was relatively more favorable or deleterious than the others in terms of final neurological outcome. Possible mechanisms for this protective effect, while not clear at present, may include depression of spinal cord metabolism, effects on SCBF, alterations in endogenous catecholamine levels, alteration of opiate receptor activity, or interaction with other potential mediators of secondary SCI (for example, prostaglandins). Hence, while anesthetics have not been shown to play a role in treating spinal cord injury, in this model the anesthetized state using the aforementioned agents seems to provide some degree of protection against its occurrence.

As noted by Schonwald et al,[32] both a sufficiently deep general anesthetic technique, employing halothane or enflurane, and regional anesthesia (subarachnoid or epidural) effectively prevented episodes of autonomic hyperreflexia. An alternative when surgical considerations would require high spinal levels (above T5) is subarachnoid block followed by light general anesthesia with endotracheal intubation and controlled ventilation.

A study[42] in dogs showed consistent statistically significant increases in lumbosacral spinal cord blood flow with a lesser, nonsignificant tendency toward increases in thoracic and cervical cord flow after subarachnoid tetracaine, as long as mean arterial pressure remained 100 mm Hg or more. The favorable effect was blocked by the addition of epinephrine to the tetracaine; in fact, a nonsignificant tendency toward decreased thoracic and cervical cord flows actually occurred. Hence, spinal anesthesia may improve cord blood flow and vasoconstrictors should not be added to the anesthetic.

Although spinal or epidural anesthetics have been considered hemodynamically unpredictable in these patients,[25] baseline hemodynamic stability as well as ablation of autonomic hyperreflexia has been verified by many other workers.[32,35] One recent study[43] showed such stability of cardiac output, stroke volume, and heart rate during cystoscopy that it was actually impossible to determine from the data alone when bladder distention and emptying had occurred. Also, no ephedrine was required during the study. These authors emphasized the importance of judicious choice of the anesthetic dosage and attention to intravascular volume as factors contributing to the recorded stability. A note of caution is warranted in patients with spinal subarachnoid block of cerebrospinal fluid circulation because a 14 per cent incidence of neurological deterioration after removal of cerebrospinal fluid or from delayed leakage through the puncture sites has been reported.[44] Continuous intra-arterial and pulmonary arterial or central venous pressure monitoring will allow safe management of any of these techniques as well as the detection and management of hyperreflexive breakthroughs.

Obstetrical management of women with spinal cord injury during labor and delivery or cesarean section, as already mentioned, is complicated by the possibility of autonomic hyperreflexia, threatening both the mother and the fetus. Although many anesthesiologists think that epidural anesthetics in these circumstances, while not needed for analgesia, are indicated for and are effective in preventing hyperreflexive episodes,[35,45,46] others fear hypotension as a potential complication. In our personal practice, epidural anesthesia with careful titration of drug dosage and maintenance of normal cardiac filling pressures is used if not otherwise contraindicated by the obstetric condition.

Techniques based on nitrous oxide, oxygen, and narcotics seem less recommendable in light of their failure to prevent hyperreflexia in two of nine patients. Regardless of the technique employed, direct-acting arteriolar dilators (e.g., nitroprusside), alpha-adrenergic blockers (e.g., phentolamine), and antiarrhythmics (e.g., lidocaine, propranolol, esmolol), new antihypertensives (e.g., labetalol and nifedipine), and atropine should be readily available.[32] The need to avoid succinylcholine is reiterated; however, the new short-acting nondepolarizing agents make this constraint clinically feasible, since they are a reasonable alternative.

The recent increased utilization of extracorporeal shock wave lithotripsy (ESWL) and the increased incidence of nephrolithiasis in spinal cord injury patients prompts consideration of the proper anesthetic management for ESWL in such patients. Five traumatic quadriplegic patients were studied during ESWL performed without either general or regional anesthesia.[47] Although some increase in blood pressure was noted in all patients, it was transient or mild in most; however, in two patients the increase was sufficient to warrant therapy for the hypertension. An effort to avoid hydronephrosis and

bladder distention was made by catheterization, ureteral stents, or percutaneous nephrostomies in most patients. Two patients with intact pinprick sensation in the skin overlying the impact area received field blocks (50 to 60 ml of 0.25 per cent bupivacaine). All of the patients received incremental intravenous doses of diazepam (2.5 mg) and fentanyl (25 μg). Total doses ranged from 25 to 200 μg of fentanyl and from 5 to 15 mg of diazepam. Because none of the patients demonstrated other signs or symptoms of autonomic hyperreflexia, they concluded that the hypertension was probably caused by another etiology, such as the translocation of blood from the peripheral to the central vascular compartment. They conclude that ESWL may be safely performed using their methodology without risking possible morbidity from general or spinal anesthesia.

There are a number of problems with this study. First, the number of patients is small and without a control group. Second, the lack of hemodynamic monitoring leaves their explanation for the central vascular overload suppositional. The etiology of autonomic hyperreflexia would have been supported by measurement of serum catecholamines during the procedure, because increased serum norepinephrine, but not epinephrine, has been found during hyperreflexive episodes.[48] Until the results of further controlled studies are available, it may be advisable to utilize an anesthetic prophylactic technique with appropriate safeguards.

In the case of incomplete spinal cord lesions, somatosensory-evoked potentials (SSEP) and motor-evoked potentials (MEP) can be useful in monitoring cord function (see below). This is true during surgery to relieve cord compression or to correct spinal deformity as well as during the acute phase of spinal cord injury when neurologic status may progressively worsen. Of possible value during surgery in patients with incomplete lesions is the observation that etomidate improved the SSEP in patients receiving neuroleptanesthesia by increasing the latency and increasing the amplitude of the short latency cortical responses.[49] A 0.3 to 0.5 mg/kg bolus of etomidate followed by a continuous infusion of 0.01 to 0.05 mg/kg/min was used. Areas of potential concern which should be resolved include the possibility that the improved amplitude may be associated with etomidate's tendency to produce myoclonic activity and its ability to produce adrenocortical suppression for 8 to 24 hours.

The clinical significance of these two drug properties when it is used on a short-term basis remains to be documented, in contrast to the known adrenal insufficiency which required treatment and influenced mortality when the drug was employed for more prolonged sedation in a critical care setting. Further study is needed before there will be widespread acceptance of this technique. However, when SSEP monitoring is considered essential but is technically nonreproducible, etomidate may provide the solution. Another recent report[50] suggests that the use of lower than usual stimulus presentation rates (1.1 to 2.1 Hz as compared with 5.1 Hz) resolved problems similar to those found in the first study and may provide an acceptable alternative solution.

PATHOPHYSIOLOGY

Spinal cord trauma results in both primary and secondary injuries. The primary injury, if severe enough, will result in functional or anatomic disruption of the cord at the scene of the accident with a correspondingly dismal prognosis. The uniformly encountered anatomic and histologic findings associated with such primary injury include direct neurilemmal and neuronal disruption and/or destruction, petechial hemorrhages, gross hematomyelia, or even total cord transection, a rare event. The areas rendered nonviable by this primary insult will develop cavitating necrosis and ultimately glial scar formation.

The observation that areas of the spinal cord not immediately destroyed by traumatic force subsequently undergo progressive hemorrhagic necrosis, edema, and inflammation at a rate proportional to the severity of the lesion has produced the concept of a secondary injury, perhaps mediated and propagated by mechanisms distinct from the initial mechanical deformation.

The extension of the lesion from the initial gray matter involvement to include the white matter is preceded by endothelial damage with platelet adhesion, platelet aggregation, microvascular occlusion, and embolization of microthrombi. On a macroscopic scale, corresponding vascular stasis, decreased spinal cord blood flow, and ischemia are noted. Axonal degeneration (hydropic and then granular), myelinolysis, cell necrosis, inflammatory infiltrate, and neuronophagia ensue. A striking feature is the finding of intra-axonal calcium hydroxyapatite crystals and mitochondrial calcification. Similar degenerative changes have been observed following in vivo exposure of rat spinal cords to calcium or calcium in the presence of an ionophore.[51]

Biochemical events coinciding with this process of progressive autodestruction include a massive translocation of calcium from the extracellular to the intracellular space; decreased Na^+, K^+-ATPase activity; the loss of intracellular potassium; activation of phospholipase A_2 leading to arachidonic acid release and its metabolism to lipid peroxides (via free radical attack), prostaglandins (via cyclo-oxygenase), or leukotrienes (via lipoxygenase); increase in total thromboxane A_2, as well as its ratio to prostacyclin; the degradation of axonal and myelin proteins by neutral proteinases; the failure of energy metabolism and protein synthesis; and hypoxia and lactic acidosis.[51,52]

The tantalizing aspect of this wealth of biochemical data is that it is possible to organize these events into a positive feedback cascade mechanism activated by the release of certain catalysts from the blood and their initial intracellular flux caused by the endothelial and neuronal membrane disruption at the initial site of maximal tissue trauma. Calcium,[53] in addition to bradykinin, thrombin, and ferrous ion,[52] has been cast in such a role. Another investigator[54] made a case for norepinephrine. The basic scheme of such a secondary injury hypothesis is an activation of membrane phospholipase A_2, yielding arachidonic acid, lipid peroxides, free radicals, prostaglandins (mostly thromboxane), and leukotrienes. These can account for membrane lipid destruction, microcirculatory thrombosis and stasis, vasogenic edema, ischemia, and chemotaxis. Calcification of mitochrondria and other intracellular sites secondary to influx through damaged membranes should have obvious deleterious effects on cellular energy metabolism and maintenance of integrity and function. Na^+, K^+-ATPase has been shown to be phospholipid dependent and very susceptible to free radical attack and lipid peroxidation[54]; this enzyme is needed to maintain normal cellular volume and ion content, membrane potential, and cellular function. Finally, the neutral proteinase, which is the predominant source of increased proteolytic activity in experimental spinal cord injury, is calcium activated.[53]

The feasibility of such secondary injury mechanisms is supported by a number of additional observations. The time course of change in tissue concentration of the various proposed mediators closely matches that of the histological, biochemical, and physiological processes already described above. In the case of calcium, neurological deficit scores have also been shown to be proportional to the extent of calcium influx, the rise in phospholipase-generated metabolites, vascular damage, and increased tissue water content.[55] In addition, as mentioned before, exposure of the spinal cord to calcium chloride solution results in similar prostaglandin (thromboxane) generation, proteolysis, and morphological changes in proportion to the solution molarity.[53]

Finally, Faden and his co-workers have demonstrated an increase in the endogenous opioid *kappa* receptor agonist dynorphin, as well as an increase in receptor binding capacity after experimental spinal cord injury in rats which correlates closely with neurological dysfunction. No change in *mu* or *delta* receptor binding was found. Since intrathecal dynorphin A, but not other opiate agonists, can produce drug-related hindlimb paralysis in the rat, it has been postulated that this opioid system may contribute to the pathophysiology of secondary spinal cord injury.[56,57]

However, caution must be exercised in equating close correlation with causation, and further investigation continues. Nevertheless, what has been clearly documented is that in the period following primary spinal cord injury, a progressive decrease in spinal cord blood flow occurs, resulting in marked ischemia associated with a morphological and biochemical cascade as detailed above.[58] The fact that this sequence may not begin for over an hour, or in some cases as much as four hours, after the primary injury suggests the possibility of pharmacological intervention to prevent or alter the ischemic sequence.[59]

The normal mean spinal cord blood flow of 40 to 50 ml/100 gm/min is partitioned in a ratio of 3:1 between gray and white matter, respectively.[60] Autoregulation of spinal cord blood flow between 60 and 150 mm Hg has been demonstrated in rats.[61] Spinal cord blood flow has been shown to vary in direct proportion (1:1) with $PaCo_2$.[62] Although conflicting results have been reported as mentioned,[63] the preponderance of researchers agree that total spinal cord blood flow decreases significantly from one to four hours after subtotal experimental injury, with most of the decrease occurring in the central cord region.[58]

Spinal cord injury in cats has been shown to abolish autoregulation with the onset of ischemia.[64] This would be expected to render the spinal cord susceptible to increased hemorrhage and edema in the face of significantly increased blood pressure, as has been shown experimentally in cats.[65] Such a hypertensive phase has been documented for three to four minutes after experimental spinal cord injury.[19,20] Spinal shock, in which endorphin-mediated parasympathetic stimulation has been implicated, would decrease spinal cord blood flow in the absence of autoregulation.

Also, vasoconstriction of resistance vessels would more readily result in ischemia. Such vasoconstriction may be secondary to some of the mediators already mentioned: a preponderance of thromboxane A_2 over prostacyclin, $PGF_{2\alpha}$, and slow-reacting substance of anaphylaxis.[51] Although the originally proposed increase in spinal cord catecholamines (as a cause of ischemia and hemorrhagic necrosis)[66,67] has not been verified by subsequent investigators, norepinephrine has been shown to significantly reduce spinal cord blood flow when the cord-blood barrier had been disrupted.[68] More recent investigations already mentioned have described a number of membrane-damaging factors, operating by way of free radical attack and lipid peroxidation, that may disrupt the cord-blood barrier and that correlate with cord edema. Norepinephrine has been shown capable of activating similar membrane-lipid peroxidation.[54] Of interest is the finding that acute ethanol intoxication (blood level of 100 mg/dl) worsens spinal cord hemorrhage and the extent of anatomical damage and impairs recovery of function.[69] Possible reasons for this include the direct effects on neuronal conduction, vascular congestion, and increased permeability (altered blood-cord barrier), increased lactate production, increased free radical peroxidation catalyzed by iron, and toxic aldehyde metabolite effects.

On a gross physiological scale, spinal cord impulse transmission, as assessed by evoked potentials, disappears immediately with complete transection and after a variable delay period in less severe lesions. Somatosensory-evoked potentials (SSEPs) studied in humans distinguished complete anatomic lesions with little or no possibility of recovery from those in patients with complete or incomplete functional deficits but could not predict the degree of functional deficit.[70] On the other hand, motor-evoked potentials (MEPs) or corticomotor-evoked potentials (CMEPs) have been shown in both rat and cat dynamic spinal cord injury models to be more sensitive indicators of the onset of injury[71] as well as good predictors of the extent of tissue damage and prognosis for functional recovery.[72,73]

RESUSCITATIVE MODALITIES IN SPINAL CORD INJURY

A number of pharmacological and physical measures have been employed in an effort to limit the progression of secondary spinal cord injury and yield improved neurologic recovery. Spinal cord injury may abolish normal autoregulation, causing spinal cord blood flow and blood volume to vary directly with perfusion pressure. Spinal cord perfusion pressure must be maintained close to the middle of the normal autoregulatory range of 60 to 150 mm Hg by cautious restoration of a normal circulating blood volume (see Cardiovascular Complications). In addition, glucocorticoids and hyperosmolar agents have frequently been used to decrease post-traumatic edema and increase spinal cord blood flow.

Mannitol draws fluid from the interstitial into the intravascular space and then promotes a net loss of fluid via osmotic diuresis. It has been shown to reduce edema following traumatic canine spinal cord injury.[74] In view of the initially low central venous pressures in the acute phase after spinal cord injury and the limited cardiac reserve, allowance must be made for the initial rise and then fall in venous return caused by mannitol.

In a canine model, improved functional recovery after spinal cord injury has been demonstrated with dexamethasone therapy.[75] Better recovery of SSEPs and partial restoration of extracellular calcium concentration have been shown in cats receiving 15 to 30 mg/kg of methylprednisolone 45 minutes after spinal cord contusion.[76] Others have found less axonal degeneration using morphometric analysis when the same steroid dose was given to rats after spinal cord injury.[77] Nonetheless, the multicenter, double-blind randomized clinical trial in humans sponsored by the National Acute Spinal Cord Injury (NASCIS) Study Group failed to find any improvement in motor or sensory neurological function one year after injury as a result of two levels of methylprednisolone therapy.[78]

Several cautionary comments regarding interpretation of this study are pointed out by the authors themselves. First, the animal studies may not accurately duplicate conditions of human spinal cord injury, not to mention interspecies differences in anatomy, physiology, or biochemistry. Secondly, both study arms, 100 mg or 1000 mg initial boluses of methylprednisolone followed by the same dose daily (4 divided doses) for 10 days, used doses below the 15 to 30 mg/kg range used in the most successful animal studies. Third, there was no placebo control; the two steroid regimens were compared with each other and then with historic outcome data. Finally, only 12 per cent of the patients started treatment within 3 hours of injury and another 20 per cent between 3 and 6 hours after injury; the remainder entered the study up to 48 hours after their injury. For these reasons, further investigation is warranted before steroids are determined not to be useful, especially when given earlier and in larger doses.

In view of the potential shortcomings in this study (NASCIS 1), the same group of investigators completed a second study (NASCIS 2),[78a] which added placebo-controlled and naloxone therapeutic arms to the original study design. The study was carried out in a prospective, randomized, double-blind manner. The study groups received one of three drug regimens: methylprednisolone plus naloxone placebo, naloxone plus methylprednisolone placebo, or methylprednisolone placebo plus naloxone placebo. Each drug or placebo was administered through separate intravenous sites by separate pumps. Methylprednisolone was administered in a bolus dose of 30 mg/kg followed by a maintenance infusion of 5.4 mg/kg/hr, while naloxone was administered in a bolus dose of 5.4 mg/kg followed by a maintenance infusion of 4.0 mg/kg/hr. Both bolus doses were given over a 15-minute period followed in 45 minutes by the maintenance infusion for 23 hours.

As compared with NASCIS 1, NASCIS 2 found that treatment with the higher 30 mg/kg regimen improved sensory and motor function as evaluated six weeks and six months after injury. This effect was statistically significant only when treatment was initiated within eight hours of injury. On the other hand, naloxone failed to influence outcome. The naloxone regimen employed was essentially identical to that employed in the Phase I study to be discussed in this section, reinforcing its negative conclusions and suggesting the need for evaluation of a higher dose regimen.

It should be noted, however, that the NASCIS 1 study excluded patients with severe associated injuries. Another investigation found that spinal cord injured patients with severe multiple trauma had more than a three-fold increase in infections, which often involved multiple organisms and foci, when they received steroid therapy for CNS trauma (4 to 20 mg of dexamethasone every 6 hours). All of the septic deaths occurred in steroid-treated patients.[79]

Although NASCIS[78a] revealed no increase in septic complications or overall morbidity and mortality and the steroid regimen used was different, a vigilant attitude with regard to possible increased susceptibility to sepsis is still warranted.

The area of opiate antagonist therapy is currently a subject of heated research and debate. Following the demonstration that the opiate antagonist naloxone improved arterial pressure and survival in hemorrhagic and septic shock, investigators studied its effect in spinal shock and in enhancing recovery from spinal cord injury.[31]

Intravenous naloxone has effectively prevented or reversed spinal shock in rat and cat cervical cord transection models—significantly increasing mean arterial pressure (MAP), increasing respiratory rate, and decreasing hypothermia.[80,81] Also, naloxone in doses of 2 to 20 mg/kg has been shown to yield significant improvement in SSEPs[82] and neurologic function.[83]

Although these and many other animal studies supported naloxone's effectiveness, a human phase I clinical trial of naloxone was less encouraging. This trial showed some clinical improvement only with the highest loading dose of 5.4 mg/kg (IV) followed by continuous hourly infusion of 75 per cent of this amount for 23 hours; however, the results fell short of statistical significance. The mortality rate was not greater than expected in similar injuries, but awareness of pain was significantly increased. A possible contributing factor limiting success may be the average interval of 6.6 hours from admission until the start of therapy.[84] Further clinical trials are needed. However, a number of animal researchers have recently challenged the effectiveness of naloxone.[85–87]

A potentially significant effect of naloxone therapy in patients undergoing general anesthesia was reported. The patient had received the 5.4 mg/kg regimen mentioned in the preceding paragraph 30 minutes before a stabilization procedure of the thoracolumbar spine was performed. Fentanyl (25 μg/kg), isoflurane (2 to 3.5 per cent) thiopental (700 mg), diaze-

pam (10 mg), morphine (15 mg), and sufentanil (0.5 μg/kg) were used during and immediately after surgery to manage hypertension and hyperventilation. This resistance to normally effective anesthetic doses was attributed to an antianalgesic and analeptic effect of the naloxone treatment.[88]

Experimental work on the possible sites and mechanisms of action of opiate antagonists has been reviewed.[31] Briefly summarized, evidence indicates that naloxone interacts stereospecifically at a central site to inhibit opiate receptor-mediated stimulation of the parasympathetic nervous system in achieving improvement of MAP and SCBF. A central outpouring of beta-endorphin following spinal cord injury has been found at the time of cord ischemia, and naloxone may antagonize its effects.

In addition, naloxone elevates peripheral dopamine levels 300 to 400 per cent, partially contributing to the hemodynamic effects of naloxone after spinal cord injury. Other catecholamine levels remain unaltered. It is postulated to be an indirect effect, possibly mediated by the central parasympatholysis.

Finally, because naloxone is effective only in dose orders of magnitude greater than those required for *mu* receptor agonist reversal, it is possible that it is acting as a receptor, perhaps the *kappa* receptor, for which it has marginal affinity. Naloxone and a specific *kappa* receptor antagonist have prevented experimental cord damage induced by dynorphin, a κ receptor agonist (see above). In fact, some evidence exists that naloxone acts through nonopioid mechanisms, involving its ability to inhibit membrane damage by free radical–induced lipid peroxidation, to act as an antioxidant, to modulate calcium fluxes, and to increase cyclic-AMP activation of prostaglandins.

Thyrotropin-releasing hormone (TRH), in addition to stimulating release of TSH from the anterior pituitary, is thought to act as a partial physiologic, not pharmacologic, opiate antagonist. It seems to reverse the behavioral and autonomic effects of opiates without antagonizing their analgesic effects. TRH has also improved recovery following experimental spinal cord injury.[88a]

Methylprednisolone sodium succinate, alpha-tocopherol (vitamin E), selenium (cofactor of glutathione peroxidase), and DMSO have been shown to be experimentally beneficial in ameliorating spinal cord injury, perhaps as a result of their shared ability to act as antioxidants or reducing agents in scavenging free radicals and interrupting lipid peroxidation reactions.[52] Protease inhibitors such as leupeptin have shown promise experimentally.[89]

Finally, it should be noted that new physiotherapeutic measures show promise in preserving and enhancing function remaining after spinal cord injury, and initial investigation of chemical and physical stimulation of axonal regeneration is showing some promising results. Functional neuromuscular stimulation has been used to create or enhance knee extension and bicycle ergometer exercises. However, limitation in skeletal strength, the deteriorated condition of the muscles, and lack of cardiopulmonary and other system adjustments to exercise have limited its success. Strength and endurance gains have been made, but relatively easy fatigability remains a problem.[90]

Recent studies have demonstrated potential effectiveness of GM-1 ganglioside[91] and a combination of triethanolamine and cytosine arabinoside[92] to markedly stimulate axonal growth in spinal cord transected rats. Continuously applied weak electrical fields achieved similar results in guinea pigs.[93] A series of investigations has shown that peripheral nerve grafts or central nervous system implants derived from the embryonal neuraxis can stimulate axonal outgrowth and may prove useful in repairing disrupted intraspinal circuits.[94]

Currently, much of this work has proven to be of limited clinical utility. Nevertheless, understanding and new directions for research, as well as more effective application of existing knowledge, are advancing at an unprecedented and encouraging pace. Prompt initiation of currently accepted therapy or experimental protocols in a specialized care center holds the most hope for preserving or restoring function.

Acknowledgment

The authors wish to thank Grune and Stratton for giving permission to use information that was previously published in Seminars in Anesthesia Vol. VI No. 4 (December) 1987, pp. 246–259.

In addition, special thanks go to James E. Cottrell, M.D., for editorial assistance and Naomi Barker for preparation of the manuscript.

REFERENCES

1. Kalsbeek WD, McLaurin RL, Harris BSH, III: The national head and spinal cord injury survey: major findings. J Neurosurg 53:S19, 1980.
2. Eisenberg MG, Tierney DO: Changing demographic profile of the spinal cord injury population: Implications for health care support systems. Paraplegia 23:335, 1985.
3. Kraus JF: A comparison of recent studies on the extent of the head and spinal cord injury problem in the United States. J Neurosurg 53:S35, 1980.
4. Woolsey, RM: Rehabilitation outcome following spinal cord injury. Arch Neurol 42:116, 1985.
5. Albin MS: Resuscitation of the spinal cord. Crit Care Med 6:270, 1978.
6. Luce JM, Culver BH: Respiratory muscle function in health and disease. Chest 81:82, 1982.
7. DeTroyer A, Estenne M, Heilporn A: Mechanism of active expiration in tetraplegic subjects. N Engl J Med 314:740, 1986.
8. Davis JN, Goldman M, Loh L: Diaphragm function and alveolar hypoventilation. Q J Med 177:87, 1976.
9. Heros RC: Spinal cord compression. In Ropper AH et al (eds): Neurological and Neurosurgical Intensive Care. Baltimore, University Park Press, 1982, pp. 231–248.
10. Luce JM: Medical management of spinal cord injury. Crit Care Med 13:126, 1985.
11. Forner JV, Llombart RL, Valledor MCV: The flow-volume loop in tetraplegics. Paraplegia 15:245, 1977–78.
12. Ledsome JR, Sharp JM: Pulmonary function in acute cervical cord injury. Am Rev Respir Dis 124:41, 1981.
13. De Troyer A, Heilporn A: Respiratory mechanics in quadriplegia. The respiratory function of the intercostal muscles. Am Rev Resp Dis 122:591, 1980.
14. Gross D, Ladd HW, Riley EJ: The effect of training on strength and endurance of the diaphragm in quadriplegia. JAMA 68:27, 1980.
15. Welphy NC, Mathias CJ, Frankel HL: Circulatory reflexes in tetraplegics during artificial ventilation and general anesthesia. Paraplegia 13:172, 1975.
16. Glenn WWL, Holcomb BEE, McLaughlin AJ: Total ventilatory support in a quadriplegic patient with radiofrequency electrophrenic respiration. N Engl J Med 286:513, 1972.
17. Sugarman B: Medical complications of spinal cord injury. Quart J Med 54:3, 1985.
18. McMichan JC, Michel L, Westbrook PR: Pulmonary dysfunction following traumatic quadriplegia. JAMA 243:528, 1980.
19. Rawe SE, Perot PL: Pressor response resulting from experimental contusion injury to the spinal cord. J Neurosurg 50:58, 1979.
20. Young W, DeCrescito V, Tomasula JJ: The role of the sympathetic nervous system in pressor responses induced by spinal injury. J Neurosurg 52:473, 1980.
21. Albin MS, Bunegin L, Wolf S: Brain and lungs at risk after cervical spinal cord transection: Intracranial pressure, brain water, blood-brain barrier permeability, cerebral blood flow, and extravascular lung water changes. Surg Neurol 24:191, 1985.
22. Meyer GL, Berman IR, Doty DB: Hemodynamic responses to acute quadriplegia with or without chest trauma. J Neurosurg 34:168, 1971.
23. Kurnick NB: Autonomic hyperreflexia and its control in patients with spinal cord lesions. Ann Intern Med 44:678, 1956.

24. Kendrick WW, Scott JW, Jousse AT: Reflex sweating and hypertension in traumatic transverse myelitis. Treatment Serv Bull (Ottawa) 8:437, 1953.

25. Desmond J: Paraplegia: Problems confronting the anaesthesiologist. Can Anaesth Soc J 17:435, 1970.

26. Evans DE, Kobrine AI, Rizzoli HV: Cardiac arrhythmias accompanying acute compression of the spinal cord. J Neurosurg 52:52, 1980.

27. Quimby CA, Williams RN, and Greifenstein FE: Anesthetic problems of the acute quadriplegic patient. Anesth Analg 52:333, 1973.

28. Troll GF, Dohrmann GJ: Anaesthesia of the spinal cord-injured patient: Cardiovascular problems and their management. Paraplegia 13:162, 1975.

29. MacKenzie, CF, Shin B, Krishnaprasad D, et al: Assessment of cardiac and respiratory function during surgery in patients with acute quadriplegia. J Neurosurg 62:843, 1985.

30. Dolan EJ, Tator CH: The effect of blood transfusion, dopamine, and gamma hydroxybutyrate on posttraumatic ischemia of the spinal cord. J Neurosurg 56:350, 1982.

31. Hamilton AJ, Black PM, Carr DB: Contrasting actions of naloxone in experimental spinal cord trauma and cerebral ischemia: A review. Neurosurgery 17:845, 1985.

32. Schonwald G, Fish KJ, Perkash I: Cardiovascular complications during anesthesia in chronic spinal cord injured patients. Anesthesiology 55:550, 1981.

33. Kuhlemeier KV, Huang CT, Lloyd LK: Effective renal plasma flow: Clinical significance after spinal cord injury. J Urol 133:758, 1985.

34. Kuhlemeier KV, Lloud LK, Stover SL: Long-term followup of renal function after spinal cord injury. J Urol 134:510, 1985.

35. Verduyn WH: Spinal cord injured women, pregnancy and delivery. Paraplegia 24:231, 1986.

36. Gronert GA, Theye RA: Pathophysiology of hyperkalemia induced by succinylcholine. Anesthesiology 43:89, 1975.

37. Tobey RE: Paraplegia, succinylcholine and cardiac arrest. Anesthesiology 32:359, 1970.

38. Claus-Walker J, Carter RE, Campos RJ: Hypercalcemia in early traumatic quadriplegia. J Chronic Dis 28:81, 1975.

39. Duckworth WC, Jallepalli P, Solomon SS: Glucose intolerance in spinal cord injury. Arch Phys Med Rehabil 64:107, 1983.

40. Sninsky CA, Martin JL, Mathias JR: Effect of lidamidine hydrochloride, a proposed alpha$_2$-adrenergic agonist in patients with gastroduodenal motor dysfunction. Gastroenterology 84:1315, 1983.

41. Ford RWJ, Malm DN: Therapeutic trial of hypercarbia and hypocarbia in acute experimental spinal cord injury. J Neurosurg 61:925, 1984.

41a. Lanier WL, Stangland KJ, Scheithauer BW, Milde JH, Michenfelder JD: The effects of dextrose infusion and head position on neurologic outcome after complete cerebral ischemia in primates: Examination of a model. Anesthesiology 66:39, 1987.

41b. Drummond JC, Moore SS: The influence of dextrose administration on neurologic outcome after temporary spinal cord ischemia in the rabbit. Anesthesiology 70:64, 1989.

41c. Cole, DJ, Shapiro HM, Drummond JC, et al: Halothane, fentanyl, nitrous oxide, and spinal lidocaine protect against spinal cord injury in the rat. Anesthesiology 70:967, 1989.

42. Kozody R, Palahniuk RJ, Cumming MO: Spinal cord blood flow following subarachnoid tetracaine. Can Anaesth Soc J 32:23, 1985.

43. Barker I, Alderson J, Lydon M: Cardiovascular effects of spinal subarachnoid anaesthesia. Anaesthesia 40:533, 1985.

44. Hollis PH, Malis LI, Zappulla RA: Neurological deterioration after lumbar puncture below complete spinal subarachnoid block. J Neurosurg 64:253, 1986.

45. McCunniff DE, Dewan D: Pregnancy after spinal cord injury: Letter to the Editor. Obstet Gynecol 63:757, 1984.

46. Spielman FJ: Parturient with spinal cord transection: complications of autonomic hyperreflexia: Letter to the editor. Obstet Gynecol 64:147, 1984.

47. Spirnak PJ, Bodner D, Udayashankar S: Extracorporeal shockwave lithotripsy in traumatic quadriplegic patients: Can it be safely performed without anesthesia? J Urol 139:18, 1988.

48. Mathias CJ, Christensen NJ, Corbett JL, et al: Plasma catecholamines during paroxysmal neurogenic hypertension in quadriplegic man. Circ Res 39:204, 1976.

49. Sloan TB, Ronai AK, Toleikis RJ: Improvement of the intraoperative somatosensory evoked potentials by etomidate. Anesth Analgesia 67:582, 1988.

50. Schubert A, Drummond JC, Garfin SR: The influence of stimulus presentation rate on the cortical amplitude and latency of introperative somatosensory-evoked potential recordings in patients with varying degrees of spinal cord injury. Spine 12:969, 1987.

51. Banik NL, Hogan EL, Hsu CY: Molecular and anatomical correlates of spinal cord injury. CNS Trauma 2:99, 1985.

52. Anderson DK, Demediuk P, Saunders RD: Spinal cord injury and protection. Ann Emerg Med 14:816, 1985.

53. Hogan EL, Hsu CY, Banik NL: Calcium-activated mediators of secondary injury in the spinal cord. CNS Trauma 3:175, 1986.

54. Kurihara M: Role of monamines in experimental spinal cord injury in rats: Relationship between Na^+, K^+-ATPase and lipid peroxidation. J Neurosurg 62:743, 1985.

55. Hsu CY, Hogan EL, Gadsden, KM Sr: Vascular permeability in experimental spinal cord injury. J Neurosci 70:275, 1985.

56. Faden AI, Molineaux CJ, Rosenberger JG: Increased dynorphin immunoreactivity in spinal cord after traumatic injury. Regulatory Peptides 11:35, 1985.

57. Krumins SA, Faden AI: Traumatic injury alters opiate receptor binding in rat spinal cord. Ann Neurol 19:498, 1986.

58. Sandler AN, Tator CH: Review of the effect of spinal cord trauma on the vessels and blood flow in the spinal cord. J Neurosurg 45:638, 1976.

59. Senter HJ, Venes JL: Altered blood flow and secondary injury in experimental spinal cord trauma. J Neurosurg 49:569, 1978.

60. Rivlin AS, Tator CH: Regional spinal cord blood flow in rats after severe cord trauma. J Neurosurg 49:844, 1978.

61. Hickey R, Albin MS, et al: Autoregulation of spinal

cord blood flow: Is the cord a microcosm of the brain? Stroke 17:1183, 1986.

62. Griffiths IR: Spinal cord blood flow in dogs. 2. The effect of the blood gases. J Neurol Neurosurg Psych 36:42, 1973.

63. Kobrine AI, Doyle TF, Martins AN: Local spinal cord blood flow in experimental traumatic myelopathy. J Neurosurg 42:144, 1975.

64. Senter HJ, Venes JL: Loss of autoregulation and posttraumatic ischemia following experimental spinal cord trauma. J Neurosurg 50:198, 1979.

65. Rawe SE, Lee WA, Perot PL: The histopathology of experimental spinal cord trauma: The effect of systemic blood pressure. J Neurosurg 48:1002, 1978.

66. Osterholm JL, Matthews GJ: Altered norepinephrine metabolism following experimental spinal cord injury. Part 1: Relationship to hemorrhagic necrosis and post-wounding neurological deficits. J Neurosurg 36:386, 1972.

67. Osterholm JL, Matthews GJ: Altered norepinephrine metabolism following experimental spinal cord injury. Part 2: Protection against traumatic spinal cord hemorrhagic necrosis by norepinephrine synthesis blockade with alpha methyl tyrosine. J Neurosurg 36:395, 1972.

68. Crawford RA, Griffiths IR, McCulloch J: The effect of norepinephrine on the spinal cord circulation and its possible implications in the pathogenesis of acute spinal trauma. J Neurosurg 47:567, 1977.

69. Anderson TE: Effects of acute alcohol intoxication on spinal cord vascular injury. CNS Trauma 3:183, 1986.

70. Chabot R, York DH, Watts C: Somatosensory evoked potentials evaluated in normal subjects and spinal cord-injured patients. J Neurosurg 63:544, 1985.

71. Levy W, McCaffrey M, York D: Motor evoked potential in cats with acute spinal cord injury. J Neurosurg 19:9, 1986.

72. Levy WJ, McCaffrey M, Hagichi S: Motor evoked potential as a predictor of recovery in chronic spinal cord injury. Neurosurg 20:138, 1987.

73. Simpson RK, Baskin DS: Corticomotor evoked potentials in acute and chronic blunt spinal cord injury in the rat: Correlation with neurological outcome and histological damage. Neurosurgery 20:131, 1987.

74. Parker AJ, Park RD, Stowater JL: Reduction of trauma-induced edema of spinal cord in dogs given mannitol. Am J Vet Res 34:1355, 1973.

75. Kuchner EF, Hansebout RR: Combined steroid and hypothermia treatment of experimental spinal cord injury. Surg Neurol 6:371, 1976.

76. Young W, Flamm ES: Effect of high-dose corticosteroid therapy on blood flow, evoked potentials, and extracellular calcium in experimental spinal injury. J Neurosurg 57:667, 1982.

77. Iizuka H, Iwasaki Y, Yamamoto T: Morphometric assessment of drug effects in experimental spinal cord injury. J Neurosurg 65:92, 1986.

78. Bracken MB, Shepard MJ, Hellenbrand KG, et al: Methylprednisolone and neurological function 1 year after spinal cord injury: Results of the Na-

tional Acute Spinal Cord Injury Study. J Neurosurg 63:704, 1985.

78a. Bracken MB, Shephard MJ, Collins WF, et al: A randomized, controlled trial of methylprednisolone or naloxone in the treatment of acute spinal cord injury. N Engl J Med 322:1405, 1990.

79. DeMaria EJ, Reichman W, Kenney PR: Septic complications of corticosteroid administration after central nervous system trauma. Ann Surg 202:248, 1985.

80. Holaday JW, Faden AI: Naloxone acts at central opiate receptors to reverse hypotension, hypothermia, and hypoventilation in spinal shock. Brain Res 189:295, 1980.

81. Holaday JW, Faden AI: Spinal shock and injury: Experimental therapeutic approaches. Adv Shock Res 10:95, 1983.

82. Flamm ES, Young W, Demopoulos HB: Experimental spinal cord injury: Treatment with naloxone. Neurosurgery 10:227, 1982.

83. Faden AI, Jacobs TP, Holaday JW: Opiate antagonist improves neurologic recovery after spinal injury. Science 211:493, 1981.

84. Flamm ES, Young W, Collins WF: A phase I trial of naloxone treatment in acute spinal cord injury. J Neurosurg 63:390, 1985.

85. Haghighi SS, Chehrazi B: Effect of naloxone in experimental acute spinal cord injury. Neurosurgery 20:385, 1987.

86. Wallace MC, Tator CH: Failure of naloxone to improve spinal cord blood flow and cardiac output after spinal cord injury. Neurosurgery 18:428, 1986.

87. Wallace MC, Tator CH: Failure of blood transfusion or naloxone to improve clinical recovery after experimental spinal cord injury. Neurosurgery 19:489, 1986.

88. Benthuysen JL: Naloxone therapy in spinal trauma: Anesthetic effects. Anesthesiology 66:238, 1987.

88a. Faden AI, Jacobs TP, Holaday, JW: Thyrotropin-releasing hormone improves neurologic recovery after spinal cord trauma in cats. N Engl J Med 305:1063, 1981.

89. Iwasaki Y, Iizuka H, Yamamoto, TY: Alleviation of axonal damage in acute spinal cord injury by a protease inhibitor: automated morphometric analysis of drug effects. Brain Res 347:124, 1985.

90. Glaser RM: Physiologic Aspects of spinal cord injury and functional neuromuscular stimulation. CNS Trauma 3:49, 1986.

91. Bose B, Osterholm JL, Kalia M: Ganglioside-induced regeneration and reestablishment of axonal continuity in spinal cord-transected rats. Neuroscience Letters 63:165, 1986.

92. Guth L, Barrett CP, Donati EJ: Enhancement of axonal growth into a spinal lesion by topical application of triethanolamine and cytosine arabinoside. Exp Neurol 88:44, 1985.

93. Borgens RB, Blight AR, Murphy DJ: Transected dorsal column axons within the guinea pig spinal cord regenerate in the presence of an applied electric field. J Comp Neurol 250:168, 1986.

94. Reier PJ: Neural tissue grafts and repair of the injured spinal cord. Neuropathol Appl Neurobiol 11:81, 1985.

Pressure Sores

17

Overview

BERIT L. MADSEN, B.A., PHILLIP W. BARTH, Ph.D., and
LARS M. VISTNES, M.D.

Pressure sores, also known as decubitus ulcers or bed sores, remain a major problem in the management of paralyzed or immobilized patients. A pressure sore is an area of damage to the skin and tissues caused by unrelieved pressure. A person with normal sensation and mobility does not develop pressure sores because the integrated sensory and motor systems cause subconscious frequent changes in position so that no tissue is ever deprived of blood flow for very long. In paralyzed or immobilized patients pressure sores usually occur in tissues near a bony prominence where pressures are the greatest. Although pulmonary infections and urinary tract infections are the leading cause of death in patients who have suffered a spinal cord injury, pressure sores are a major cause of morbidity and increased health care expenditures for these patients.

INCIDENCE

Pressure sores are an extremely common problem for spinal cord injured or otherwise immobilized patients. In a retrospective study of spinal cord injuries, it was found that 60 per cent of patients having complete cervical cord injury developed a pressure sore; of these patients, the majority developed multiple sores. In addition, 50 per cent of paraplegics developed at least one pressure sore.[1] Even in the general hospital population pressure sores are a problem. A recent survey of a university hospital population (excluding the obstetric, ophthalmic, and psychiatric patient populations) identified 4.7 per cent of the patients to have sores and another 12.3 per cent to be at risk of developing sores caused by prolonged immobility. In addition to immobility, factors associated with the presence of pressure sores in

this hospital population were fecal incontinence, hypoalbuminemia, and fractures. Although these risk factors may reflect the chronicity of disease in the patient population, these factors were predictors of the development of sores in the "at risk" population.[2]

Not only do pressure sores contribute to patient morbidity, they also represent considerable expense. The financial cost of pressure sores is difficult to analyze separately from the cost of underlying medical or surgical problems but would have to include the direct medical costs of treating the sore as well as income lost during a prolonged period of treatment and rehabilitation often required to heal a pressure sore. In the general hospital population, the presence of a pressure sore is associated with prolonged hospitalization independent of underlying diseases.[2] Furthermore, it has been estimated that one fourth of the medical costs associated with spinal cord injuries are incurred as a result of treating pressure sores.[1]

ETIOLOGY

It is generally accepted that pressure sores are caused by prolonged pressure, usually over a bony prominence. Prolonged pressure leads to ischemia, mechanical damage, and subsequent tissue necrosis. Most studies have shown that an inverse relationship exists between the pressure and the duration required to produce a pressure sore. A high pressure in a tissue will produce a pressure sore with only a short duration. During normal activities such as lying, sitting, or leaning against another surface, relatively small volumes of tissues are compressed between a bony prominence and the external surface. Since nearly all the body weight is supported by the skeleton, extremely high pressures can be generated in the tissues compressed between the weight-bearing bone and the external surface. People with normal sensation and mobility subconsciously sense the prolonged pressure in the tissues and subconsciously shift their weight even while asleep. Patients with spinal cord injuries are unable to shift their weight subconsciously; they must consciously move or rely on an assistant to move them. Other factors that are associated with the breakdown of injured tissues include friction, shear forces, elevated temperature, sepsis, accumulation of metabolic waste products, altered lymph drainage, advanced age of the patient, malnutrition, atrophy of the underlying tissues, and contamination by urine and feces.

Numerous investigators have studied aspects of pressure sore development using various systems including animal models (pigs, dogs, and rats), synthetic tissue models, computer models, and noninvasive measurement in human subjects. As a result of the efforts of many investigators, the study of pressure sores has become advanced and technical; yet the body of data on pressure sores is not unified and has not been put into clinical practice. Animal studies have led to the understanding of the basic etiologic factors in pressure sores, but animal data are difficult to translate to the condition in the human patient. Animal skin and tissue differs from human in many important ways. In animal models tissue pressures can be measured invasively, a better reflection of the risk for tissue damage than pressures measured at the skin-support surface interface. However, neither the measurement of forces inside the tissue nor at the interface of skin and supporting surface is always accurate, because the introduction of a measuring device perturbs the system itself. Shear forces and friction as etiologic factors in the development of pressure sores are difficult to quantify due to a lack of direct measurement techniques.

Although most studies show that an inverse relationship exists between pressure and duration, the exact thresholds of pressure and duration to produce tissue damage vary with the type of experiment conducted. However, it is generally accepted that a pressure exceeding 32 mm Hg,[3] the tissue capillary pressure measured by a microinjection technique, will occlude blood flow in that tissue and lead to ischemia if unrelieved. The exact contributions of other factors such as sepsis, contamination by urine and feces, and malnutrition to pressure sore development cannot be quantified.

Experimental Studies

In one of the earlier studies of pressure sore etiology in dogs, Kosiak applied a known force to the skin using an inverted syringe driven by compressed air over the femoral trochanter and ischial tuberosity of dogs and measured the applied pressure. Pressure in the tissues directly under the force applicator was measured using constant saline infusion through a needle connected to a pressure transducer. Kosiak reported that a regimen of 500 mm Hg for two hours or 150 mm Hg for 12 hours was necessary to produce sores, but that a pressure of 70 mm Hg for two hours was enough to produce microscopic changes in the tissues. Microscopic changes included a decrease or loss of cross-striations of myofibrils, hyalinization of fibers, neutrophilic infiltration, and phagocytosis by neutrophils and macrophages. An inverse relationship between pressure and duration was clearly established in these experiments.[4]

In a subsequent experiment, Dinsdale applied pressure to the skin overlying the posterior iliac spine of both normal and paraplegic pigs and in addition studied the effects of friction in the development of pressure sores. The pressure application system consisted of a ball-bearing axle with two parallel metal bars of equal length. A metal square was placed at the distal end of the lower bar for pressure application. Weights placed at the distal end of the upper bar provided the force to generate the pressure on the pig. Friction was applied using a linear force system that dragged a metal webbing across the skin. Applied pressure was monitored using a push-pull strain gauge. Internal pressures were not monitored. Dinsdale reports that seven days after one three-hour application of 480 mm Hg to paraplegic pigs, no ulceration was noted. However, with the addition of friction, this regimen did produce visible pressure sores. In addition, Dinsdale showed that daily pressure application of as little as 45 mm Hg with friction for three 90-minute intervals produced pressure sores. Without applied friction, pressure sores did not appear until pressures exceeded 290 mm Hg. Dinsdale considered only skin ulceration as evidence of pressure damage and does not report biopsy results. On the basis of Kosiak's earlier work and later studies by Nola and Vistnes, it is possible that deeper tissue damage did exist in Dinsdale's pigs even though no skin ulceration was evident.[5,6]

Nola and Vistnes applied a regimen of 100

to 110 mm Hg for six hours a day to various sites on Sprague-Dawley rats in order to determine the differential response of skin and muscle to pressure.[6] Pressure was applied using a system patterned after that of Kosiak. The delivered pressure was measured using a water-filled bladder attached to a pressure transducer. When pressure was applied over the greater trochanter, gross skin ulceration was present in all the rats within 48 to 72 hours. The same regimen applied to the biceps femoris overlying the tibia produced no skin ulceration but did produce a moderate amount of muscle fiber necrosis. In addition, rats that had undergone a gluteus maximus flap transposition over one trochanter had skin ulceration on the skin-only side and significant muscle fiber necrosis with only moderate skin ulceration on the side that had undergone muscle flap transposition. Nola and Vistnes concluded that muscle fibers are more sensitive to the ischemic effects of prolonged pressure than skin by itself. However, an underlying muscle flap also seemed to shield the overlying skin from the effects of pressure.

A study by Daniel substantiated the conclusion that muscle is more sensitive to pressure and showed that the initial pathologic changes in response to pressure first occur in the muscle layer overlying the bony prominence and spread outward. In this study a computer-controlled pressure applicator was used to apply a constant pressure ranging from 30 mm Hg to 1000 mm Hg for periods of two to 18 hours over the greater trochanter of small Poland-China pigs. The transmitted pressure was measured using a catheter transducer. The pressure sites were evaluated both visually and by full-thickness biopsy seven days after pressure ap-

plication. Daniel found that the initial damage was first recorded in the deep muscle layers with progression outward. To produce only muscle damage, 500 mm Hg for a duration of four hours or 100 mm Hg for 10 hours was sufficient. In order to produce muscle and deep dermis damage, it was necessary to apply either 800 mm Hg for 10 hours or 200 mm Hg for 15 hours. Finally, skin ulceration appeared only after experiments of longer duration—600 mm Hg for 11 hours or 200 mm Hg for 16 hours.[7,8]

Surface Pressure Distribution

In the experimental studies mentioned, pressure was applied to the surface of the animal and was measured at the interface between the skin and applicator. The occurrence of pressure sores was then documented for various protocols of pressure, friction, and duration. However, pressure sores normally develop from unrelieved pressure exerted by the body's own weight over a bony prominence. It is therefore more realistic to consider the distribution of pressures both internally and externally in the lying and sitting positions rather than with the application of external force.

Several studies of the external or surface distribution of pressure in the sitting and lying positions indicate that at the bony prominence, the pressures exceed the capillary pressure (32 mm Hg), and ischemia of the underlying tissues would be expected if pressure was unrelieved. In a study of 12 paraplegic patients instrumented with small electrical pressure transducers and thermistors taped to the skin under the ischial tuberosities, Patterson and Fisher found that during a day of normal activ-

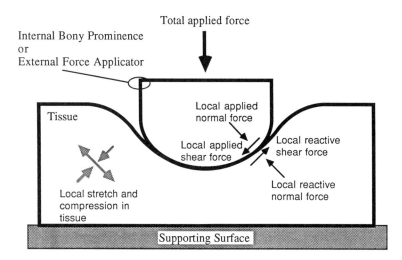

Figure 17–1. Applied load forces and reactive tissue forces. Net loading is vertical, but local surface force may be dominated by either normal force or shear, internal forces in tissue balance locally.

ities the subjects sat for 91.8 per cent of the time with pressures exceeding 30 mm Hg and 53.5 per cent of the time with pressures exceeding 90 mm Hg. The average interval that the subjects sat with unrelieved pressures was 30 minutes. Some subjects sat as long as one hour without pressure relief. Four of the 12 subjects in this study did have a history of pressure sores. None of the subjects had developed pressure sores up to six months after the completion of this study.[9]

Lindan used a bed of compressible nails to measure the external distribution of various nonparaplegic subjects classified as obese, normal-weight, and underweight in the supine, sitting, and prone positions. In the supine position the maximum pressures recorded were 50 to 60 mm Hg near the ischial tuberosities and the heels. The underweight subjects experienced the largest area of high pressure, indicating that decreased weight may actually increase the risk of developing pressure sores. In the sitting position, maximum pressures of 60 to 100 mm Hg were noted near the ischial tuberosities. Lindan reported that limitations to his methods such as nail wedging and limited compressibility could have led to underestimation of the pressures recorded in this experiment.[10]

In one of the more recent observations of surface pressures, Bennett developed a multisensor device to measure pressure and shear force using cantilevered strain gauges and to measure blood flow by a photoplethysmographic sensor. This assembly of sensors was embedded within a small aluminum cylinder and placed under the ischial tuberosities of seated paraplegic, geriatric, and normal young subjects. Bennett reported that the pressures measured under the ischial tuberosities in all groups were equal although significantly above the 32 mm Hg tissue capillary pressure. However, paraplegic and geriatric subjects had significantly higher shear stresses under the ischial tuberosities and a corresponding decrease in blood flow at that site compared with the normal young subjects.[12,13]

Surface pressure measurements on patients with spinal cord injuries and normal subjects have been conducted to evaluate various support systems: waterbeds, airbeds, cushions, and special seats. Separate studies[14-17] indicated that with the exception of flotation beds and an alternating drop seat, no support system was able to reduce the pressure measured at the skin surface below 32 mm Hg. In most cases the pressures were significantly above 32 mm Hg. Furthermore, some devices that are in-

tended to reduce pressures may actually compromise blood flow. Klemp conducted a study of subcutaneous blood flow using the ^{133}Xe rinsing method during alternating pressure on a two-channel air-filled antidecubitus mattress. Klemp reports that circulation was actually compromised below the control level seen on a standard hospital mattress during the inflation of the antidecubitus mattress. Furthermore, the period of reactive hyperemia normally following a period of decreased blood flow was cut short due to the four-minute cycling of inflation and deflation. The average tissue perfusion was in fact less using the antidecubitus mattress than on the standard mattress.[18]

Tissue Pressure Distribution

It is vital to realize that the formation of pressure sores due to ischemia is not only a function of the external pressure recorded at the skin and of the duration of pressure but also a function of how the pressure is distributed within the tissues. A bony prominence that bears most of the patient's weight will exert force on the tissues compressed between the bone and the supporting surface, leading to very high internal pressures. The internal pressures will be highest at the bony prominence and decrease as the force is distributed through the soft deformable tissues between the bone and the supporting surface. The distribution of pressures resembles a cone with the apex at the bone and the base at the skin. Another factor that must be taken into account is shear force. Shear forces can be more significant than pressure by itself in the dermis where capillaries run perpendicular to the skin and near the bone where nutrient vessels pierce the fascia also in a perpendicular manner. Shear forces alone or in combination with pressure significantly compromise circulation in tissues. The tissue pressure distribution and shear forces help to explain why some patients develop pressure sores even though clinically measured pressures at the skin surface are less than those expected to produce sores.

Theoretic analysis and empirical testing of deformation and stresses in a gel simulation of the soft tissues of a sitting person provide a basis for evaluating and manipulating pressure and shear distributions in various conditions of load, posture, and support surface characteristics.[12,13,19,20] According to these models, soft tissues under a bony prominence are flattened and pushed away from the center of the prominence. According to Bennett's model, the ap-

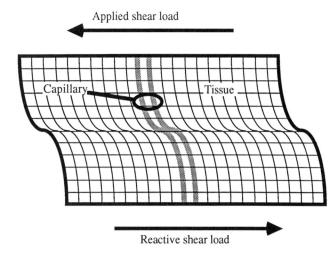

Applied shear load

Capillary

Tissue

Reactive shear load

Figure 17–2. Occlusion of a capillary by pure shear loading.

plied force per radius of contact (i.e., the weight of the person as transferred through the skeleton to the tissue under the weight-bearing bony prominence) will be countered by reactive normal forces and shear forces in the tissue. The highest forces will be directly under the bony prominence and will decrease with distance from the prominence. Furthermore, as tissue thickness decreases, normal tissue force will approach the applied force and shear forces will diminish. Since cushions are effectively like adding tissue thickness, one would expect that normal tissue forces would diminish but that shear forces would increase. This is a difficult hypothesis to prove in vivo since there are no instruments to measure shear forces directly. Reddy and his associates used a model of a buttock to aid in the design of seat cushions noted that the thickness, geometry, and material of the cushion greatly affected the stresses calculated from photographs of the tissue model deformed by sitting on the cushion.[20] Thick cushions of medium-density foam produced the lowest calculated compressive and shear stress in the simulated buttock. Reddy also noted that the point of highest pressure is directly beneath the core of a simulated bony prominence and the area of highest shear stress is just lateral to the core of the prominence.

Actual tissues are neither as isotropic nor as homogeneous as those used in these simulations, nor are the bones and overlying tissues as regularly shaped. In addition, tissue properties such as elasticity and compressibility are not accurately simulated by gel or foam rubber. Few groups have studied the in vivo pressure distribution in tissues subjected to loading; however, these studies yield valuable informa-

tion on the development of pressure sores. Three basic techniques for measuring tissue pressure exist: an intratissue balloon method, the needle method, and fluid equilibration methods using an implanted capsule or wick. Each of these methods has advantages and disadvantages but no method is really perfect for measuring tissue pressures. The wick and capsule methods can distinguish between interstitial fluid pressures and total tissue pressures but are more cumbersome to use than the needle method or intra-tissue balloon method.

A variation of the needle method was used by Le[21] to measure the distribution of tissue pressures near the trochanter of an anesthetized pig lying in the lateral position on a table. The pressure probe assembly consisted of a silicon pressure sensor and a hypodermic needle, together with a high-resistance fluid injection system. A constant slow flow of fluid produced a fluid column between the needle tip and the pressure sensor. Pressure was measured at the tip of the needle. The needle was inserted in the anesthetized pig using a grid pattern of holes drilled into a plastic support surface. The position and depth of insertion were varied in order to examine the pressure profile under the trochanter. Surface pressure measurements were obtained using an air-filled bladder connected to a manometer.

Pressure distributions were sampled in several horizontal and vertical planes within the tissue underlying the trochanter. The pressure in the tissues peaked directly under the trochanter and decreased with distance from the pominence. Pressures as high as 270 mm Hg were measured directly beneath the bone at a depth of 1.25 cm under the skin, while the surface pressures were only 47 mm Hg. The pressures varied nonlinearly with depth depending on type of tissue. Postoperative dissection of the tissues under the trochanter correlated pressure changes with the thickness of different tissue layers where the pressure changes occurred. Pressure was observed to increase from the surface into the dermis, to decrease in the superficial fascia, and then to increase again inside the muscle layers. The local decrease in pressure was a measurement artifact caused by space between the layers, which provided little resistance to flow preventing the catheter system from sensing pressures in this area. This experiment proved that although the externally measured pressures under a weight-bearing bone were low (25 to 33 mm Hg), internal pressures were three to five times higher and significantly above the tissue capillary pressure. Therefore, external pressure measurements are not indicative of internal pressures and may not reflect the true risk of developing a pressure sore.

The main points that have been learned in this and other experiments about the causes of pressure sores are:

1. There is an inverse relationship between pressure and duration.
2. Friction and shear forces are important factors in pressure sore development.
3. Tissue damage due to pressure occurs first at the bone and progresses toward the skin.
4. Pressures are highest near the weight-bearing bone and lowest at the skin.
5. Pressures recorded at the sitting surfaces under paraplegic patients are over 32 mm Hg (tissue capillary pressure).
6. Cushions and beds designed to relieve pressures do not always work.

PREVENTION

Although the preceding discussion illustrates some important concepts regarding the causes of pressure sores, the most important element to realize about pressure sores is how to prevent them. The only way to prevent pressure sores is to relieve continued excessive pressure, which is easier said than done. The general principle is to distribute the body weight over as great an area as possible. Numerous devices exist on the market for the prevention of pressure sores. Most cushions and beds have been evaluated by observance of the responses of pa-

tients who have used them. These clinical trials have not been well controlled. In addition, the needs of each paralyzed patient are different according to the level of injury, neurologic deficits, and personal preferences. One support system does not work for everyone.

Studies have shown that the best beds for pressure sore prevention are flotation beds, because they distribute the patients' weight over the greatest surface area, reducing the average surface pressure to 20 mm Hg.[15,17] Furthermore, the bouyancy of the beds prevents compression of internal tissues. The sheet covering a flotation bed must not be too tight, otherwise tenting can negate the pressure-relieving properties of the bed. Care must be taken if cushions or cut-out pads are used for the redistribution of pressure in bed or in a wheelchair because although local pressure may be reduced, shear forces may increase. As discussed previously, shear forces are very detrimental to blood flow. The most effective way to ensure adequate tissue blood flow is to have the patients reposition themselves or the caregiver reposition the patient every 30 minutes. Reminder devices or automated drop seats may be helpful for some patients. It is also important to correct other factors that contribute to pressure sore development, such as poor nutrition, infection, and contamination by urine and feces. Part of the rehabilitation efforts for all patients at risk for pressure sores should be the frequent inspection of body parts for evidence of tissue damage. Patients should receive instruction about the causes and prevention of pressure sores. In some patients, the elimination of flexor spasm is important in reducing the risk of pressure sores, especially in the trochanteric region. Intrathecal administration of phenol eliminates flexor spasms but should be used only in patients in whom there is absolutely no hope of regaining neurologic function.

TREATMENT

When a pressure sore occurs it can be treated either medically or surgically depending on the chronicity, position, and size of the sore. Whichever treatment is chosen, all pressure must be immediately removed and the skin kept clean and dry. A bed consisting of glass beads supported by columns of air is considered the best treatment because it redistributes the patient's weight over a large area and also helps to keep the sore dry. Waterbeds are also effective at promoting healing.

Nonsurgical Treatment

Local therapy of the pressure sore is the same whether for definitive treatment or to prepare for surgery. Local treatment involves debridement of necrotic tissues, control of sepsis, and the promotion of epithelialization. Debridement should be done every other day. Between debridements, a dressing that promotes the elimination of necrotic tissues can be used. Gauze soaked with Dakin's solution, hydrogen peroxide, and 0.5 per cent silver nitrate is commonly used to pack the wound in a wet-to-dry manner. Local antibiotic treatment is usually sufficient unless systemic infection is present. Pressure should be kept off the injured tissues. When the wound is clean, healing can be further enhanced with the use of a skin graft, provided that a vascular bed is available to accept the graft. Although an autogenous split-thickness graft is preferable, an allograft or xenograft can also be effective. Once a pressure sore has healed, it is most important to prevent further sores. The circumstances leading to the development of the pressure sore should be investigated. Patient, family, and nursing education should be vigorous.

Surgical Treatment

The surgical treatment of pressure sores takes several forms. Sores that have granulated can be closed with a split-thickness skin graft; more troublesome sores should be excised, the underlying bony prominence reduced, and the wound closed with a skin flap. Pressure sores in certain patients can be prevented by transposition of a skin flap that has sensation over the insensate area. In cases in which bone reduction is desired, the sore is excised with the surrounding damaged tissue and the underlying bursa. The bony prominence is removed along with the periosteum. Any heterotrophic bone should also be removed. A pressure sore with bone in the base must be covered with a skin flap. In the sacral area, flaps can be turned from the gluteus maximus; in the trochanteric area, the fascia lata or tensor fascia lata is used; while in the ischial area, the biceps femoris can be divided in the distal thigh and folded back to cover the defect. The rotated flap should be large in order to provide optimal blood supply and to allow placement of the suture lines away from the original ulcer site. Hemostasis should be meticulous and the wound should be drained postoperatively in order to prevent hematoma formation and subsequent calcification. Postoperatively, pressure should be kept off the wound by use of a Stryker frame or flotation bed.

CONCLUSIONS

Pressure sores are a serious and common problem in the management and rehabilitation of patients with spinal cord injuries or other

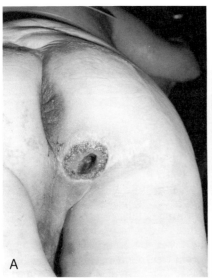
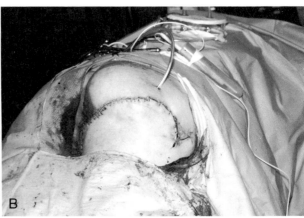

Figure 17–3. *A*, and *B*, A deep ischial pressure sore before and after placement of a full thickness flap.

conditions affecting sensation and mobility. Studies indicate that there is an inverse relationship between the magnitude of pressure and the duration of unrelieved pressure to produce a sore. Other etiologic factors include shear forces, malnutrition, sepsis, incontinence, and advanced age of the patient. The data presented in the earlier discussion indicate that tissue pressure increases with proximity to a weight-bearing bony prominence. Pressures near such a bony prominence occlude capillary flow in the surrounding tissues causing ischemia and subsequent pressure sores if unrelieved. This information substantiates the clinical observation that pressure sores often start at the bone and spread outward toward the skin.

Prevention is the key to managing pressure sores and involves the education and interaction of patient, physician, and caregivers. The importance of frequently shifting sitting and lying positions cannot be overemphasized. Many devices, including pads, cushions, and beds, exist to help prevent sores, but data proving efficacy are often scant, and no one device will work for all patients. The specific needs of each user have to be assessed in determining the best device to prevent sores. Very few of the available devices are adequate substitution for physically shifting the patient's weight off the bony prominence. Treatment of sores can be conservative medical management or more frequently involves placement of a skin graft; with more extensive sores, treatment involves excision of the bone with transposition of a full-thickness flap to close the ulcer. Treatment is often lengthy and costly.

REFERENCES

1. Richardson RR, Meyer PR: Prevalence and incidence of pressure sores in acute spinal cord injuries. Paraplegia 19:235, 1981.
2. Allman RM, Laprade CA, Noel L: Pressure sores among hospitalized patients. Ann Intern Med 105:337, 1986.
3. Landis EM: Micro-injection studies of capillary blood pressure in human skin. Heart 15:202, 1962.
4. Kosiak M: Etiology of decubitus ulcers. Arch Phys Med Rehabil 42:19, 1961.
5. Dinsdale SM: Decubitus ulcers: Role of pressure and friction in causation. Arch Phys Med Rehabil 55:147, 1974.
6. Nola GT, Vistnes LM: Differential response of skin and muscle in the experimental production of pressure sores. Plast Reconstr Surg 66:728, 1980.
7. Daniel RK, Priest DL, Wheatly DC: Etiologic factors in pressure sores: An experimental model. Arch Phys Med Rehabil 62:492, 1981.
8. Daniel RK, Priest DL, Wheatly DC: Pathophysiology of pressure sores. Plastic Surgical Forum: Proceedings of the American Society of Plastic and Reconstructive Surgeons 4:15, 1981 (summary).
9. Patterson RP, Fisher SV: Pressure and temperature patterns under the ischial tuberosities. Bull Pros Res 17:5, 1980.
10. Lindan O, Greenway RM, Piazza JM: Etiology of decubitus ulcers: An experimental study: Arch Phys Med Rehabil 42:774, 1961.
11. Bennett L: Transferring load to flesh. Part V. Experimental Work. Bull Pros Res 10-19:88, 1973.
12. Bennett L, Lee BY, Trainor F: Shear versus pressure as causative factors in skin flow occlusion. Arch Phys Med Rehabil 60:309, 1979.
13. Bennett L, Lee BY, Trainor F: Skin stress and blood flow in sitting paraplegic patients. Arch Phys Med Rehabil 65:165, 1984.
14. Holley LK, Long J, Stewart J, Jones RF: A new pressure measuring system for cushion and beds—With a review of the literature. Paraplegia 17:461, 1979.
15. Wells P, Geden E: Paraplegic body-support pressure on convoluted foam, waterbed, and standard mattresses. Res Nurs Health 7:127, 1984.
16. Houle R: Evaluation of seat devices designed to prevent ischemic ulcers in paraplegic patients. Arch Phys Med Rehabil 50:587, 1969.
17. Siegel R, Vistnes LM, Laub DR: Use of water bed for prevention of pressure sores. Plast Reconstr Surg 51:31, 1973.
18. Klemp P, Staberg B, Munkvad M: Subcutaneous circulation in pressure regions while lying on an air mattress designed to prevent pressure sores. Ugeskr Laeger 145:559, 1983.
19. Chow WW, Odell EI: Deformations and stresses in soft body tissues of a sitting person. J Biomech Eng 100:79, 1978.
20. Reddy N, Patel H, Cochran GVB: Model experiments to study the stress distributions in a seated buttock. J Biomech 15:493, 1982.
21. Le KM, Madsen BL, Barth PW: An in-depth look at pressure sores using monolithic pressure transducers. Plast Reconstr Surg 74:747, 1984.

Pressure Sores:
Nursing Aspects and Prevention

ROBERTA S. ABRUZZESE, Ed.D., R.N., F.A.A.N. _____

Pressure sores are one of the most pervasive complications of spinal cord injured patients. Forty to 60 per cent of patients with spinal cord injury develop pressure sores.[1] The most common sites of pressure sore development are the sacrum, trochanter, and ischium. Immobility and lack of innervation are usually postulated as the reasons for the high percentage of ulceration among these patients. However, the prevalence of pressure sores resistant to healing and the frequency of these breaking down again after skin grafts indicate far more complex problems. A holistic approach to patient care explores the psychosocial as well as the physiologic ramifications of spinal cord injury with all the members of the health care team—physician, surgeon, nurse, physical therapist, dietitian, and rehabilitation specialist—supported by an effective system that encompasses protocols, equipment, and supplies. Prevention of pressure sores needs to be the major goal of therapy. If this fails, the goal becomes not only to heal the pressure sores but also to ensure that they will not recur. To achieve these goals requires a knowledgeable health care team to mobilize resources for skin care of spinal cord injured patients.

IMPORTANCE OF THE PROBLEM

There are misconceptions about the incidence, prevalence, and severity of pressure sores and the costs that they add to treatment of spinal cord injured patients from acute phase through rehabilitation. The increased cost is partially related to the additional days of hospital stay that treating pressure sores adds to those already required by the spinal cord injury. The variance in healing time of stage I sores relates to the underlying pathology. Some stage I sores are merely reddened areas of the epidermis that will dissipate when pressure is relieved; other stage I sores are like the tip of an iceberg—70 per cent of their mass is hidden. It has been shown that the destruction of tissue begins at the interface of the bone and soft tissue, with only a reddened area appearing at the epidermis. The healing of the ulcer with the "tip of the iceberg" phenomenon depends on the extent of deep tissue trauma.

The variance of healing for stage IV sores is related to involvement of muscle and bone, osteomyelitis, systemic infection, undermining of tissue, and large area of necrosis. Sometimes stage IV sores are chronic, with fixation in the inflammation stage of healing. Ordinarily a wound progresses from inflammation to regeneration to remodeling.[3] Chronic ulcers seem unable to progress beyond the inflammatory stage; one theory of etiology postulates that pericapillary fibrin prevents perfusion of the sore perimeter and contributes to its stasis.[4] Other theories posit that growth factors play an active role in accelerating healing,[5] although more than 10 years of research on growth factors have resulted in little clinically significant increase in the rate of healing.

The acceleration of healing may not be as easily promoted as is the decrease of sores that progress from stage I to stage IV. Rubin, Dietz, and Abruzzese found that attention to the problem of pressure sores had a profound influence on their severity.[6] In their nine-month survey of pressure sores in an acute care hospital, the severity of sores decreased dramatically from a mix of all stages to the rare existence of sores at stage III or IV. If pressure sores cannot be totally prevented in chronically ill patients, spinal cord injured patients, and terminally ill patients, their severity can be minimized. The present cost-conscious era in health care resulting from fixed prospective payment systems rewards reduction in severity of pressure sores so that patients do not become "outliers" using nonreimbursable hospital days. More emphasis on prevention and providing rewards for health care teams can aid in diminishing the severity of sores or in preventing them entirely.

Prevention strategies can greatly change the percentage of sores that progress to stage IV (Table 17–1). By 1999 only 3 per cent of sores should progress to stage IV, 5 per cent to stage III, 67 per cent to stage II, and 25 per cent to stage I. This contrasts sharply with the 1986 estimation by Find/SVP that 11 per cent of sores progress to stage IV, 17 per cent to stage III, 57 percent to stage II, and 15 per cent to stage I. The net effect of prevention strategies should be that fewer spinal cord injured patients will require costly, time-consuming treatments for stages III and IV pressure sores. The same is true for the general population. With patients

TABLE 17-1. Severity of Pressure Sores and Healing Time

Stage	1986	1999	HEALING TIME
I	15%	25%	14 days
II	57%	67%	45 days
III	17%	5%	90 days
IV	11%	3%	120 days

*Estimates are an average, with some sores healing in fewer days and some in more.

living longer and having more concurrent health problems, it could be expected that the total number of patients with pressure sores will increase, but their severity would not progress to the dangerous status of stage III or IV as now commonly occurs.

Financial Costs

The cost of pressure sores is directly related to the severity of the sore. Of the 6.5 billion dollars estimated spent per year for the treatment of pressure sores, only 640 million is attributable to the cost of products.[2] The larger amount results from treatment time by health care professionals. Not all these costs are reimbursed by third party payers or by federal and state governments. With prospective payment systems (PPS) in place in most hospitals since October 1, 1983, the development of pressure sores is viewed as a preventable complication that extends the length of stay. Since pressure sores are considered preventable, there is no payment for the extra days required for healing.

The PPS pays a specific amount for each diagnostic related group (DRG) with pressure sores placed in the following categories: No. 263, surgical–skin grafts and/or debridement for skin ulcers or cellulitis with age less than 69 and/or no complications or co-morbidities; No. 264, surgical–skin grafts and/or debridement for skin ulcer or cellulitis with age greater than 70 without complications or co-morbidities; and No. 271, medical skin ulcers. The amount of reimbursement and assigned length of stay for these DRGs, as for all others, are updated annually and published in the Federal Register. One fact in relation to payment that seems clear is that the cost of treating pressure sores is far greater than the amount of reimbursement that agencies receive. The most reliable statistics relate to medicare patients with primary and secondary diagnosis of pressure sores. The cost of their care for 1986 was

$417.7 million; the reimbursement was $214.2 million (Medical Technology and Practice Patterns Institute, 1988, personal communication). Therefore, about 51 per cent of the cost of care is reimbursed.

Extrapolating these figures to spinal cord injured patients who develop pressure sores is realistic. Each year approximately 8000 to 10,000 people are admitted with new spinal cord injury. Most are men under 30 years of age, and 40 to 60 per cent can be expected to develop pressure sores.[1] Their already long hospital and rehabilitation stay is increased by 90 to 120 days by the complication of pressure sores, which often progress to stage III or IV. Often the institution receives almost no additional payments for the lengthened stay attributable to preventable pressure sores.

In addition to the loss of reimbursement for the added expenditures for pressure sores, the institution incurs another cost, often referred to as *opportunity cost*. This is the loss of income that could have been generated if beds occupied by patients with pressure sores had been occupied by patients with other diagnoses that are reimbursable. Hibbs estimated that the case of one patient with a grade IV pressure sore and a hospital stay of 180 days denied the hospital payment from 21 other patients who had the standard length of stay.[7] If 28 per cent of patients with pressure sores are at stages III and IV levels of severity,[2] the number of beds occupied by these patients is considerable. Concomitantly, the loss of income for the institution is staggering. It follows that prevention of pressure sores is the only true way to reduce costs and increase income.

Human Costs

The financial costs of pressure sores are far outweighed by the human costs in terms of the psychological, physiologic, and social effects. The psychological effects are the greatest when the patient has a stage IV draining, foul-smelling sore. Although spinal cord injured patients can deny the existence of sores they cannot feel, they can seldom deny the foul odor, the extra time health care personnel spend treating the ulcer, or the aversion and sense of disgust often nonverbally conveyed by the staff. Self-image is changed in a negative way when patients must view themselves as abhorrent to the very people who must care for them. Sometimes this results in accusations of noncaring. The staff and family are accused of not caring for the patient and not answering calls for help.

The patient is accused of not caring enough to assist in prevention of pressure sores, is labeled a "problem" patient, and is dismissed as impossible to help. In reality the anger of the patient may be directed at life, at fate, at the accident, or at circumstance that resulted in spinal cord injury and that will produce enormous changes in the future. There is a painful struggle to accept a changed body with all the ramifications of redefining how life can be satisfying. This is a large task, requiring coping skills of a high order. This patient needs the assistance of all on the health care team.

Another psychological aspect of pressure sores that is receiving more attention is that of the "lived experience." This means the experience of the pressure sore for the individual patient: the ways the pressure sore affects the person's life, how social relationships are changed, and what is possible for the future. The lived experience of pressure sores is related to the personality of the patient—personality understood as the totality of unique and characteristic aspects of each person.[8] These characteristics are exhibited in response to the problem of having a pressure sore. Patients with a dependent, demanding personality become angry at the slightest indication that their needs are not being met. Their fears of abandonment are exacerbated by delays in meeting their requests. They depend on others to prevent the pressure sores. They must be helped to understand their own role in taking care of themselves and in preventing sores. Only when they are assured of the attention of others can they relinquish fear and take ownership of their role in healing and prevention.

On the other hand, the orderly, controlled personality wants to know and be in control of all aspects of care. These patients usually are well read and have a knowledge of medical terminology, treatment principles, and outcome projections; they may question everything. The pressure sore represents a loss of control or a neglect on their part or on the part of caregivers. Their reaction is that they must be alert that this does not happen again. These patients can cause a sense of frustration in caregivers; their need to control can be utilized for healing and prevention of recurrence. Caregivers can assist by good communication—providing detailed physiologic explanations for treatments and sharing projected outcomes.

This behavior contrasts sharply with that of the long-suffering personality whose hallmark is misery. These patients use the pressure sore as a means of getting attention for their many afflictions. This person is always engaged in a "pity party" and wants everyone to verify that the problems are awful. Staff can assist the patient to use the treatment and prevention strategies as one more "suffering" that must be a part of life and thus engage the patient in healing the sore without calling attention to the positive aspects. Because these patients fear that if they have no problems, no one will pay attention to them, it is important for caregivers to provide as much attention when the sore is healed as they did when it was present.

Patients provide many clues as to the meaning of pressure sores in their lives. For some patients, the nurses' visit to the home to treat the pressure sore is an opportunity for a social visit. For other patients, hospitalization is an escape from an unsatisfying home life. Neglect of self and lack of cooperation in preventing the recurrence of pressure sores may indicate anger turned against the self or a death wish, which is a cry for help in coping with the consequences of spinal cord injury.

In counting the human costs of pressure sores, the physiologic aspects are sometimes poorly understood, especially in relation to pain and to the hazards of immobility. In the literature related to pressure sores there is seldom mention of pain associated with pressure sore treatment. This contrasts sharply with the literature related to burns, in which pain is a major concern of treatment and nursing care. Is pain not a factor in stages II and III pressure sores, which roughly compare with second and third degree burns? For the spinal cord injured patient in the early phases of injury, generalized pain (which is associated with the traumatic injury that affected the spinal cord) is treated with narcotics. By the time pressure sores appear in the sacrum, ischium, or trochanter, denervation to these areas precludes physiologic pain, although the psychological pain of loss may mimic physiologic pain.

The physiologic hazards of immobility include an increase in bacteria in the nares and bloodstream with a concomitant decrease in circulating immunoglobulin G (IgG), which comprises 75 per cent of normal antibodies. During the first 10 to 20 days of immobilization the white blood cells are less active in encapsulating microorganisms, which can lead to susceptibility to infections. The timing of this decrease in white blood cell activity has a negative effect because pressure sores usually develop within two to nine days after hospitalization. White blood cells, needed to counteract the physiologic process of tissue ischemia, are not available. At a time when optimal nutrition is needed for cell vitality, immobility leads to a decrease in appetite, a diminution in the ability of insulin to lower blood glucose levels, a decrease in circulating blood volume, decreases in rate and depth of respirations, and possible cardiac problems related to an increase in circulating calcium. These changes in respiration and nutrition further compromise tissues that are susceptible to breakdown from the unaccustomed pressure and stress of bedrest.[9]

The third area of human cost is related to altered social relationships. The two major areas of concern are changes in family relationships and in financial responsibilities. Family relationships are altered when the usual role of an independent man or woman is replaced by a dependent role. Young adults are just beginning their process of becoming independent and with spinal cord injury must regress to an unwanted stage of dependency on parents. A young husband must forfeit his role of principal or equal breadwinner to his wife, who must now assume the dominant financial responsibility. The stereotype of the strong father as role model for his children must be replaced by an androgynous view of the possible roles of men and women. These role changes cause confusion and unrest at a time when all energy should be directed toward making the most of whatever functional ability is left for the spinal cord injured patient.

CAUSES OF PRESSURE SORES

Pressure sores are injuries to the dermis and underlying tissue caused by vascular occlusion with insufficient transport of oxygen and nutrients to tissues beyond the occlusion plus impairment in transport of waste products away from damaged tissues. Although the term pressure sore is usually limited to occlusion from external sources such as bed or wheelchair support systems, the results of occlusion are equally damaging if the occlusion is due to sickled cells, diabetic atherosclerosis, or venous insufficiency. Once an unblanchable erythematous area appears on the skin, the factors of shear, moisture, limited mobility, reduced activity, malnutrition, dehydration, and general state of health contribute to the magnitude of the problem.

Pressure

The term pressure sore is widely used because pressure that exceeds 32 mm Hg is generally recognized as the major contributing factor in subsequent dermal injury. The early studies of Lindan,[10] Kosiak,[11] and Bush[12] established that tissues were not only damaged by sustained pressures of 32 mm Hg or more but also that the longer the pressure is applied the more extensive is the tissue destruction. Husain[13] (1953) noted that prolonged low pressures were more damaging to tissue than high pressures of short duration. Tissue ischemia leads to acidosis, increased capillary permeability, extravasation, and vascular thrombosis.[14] The most damage occurs when circulation is restored and reperfusion of tissues occurs. The reintroduction of oxygen free radicals (superoxide anion, hydroxl radicals, and hydrogen peroxide) results in endothelial swelling, extravasation, and microvascular occlusion.[15] The reversal of this process may depend on the scavengers of peroxide or inhibitors of enzymes involved in producing superoxides.

Little attention is paid to the period immediately following the relief of pressure even though most institution-acquired pressure sores develop two to nine days after admission. A careful health history related to the cause of nonblanchable reddened areas would provide a clue to the hidden underlying tissue damage. Pressures are higher at the interface of bones and soft tissues than at the surface of the skin. Fat and muscle layers are more susceptible to tissue anoxia than is the dermis. Often the small reddened area on the surface of the skin is only the tip of the iceberg, with a cone-shaped area of deeper tissue necrosis.[16]

Shear

The importance of shear in relation to pressure as a causative factor in pressure ulcer development is receiving more attention through the research of Bennett and Lee.[17] They have demonstrated that trauma related to shear increases as the diameter of the pressure inducer decreases. The combination of compressive stress and vertical shear stress needs to be taken into account when the relative harm resulting from pressure is judged. Lowthian[18] estimated that 40 per cent of patients admitted to long-term care were at risk for developing pressure sores on sacrum and heels due to shear forces. In these cases, shear was exerted by patients sliding down as the head of the bed was raised. The blood supply to the skin is compromised by stretching and/or tearing of the blood vessels of the subcutaneous fat and superficial fascia.[19] Resulting pressure sores in the sacral area are long and narrow as contrasted with dermal sores resulting primarily from pressure, which are round or oblong in shape.

Moisture

The deleterious effects of pressure and shear are exacerbated in the presence of unrelieved moisture. Whether the moisture results from incontinence or sweating, the physiologic effect is an interference of the skin's ability to transmit insensible water vapor. Of the 400 gm of insensible moisture vapor transmitted through the skin during one day, 200 gm comes from the back, buttocks, and dorsal part of the legs. Flam[20] explains that " . . . this moisture must be removed to prevent overhydration of the stratum corneum and subsequent loss of mechanical strength, an increase in permeability to external solutions, and . . . under occluded conditions, an increase in microflora and an increase in pH." Temperature regulation is compromised by preventing the loss of heat through convection and radiation. The change in the normal flora and the maceration of the epidermis expose the dermis to invasion by bacteria. In areas in which skin touches skin, as the gluteal folds or under pendulous breasts, the epidermis is further eroded by friction.

Norton and colleagues[21] observed that the existence of incontinence was the single best predictor of patients most likely to develop pressure sores. Linked with limited mobility and activity, the spinal cord injured patient is at high risk for developing pressure sores. Even the small shifts of weight that occur during sleep to reposition weight from bony prominences and restore circulation are no longer automatic.

Nutrition and Hydration

The spinal cord injured patient can neither prevent nor heal pressure sores without adequate nutrition and hydration. Natow[22] recommends a diet high in protein and carbohydrates and moderate in fat, vitamin C, and zinc. Hypoproteinemia increases the susceptibility to development of pressure sores through edema and loss of elasticity, resiliency, and vitality of tissues. Edema decreases diffusion of nutrients and oxygen from capillaries to cells. Protein deficiency also compromises neoangiogenesis, fibroblastic proliferation, proteoglycan and collagen synthesis, and wound remodeling.[23]

There is some uncertainty as to the best method for monitoring protein levels. The most commonly used test is serum albumin with the desired range 3.5 to 5 ml. Holmes and colleagues found in their study of 36 patients that only 16.6 per cent of those with albumin levels over 3.5 gm/dl developed pressure sores while 75 per cent of those whose levels were below 3.5 gm/dl developed sores.[24] Other tests used are serum transferrin and total lymphocyte count. Serum transferrin is the preferred test for protein sufficiency because transferrin has a half-life of 8.8 days as opposed to serum albumin, which has a half-life of 23 days. Transferrin then would be a more sensitive indicator of protein depletion. The normal value of transferrin is above 200 mg/dl; values between 200 and 150 mg/dl are considered mild depletion; values between 150 and 100 mg/dl are considered moderate depletion; and values below 100 mg/dl are considered severe depletion. Kaminski and colleagues agree that decreased serum albumin is a late manifestation of protein deficiency and serum transferrin is more discriminating in severe malnutrition.[26] However, for less than severe malnutrition they warn that serum transferrin levels may vary over a wide range even in the presence of clinically obvious malnutrition.

Of the recommended vitamins, the role of vitamin C in prevention or healing of pressure sores is the best understood. The lack of vitamin C interferes with fibroblast function and collagen formation as well as resistance to infection. If vitamin C is decreased to scorbutic levels, wounds heal by contraction rather than by the formation of collagen.[23] Freiman and colleagues note that vitamin A also plays a role in epithelialization and collagen formation, although its effects are poorly understood.[27]

Other elements needed to prevent pressure sores or to heal those already existing are iron and zinc. Iron in the form of divalent ionic iron is needed for hydroxylation of lysine and proline and thus affects collagen synthesis. Whether or not iron also plays a role in wound healing through anemia is debatable. There may be other factors such as hypovolemia, elevated blood viscosity, or vasoconstriction which are more influential than decreased amounts of iron.[23] Zinc's role in wound healing seems related to its role with the enzymes RNA and DNA and other transferases. Lack of zinc may also be detrimental to the metabolism of vitamin A.

In addition to nutrition, adequate hydration is a concern in the prevention of pressure sores. Institutions with their air conditioning in summer and their often too-dry air in winter hasten the evaporation of water from the surface of the skin. The practice of bathing patients daily and inadequate removal of soap also contribute to the loss of natural skin oils. In addition, most people do not drink the recommended eight glasses of water per day. If appetite is decreased by bedrest and institutional food, drinking adequate fluids each day is even further neglected. Dehydration can increase susceptibility to shear and friction of bed linens and facilitate pressure sores.

General State of Health

Adequate hydration and nutrition, along with mobility, activity, continence, and prevention of pressure and shear, contribute to the general state of health and minimize the spinal cord injured patient's likelihood of developing a pressure sore. Concomitant health problems such as diabetes, sickle cell anemia, cardiovascular problems, anemias, cancer, or AIDS will increase the risk level for the spinal cord injured. These health problems must be considered when planning care in order to either prevent the formation of pressure sores or to minimize the severity of any that develop.

PREVENTION

Because prevention of pressure sores is the ultimate aim, an efficient skin care program needs to be in place. An efficient system is one which involves the entire health care team—physician, nurse, dietitian, social worker, physical therapist, pharmacist—in a consistent program. The entire health care team should be held accountable so that time is not wasted in casting blame. If all team members take responsibility for prevention and care, they will be more likely to notice incipient signs of pressure sores and to institute a vigorous prevention program. The program needs to be simple so that all can be oriented quickly and time is not wasted on explaining complicated directions or completing multiple forms. The more difficult the directions are and the more paperwork involved in reporting or initiating a prevention program, the less likely it is that the program will be implemented. The system should be efficient in the use of time and materials. There is no reason for a good skin care program to be costly or to be predicated on such elements as hiring extra personnel for turning patients. There are many inexpensive support surfaces—high-density foam or air mattresses—which can be used immediately when high-risk patients are admitted. The program needs to be effective in preventing sores from forming or in keeping an already formed sore from progressing to a more advanced stage. No skin care program will succeed without support from administrative officials and from physicians. Supportive administrative officials will provide for availability of supplies, for rewarding of personnel active in prevention of sores, and for consistent performance of protocols carried out on each shift. They will not allow nurses or physicians to change treatments from day to day; consistency of treatment has been demonstrated as an important factor in prevention and healing.[28] If physicians support the skin care program, they will encourage nurses to be vigilant in assessing erythematous skin areas and take an active part in developing and implementing treatment protocols.

An example of an efficient system supported by a health care team is NAMP, developed by Lidowski.[29] Since Lidowski's work has been in a long-term care institution, this system is particularly meaningful for the spinal cord injured. The system includes:

N   Nutritional support
A   Assessment and accountability
M   Management by moist wound healing
P   Protocols for prevention and protection

Nutritional support begins on admission and continues at a vigorous pace if the patient has a pressure sore. Dietary interventions are linked to the severity of the pressure ulcer using the staging process of the International Association for Enterostomal Therapy standards.[30] The protocols as developed by the dietitian and approved by the skin care team are shown in Table 17–2.

Assessment and accountability are considered the second key element in the NAMP system. The assessment includes both the initial evaluation on admission and periodic re-evaluation. For the spinal cord injured patient, formal weekly reassessment by a registered nurse is considered a minimum standard with daily informal assessment during bedbath. The initial and the weekly formal assessments involve the use of a form that lists high-risk variables such as mobility, activity, continence, nutrition, hydration, mental status, and general state of health. Accountability requires that each person coming into contact with the patient take responsibility for the well-being of

TABLE 17–2. Ulcer Stage and Nutritional Phase

STAGES	NUTRITION PHASE
Stage I Erythema not resolving within 30 minutes of pressure relief. Epidermis remains intact. Reversible with intervention.	Prevention phase 1. Start nutritional profile and laboratory evaluation. 2. Develop nutritional care plan. 3. Complete dietary assessment sheet. 4. Start supplement if 100% of RDA not met.
Stage II Partial-thickness loss of skin layers involving epidermis and possibly into dermis. Blister with erythema and/or induration. Wound base moist and pink.	Transitional Phase 1. Evaluate laboratory values. 2. Reassessment by registered dietitian. 3. Increase calories, protein, vitamin C, and zinc.
Stage III Full-thickness tissue loss extending through dermis to involve subcutaneous tissue. Shallow crater may be covered with eschar. May include necrotic tissue, undermining, sinus tract, exudate, or infection. Wound base is usually not painful.	Critical Phase 1. Evaluate laboratory data. 2. Reassessment by RD. 3. Increase calories, protein, vitamin C, and zinc. 4. Evaluate hydration and replace fluids 5. Reevaluate PRN or weekly.
Stage IV Deep tissue destruction extending through subcutaneous tissue to fascia and may involve muscle layers, joint or bone. Presents as deep crater. May include necrotic tissue, undermining, sinus tract formation, exudate and infection. Wound base is usually painful. (International Association for Enterostomal Therapy standards of care 1987).	Challenge Phase 1–5 as above for critical phase 6. Evaluate renal function 7. Evaluate dietary needs frequently.

Reprinted with permission from Ratra, I: in Lidowski, H: NAMP: A system for preventing and managing pressure ulcers. Decubitus 1 (1), p. 30.

that patient. No one says, " . . . skin care is not my responsibility—let the nurse do it." Each person realizes that having skin care is a basic patient right as are having air to breathe and food to eat and that everyone shares as needed in the provision of that right. Lidowski emphasizes the importance of this attitude for a successful skin care program and an efficient milieu for long-term care.[29]

Management by moist wound healing is the agreed-upon treatment of choice with the NAMP system. Moist wound healing gained prominence in the 1980s as a therapy for effective healing of pressure sores. The skin care team has written protocols for the type of dressing to be used for each stage of a pressure sore. Consistency of treatment and research protocols documenting the continued success of therapy has proven valuable. Operations for amputations and skin flaps have decreased dramatically in institutions in which strict adherence to moist wound healing has been adopted.

No prevention or treatment of pressure sores is effective without protocols for prevention and protection. The protocols include the frequency of assessment, the standard items available for bed and wheelchair support systems, procedures for treatment for each stage of pressure sore, guidelines for mandatory consultation from the skin care team, debridement op-

tions, and the program included in the general orientation of all new staff. These well-developed protocols serve as a reference to protect patients from lack of knowledge or inconsistent care from new personnel. Protection of patients from harming themselves with inadequate shifting of weight or incorrect positioning off pressure-prone areas is also emphasized in the NAMP system. Padded bed rails, foot boards, and overhead trapeze for ease of moving up in bed are considered basic protection.

Assessment Scales

A component of an efficient skin care program is a nursing assessment scale, to be used at admission and at formal weekly reassessments thereafter. Although assessment scales vary from institution to institution, all should have certain common characteristics. First, they should be easy to use by the nursing staff and require a minimum amount of orientation. In this era of nursing shortage, intensely ill patients, and shortened length of hospital stay there is no time for excessive paperwork. Assessment forms should contain all the necessary data on the form itself and not require the reading of several pages of instruction. Second, the variables on the assessment form should be those high-risk factors validated in the literature as being most influential in the development of pressure sores. In addition, the form should be adapted for evaluation of the patients most frequently admitted to the individual institution. Third, the assessment form should serve as a guide for nursing care. For each variable indicating high risk, skin care protocols should specify measures approved for counteracting the risk factor.

The variables listed on assessment forms are derived from the basic assessment scale used by Norton for long-term care.[21] Norton devised a four-point scale for the variables physical condition, mental condition, activity, mobility, and incontinence, with a score of 20 indicating no risk and a score of 5 indicating high risk. Other assessment scales have reversed the scoring so that a low score indicates low risk and a high score indicates high risk. Other variables derived from the literature are also added to presently used assessment scales. Common variables used are (1) patient characteristics of nutrition, hydration, age, medications, sensory perception, general state of health, and arteriolar pressure, and (2) exposure to moisture, friction, and shear. The aim when including variables is to have mutually exclusive categories which can be easily evaluated and will direct patient care planning in terms of prevention.

The scales by Knoll Pharmaceuticals,[28] Gosnell,[31] and Braden[32] have received extensive examination in terms of validity and reliability studies. Recent research by Towey and Erland on the predictive validity and reliability of the Knoll scale (Fig. 17–4) found that the scale was an accurate predictor of long-term patients who developed pressure sores by the 14th day of admission but not for those who developed ulcers at the 28th day.[33] The deletion of the variables nutritional intake, fluid intake, and predisposing factors increased the tool's reliability. This finding may indicate that the methods of measuring fluid and food intake

ASSESSMENT OF DECUBITUS ULCER POTENTIAL					
NAME	#	AGE	DATE		
DIAGNOSIS					
M.D.		RISK SCORE			
PARAMETERS	0	1	2	3	SCORE
General state of health	Good	Fair	Poor	Moribund	
Mental status	Alert	Lethargic	Semi-comatose	Comatose	
			Count These Conditions as Double:		
Activity	Ambulatory	Needs help	Chairfast	Bedfast	
Mobility	Full	Limited	Very limited	Immobile	
Incontinence	None	Occasional	Usually of urine	Total of urine and feces	
Oral nutrition intake	Good	Fair	Poor	None	
Oral fluid intake	Good	Fair	Poor	None	
Predisposing diseases	Absent	Slight	Moderate	Severe	
(Diabetes, neuropathies, vascular disease, anemias)					

The higher the score, the greater is the potential to develop decubitus ulcers.
Partients with scores about (12) should be considered at risk.

NEXT DATE FOR REEVALUATION _____

©Knoll Pharmaceuticals

Figure 17–4. Assessment form, Knoll Pharmaceuticals, 1978. Used with permission.

and predisposing health factors need to be changed. The original validity and reliability studies used the opinion of the patient's nurse for the adequacy of food and fluid intake.[28] Nutrition and hydration are commonly recognized as crucial factors in preventing and healing pressure ulcers. Further studies need to use serum albumin, serum transferrin, total lymphocyte count, weight loss, creatinine height index, and/or anthropometric measurements as indicators of adequate nutrition. Adequate hydration might be measured by skin turgor, acid-base balance, fluid intake, and urine output. The finding that the variable of predisposing diseases was not predictive of those who developed pressure sores by day 14 may be related to the study population at a long-term care institution, in which most patients could be expected to have vascular disease. On the other hand, Constantian and Jackson in a retrospective study of 280 patients also found that patients with diabetes mellitus, alcoholism, cancer, peripheral vascular disease, or anemia had no higher risk for developing pressure sores than did patients without those predisposing diseases.[34]

For greater predictive validity the ideal assessment scale would have discrete variables without overlapping categories. For example, on the Knoll scale and the Gosnell scale the variable of mental status is measuring whether the patient is alert, lethargic, semiconscious, or comatose. This measurement is important as it relates to ability to move freely around in bed or the ability to be up in a wheelchair or ambulating. This relates to the hazard of immobility and is already measured by the variables of mobility and of activity. Similarly on the Braden scale, the variable of sensory (perception) is measuring consciousness and response to painful stimuli. This is of interest in relation to pressure sores as it relates to mobility and activity, which have their own variables on the Braden scale. One could argue that sensory perception is especially important in relation to the spinal cord injured because some authors[14,35,36] have indicated that denervation predisposes to pressure ulcer formation. However, others[34,36a] have found that there is no difference directly related to denervation of muscles. The predisposing factor is prolonged pressure related to lack of mobility or activity or both. The variable that needs measuring is the patient's psychological status relating to such factors as self-care, hope, and coping with stress—the psychological aspects discussed previously. The recommendation is that the de-scriptors for the variable mental status be changed to measure psychological aspects rather than aspects related to mobility and activity.

Whichever assessment scale is used, its primary benefit appears to be that it serves as an indicator of the importance of preventing pressure sores. A study of the usefulness of an assessment scale to specify nursing care revealed that when using case studies, nurses without an assessment scale were just as able to specify nursing care to prevent pressure sores as were nurses using an assessment scale.[37] This seems to indicate that the knowledge of prevention of pressure sores is fairly widespread among nurses. The magnitude of the pressure sore problem is not related to a lack of knowledge of prevention but rather to factors within the nursing care settings which mitigate against prevention. Some of these may be a lack of reward from administration and physicians for nurses' time spent on prevention measures or a lack of equipment and supplies such as pressure-relieving support systems for patients at risk who have not yet developed pressure sores. A valid and reliable assessment scale is most useful when it is incorporated into a comprehensive skin care program.

Severity Staging

Just as an assessment scale is necessary to determine potential to develop pressure sores, so a severity scale is necessary in evaluation of those that are pre-existing. Shea presented a scale ranging from I to IV which specifies the levels of skin breakdown.[38] Grade I is a partial thickness ulcer resembling an abrasion; grade II is a full-thickness ulcer through the dermis to the subcutaneous fat; grade III is deep, foul-smelling, and infected; grade IV is the ulcer complicated by muscle and bone involvement. The International Association of Enterostomal Therapy[31] published a recommended severity-staging system that differs from Shea's. Stage I is erythema not resolving within 30 minutes. Stage II is partial thickness; stage III is full thickness; and stage IV is deep tissue destruction. Oot-Giromini[39] proposes grades which begin with stage O indicating intact skin with no redness; stages I through IV resemble the stages proposed by IAET. The State of California Department of Health in its licensing procedure memo No. 46, May 1977, presents a staging system similar to IAET's but lacking in some specificity of descriptors. Until there is a nationally recognized standardization of definitions, it is advisable to chart detailed descriptions as well as the grade of the sore.

In addition to the risk assessment score and the stage of the sore, other factors that need to be documented are location, size, sinus tract formation, necrotic tissue present, eschar, exudate, pain and signs of infections such as induration, edema, odor, crepitus, temperature, and cellulitis. Since all pressure sores are contaminated, culture and sensitivity screening is important only if there are systemic signs of infection.

TREATMENTS OLD AND NEW

Treatment depends on the severity and location of the sore and takes into account the total profile of the patient. The emphasis is on treating the whole person rather then just treating the sore, so that once healed it will not recur. Only if the patient takes responsibility for skin health will sores remain healed. All must be convinced that prevention of sores and not treatment is the ultimate primary goal. The primacy of prevention is reflected in the use of air-fluidized beds and low air loss beds to prevent pressure sores from progressing to stages III and IV rather than using these technologies only with sores in stages III and IV. The methods of treatment have changed over the years as prevention has received more attention and resulted in greater sophistication in support systems for beds and wheelchairs. The following compares some old and new treatment principles with the recognition that not all the old treatments are made obsolete by the newer treatments.

1. *Old:* Keep it dry; *New:* Keep it moist. A major shift in the treatment of pressure sores is to moist wound healing. Before this decade, the aim of most treatments was to keep the sore dry. Heat lamps, fans, and uncovered wounds allowed the sore to dry out. A large black eschar was considered protective and useful for healing as it prevented the loss of fluid and exposure to pathogens. Winter pointed out that exposing the dermis to dehydration prevents healing by destroying epidermal remnants that initiate healing.[40] Under a scab, epidermal regeneration occurred in 18 hours while in a moist environment dermal regeneration occurred in 6 hours. Minimum requirements for healing are a rich supply of oxygen and glucose plus a moist, protein-rich environment into which cells can migrate. An intact blister provides this environment; so does a transparent film dressing. Ointments also provide a moist healing environment.

2. *Old:* Absorb drainage with packing; *New:* Absorb drainage with hydroactive dressings and granules. One problem with transparent film dressings as with blisters is the collection of excessive fluid. Previous treatments involved packing of sores with gauze saturated with bactericidal solution. The bactericidal saturation fluid was toxic to newly forming epithelial cells as well as to unwanted organisms. The removal of the packing also mechanically removed many epithelial cells. Newer methods of treatment involve the use of hydrocolloid dressings and absorbant granules. Excessive moisture is absorbed while a moist environment is retained for rapid proliferation of epithelial cells. One problem inherent in the use of occlusive dressings is the interaction of the dressing with wound fluid, which causes an accumulation of yellow viscous exudate resembling pus. This detritus can be easily removed by irrigation with normal saline to reveal healthy granulation tissue beneath. Hydroactive occlusive dressings promote physiologic debridement. As the necrotic tissue is loosened from healthy tissue, the wound may increase in size and depth. This is expected just as in any debridement; the removal of necrotic tissue does increase the size and depth of the sore. The key to whether the sore is better or worse is the quality of the base of the sore. A red base indicates active angiogenesis and impending epithelialization and closure of the sore. Treatment with occlusive hydroactive dressings should not be terminated in the presence of the yellow exudate nor in the presence of foul odor. This is an expected finding with liquefaction of necrotic tissue. This method of debridement is far superior to mechanical debridement because the skin itself can demarcate healthy and necrotic tissue. In mechanical debridement, healthy tissue is removed as well as necrotic tissue. All sores are contaminated and cultures are not indicated unless there are clinical signs of infection such as cellulitis and fever. The newer hydroactive occlusive dressings generate much less yellow material and odor and are more acceptable aesthetically.

3. *Old:* Irrigate forcefully with bactericidal solutions; *New:* Use gentle irrigation with physiologic solutions. Povidone-iodine 1 per cent, acetic acid 0.25 per cent, hydrogen peroxide 3 per cent, and sodium hypochlorite 0.5 per cent are among the solutions used to irrigate pressure sores. The principle is to use an agent toxic to bacteria in the wounds. Formerly it was gen-

erally accepted that these solutions were effective.[41,42] More recent studies have shown that the strength of the solution toxic to bacteria was also toxic to newly forming cells in the pressure sore.[43-45] Lineaweaver and colleagues also found that wounds irrigated with povidone-iodine were significantly weaker than wounds irrigated with saline or other topical agents or wounds that were not irrigated.[44] For routine cleansing, physiologic saline solutions are recommended with a bulb syringe or large-caliber needle on a syringe. Small-gauge needles or waterpiks deliver the irrigating solution at high pressure and may damage newly forming cells.

4. *Old:* Wet to dry dressings changed frequently; *New:* Occlusive dressings changed infrequently. An age-old method of debridement for pressure sores is the wet-to-dry dressing. Typically a gauze dressing is saturated with bactericidal solution packed in the sore and allowed to dry. During removal of the dressing necrotic tissue displacement causes bleeding in the wound bed, which formerly was considered therapeutic.[46] As of this writing it is recognized that during the removal of the dry dressing newly forming epithelial cells are also removed. Furthermore, changing dressings several times a day is expensive in both material and the nurses' time for the procedure. Newer methods seek to conserve the nurses' time by decreasing the frequency of dressing change. Hydrocolloid dressings can be left in place from five to seven days unless there is leakage of exudate. Even though the hydrocolloid dressing is more expensive initially, the time saved by fewer dressing changes and increased healing time results in savings for the institution. Fellin[47] estimated that the use of occlusive dressings resulted in costs seven times lower than for wet to dry dressings.

5. *Old:* Blunt surgical debridement; *New:* Laser debridement. The aim of debridement is to rid the pressure sore of devitalized tissue. The removal of necrotic tissue leads to proliferation of healthy tissue and eventual re-epithelialization and contraction. Surgical debridement in the operating room is used for deep, extensive pressure sores. To ensure the removal of all dead tissue, debridement extends into healthy tissue and causes bleeding. A new technique that holds promise of generating less bleeding is laser debridement. The laser cauterizes and sterilizes the ulcer so that it is prepared for primary closure or flap closure if necessary. For 200 laser debridements since 1983 at Los Alamitos Medical Center, 85

per cent have shown no signs of recurrence. Usually laser treatment is performed for sores at stage III or IV.[48]

6. *Old:* Extensive skin flaps to close large ulcers; *New:* Skin expanders to provide skin for closure. Surgical procedures to close large pressure sores over the sacrum, ischial tuberosities, or trochanters are not uncommon for spinal cord injured patients. Lee and Thoden noted that myocutaneous rotation flaps, conventional rotation flaps, and primary closure are most often used to cover large pressure sores that do not heal by medical treatment.[49] Sometimes, a temporary closure with a split-thickness skin graft is used to prevent protein loss through exudate and to protect the ulcer.

A new technique described by Fuerry uses expanded skin adjacent to the wound for skin coverage.[50] This technique was used in plastic surgery by Neuman[51] and Radovan[52] and is being used for closure of pressure ulcers. The procedure for skin expanders is to insert a balloon under the skin to be expanded; the balloon is filled once a week with increasing amounts of saline until the skin is of the desired expansion. An incision is then made, the balloon is removed, the skin is stretched over the sore and sutured in place.

SUMMARY

For spinal cord injured patients all improvements in treatment of pressure sores are welcome. What is more welcome is the increased attention to prevention, involvement of the entire health care team, establishment of effective skin care programs, and emphasis on holistic individualized care of each spinal cord injured patient.

REFERENCES

1. Nawoczenski, DA (1987). Pressure sores: Prevention and management. In L. E. Buchanan & D.A. Nawoczenski, Spinal Cord Injury (101–121). Baltimore: Williams & Wilkins.
2. Find/SVP. (1986). The Market for decubitus ulcer treatment products, drugs and devices. New York: Find/SVP.
3. Hunt, TK & Dunphy, JE (1979). Fundamentals of Wound Management. New York: Appleton-Century-Crofts.
4. Falanga, V & Eaglstein, WH (1986). Management of venous ulcers. AFP Practical Therapeutics, 33 (2), 274–286.
5. Knighton, D, Ciresi, K, Fiegel, F, Austin L, & Butler, E (1986). Classification and treatment of chronic nonhealing wounds: successful treatment with au-

tologous platelet-derived wound healing factors. Annals of Surgery, 204, pp. 322–330.

6. Rubin, CF, Dietz, RR, & Abruzzese, RS (1974). Auditing the decubitus ulcer problem. American Journal of Nursing, 74, 1820–1821.

7. Hibbs, P (1988). The economics of pressure ulcer prevention. Decubitus, 1(3), 32–38.

8. Silverman, JJ (1980). Emotional care of the cord-injured and chronically ill patient. In M. B. Constantian (Ed.), Pressure Ulcers: Principles and Techniques of Management (47–66), Boston: Little, Brown and Co.

9. Rubin, M (1988, January). The physiology of bedrest. American Journal of Nursing, 88, 51–56.

10. Lindan, O (1961). Etiology of decubitus ulcers: An experimental study. Archives of Physical Medicine and Rehabilitation 42, 774–783.

11. Kosiak, M (1961). Etiology of decubitus ulcers. Archives of Physical Medicine and Rehabilitation 42, 19–29.

12. Bush, CA (1969). Study of pressure, on pain under ischial tuberosities and thighs during sitting. Archives of Physical Medicine and Rehabilitation 50, 207.

13. Husain, T (1953). An experimental study of some pressure effects on tissues, with reference to the bed-sore problem. Journal of Pathology and Bacteriology 66, 347–358.

14. Sather, MR, Weber, CE, & George, J (1977). Pressure sores and the spinal cord injury patient. Drug Intelligence & Clinical Pharmacy, 11, 154–169.

15. Parish, LC & Witkowski, JA (1987). The decubitus ulcer: Reflections of a decade of concern. International Journal of Dermatology, 26, 639–640.

16. Alterescu, V & Alterescu, K (1988). Etiology and treatment of pressure ulcers. Decubitus, 1 (1), 28–35.

17. Bennett, L & Lee, BY (1988). Vertical shear existence in animal pressure threshold experiments. Decubitus, 1 (1), 18–24.

18. Lowthian, PT (1975). Underpads in the prevention of decubiti. In R. M. Kenedi, J. M. Cowden, & J. T. Scales (Eds.), Bedsore Biomechanics (141–145) Baltimore: University Park Press.

19. Parish, LC, Witkowski, JA, & Crissey, JT (1983). The Decubitus Ulcer. New York: Masson.

20. Flam, E (1987). Optimum skin aeration in pressure sore management. Proceedings 40th Annual Conference on Engineering in Medicine and Biology, Niagra Falls, NY, September 10–13, p. 84.

21. Norton, D, McLaren, R, & Exton-Smith, AN (1962). An investigation of geriatric nursing problems in hospitals. London: National Corporation for the Care of Old People.

22. Natow, AB (1983, July). Nutrition in prevention and treatment of decubitus ulcers. Topics in Clinical Nursing, 5, 39–44.

23. Pollack, SV (1979). Nutritional factors affecting wound healing. Journal of Dermatologic Surgery and Oncology, 5 (8), 615–619.

24. Holmes, R, Macchiano, K, Jhangiani, SS, Agarwal, NR, & Savino, JA (1987, October). Combating pressure sores—nutritionally. American Journal of Nursing, 87, 1301–1303.

26. Kaminski, MV, Pinchcofsky-Devin, G, & Williams, SD (1989) Nutritional management of decubitus ulcers in the elderly. Decubitus, 2(4), 20–30, 1990.

27. Freiman, M, Seifter, E, Connerton, C, & Levenson, SM (1970). Vitamin A deficiency and surgical stress. Surgical Forum, XXI, 81.

28. Abruzzese, RS (1985). Early assessment and prevention of pressure sores. In B.Y. Lee, Chronic Ulcers of the Skin (1–19). New York: McGraw-Hill.

29. Lidowski, H (1988). NAMP: a system for preventing and managing pressure ulcers. Decubitus, 1 (2), 28–37.

30. International Association for Enterostomal Therapy. (1987). Standards of Care: Dermal Wounds: Pressure Sores. Irvine, CA: The Association.

31. Gosnell, DJ (1987). Assessment and evaluation of pressure sores. Nursing Clinics of North America, 22, 399–416.

32. Bergstrom, N, Braden, BJ, Laguzza, A, & Holman, V (1987). The Braden scale for predicting pressure sore risk. Nursing Research, 36, 205–210.

33. Towey, AP & Erland, SM (1988). Validity and reliability of an assessment tool for pressure ulcer risk. Decubitus, 1 (2), 40–48.

34. Constantian, MB & Jackson, HS (1980). Factors affecting pressure ulcer development. In M. B. Constantian (Ed.), Pressure Ulcers: Principles and Techniques of Management (143–148). Boston: Little, Brown and Company.

35. Robinson, CE (1978). Decubitus ulcers in paraplegics: Financial implications. Canadian Journal of Public Health, 69, 199.

36. Guttman, L (1976). The prevention and treatment of pressure sores. In RM Kenedi, J. M. Cowden, & J. T. Scales (eds.), Bedsore Biomechanics (153–159). Baltimore: University Park Press.

36a. Moolten, SE (1977). Bedsores. Hospital Medicine, 83–103.

37. Abruzzese, RS (1982). The effectiveness of an assessment tool in specifying nursing care to prevent decubitus ulcers. PRN: The Adelphi Report, 43–61.

38. Shea, JD Pressure sores: classification and management. Clinical Orthopedics 112, 89–100.

39. Oot-Giromini, B (1986). Treatment standards for pressure sores. Gaymar Industries Conference—Pressure Ulcers: A Team Approach.

40. Winter, GD (1976). Some factors affecting skin and wound healing. In R. M. Kenedi & J. M. Cowden (Eds.), Bedsore Biomechanics (47–54). Baltimore: University Park Press.

41. Gilgore, A (1978). The use of povidone-iodine in the treatment of infected cutaneous ulcers. Current Therapy Research, 23, 843–848.

42. Lee, BY, Trainor, FS, & Thoden, WR (1979, July). Topical application of povidone-iodine in the management of decubitus and stasis ulcers. Journal of the American Geriatrics Society, 27, 302–306.

43. Rodeheaver, G, Bellamy, W, Kody, M, Spatafora, G, Fitton, L, Leyden, K, & Edlich, R (1982). Bactericidal activity and toxicity of iodine-containing solutions in wounds. Archives of Surgery, 117, 181–186.

44. Lineaweaver, W, Howard, R, Soucy, D, McMorris, S, Freeman, J, Crain, C, Roberston, J, & Rumley, T (1985). Topical antimicrobial toxicity. Archives of Surgery, 120, 167–270.

45. Zamora, JL (1986, March). Chemical and microbiologic characteristics and toxicity of povidone-iodine solutions. The American Journal of Surgery, 151, 400–406.

46. Michocki, RJ & Lamy, PR (1976). Care of decubitus ulcers. Journal of the American Geriatric Society 24, 217–224.

47. Fellin, R (1984, February). Managing decubitus ulcers. Nursing Management, 15, 29–30.

48. Ginsburg, SB (1988). Surgical skin grafts and closure

laser therapy. Lecture at The Symposium on Advanced Wound Care, Long Beach, April 12, 1988.

49. Lee, BY & Thoden, WR (1985). Surgical management of pressure sores. In BY Lee, Chronic Ulcers of the Skin (147–170). New York: McGraw-Hill.

50. Fuerry, J (1986). Surgical interventions for pressure ulcers: Skin expanders. Lecture at Pressure Ulcers: A Team Approach Conference, Buffalo, August 15, 1986.

51. Neuman, CG (1957). The expansion of an area of skin by progressive distention of a subcutaneous balloon: Use of the method for securing skin for subtotal reconstruction of the ear. Plastic and Reconstructive Surgery 19:124–130, 1957.

52. Radovan, C (1984). Tissue expansion in soft-tissue reconstruction. Plastic and Reconstruction Surgery, 74, 482–492.

18 Plastic Surgery for Pressure Sores

BOK Y. LEE, M.D.

Pressure sores are a common occurrence and continue to be a vexing problem. Such lesions not only affect the patient but also the community as a whole and the health care team. The patient's overall rehabilitation program is delayed, his overall health is jeopardized, and he is separated from his family; the community bears the direct and indirect costs of treatment; and the health care team must weather the implications of neglect, mismanagement, and poor nursing care.[1] Although pressure sores may be seen in any patient immobilized for a prolonged period of time, the spinal cord injured patient is particularly at risk.

Pressure sores are no less problematic today than they have been in the past. They have been observed in Egyptian mummies,[2] and Fabricius attributed the formation of pressure sores to a "pneuma" that was a consequence of severed nerves and loss of blood supply.[3] Brown-Sequard reported in 1852 that pressure and moisture were important factors in the development of pressure sores, and in 1873 Paget defined pressure sores, which he termed "bedsores," as the "sloughing and mortification or death of a part produced by pressure."[3] In 1879, Charcot stated his view of the cause of what today are called pressure or pressure ulcers and expressed the idea of pressure sores being "natural" and an "inevitable" complication seen in spinal cord injured patients with no possibility of treatment.[3] He believed that an injury to a nerve released a neutrotrophic factor that led to tissue necrosis. This theory was the forerunner of an era of "therapeutic nihilism."[3] This therapeutic nihilism was present as late as 1940, as evidenced by Munro's suggestion that a disturbance of the autonomic nervous system altered the peripheral reflexes of the skin and predisposed the patient to ulceration.[3] Munro was opposed to any form of

surgical intervention because he believed that progressive ulceration was a natural consequence of the condition.[3] Although disturbance of the autonomic nervous system does occur in some spinal cord injured patients, the direct role of such disturbances in the development of pressure sores has not been substantiated.[2]

These theories of Charcot and Munro overshadowed such enlightened observations[3] as that of Van Gehuchter, who reported that the wasting of muscle and atony were more important causes than loss of sensation; Kuster's work on bacterial infection of acute sores; Marie and Baussing's work showing that any debilitated patient could develop bedsores and that such lesions were indeed treatable; and the work of Ascher on the importance of secondary infection of damaged tissue in the extension of the pressure sore.[3]

It was not until World War II that reports of successful surgical treatment of pressure sores were seen. The history of the surgical management of pressure sores can be said to have begun in 1938 with Davis's idea for use of pedicle flaps in the treatment of pressure sores.[4] Scoville in 1944[3] and Lamon and Alexander in 1945[5] reported the first successful excision of a sacral ulcer and primary closure in patients receiving parenteral administration of penicillin. In 1945, good results in patients with sacral ulcers treated by rotation flaps were reported by White et al.[6] In 1947, Kostrubola and Greeley[7] advised the removal of bony prominences beneath the ulcer and the use of muscle flaps for padding. Although great strides have been made in the treatment of pressure sores from the days of therapeutic nihilism and the belief that they were a natural consequence in incapacitated patients, the best mode of treatment continues to be prevention.

223

COMPLICATIONS OF SPINAL CORD INJURY

In addition to the development of pressure sores, spinal cord injured patients are at risk for life-threatening complications that can involve a number of organ systems.

A frequent complication of spinal cord injury is *urinary tract* problems.[3] The use of indwelling catheters, excessive calcium mobilization due to the lack of stress on bone, and bacilluria lead to calcification in the urinary tract. This can be managed by a low calcium diet and the use of urine-acidifying agents, and antiseptics that can increase the solubility of calcium and keep the urine free of bacteria; a high fluid intake helps to produce an adequate flow of urine, and some patients can train themselves not to require the use of a catheter.

The generalized inactivity of the *gastrointestinal tract* and the patient being bedridden frequently lead to constipation.[3] A high residue diet and the use of stool softeners are helpful. Patients can usually regulate themselves for evacuation every 48 hours with the use of a suppository; enemas should be used if impaction develops. Also relating to the gastrointestinal tract, a negative nitrogen balance can result in atrophy of the muscles.

In about 25 per cent of spinal cord injuries, significant *heterotrophic ossification* can occur, the most common locations being the flexor muscles of the elbows, the knees, and the hips. The occurrence of heterotrophic ossification, which can lead to significant loss of function and the consequent decalcification and general demineralization of bone, places the spinal cord injured patient at high risk for fractures, particularly of the long bones of the extremities, which are delayed in healing. The maintenance of function in the presence of heterotrophic ossification is probably best done through passive motion.[8]

Contracture can develop rapidly if preventive measures are not begun.[3] Spinal cord injured patients require frequent and regular full range-of-motion exercise.

Psychologic problems in the form of mental depression, self-pity, lack of motivation, and suicidal tendencies are a common occurrence. Particularly problematic is a lack of motivation due to depression that can lead to a failure of the rehabilitation program, chronicity of pressure sores, sepsis, and even death.

The level of the injury to the spinal cord determines the patient's *sexual capibilities.*[9,10] Women with spinal cord injuries, in general, remain fertile and capable of childbearing. Upper motor neuron lesions in men generally result in a potent but sterile patient, while lower motor neuron lesions generally result in an impotent but fertile patient.

Thromboembolism is a common problem due to immobility leading to venous stasis, a causative factor in the formation of venous thrombosis. This topic is discussed in detail elsewhere in this volume.

PATHOPHYSIOLOGY

Pressure sores develop as a result of an active metabolic and inflammatory process that begins when sufficient pressure is applied to the skin to overcome the normal capillary pressure of 32 mm Hg at the arterial end.[11] This results in tissue anoxia and cellular death.[12-14] The removal of pressure can reverse the process. Dinsdale[15] reported that a constant pressure of 70 mm Hg for two hours caused irreversible damage to the tissues, but pressure up to 240 mm Hg could be sustained if the pressure was relieved intermittently. Kosiak[13,14] also showed that the application of 70 mm Hg pressure for two hours produced pressure sores, but that if the pressure was relieved every five minutes, tissue effects were minimal. The discomfort associated with a prolonged application of pressure would cause the normal person to move in order to relieve the pressure. Obviously, the spinal cord injured patient is unaware of the associated discomfort of prolonged pressure application and also is unable to move to relieve the pressure.

Although the first clinical sign of impending necrosis is inflammation, it is very likely that necrosis of the subcutaneous tissue and fat and the underlying muscle has already occurred, and over a larger area than apparent from the area of skin loss.[16] Also, muscle is more susceptible than skin to pressure injury.[17] Indeed, in normal human weight-bearing positions over bony prominences, muscle is seldom seen to be interposed between bone and skin.[18] The distribution of pressure points in humans lying prone and supine and in the seated position has been documented (Figs. 18–1 and 18–2).[19] The regions of highest pressure in the supine position include the sacrum, buttocks, heel, and occiput (40 to 60 mm Hg of pressure). The knees and chest receive the most pressure in a prone position (approximately 50 mm Hg). In the seated position, a hard surface provides for less distribution of pressure and thus produces

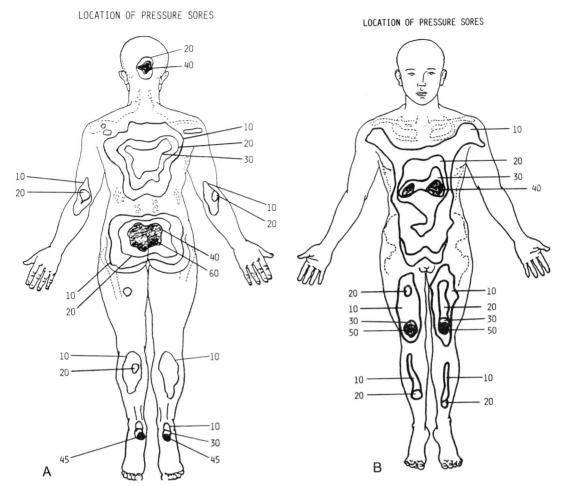

Figure 18–1. *A*, The regions of highest pressure for the supine patient. *B*, The regions of highest pressure for the prone patient.

higher pressures. Seated, pressures of 40 to 60 mm Hg are seen at the ischial tuberosities and the thighs when the feet are dangling free; pressures at the ischial tuberosities rise to about 100 mm Hg when the feet are supported.

Normal capillary hydrostatic pressures vary from 15 to 30 mm Hg and, in areas over bony prominences, from 40 to 75 mm Hg.[11] The pressure is transmitted from the skin to the underlying bone and compresses all the underly-

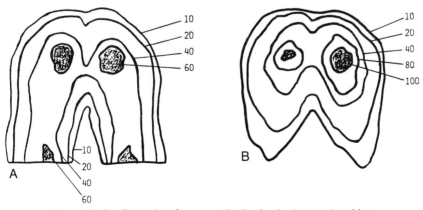

Figure 18–2. Examples of pressure distribution in the seated position.

ing tissue; the greatest pressure is over the bone and gradually decreases towards the surface. Thus, because of the greater pressure over the bony prominence and the greater susceptibility of muscle to pressure injury, the greatest extent of necrosis is at the bony interface and not at the surface. It has been shown that relieving pressure for as short a period of time as five minutes allows tissues to withstand greater pressures.[13,14] Husain[12] has confirmed the relationship between intensity of pressure and duration of application: low pressures for long periods produce more damage than high pressures for short periods.

Shear pressure is also an important contributing factor.[20,21] Dinsdale[15] concluded that friction was additive to pressure in producing ulceration of the skin. He showed that shear did not stretch and compress muscle-perforating vessels to lead to ischemia but that it contributed to skin ulceration by a direct application of mechanical forces to the epidermis.[15] Shear pressure is manifested whenever the patient is pulled up in the bed or when the head of the bed is elevated.

Other factors contributing to the formation of pressure sores include heat in the form of fever that increases the demand for oxygen, which may already be compromised by compression; moisture in the form of sweat, urine, and feces that reduces the skin's resistance and predisposes it to maceration; and a negative nitrogen balance, hypoproteinemia, anemia, and weight loss that predispose to infection of the pressure sore.[22]

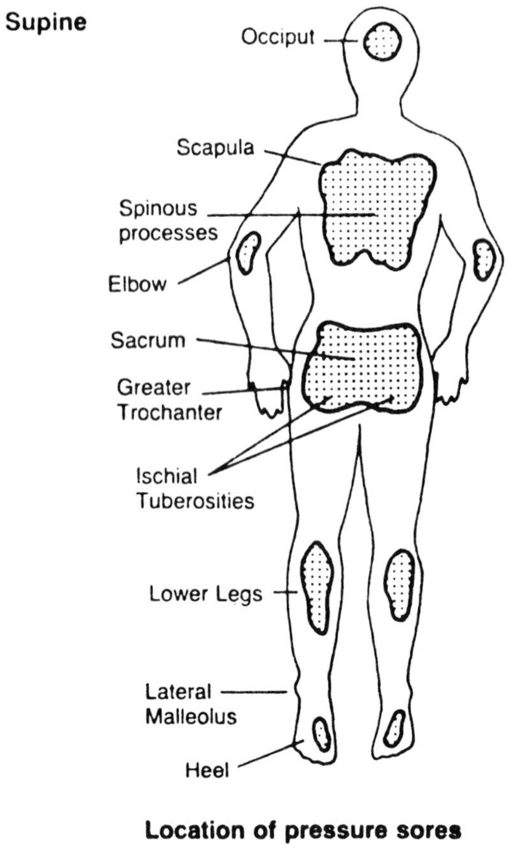

INCIDENCE AND SITES OF FORMATION

The incidence of pressure sore formation is increasing as the life span of the spinal cord injured patient is prolonged with improved medical care and antibiotics. This longer life span increases the patient's at-risk time for pressure sore development. Prior to 1940, spinal cord injury was associated with a 61 per cent mortality rate within the first two months of injury and 81 per cent within two years of injury; after World War II, the mortality rate decreased to 3.8 per cent and 7.8 per cent, respectively.[23] An increase in the incidence of ischial ulceration is evidence of the patient being moved from a bed-ridden position to movement in a wheelchair.[3]

Most pressure sores occur in the lower part of the body (96 per cent), followed by the hip

Supine

Location of pressure sores

Figure 18–3. Areas at risk for development of pressure sores.

and buttocks (67 per cent) and the lower limbs (29 per cent)[24]; however, any part of the body is at risk (Fig. 18–3). Some areas are easier to protect. For example, heel pads can prevent ulceration of the foot, and a patient in the prone position also limits the areas at risk to ones that are easy to care for: anterosuperior iliac spine, knees, and elbows.[3]

In spinal cord injured patients, the incidence of pressures at the ischial tuberosity has been shown to range from 5 per cent to 8 per cent annually[2] with 25 per cent to 85 per cent having an ulcer at some time.[25] From 3 per cent to 4.5 per cent of spinal cord injured patients develop sores while hospitalized,[24,26] and from 7 per cent to 8 per cent of deaths in paraplegics are due to pressure sores.[15]

PREVENTION

The key to prevention of pressure sores is patient and physician awareness of developing signs and symptoms. A clinically useful outline

TABLE 18–1. Assessment of Stage of Pressure Sore Development[27]

Hyperemia	Stage I	Seen within 30 minutes of application of pressure as a redness of the skin that disappears within one hour after removal of pressure
Ischemia	Stage II	Observed with continuous pressure of 2 to 6 hours' duration; redness of ischemia requires 36 or more hours to disappear after removal of pressure
Necrosis	Stage III	Characterized clinically by a blueness of the skin or a hard lump after more than 6 hours of pressure; does not disappear after pressure removal
Ulceration	Stage IV	Observed within 2 weeks as ulceration and infection; may progress to involve bony prominences

TABLE 18–2. Grading of Pressure Sore Development from the National Spinal Cord Injury Data Collection Center[28]

Grade I	Pressure sore limited to superficial epidermal and dermal layers
Grade II	Pressure sore extends into adipose tissue
Grade III	Pressure sore involves all superficial structures as well as underlying muscle
Grade IV	Pressure sore has destroyed all soft tissues down to and including bone and/or joint structure

for assessing the stages of development and the appropriate care is presented in Table 18–1.[27] Pressure sores can also be graded using the system from the National Spinal Cord Injury Data Collection Center (Table 18–2).[28]

Basic skin care in spinal cord injured patients has been reviewed by Ungar[29] and includes elimination of particulate matter from the bed, reduction of excess moisture, alternation of position, and limitation of skin soilage through the combination of good nursing care and an indwelling catheter or even urinary or fecal diversion procedures, if necessary.[2]

Proper positioning of the patient is essential for uniform pressure distribution and relieves

spasticity.[30] Additionally, numerous devices for weight distribution have been developed including pads for chairs and beds and specifically designed beds. Houle[31] has found, however, that such padding for seats and beds does not reduce ischial pressure below capillary pressure and is therefore not a substitute for alternating pressure. A number of beds have been developed that reduce pressure to 15 to 30 mm Hg. They include air-fluidized beds, mud beds, and low–air loss beds (Figs. 18–4 and 18–5). If used properly, these beds can maintain pressure below capillary arterial pressure.[2] Other methods include the Stryker frame, circle electric bed, ripple mattresses, and rocking beds, all based on Kosiak's theory that tissue tolerates higher levels of pressure if there are intermittent periods of relief.[13,14]

SURGICAL MANAGEMENT

The surgical management of pressure sores is difficult. The traditional approaches of conven-

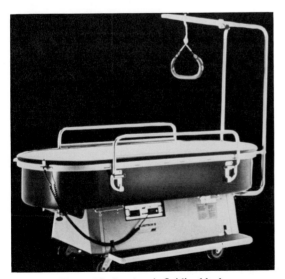

Figure 18–4. An air-fluidized bed.

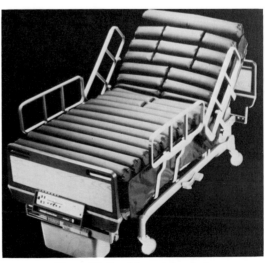

Figure 18–5. A low–air loss bed.

228

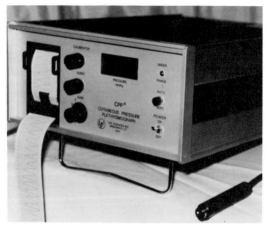

Figure 18–6. The cutaneous pressure plethysmograph.

Effect of Pressure on Skin Blood Flow

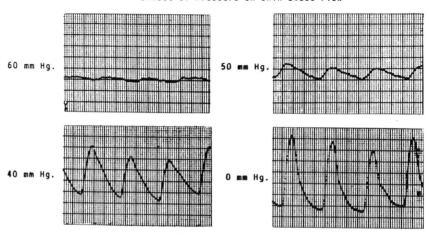

60 mm Hg.   50 mm Hg.

40 mm Hg.   0 mm Hg.

Figure 18–7. Effect of pressure on skin blood flow.

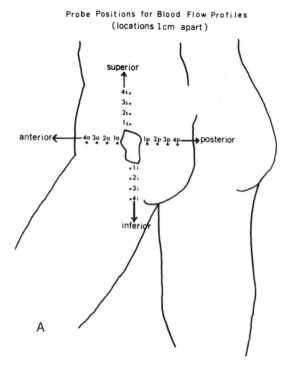

Probe Positions for Blood Flow Profiles
(locations 1cm apart)

A

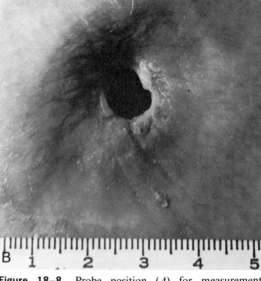

Figure 18–8. Probe position (*A*) for measurement around an ulcer (*B*).

tional rotation flap and primary closure yield less than optimal results. In a series of 374 surgically managed pressure sores reported by Conway and Griffith,[32] multiple procedures were required to achieve successful healing in 148 ulcers.

A number of techniques are available to the surgeon managing a patient with pressure sores; use of the appropriate technique for each patient is crucial. Much morbidity can be avoided through the use of a technique for assessing the healing potential of pressure sores. The cutaneous pressure plethysmograph (Fig. 18–6) is a vascular diagnostic instrument that senses the flow of blood in the skin to various

skin-bearing pressures using a hand-held probe. With the application of incremental pressures, the blood flow waveform is gradually reduced and obliterated at a critical pressure. The technician gradually reduces the pressure until the waveform reappears (Fig. 18–7). The probe can be applied to any skin surface area (Fig. 18–8) and provide a systematic quantitative analysis of cutaneous pressure (Fig. 18–9).

Surgical techniques may be inappropriate for some patients. For example, split-thickness skin grafts are not for definitive treatment but are of value in patients unable to undergo immediate flap repair. Excision and closure are only functional in temporarily closing the skin

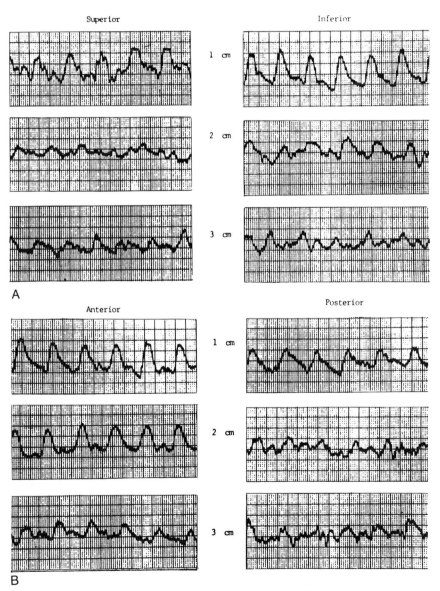

Figure 18–9. *A* and *B,* Systematic quantitative analysis at selected measurement sites.

defect, because increased tension at the suture line will often lead to a recurrence of the lesion. These flaps require a lengthy procedure with numerous stages. Perhaps the best approach is the use of a myocutaneous flap.

The myocutaneous rotation flap is a single unit of skin and underlying muscle that is transferred to cover a defect. The use of a myocutaneous rotation flap is advantageous because it brings a new blood supply to an avascular area while providing bulk for filling defects or covering bone grafts and also it supplies a mass of tissue to cushion a pressure-bearing area.

We have recently reviewed our experience with a total of 142 surgical repairs of pressure sores in 70 patients.[33] The ischium was most frequently involved (47 per cent), followed by the sacrum (27 per cent), trochanter (23 per cent), and calcaneus, hips, ribs, thorax, and thigh (each 1 per cent). Short-term success (i.e., no need for additional surgery during the first posterior month) was similar for all procedures; long-term success was greatest for the myocutaneous rotation flap.

SUMMARY

Pressure sores remain a difficult problem. Pressure shear forces, friction, and moisture all contribute to the formation of a pressure sore. Operative management is difficult because no one procedure is appropriate for all patients. The use of the cutaneous pressure photoplethysmograph is of value in noninvasive assessment of the healing potential of a pressure sore and in assisting the surgeon in proper patient selection. The myocutanous rotation flap is advantageous in providing a healthy vascular supply and cushioning over the pressure-bearing area.

REFERENCES

1. Bereck K: Treatment of decubitus ulcers. Nurs Clin North Am 10:171, 1975.
2. Snively SL, Tebbetts JB: Pressure sores (overview). Selected Readings in Plastic Surgery 3:1, 1986.
3. Vasconez LO, Schneider WJ, Jurkiewicz MJ: Pressure sores. Curr Probl Surg 14:1, 1977.
4. Davis JS: Operative treatment of scars following bedsores. Surgery 3:1, 1938.
5. Lamon JC, Alexander E: Secondary closure of decubitus ulcers with the aid of penicillin. JAMA 127:396, 1945.
6. White J, Hudson AH, Kenward H: Treatment of bedsores by total excision with plastic closure. Navy Medical Bulletin 45:454, 1945.
7. Kostrubola, JC, Greeley PW: The problem of decubitus ulcers in paraplegics. Plast Reconstr Surg 2:403, 1947.
8. Hassard GH: Heterotrophic bone formation about the hip and unilateral decubitus ulcers in spinal cord injury. Arch Phys Med Rehabil 56:355, 1975.
9. Talbot H: Sexual function in paraplegia. J Urol 73:91, 1955.
10. Zeitlin A, Cottrell T, Lloyd F: Sexology of the paraplegic male. Fertil Steril 8:337, 1957.
11. Landis E: Studies of capillary blood pressure in human skin. Heart 15:209, 1930.
12. Husain T: An experimental study of some pressure effects on tissues with reference to the bedsore problem. J Pathol Bacteriol 66:347, 1953.
13. Kosiak M: Etiology and pathology of decubitus ulcers. Arch Phys Med 40:62, 1959.
14. Kosiak M: Etiology of decubitus ulcers. Arch Phys Med 42:19, 1961.
15. Dinsdale SM: Decubitus ulcers: Role of pressure and friction in causation. Arch Phys Med Rehabil 55:147, 1974.
16. Shea JD: Pressure sores. Clin Orthop 112:89, 1975.
17. Keane FX: The function of the rump in relation to sitting and the Keane reciprocating wheelchair seat. Paraplegia 16:390, 1978–1979.
18. Daniel RK: Muscle coverage of pressure points: The role of myocutaneous flaps. Ann Plast Surg 8:446, 1982.
19. Lindan O, Greenway RM, Piazza JM: Pressure distribution on the surface of the human body: Evaluation in lying and sitting positions using a "bed of springs and nails." Arch Phys Med Rehabil 46:378, 1965.
20. Reichel S: Shearing force as a factor in decubitus ulcers in paraplegics. JAMA 166:762, 1958.
21. Bennett L, Kavner D, Lee BY, Trainor FS: Shear versus pressure as causative factors in skin blood flow occlusion. Arch Phys Med Rehabil 60:307, 1979.
22. Mulholland JH, Tui C, Wright AM, et al: Protein metabolism and bedsores. Ann Surg 118:1015, 1943.
23. Taylor RG: Spinal cord injury: Its many complications. Am Fam Physician 8:138, 1973.
24. Petersen NC, Bittmann S: The epidemiology of pressure sores. Scand J Plast Reconstr Surg 5:62, 1971.
25. El-Toraen I, Chung B: The management of pressure sores. Dermatol Surg Oncol 3:507, 1977.
26. Manley MT: Incidence, contributing factors, and cost of pressure sores. S Afr Med J 53:217, 1978.
27. Edberg EL, Cerny K, Stauffer ES: Prevention and treatment of pressure sores. Phys Ther 53:246, 1973.
28. Staas WE, LaMantia JG: Decubitus ulcers and rehabilitation medicine. Int J Dermatol 21:437, 1982.
29. Ungar GH: The care of the skin in paraplegics. Practitioner 206:507, 1971.
30. Reuler JB, Cooney TG: The pressure sore: Pathophysiology and principles of management. Ann Intern Med 94:661, 1981.
31. Houle RJ: Evaluation of seat devices designed to prevent ischemic ulcers in paraplegic patients. Arch Phys Med Rehabil 50:587, 1969.
32. Conway H, Griffith BH: Plastic surgery for closure of decubitus ulcers in patients with paraplegia. Am J Surg 91:9, 1956.
33. Lee BY, Shaw WW, Madden JL, et al: Surgical management of pressure sores. Contemporary Orthopaedics 5:49, 1982.

19 Reconstructive Surgery for the Upper Limb and Hand in Traumatic Tetraplegia

DOUGLAS W. LAMB, M.B., Ch.B., F.R.C.S.E.

Complete injury of the spinal cord in the cervical area usually occurs in sporting injuries or vehicular accidents. The patients are commonly young men. As a result of the improvements in initial management most will survive, have a life expectancy of 20 to 30 years, and be confined permanently to a wheelchair. Most injuries affect the lower cervical spine, and there will be impairment of the function of the upper limbs to some extent. Zancolli found that three-quarters of the patients in his series had survival of the sixth cervical neural segment.[1] In a group of 300 patients with cervical cord damage (studied by the author) two-thirds also came into this category, when the patient has good shoulder abduction and elbow flexion and the main functional deficits are inability to extend the elbow and loss of active flexion and extension of thumb and fingers and all intrinsic muscle activity.

Patients who have cord damage at a higher level can rarely be helped by reconstructive surgery. If they survive they will be dependent for any functional benefit on aids and gadgets, usually of a sophisticated type. Their management, while important, is beyond the scope of this chapter.

The commonest cause of severe bilateral upper limb paralysis in the western world is cervical cord injury; its frequency in the rest of the world is only exceeded by leprosy. As a result of such injury a significantly large group of young people is left with impaired ability for activities of daily living. It is incumbent upon those responsible for their care that every effort be made, through reconstructive surgery to the upper limb and hand, to improve control of the limb and to provide grasp and release of the hand.

Although there have been many communications in the literature over the past 20 years on the potential benefits of judiciously chosen and applied reconstructive surgery,[1-11] a considerable lack of knowledge remains about its possible benefits in many spinal injury units. There have now been three International Conferences on the surgical management of the upper limb in tetraplegia.[12,13] The Third Conference has recently been completed in Gothenberg, and the proceedings should be published in the near future.

Patients who are tetraplegics are aware of the benefits which are obtainable from reconstructive surgery. They meet one another in spinal injury units and sporting and social occasions and discuss the benefits they have obtained. It has been the author's experience that they make their way to units that can provide this service and are often prepared to travel long distances. Moberg[4] has reported the findings of Hansen and Franklin[14] of their survey of a group of young tetraplegics. Three out of four considered the loss of upper limb function to be their main disability.

EARLY MANAGEMENT OF THE UPPER LIMBS [6,9,7,15,16]

The importance of preventing joint contractures cannot be overemphasized. Adduction contractures of the shoulder, flexion contractures of the elbow, extension contractures of the metacarpophalangeal joints, and contractures of the thumb web are seen not infrequently. In order to allow the maximum possible recovery of upper limb function, either as a result of spontaneous root escape or reconstructive surgery, it is essential that these contractures be prevented. All paralyzed joints should be positioned carefully and put through a regular gentle passive range of movement several times daily. Orthoses are not usually required but can be kept in reserve if there is any sign of contracture development.

An early accurate assessment of remaining muscle power in the upper limbs must be made. A muscle chart evaluation should be repeated at not less than monthly intervals over the first six months following injury. So long as there is recovery of muscle power in any muscle groups, reconstructive surgery should not be contemplated. However, if at the end of six to nine months the muscle chart remains constant from the initial assessment, consideration should be given to reconstructive surgery. In tetraplegia the main indications for reconstructive surgery by tendon transfer or a combination of transfer and tenodesis are to restore elbow extension, thumb and finger movements, and a key type of pinch of the thumb against the side of the index finger.

Tenodesis and arthrodesis by themselves are rarely of value in the management of the paralytic hand in tetraplegia. Such surgical procedures as described in the past[17–19] are not now indicated. The emphasis in surgical reconstruction is on the use of properly selected and carefully applied tendon transfers.

Although most tetraplegic patients are candidates for some form of reconstruction, their remaining muscle power is so crucial that any surgical procedure must not be associated with loss of function. Careful assessment of activities of daily living is necessary, and the strength of grasp, pinch or key grasp should be evaluated. While the remaining muscle power and the possibilities of tendon transfers that it affords are prime considerations, there are other factors that affect patient selection for operation.

SPASTICITY. Upper limb spasticity is uncommon in the complete cervical injury unless complicated by pressure sores or urinary infection. Tendon transfers should be avoided in the presence of considerable spasticity.

PAINFUL PARESTHESIAS. The patient who has painful paresthesias is unlikely to make use of any function provided by tendon transfer; however, it is rare for this to be a problem.

IMPAIRED SENSATION. Moberg has emphasized the importance of the sensory side as assessed by two-point discrimination in relationship to reconstructive surgery and improvement in function.[4] This must be carried out with great care by an experienced examiner using gentle pressure of the two points of a paper clip. He considers that there is a strong association between two-point discrimination on the pads of fingers and the position sense at the finger joints and that the test is a measure of proprioception.[3] A threshhold of less than 10 ml on the pad gives useful proprioception. Results of this test should be recorded in the tetraplegic, particularly on the thumb and the index and long fingers. In practice, all patients who are likely to benefit from tendon transfers will have sensation in the thumb and index finger sufficient to make the hand useful.

FIXED CONTRACTURES. Flexion contractures of the elbow occur very readily in those who have no active elbow extension. Full passive extension of the elbow must be restored before tendon transfer can be successful. This may be achieved by serial stretching with plaster or thermoplastic splints. If this fails to correct the contracture, lengthening of the biceps tendon and possibly of the brachialis tendon and anterior capsulotomy of the elbow can be carried out to restore full passive correction. Restoration of active elbow extension by tendon transfer can then be successful. If the biceps is active in the absence of function of the pronator and supinator muscles, then not only fixed flexion contracture of the elbow but also a supinated contracture may develop.[20,21] Ejeskar[22] considers that the presence of a fixed flexion/supination contracture at the elbow is a good indication for a biceps to triceps transfer to restore active elbow extension (see later).

Contractures of the wrist (usually dorsiflexion due to the unopposed activity of the radiocarpal extensors), of the finger joints, and of the thumb can occur easily and must be avoided by careful attention to positioning, gentle passive stretching, and suitable splinting as required.

The presence of fixed contractures render useful reconstructive procedures quite impossible.

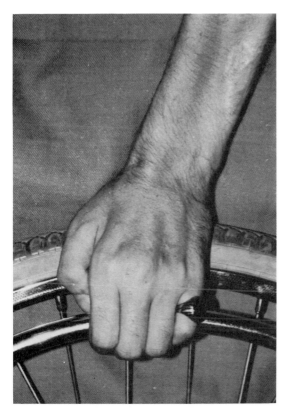

Figure 19–1. The importance of the positioning of the thumb for gripping the rim of the wheelchair.

CONSIDERATION OF METHODS OF FUNC-
TIONAL ACTIVITY. The method of transfer of
patient from bed to wheelchair and back and
the way in which the patient places the hand
for propulsion of the wheelchair and for various attempted self-care activities must be assessed carefully by the surgeon. Any operative
treatment must not change the pattern of these
to such an extent that the patient is unable to
manage. This is particularly important when
any surgical procedure is contemplated that
would make it difficult to place the thumb
around the rim of the wheelchair (Fig. 19–1) or
prevents the hand from being positioned in a
flattened way for transfer.

TIME FROM INJURY. Experience has shown
that this is a most significant factor to be taken
into account. It is of course important not to
carry out any tendon transfers until no further
spontaneous recovery is taking place. On the
other hand, one does not want to wait so long
after injury that the patient has returned home
from the hospital environment and does not
wish to go back for further treatment. Of even
greater significance is the situation of those patients, several years after injury, who have

adapted to methods of doing things to the best
of their ability but who, having seen patients
with successful improvement following operation, wish to consider operation themselves.
The benefits of tendon transfer seem to be
much less satisfactory in these circumstances,
as these patients have developed numerous
tricks and substitutions that it is unwise to
alter.

Moberg has warned about the precautions
necessary in this field of surgery which is very
specialized; much experience, difficult to obtain, is required in order to make correct decisions.[4,23] Because of the limited muscle resources available to the patient, mistakes can
be detrimental. Patients know each other and
often meet regularly; any failure following surgery may prevent others from accepting the opportunity of a better quality of life. While the
surgeon is able to tell the patient what can be
done, the decision to accept operation must be
that of the patient and will be influenced by the
results obtained in those around him.

For the surgeon it is necessary to distinguish
between science and art. Skill in the first can be
obtained by reading and attending meetings,
but the art of applying the right procedure to
the right patient at the right time can be gained
only be experience. An operation on the occas-
sional patient is not enough to gain this experience.

AIMS OF SURGERY

There are two main aims of the surgeon in
the tetraplegic which can be gained by tendon
transfers: restoration of elbow extension and
restoration of grasp.

Restoration of Elbow Extension

Loss of elbow extension is a very significant
functional loss. The patient is unable to use the
arms to stabilize the body when sitting or transferring from bed to chair. The arm cannot be
sustained overhead in the extended position
and the elbow will buckle as soon as it is elevated. This makes it difficult to reach out for
objects or to reach up to a shelf or to a hook
for clothes. Even if grasp could be provided
subsequently for the patient, it would not be
possible to take advantage of this in reaching
up to a trapeze for transfer in bed. Moberg was
the first to realize the significance of this to the
patient.[24] He has stressed that even if nothing
can be done to improve hand function, resto-

ration of active elbow extension to the patient is valuable and becomes even more valuable if hand function can be improved as well. The operation that Moberg has devised is to take the posterior third of the deltoid muscle as the motor and elongate this by free tendon grafts into the triceps near the olecranon.[4,24,25]

Surgical Procedure [2,4,24,26]

With the patient lying on the side, an incision is made along the posterior border of the deltoid muscle to its insertion. The flaps are raised along the superficial surface of the muscle enclosed by its sheath of fascia. The fascia is divided and the muscle exposed to its insertion. Because there is no clear defining line between posterior and middle thirds this must be judged by the surgeon and separated in the line of the muscle fibers. The muscle is divided to its tendinous insertion into the humerus. It is important to take a strip of the insertion with adjacent periosteum to provide good fixation for the tendon grafts. The muscle is separated proximally until the neurovascular bundle can be seen and felt. By subperiosteal dissection and freeing of the posterior deltoid far proximally, five centimeters of active gliding of the tendon will be produced.[27] A separate L-shaped incision is made over the posterior triceps near its insertion. The skin flap and deep fascia are elevated off the surface of the triceps to expose the tendon. Free tendon material is readily available from the foot. The extensor digitorum longus is harvested through a series of transverse incisions from the metatarsophalangeal joints up to the musculotendinous junction. Freehafer has described use of the tibialis anterior.[28] The plantaris tendon can be removed with a Brand stripper and used in addition. The tendons used by Moberg and Freehafer are free grafts and require a new blood supply. This is the main reason for the extensive period of postoperative immobilization with the elbow fully extended as recommended by Moberg.

Castro-Sierra and Lopez-Pieta advised a new technique to try and reduce the period of immobilization.[29] At the common level of cervical injury which leads to paralysis of elbow extension, the patient usually has survival of the radiocarpal extensor muscles to dorsiflex the wrist, but the extensor carpi ulnaris is paralyzed. Since 1987 I have used the tendon of the paralysed extensor carpi ulnaris to weave between the deltoid and triceps. The musculotendinous unit is freed through a series of short

transverse incisions and left attached at its extensor origin. While initially the tendon was woven through the lower triceps and up to the deltoid, a recent successful modification is to take the tendon through the olecranon to get firm fixation at that point and then to the deltoid. The advantage of this procedure, in addition to getting firm fixation at the lower end, is that there is some blood supply coming into the muscle through its origin. Because of this it has been our practice to start mobilizing the elbow three weeks after operation.

Any of these tendons are usually long enough to stretch from the tendon insertion of the deltoid to the triceps and be doubled back. They are threaded through the deltoid tendon insertion and related periosteum and sutured firmly. A tunnel is made from proximal to distal using the tendon passer, and the tendons are pulled through to the distal wound. Each tendon is then passed through a series of vertical incisions in the aponeurosis over the lower triceps and fixed firmly by suture. With the tunnel passer, the tendons are then returned and sutured under maximum tension to the posterior third of deltoid with the elbow in full extension and the shoulder adducted. It has been my experience that the operative detail should be adhered to strictly for best results. The arm is held to the side of the body postoperatively by a plaster shell over the shoulder and down the back of the upper limb with the elbow in full extension. Moberg has advised that this position should be maintained for six weeks postoperatively and then gradual mobilization of the elbow introduced under strict physiotherapy supervision.[4,24] He recommends that 15 degrees of flexion should be allowed each week until a right angle of flexion has been regained. The arm is maintained in the acquired degree of flexion by a posterior plaster slab and immobilized again with the elbow fully extended at night. Despite the prolonged postoperative period, all our patients have returned for operation on the other side. All patients have regained active flexion of the elbow enabling them to reach mouth and face, and have been able to extend the elbow against gravity. In most patients full elbow extension while holding a 4 lb weight is achieved (Fig. 19–2). When a patient is lightly built, the strength of the elbows following operation is such that the arms can be readily used to assist movement in bed and transfer to a wheelchair.

Moberg reports 75 deltoid to triceps transfers.[23] In one no elbow extension was obtained and in two others very limited function was ob-

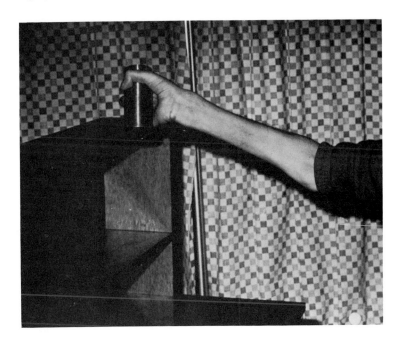

Figure 19–2. After deltoid to triceps transfer, the elbow can be extended fully and a 9 lb weight lifted up to a shelf.

tained. One patient had impaired deltoid function following operation. In my series all patients asked for surgery on second side, and on a follow-up review, not less than a year after the second operation, all patients stated that they had considerable benefit from the ability to elevate the arm overhead, to put objects onto a shelf or a hook, and to stretch and reach for objects on a table.[30] Patients should be encouraged to make full use of elbow extension and to practice regularly at maintaining the range of movement, otherwise the transfer may stretch and become weakened. A three-month period of restoring movement following operation is considerable, and many patients have already spent up to a year in the hospital after their injury. At this stage they are often ready to go home and are reluctant to come back for a period of several months. When the strength of the elbow extension is thought to be inadequate clinically or after an initial good result may have stretched out and decreased in power, a revision technique described by Moberg can be used.[13] A 4 mm thickness slice of the olecranon is raised off the posterior part, displaced distally by 2 to 2.5 cm, and fixed in its new position with a screw.

Zancolli uses the biceps to triceps transfer if the supinator is working and reports good results[31]; however, these do not seem to have been replicated by others. Ejeskar, in a small group of patients in whom the biceps has been transferred, has found the results disappointing. Nearly half of these patients do not have active elbow extension.[21,22] However, he believes that the operation is indicated, particularly in the patient with a supinated elbow contracture. The results do not appear to be as reliable as after deltoid to triceps transfer.

Bilateral loss of active elbow extension is quite disabling and its effects have been underestimated. Restoration of elbow extension (Fig. 19–2) gives the ability to stretch out the arm against gravity and increases the functional range available to the hand.[24–26,30]

Restoration of Grasp [8,7,23,24,30,32,33]

Many operations have been described. It is better to provide a simple grip than a complicated one that is weaker. The aim is to provide grasp to each hand so that both hands can be used independently; it is sometimes possible to provide a different pattern of grasp for each hand. An early procedure consisted of tenodesis of the long flexors into the lower radius.[18,19] This simply provides a fixed hook grip. It is far inferior to the function provided by good tendon transfers and is not indicated. Most attempts to provide grasp in the hand of the tetraplegic patient have utilized tendon transfers. However, the surgeon is limited by the number of active tendons that are available. This is particularly the case in the common level of cervical injury in which the only active muscles below the elbow are the radial carpal extensors and the brachioradialis. Available active dorsiflexion of the wrist is of supreme importance to the patient, and there is no justification to fuse the wrist. Mobility of the wrist is of primary importance. On active dorsiflexion of the wrist in a patient with a lesion at this level, the fingers are pulled into the palm of the hand by the tenodesing effect of the long flexors. This cannot be maintained against resistance to provide a strong grip. The possibility of improving upper limb function by tendon transfers should always be considered in these cases. Even at this level there are sufficient motors to provide active flexion of the digits; at a lower level of spinal damage, if C7 segment is preserved there may be active extension of the digits, and other active tendon function may be available which can be utilized for transfer. A knowledge of the possible procedures is of vital importance. It must be stressed that the selection of patients, the care with which the procedure is carried out, and the standard of postoperative management are all essential to successful results. Selection of patients with poor motivation or a series of operations which have been carelessly chosen or badly performed can lead to poor results and apathy or opposition to surgical treatment among other patients and their doctors.

Lipscomb et al[2] described the use of a two-stage tendon transfer procedure to provide flexion and extension of the digits.[2] However, my attempts to provide both active flexion and extension with the limited number of motors available at this level were not found to be satisfactory. There is a tendency for clawing of the fingers to develop as a result of overactivity of the extensors at the metacarpophalangeal joints and of the flexors at the interphalangeal joints. Other authors have found similar problems developing after attempts to restore both active flexion and extension of the fingers. House et al[33] transfers the extensor carpi radialis longus into the long flexors and tries to prevent overaction by tenodesing the extensor digitorum communis into the lower end of the radius.[33] A tendency to clawing at the metacarpophalangeal joints which develops after this procedure is controlled by routing a free tendon graft along the lumbrical canal. A similar effect can be obtained by the use of the "lasso" superficial transfer of Zancolli.[31] This procedure has been utilized by Beasley, who carries out a complex series of procedures.[35] Extensor carpi radialis longus is transferred into the profundi and the full action of this transfer is concentrated on the proximal interphalangeal joints by fusing the terminal joints in 10 to 15 degress of flexion. All thumb joints are also fused as will be described in the section on

management of the thumb. The "lasso" procedure is carried out with the superficialis and active flexion at the metacarpophalangeal joints obtained by transfer of the brachioradialis into the superficialis above the wrist, thus controlling any tendency to clawing. Active finger extension is obtained by transfer of the pronator teres to the extensor digitorum communis. Although posting of the thumb may make the use of the hand for wheelchair propulsion more difficult, Beasley has demonstrated good results.[35] These complex procedures should be performed only by a surgeon experienced in tendon surgery.

I prefer to provide flexion of the fingers and lateral key pinch of the thumb by transfer of the extensor carpi radialis longus (ECRL) into the profundi and brachioradialis into the flexor pollicis longus (FPL).[6-8,30] Full active dorsiflexion of the wrist must be maintained to get maximal benefit from these transfers. Preoperative assessment of the power of both radial carpal extensors is necessary. The transfer of ECRL is synergistic but is dependent on the maintenance of a full range of active dorsiflexion of the wrist to provide full finger flexion (Fig. 19–3A). Extension of the fingers is obtained by dropping the wrist and taking advantage of the passive tenodesis effect of the long extensors (Fig. 19–3B). When active dorsiflexion of the radial carpal extensors is weak the brevis can be reinforced by transfer of the brachioradialis (BR).[24,36] It must be remembered that BR is a flexor of the elbow and before it is utilized for transfer there should be antagonistic action of elbow extension. This is one of the reasons that restoration of elbow extension should be carried out before any reconstructive surgery is done on the hand. BR is also valuable for transfer into the thumb flexor[6,7,16] or finger flexors.[37] It is necessary for the muscle to be stripped from its extensive fascial attachments in the lower forearm and freed up to the musculotendinous junction. With both ECRL and BR there is a high neurovascular hilum. It must be remembered that the lateral cutaneous nerve of the forearm and the sensory branch of the radial nerve, both bringing important sensation to the radial side of the forearm and thumb area, are closely related to the BR and should be carefully preserved. Following transfer of the ECRL to the finger flexors and the BR to FPL there may be some stretching at the site of tendon junction. Ejeskar utilizes stainless steel sutures as markers on each side of the tendon junction.[22] Postoperative x-ray examination may show that the markers have separated;

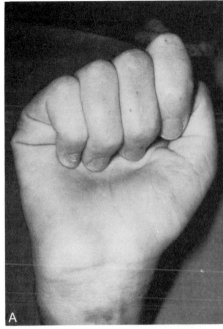
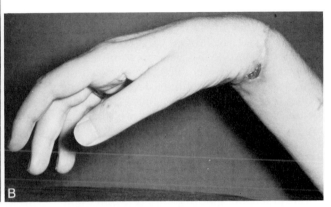

Figure 19–3. *A*, Full flexion of the fingers into the palm obtained with the wrist dorsiflexed following transfer of the tendon of extensor carpi radialis longus into the profundi. *B*, After tendon transfers to restore grasp, "dropping" the wrist allows the passive pull of the digital extensors to straighten fingers and thumb and release objects held in the hand.

elongations of up to one centimeter were not uncommon. Greater separation resulted in significant loss of movement and impairment of grip strength and justified re-exploration.

Operative Technique

This operation is carried out through a series of transverse incisions which leaves minimum scarring (Fig. 19–4). Because the patient usually has extensive respiratory paralysis and is prone to chest infection, a Biers intravenous block has proved adequate. Recently the use of cervical thoracic epidural anesthesia has been described for use in the tetraplegic patient.[38] This provides selective sensory block and allows active movement of the wrist to aid in adjustment of tendon tension at operation.

A transverse incision centered on the radial styloid extends dorsally to expose the insertion of the radial carpal extensors. The extensor carpi radialis longus is divided near its insertion, its stump is attached to the brevis, and the retinaculum is closed. The fascia anterior to

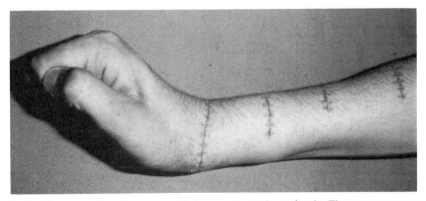

Figure 19–4. The tendon transfers were carried out one month previously. The transverse scars are well healed and will soon be inconspicuous. With the wrist dorsiflexed, the fingers are semiflexed and the thumb flexed against the side of index.

the radial styloid is divided; the abductor pollicis longus and extensor pollicis brevis tendons are identified and retracted dorsally to expose the insertion of the brachioradialis, which is freed and stripped proximally. Fascial attachments are extensive and must be freed under direct vision. The nerves related to the muscles as already described should be visualized and protected during its dissection.

Both tendons can now be freed proximally through a series of short transverse incisions until the muscle bellies are exposed. Through the anterior part of the distal incision the superficial flexors are identified and retracted radially to expose the profundi. The three ulnar profundi are usually closely joined and easily identified; however, the index profundus is usually lying separately.

The FPL and the profundi are now ready to receive the transfer of the BR and ECRL to the volar part of the wrist. The ECRL is orientated toward the profundi and passed obliquely through these tendons in series. It is important to obtain the correct tension of the transfer so that when the wrist is fully dorsiflexed the fingers should be semiflexed and when the wrist is flexed the fingers should be fully extended. There must be no flexion contracture of the interphalangeal joints when the wrist is flexed. The ECRL is fixed to the recipient profundus tendons individually by mattress sutures to avoid any "lag" of a finger into flexion subsequently.

The BR tendon is shorter and is woven two or three times through the upper part of the tendon of the FPL. The correct tension is such that when the wrist is fully dorsiflexed the interphalangeal joint of the thumb is flexed to about 30 degrees, with the tip of the thumb lying against the side of the index middle phalanx. When the wrist flexes the interphalangeal joint of the thumb should be fully straight. It is important that the transfer should not be too tight. I have reported the results of this operation over a 25-year period.[30] Four patients (operated on in the early period while the operation was being developed) believed that they had little functional benefit from the procedure but had lost no function possible before the operation. The others reported improved function and usually requested an operation on the other hand. Originally the wrist was immobilized in the neutral position with a plaster slab for three weeks with passive movement of the fingers allowed under supervision of the therapist. However, it has been found that full dorsiflexion of the wrist is better maintained by early active movement and, provided that the site of the tendon junction has been fixed firmly, this has proved very effective. On two occasions the transfer of the BR to the thumb stretched out later. The patient soon gets active flexion of the fingers and thumb but this will not reach full range and power before three to four months after the operation. With the lack of active antagonist extensor power there may be a tendency for the transfers to overreact. Provided that they are not fixed too tight, it is

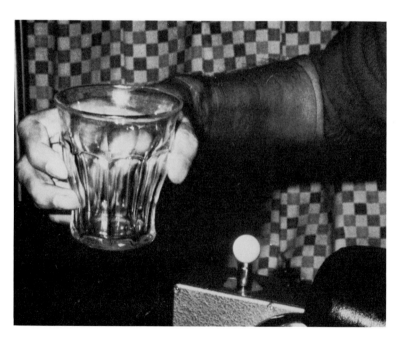

Figure 19–5. A good grasp of the hand round a tumbler following the tendon transfers described.

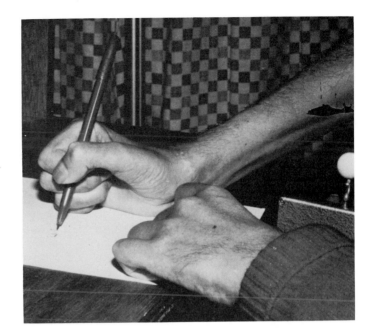

Figure 19–6. A pencil can be gripped firmly between the thumb and side of index.

rare for flexion contractures to develop. The patient must continue to stretch the fingers and thumb regularly, and the use of night splints for some months after operation is wise. The thumb tends to flex into the palm of the hand when the wrist is dorsiflexed and may obstruct finger flexion. This can be prevented by resting the thumb on a flat surface while initiating flexion of the fingers and then allowing the thumb to come in against the side of the index finger. It has not been thought necessary to carry out any tenodesis of the thumb extensors.

Examples of some results in function following operation are shown in Figures 19–5 and 19–6. The examples shown are of patients without any active digital extension. However, even better function is obtained by the operation when the digital extensors are active.

MANAGEMENT OF THE THUMB

In the earlier procedures an attempt was made to provide pulp pinch between thumb and index and long fingers.[2] This is difficult to obtain by tendon transfer except in the lower cervical cord injuries, where there are more motors available to provide an opposition type of transfer. However, the thumb can be posted in the abducted opposed position by fusion of the carpometacarpal joint. This has been practiced by experienced surgeons.[1,33–35,39] In addition, Beasley advocates fusion of the metacarpophalangeal and interphalangeal joints and

puts a bone graft between the 1st and 2nd metacarpals so as to hold the thumb firmly in the abducted position where it provides good pinch between the thumb and index and long fingers.[35] Fixing the thumb in this way has the disadvantage that it may get in the way of activities such as propelling the wheelchair, may obstruct flexion of the index and long fingers into the palm, and may prevent the heel of the hand from being flattened while supporting the body for transfer. Most surgeons experienced in the management of the tetraplegic now think that the best thumb function is provided by a key pinch so that the thumb is brought against the side of the middle phalanx of the index finger to provide grip. There are several ways in which this grip can be given. Provided that there is good active dorsiflexion of the wrist, tenodesis of the flexor pollicis longus into the lower radius accompanied by stabilization of the interphalangeal joint is one way.[24,40,41] The tendon is passed through a drill hole in the lower radius so that when the wrist is dorsiflexed the thumb is brought firmly against the side of the index finger. When the wrist drops into flexion the thumb is pulled away from the index, allowing smaller objects to be picked up between thumb and index. As the wrist is dorsiflexed the grip becomes stronger. The object is released by dropping the wrist. Fixation of the interphalangeal joint with a small Steinmann pin[24] is sometimes difficult, and the pin may work out or break.[42] A threaded pin gives better fixation. I use a polypropolene peg to stabilize the joint. While the tenodesis grip may be effective, initially, there is a tendency for the grip to loosen as the tendon stretches. Moberg has modified the procedure by routing the flexor tendon across the base of the palm and through Guyon's canal before it passes through the radius. This gives a more secure fixation of the tendon and a better line of pull for it to be effective. House has found it difficult to control the position and function of all three joints of the thumb by FPL tenodesis with stabilization of the interphalangeal joint and combined the procedure with fusion of the carpometacarpal joint in about 20 to 25 degree extension and 40 to 45 degree abduction.[34] He either tenodeses the FPL according to the method described by Moberg or transfers the BR to the FPL to maintain active flexion of the interphalangeal joint. To prevent the thumb flexing into the palm and interfering with finger flexion he tenodeses the extensor pollicis longus to the extensor retinaculum near Lister's tubercle. This provides extension of the thumb when the wrist is allowed to drop into flexion for release of objects.

In order to strengthen thumb grip, House describes an adduction-opponens plasty procedure involving rerouting of one of the paralyzed superficialis tendons around the ulnar side of the palmar fascia and inserting it into the tendon of the abductor pollicis longus.[33] Transfer of an active pronator teres, BR, or flexor carpi radialis can be used to motor this transfer. House states that fusion of the basal joint of the thumb has not interfered with transfers from bed to chair. He considers the thumb posture to be very satisfactory cosmetically, and it has restored effective lateral pinch in his patients.

It is not necessary for both an adduction-opponens plasty and fusion of the carpometacarpal joint to be carried out at the same time. House and Shannon have compared a small series of patients in whom an adduction-opponens plasty was carried out on one hand and a carpometacarpal fusion on the other.[39] Both procedures gave the patients satisfaction, some preferring one type of thumb action and others the second type. There was a slight preference for the tendon transfer control of the thumb. An average grasp of 7 kilograms of power and a pinch grip of about 2 ½ kg is obtained. The reason for the preference of the tendon transfer was that the thumb could be adapted to varying sizes of objects whereas following carpometacarpal fusion only small objects could be grasped.

Hentz et al also recommended the reconstruction of key pinch, particularly for patients lacking functional active wrist flexion.[10] They also recommended transfer of the FPL tendon through Guyon's canal. In their view the stability of the ligaments of the carpometacarpal joint of the thumb will determine whether an adduction-plasty as described by House or a fusion of the carpometacarpal joint should be performed.

They also advocate transfer of the extensor carpi radialis longus into the finger flexors, but, unlike the procedure which I have described, they prefer to put the ECRL not into the profundus of index and middle but into the superficialis of ring and little so as to avoid excessive flexion of the ulnar two fingers which they have observed following transfer into the profundi of those two fingers.

For the reasons already stated, I prefer to avoid fusion of the carpometacarpal joint of the thumb and maintain mobility at the base of the thumb to allow adaptation to objects of varying sizes and to allow the hand to be flattened for transfer activities. Active flexion of the interphalangeal joint of the thumb is achieved by transfer of the BR into the FPL, which provides a key pinch against the side of the index finger (Figs. 19–4 and 19–7). There are certain disadvantages from this procedure when the wrist is dorsiflexed in an attempt to provide grasp as there is a tendency for the thumb to flex into the palm and obstruct the flexion of the fingers. Patients can learn readily to hold the thumb against a flat surface such as a chair, table, or bed, and, while the wrist is being dorsiflexed, allow the fingers to flex into the palm and then to release the thumb and allow it to come against the side of the index.

Preoperative assessment is important in deciding which procedure to carry out. In those patients who have hypermobile metacarpophalangeal joints it is wise to tenodese the extensor pollicis longus in the way that House has described.[34] In six patients, transfer of the BR to the FPL has been done on one hand and Moberg tenodesis with stabilization of the IP joint on the other. The patients were pleased with both procedures and found that each type of thumb reconstruction is valuable for differing functions.

Keeping these different methods in mind, the surgeon can decide which is the most appropriate for each individual patient considering the type of hand and the laxity of ligaments and mobility of joints. The simple procedures already described have been found to be well

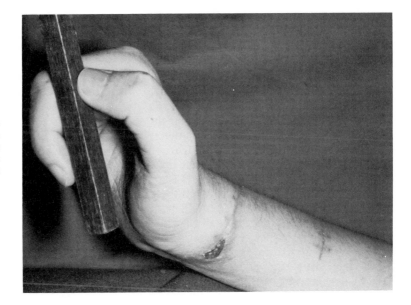

Figure 19–7. A good grip between index finger and thumb following tendon transfers. The strength of the grip is due to maintaining full dorsiflexion of the wrist.

accepted and the results appreciated by patients.[30]

There have been few complications following tendon transfer. Powerful finger flexion following transfer of ECRL to FDP has been routine (Figs. 19–1 and 19–3A). Provided that there is careful postoperative management and the patient is warned about the importance of stretching the fingers, flexion contractures have been very uncommon. Clawing of the metacarpophalangeal joints of the fingers has also not been a problem, although this complication has been reported by other surgeons. Active flexion of the thumb by transfer of the BR to the FPL is usually strong and effective for side key pinch (Fig. 19–4). It is important that at the time of operation the transfers should not be too tight. The correct tension is such that when the wrist is fully dorsiflexed the fingers are semiflexed and the thumb flexes 30 degrees at the interphalangeal joint and the tip is lying against the side of the middle phalanx of the index. On moving the wrist into flexion, the fingers and thumb should be completely straight owing to the natural passive pull of the extensors.

To provide strong grasp it is essential that full dorsiflexion of the wrist be maintained. Any adherence of the tendon transfer in its new pathway will not only restrict flexion of the fingers but also lead to flexion contractures. This can be avoided by good postoperative care. As with most reconstructive surgery around the hand and upper limb, success will depend on several factors:

1. Careful assessment by the therapist of the functional capabilities of the patient before operation. On completion of the surgical program the same tests should be carried out. It is important to ensure that no previous function has been lost.

2. Selection of a patient with motivation, drive, and desire to have improved function.

3. The choice of the appropriate surgical procedure and the care with which it is carried out.

4. Skillful postoperative nursing in patients prone to respiratory infections.

5. The therapist spends most time with the patient in the postoperative period and becomes the confidante and friend of the patient. Without skilled, dedicated, enthusiastic therapy staff constantly stimulating and encouraging the patient, this difficult surgery will fail.

SPECIFIC POSTOPERATIVE CARE BY THE THERAPIST

After Restoration of Elbow Extension

The arm is immobilized by the side of the body with the elbow in full extension. Shoulder movement must be avoided by strapping the arm to the side. The patient is usually in bed for a few days after the operation with the arm lying by the side. As soon as the patient's general condition allows transfer to the wheelchair, this is encouraged. However, with the arm in a vertical position and the hand dependent there is a tendency for edema to develop in the hand; this must be watched for and controlled.

Six weeks after operation the patient is allowed to begin moving the elbow under the supervision of the therapist and to increase flexion by 15 degrees a week. Any attempt to push this more quickly is likely to lead to loss of ability to get full extension. After every increase in flexion a plaster slab or orthoplast splint is made to hold it in this position. Under the supervision of the therapist the arm is taken out of the splint and attempts to gain full active extension allowed. The elbow is again immobilized in full extension at night. This is a slow program of not less than 12 weeks but the value of the procedure is emphasized by the patient's request for the other side to be dealt with similarly. Attempts to shorten the period of immobilization are natural and the procedure described of using the extensor carpi ulnaris tendon has proved satisfactory over the past few years. Despite the prolonged period with the elbow extended we have seen no patient in whom active elbow flexion has not been regained so that the patient can get hand to face and mouth.

The strength of the active extension of the elbow (i.e., its ability to hold the arm against gravity and the weight of any object being held in the hand) varies, but it is usually possible for the patient to stabilize the body in the sitting position, to push a wheelchair, and to reach upward. The power is insufficient usually for heavily built patients to push themselves up from bed or chair but in some slight patients this has been possible. An advantage to patients has been control of the elbow while swimming and in sports such as table tennis, which require active extension of the elbow.

After Tendon Transfers to Improve Hand Grasp

It is usually advisable to immobilize wrist or hand for three to four weeks after tendon transfer. Following transfer of the radial carpal extensor to finger flexors and BR to FPL, it has been my practice to immobilize the wrist in slight flexion by a dorsal plaster slab. It was found that it often took several weeks or even months before strong active dorsiflexion was regained and during this period the tendon transfers might get stuck in their new pathway. It is now my practice not to immobilize the wrist completely. A plaster backslab or an orthoplast splint is applied after operation holding the wrist in a neutral position, but the fingers are not immobilized. The patient is warned that the hand must not be used for

transfer or for wheelchair propulsion until at least four weeks after the operation. Under the supervision of the therapist passive movements of the fingers are encouraged to prevent the transferred tendon from becoming adherent. Also the wrist support can be removed several times a day to allow the patient passive and active assisted movements, with the effects of gravity minimized initially. It is remarkable how quickly the transfer of the ECRL to profundi seems to become effective, particularly when early dorsiflexion of the wrist is allowed (see Fig. 19–3). Between therapy sessions the wrist should be immobilized. The therapist is encouraged to carry out full passive range of wrist and finger movement, taking care not to extend wrist and fingers at the same time. Active flexion of fingers and thumb often develops within a few days of operation, and the patient is encouraged to pick up objects of varying sizes. While it is easy under the supervision of the therapist to prevent joints from becoming contracted, the patient must be encouraged to maintain the same discipline after discharge home. Night splintage holding the fingers in an extended position is advisable for some months after operation. Some patients who live near the hospital can be treated on an outpatient basis. Those who have come from a distance should be reviewed at not longer than three-month intervals to make sure that the progress is being maintained.

Provided that the patient has been well motivated and is not expecting too much, the results can be gratifying.

SUMMARY

The indications for reconstructive surgery of the upper limb in the tetraplegic are described. Restoration of elbow extension and of grasp to the hand are possible by tendon transfer, and the benefits they give to the tetraplegic patient can be of the greatest value. The factors that will influence the quality of the result must be taken into account.

REFERENCES

1. Zancolli E: Surgery for the quadriplegic hand with strong wrist extension preserved. Clin Orthop 12:101, 1975.
2. Lipscomb PR, Elkins EC, Henderson ED: Tendon transfers to restore function of hands in tetraplegia. J Bone Joint Surg 40A:1071–1080, 1958.
3. Moberg E: Reconstructive hand surgery in tetraple-

gia, stroke and cerebral palsy. Some basic concepts in physiology and neurology. J Hand Surg 1:29, 1976.

4. Moberg E: The Upper Limb in Tetraplegia: A New Approach to Surgical Rehabilitation. Stuttgart, Thieme, 1978.

5. Lamb DW: Chapter in "The Practice of Hand Surgery" 2nd ed. Blackwell Medical Publishing, Oxford and Edinburgh, in press.

6. Lamb DW: The management of upper limbs in cervical cord injuries. Proceedings of Symposium. Morrison and Gibb, Royal College of Surgeons, Edinburgh, 1963.

7. Lamb DW, Landry RM: The hand in quadriplegia. Paraplegia 7:118, 1972.

8. Lamb DW: Chapter 10. The Paralyzed Hand. (Ed. D.W. Lamb). New York, Churchill Livingstone, 1987.

9. Freehafer AA: Care of the hand in cervical spinal cord injuries. Paraplegia 7:118, 1969.

10. Hentz VR, Hamlin C, Keoshian LA: Surgical Reconstruction in Tetraplegia. Presented at 3rd International Conference, Gothenberg, 1988.

11. Hentz VR, Brown M, Keoshian LA: Upper limb reconstruction in quadriplegia: Functional assessment and proposed treatment modifications J Hand Surg 8:119, 1983.

12. Moberg E, Lamb DW: Surgical rehabilitation of the upper limb in tetraplegia. Proceedings of the International Conference in Edinburgh on The Hand 12:209, 1980.

13. Moberg E, McDowell CL, House JH: Third International Conference on Surgical Rehabilitation of the Upper Limb in Tetraplegia (quadriplegia). J Hand Surg 14:1064–1066, 1989.

14. Hansen RW, Franklin WR: Quoted from Moberg E. The upper limb in tetraplegia, p 2. Stuttgart, Thieme, 1978.

15. McDowell CL: Tetraplegia, early stages of treatment of the upper extremity. In Hunter et al: Tendon Surgery in the Hand. St. Louis, CV Mosby, 1987.

16. Waters RL, Moore KR, Graboff SR, Paris K: Brachioradialis to flexor pollicis longus tendon transfer for active lateral pinch in the tetraplegic. J Hand Surg 10A:385, 1985.

17. Nickel VL, Perry J, Garrett AL: Development of useful function in severely paralysed hands. J Bone Joint Surg 45A:933, 1963.

18. Street DM, Stanbaugh HT: Finger flexor tenodesis. Clin Orthop 13:155, 1959.

19. Wilson JN: Providing automatic grasp by flexor tenodesis. J Bone Joint Surg 38A:10, 1956.

20. Freehafer AA: Flexion and supination deformities of the elbow in tetraplegics. Paraplegia 15:221, 1977.

21. Ejeskar A, Dahllof AR: Results of reconstructive surgery in the upper limb of tetraplegic patients. Paraplegia 26:204–208, 1988.

22. Ejeskar, A: Paper read at 3rd International Conference on Tetraplegia, Gothenberg, 1988.

23. Moberg E: Upper limbs surgical rehabilitation in tetraplegia. In McCollister, (ed) EVARTSC. Surgery of the muscular skeletal system. New York, Churchill Livingstone, 18:471, 1983.

24. Moberg E: Surgical treatment for absent single hand

grip and elbow extension in quadriplegia. J Bone Joint Surg 57A:196, 1975.

25. De Benedetti M: Restoration of elbow extension power in the tetraplegic patient using the Moberg technique. J Hand Surg 4:86, 1979.

26. Raczka R, Braun R, Waters RL: Posterior deltoid and triceps transfer in quadriplegia. Clin Orthop 187:163, 1984.

27. Lacey SH, Wilber RG, Peckham PH, Freehafer AA: The posterior deltoid to triceps transfer: Clinical and Biomechanical Assessment. J Hand Surg 11:542–547, 1986.

28. Freehafer AA, Vonhaam E, Allen V: Tendon transfers to improve grasp after injuries of the cervical spinal cord. J Bone Joint Surg 56A:951, 1974.

29. Castro-Sierra A, Lopez-Pieta A: A new surgical technique to correct triceps paralysis. The Hand 15:42, 1983.

30. Lamb DW, Chan KM: Surgical reconstruction of the upper limb in traumatic tetraplegia. J Bone Joint Surg 65B:291, 1983.

31. Zancolli E: Structural and dynamic bases of hand surgery. Philadelphia, JB Lippincott, pp. 229–262, 1979.

32. Freehafer AA: Tendon transfer to improve grasp in patients with cervical spinal cord injury. Paraplegia 13:15, 1975.

33. House JH, Gwathmey LW, Lundsgaard DK: Restoration of strong grasp and lateral pinch in tetraplegia due to cervical spinal cord injury. J Hand Surg 1:152, 1976.

34. House JH: Reconstruction of the thumb in tetraplegia following spinal cord injury. Clin Orthop 195:117, 1985.

35. Beasley RW: Surgical treatment of hands for C5-C6 tetraplegia. Orthop Clin North Am 14 : No.4, 1983.

36. Freehafer AA, Mast WA: Transfer of the brachioradialis to improve wrist extension in high spinal cord injury. J Bone Joint Surg 49A:648, 1974.

37. Failla JM, Peimer CA: Presented 3rd International Conference on Tetraplegia. Gothenberg, 1988.

38. Allieu Y: Cervical Thoracic Epidural Anaesthesia. Paper read at 3rd International Conference on Tetraplegia, Gothenberg, 1988.

39. House JH, Shannon MA: Restoration of strong grasp and lateral pinch in tetraplegia. A comparison of two methods of thumb control in each patient. J Hand Surg 10A:21, 1985.

40. Hiensche DL, Waters RL: Interphalangeal fixation of the thumb in Moberg's key grip procedure. J Hand Surg 9A;13, 1985.

41. McDowell CL: Tetraplegia. In Green DP (ed): Operative Hand Surgery 2:1109–1127, University Microfilms, Inc., 1982.

42. Smith AG: Early complications of key grip hand surgery for tetraplegia. Paraplegia 19:123, 1981.

43. Lamb DW: Paper read at 3rd International Conference on Tetraplegia. Gothenberg, 1988.

44. Moberg E: The role of the cutaneous absence precision sense, kinaesthesia and motor function of the hand. Brain 106:1, 1983.

45. Zachary RB: Results of nerve suture. In Sedden: Peripheral Nerve Injuries. London, H.M. Stationery Office, 1954.

The Role of Mattresses and Beds in Preventing Pressure Sores

THOMAS A. KROUSKOP, Ph.D.

Tissue pressure management, the prevention of pressure sores, should begin immediately after a person is admitted to an institution. The viability of the person's skin can be jeopardized if care is not taken to ensure that the bed surface provides pressure relief over the bony prominences and protection from shear or abrasive forces. While there is much debate on the roles of pressure and shear in the origin of pressure sores that develop during sitting, controlling the shear generated when the body slips on the bed surface during a shift to the sitting position is critical in protecting the skin.

When the tissue is idealized as in Figure 20–1, it is obvious that much of the vascular network near the surface of the tissue is oriented vertically, while in the deeper tissues, more of the vascular system is oriented parallel to the tissue surface. When this system is loaded with forces acting parallel to the skin surface, abrasive or shear forces, the vessels near the surface collapse at loads up to 10 times smaller than the deeper vessels. When loads are applied perpendicular to the surface pressure-like loads, the deeper vessels collapse at load levels up to 8 times smaller than the vessels near the surface. Thus, to effectively prevent soft tissue breakdown, it is necessary to control pressure, shear, and pressure gradients.

SELECTING A SUPPORT SURFACE

Inadequate management too often results from the incorrect assumption that if tissue pressure is kept below 32 mm Hg, the average value of capillary pressure for healthy adults reported in physiology texts, pressure sores will not form. This simplistic view is inconsistent with the results of many research studies. Bennett and co-workers[1] have measured capillary pressures in the buttocks of seated geriatric subjects, who had peripheral vascular disease, as low as 8 to 12 mm Hg. The physics of the support problem, i.e., the weight of a person's body divided by the projected area available to support the body, precludes the possibility of having all pressures less than 10 mm Hg.

Although lack of blood flow to a region can cause tissue death, the experimental time required for such damage to occur seems to be much longer than the actual time associated with tissue breakdown in clinical environments.[2-3] In the clinical situation, a significant factor in the development of soft tissue breakdown appears to be the flow of interstitial fluid out of the region and the subsequent microvascular damage that occurs.[4] Interstitial fluid flow is controlled by pressure gradients across the tissue and the resistance of flow offered by the soft tissue matrix.

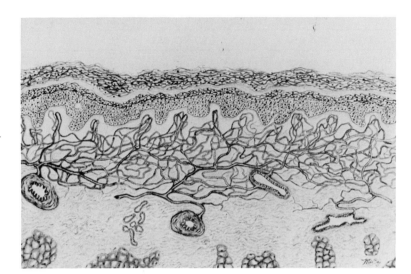

Figure 20–1. An idealized representation of tissue.

Support of the recumbent body should provide stability for the skeleton, distribute body weight over the maximum area to reduce tissue pressure, and control shear forces that are generated on the skin surface. These conditions require ingenuity and judicious use of materials. In the lying posture, tissue pressures must be kept as low as possible because the hydrostatic pressure present when a person sits no longer maintains flow of blood and lymph in the tissue. Moreover, the variability of tissue shape is more exaggerated when a person is in a lying position than when sitting. This phenomenon leads to the need for a support surface capable of large deformations without large restoring forces or shears.

The deformation requirements for a bed support surface are dictated by the differences in elevations between the lumbar areas of the back and the coccygeal region when the person is supine, and the differences between the waist and trochanters when the person is lying on his side. If the support surface is not able to accommodate deformation of a magnitude permitting prominent areas to sink into the support, the area available for weight bearing is reduced in the region and the pressures tending to impede the transport phenomena are increased.

The perfect support surface to alleviate the problems associated with pressure sores would have the following characteristics:

1. Minimizes pressure under the bony prominences
2. Controls distribution of body weight
3. Provides stability for sitting and transfers
4. Provides ease of motion for weight shifting
5. Stabilizes temperature optimally

6. Permits air exchange and controls excessive moisture
7. Does not impede independence
8. Durable, does not "bottom out"
9. Affordable

Unfortunately, no support surface satisfies all of these criteria for every potential user. Therefore, it is necessary to research available products so that an optimal support system can be selected for each patient.

When selecting a support surface for an individual, there are seven criteria that have been found to be useful. These criteria are:

1. The effectiveness of the product in reducing peak pressure, controlling shear, and reducing pressure gradients;
2. The attendant care available to the patient;
3. How long the product is to be used;
4. The financial resources available to the patient;
5. Whether the person has sensation;
6. The physical size of the user;
7. Whether the individual has bowel and bladder continence.

There are four basic groups of static mattress overlays: foam, gel, water, and air-filled systems. Each type of system has inherent advantages and disadvantages that are summarized in Table 20–1.

SUPPORT SURFACE EVALUATIONS

When the user has significant complications, or an extremely high risk of developing pressure problems, or quality nursing care cannot be assured, it may be advantageous to consider

TABLE 20–1. Characteristics of Support Systems

TYPE	ADVANTAGES	DISADVANTAGES
Air filled	1. Lightweight 2. Cleanable	1. Subject to puncture 2. Not easily repairable 3. Air pressure must be checked against leakage and for proper regulation
Water filled	1. Cleanable 2. Relatively inexpensive	1. Heavy 2. Subject to puncture
Flotation gel	1. Adjusts to body's movement 2. Simulates body fat tissue to provide more padding between patient and bed surface	1. Heavy 2. Difficult to transfer 3. Must be stored flat
Polymer foams	1. Very readily available 2. Large variety of types 3. Inexpensive 4. Lightweight 5. Easily transferred 6. Can be cut into any size, shape, thickness 7. Can be modified	1. Wear out more quickly than other materials 2. Not cleanable 3. Affected by changes in climate and temperature 4. Should not be used or stored in sunlight

one of the dynamic air flotation bed systems. There are two types that are popular: the low air loss bed and the air-fluidized bed. Depending on the needs of patients who are placed on the beds and the availability of service personnel to maintain them mechanically, one type will generally be more suitable than the other.

The advantages of the air-fluidized bed include ease of operation, relative immunity to power failure, and control of skin maseration. Its primary limitations are heavy weight and limited positioning and posturing of the patient without the use of cushions.

Because the low air loss beds are comfortable, control skin maceration, and enable change in posture easily, these are the products of choice in certain situations. However, use of these products requires personnel who can adjust the air flow in order to make them effective pressure reduction tools. Another disadvantage is the need for back-up power; the air bags deflate if the power fails and no longer provide protection.

It should be noted that in testing these beds in the Rehabilitation Engineering Program at TIRR, the interface pressure readings on all of the air-fluidized beds and low air loss beds were found to be equivalent when care was taken to adjust the low air loss products.[5] Without proper adjustment, these products may provide less protection than the static systems.

While fluidized beds or air flotation systems are effective solutions to preventing pressure sores, often they are neither practical nor cost-effective. For this reason, use of foam overlays, commonly with a convoluted surface, has become a universal, convenient method of attempting to reduce the risk of pressure sores while increasing patient comfort. Used over a conventional hospital mattress, disposable foam overlays have also proved hygienic. Foam overlays also minimize the incidence of skin maceration. This problem has been associated with impermeable plastic mattress covers, which, for reasons of hygiene and durability, have become mandatory in the construction of modern hospital mattresses.

Since these highly complex systems cannot be justified for many patients and these people must rely on mattress overlays and mattresses to manage soft tissue loading, an evaluation of representative products was conducted at TIRR.

To evaluate the effectiveness of commercially available support surfaces in redistributing weight to minimize interface pressures, 12 support surfaces, either overlays or beds, were compared on the basis of the results found after evaluation with the Texas Interface Pressure Evaluator (TIPE) pressure measurement system.[6] The TIPE system consists of a display unit, interconnecting cable, and an extra-large plastic sensor pad. The pad contains a matrix of 144 pneumatically activated switches, each of which is in turn monitored by a light-emitting diode (LED) readout on the display unit. During use, the pad is placed between the patient and the surface being evaluated. It is then inflated with a rubber pressure bulb to open all switches and thus turn off all LEDs. The pad pressure is then reduced slowly by opening a relief valve. As the load caused by the body exceeds the pressure holding a particular switch open, the switch closes and the corresponding LED is illuminated on the display matrix. By noting the pressure on the gauge as each light or group of lights illuminate, one can use the TIPE to locate the points of maximum pressure, the pressure gradient, and the body area being loaded.

Each support surface was tested according to the manufacturer's request, thus the testing conditions were not perfectly uniform.

The interface pressures generated by persons lying on the overlays or beds were evaluated under five different pressure points: the back of the head, the scapulae, the sacro-coccygeal area, the trochanters, and the heels. Two surfaces, the Rochester Modular Waterbed which required no testing beneath the head and the Span-America Geo-Matt, were tested at less than the typical number of locations. The number of subjects, too, was variable according to the manufacturer's needs, although most required 10 subjects.

The Huntleigh Technology Alpha-Care Bed was tested in both its inflation and deflation stages, although only the deflation readings were used for classification purposes. In addition, it was noted that the internal pressures of the Huntleight overlay must be reset for each patient.

All subjects were randomly selected from the population available at The Institute for Rehabilitation and Research. The subject population was categorized by gender and body build. Body build is defined in terms of the age, height, and weight of the individual.[7] The subjects were tested while recumbent in the supine and lateral positions so that pressures could be monitored under the scapulae, sacro-coccygeal area, and either right or left trochanters.

Subjects wearing loose-fitting clothing were instructed to remove their belts and shoes before being evaluated. Subjects wearing clothing with double seams (e.g., jeans or tight clothes) changed into a surgical scrub suit before the test session. The transducer pad was then placed between the mattress and the areas of the subject's body being monitored. Bony prominences were palpated and the corresponding LEDs were noted on the data collection form as location references. The magnitude of the maximum pressure at each bony prominence was then recorded. To improve the reproducibility and the accuracy of the pressure measurements, the maximum pressure readings was taken three times and the average of the three readings were recorded for each bony prominence.

Standardization in the lateral recumbent position for all subjects was achieved by using a gonimeter to position the hips at 45 degrees of flexion. The trunk was positioned perpendicular to the support surface and parallel of the long axis of the mattress. Each subject was instructed not to move while the readings were being taken. While scapular and sacral pressure measurements were made, the subjects' arms were placed flat along their sides.

Results of the study were based on an analysis of the peak pressures measured under the bony prominences on all the support surfaces.

Figures 20–2 through 20–4 illustrate the mean peak pressures and associated standard deviations of the maximum pressure measurements under the trochanter, sacrum, and scapulae for each of the commercially available mattress overlays. For the Lapidus, Gaymar, and Huntleigh products, both the high and low

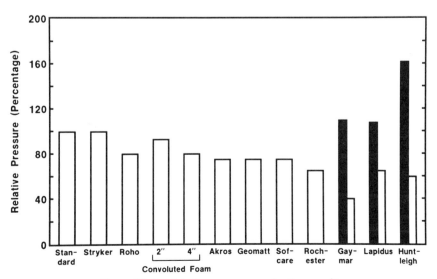

Figure 20–2. Interface pressures under the scapula.

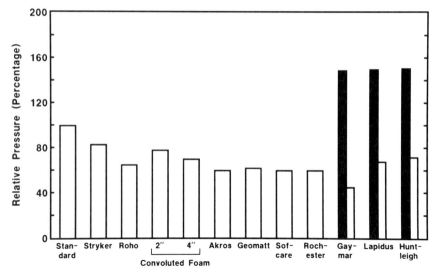

Figure 20–3. Interface pressures under the sacro-coccygeal areas.

readings in the cycle are represented on the graphs.

On all mattresses, maximum pressure under the trochanter and sacrum were generally lower for women than for men. There was no difference in scapular pressure readings between men and women. Very similar pressure curves were seen for thin, average-weight, and heavy subjects, with all the trends remaining the same. In fact, the relative effectiveness of each of the overlays was independent of the body build of the user.

Without extensive invasive laboratory testing there is no way to tell whether blood flow is being maintained in the muscles and

whether interstitial fluid is being pushed out of the region supporting the body. Making such interstitial pressure measurements in the clinical environment is impractical at this time. What can be done currently, however, is to evaluate the soft tissue stresses generated when a person is supported on various products and select a device that produces the lowest peak pressures while providing low pressure gradients over the support areas. Interface pressures and their distribution over the support surface provide data that can be used to select the most appropriate support surface for an individual. Experience at The Institute for Rehabilitation and Research (TIRR) suggests that selecting an

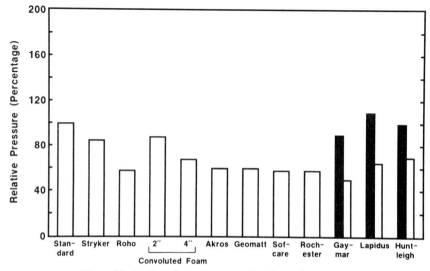

Figure 20–4. Interface pressures under the trochanters.

optimal support surface is impossible without evaluation of each individual. By collecting interface data on reasonably sized samples of people, however, it is possible to select two to four products that will be within 10 per cent of the optimum for at least 95 per cent of the population.

Experience at TIRR also has shown that even minor muscle contractions and changes in posture can lead to variations of 8 to 12 mm Hg in interface pressure. Spasticity in muscles can change peak interface pressures as much as 45 mm Hg. Wrinkles in sheets or clothing are responsible for pressure differences of up to 30 mm Hg. Thus, when considering the load redistributing effectiveness of a support surface, the professional must remember that pressure differences of less than 10 mm Hg when measured with a TIPE system are insignificant.

Therefore, when selecting a support surface, differences in interface pressures of less than 10 mm Hg as measured with the TIPE should be considered to provide equally effective pressure redistribution for care purposes, and selection should be based on other factors.

PATIENT DIAGNOSIS AND LIFESTYLE CONSIDERATIONS

Although the primary factors determining the selection of a pressure relief device may be the magnitude of the pressure and the pressure distribution pattern, other factors contribute significantly to the effectiveness of pressure relief devices. The first of these is the patient's diagnosis. Is the person's disability secondary to disease, trauma, or immobility due to aging? Does the person have intact, absent, or diminished sensation in the anatomic areas vulnerable to breakdown?

The number of hours spent on the support surfaces and the scheduling pattern of those hours are also important considerations when deciding on a device. Does the person sit for one long extended period or does he sit for shorter periods with rests in between each sitting period? What types of activities does he perform? These may include self-care, vocational, educational, homemaking, recreational, and social activities. Each activity will vary the patient's position and each will exert different levels of pressure and stress on the soft tissues.

Another factor that should be considered when selecting a pressure relief system for a person with a physical disability is the usage environment of the equipment. The climate,

level of pollution, humidity, and the patient's continence will have an effect on some of the materials of which pressure relief devices are made. Some of the foams are affected by severe changes in temperature. These devices also retain odors and cannot be washed or adequately cleaned.

The self-sufficiency of a person's living arrangement is another important consideration in selection. Does the person live alone and is he totally independent or is he assisted by family members, friends, attendants, or nurses? If the support system is very heavy or requires frequent maintenance, it would be inappropriate for the person who does not have access to assistance.

Long- and short-term tissue histories are excellent indicators of the effectiveness of pressure relief devices. Has the person ever had pressure sores or surgery to correct a pressure sore? Moreover, body build has been shown to influence pressure distribution in the person seated in a wheelchair. Thinner persons have higher pressures more frequently under bony prominences than do individuals of average or heavier weights. For this reason, thinner persons may "bottom out" on the softer cushions.

SUMMARY

Special care must be taken when evaluating the marketing claims of manufacturers of products designed to reduce pressures. Differences in average pressures of less than 8–9 mm Hg., unless they represent averages based on a very large sample, should be viewed with great skepticism. Also, the standard deviation (SD), a measure of the scatter in the data, should be reviewed. Pressure data with small standard deviations are preferable to those with large SD. With a small SD, the probability is greater that the average value represents the reading that will be obtained with any given individual.

It must be recognized that optimal application of technological advances requires exercising considerable judgment. Technology is an alternative form of assistance that can provide disabled people with quality care while reducing the need for attendant care.

REFERENCES

1. Bennett L, Kavner D, Lee et al: Shear vs pressure as causative factors in skin blood flow occlusion. Arch Phy Med Rehab 60:307, 1979.
2. Larsen JB, Holstein P, Lassen NA: On the pathogene-

sis of bedsores, skin blood flow cessation by external pressure on the back. Scand J Plast Reconstr Surg 13:347, 1979.

3. Kosiak M: Etiology and pathology of ischemic ulcers. Arch Phys Med Rehab 40:62, 1959.

4. Reddy NP, Cochran GVB, Krouskop TA: Interstitial flow as a factor in decubitus ulcer formation. J Biomechanics 14:879, 1981.

5. Krouskop TA, Williams R, Krebs M: The effectiveness of air flotation beds in lowering pressures under the recumbent body. Care, Science and Practice 4:9, 1984.

6. Krouskop, TA: A Guide for Using the Texas Interface Pressure Evaluator. Tee-Kay Applied Technology, Stafford, Texas, 1983.

7. Geigy JR: Average weights for adults. *In* Diem K., (ed): Scientific Tables. 6th ed. Geigy Pharmaceuticals, 1962.

21 Patient-Responsive EMG-Controlled Electrical Stimulation to Facilitate Unbraced Walking of Paraplegics*

DANIEL GRAUPE, Ph.D., and KATE H. KOHN, M.D.

It has been known that functional electrical stimulation (FES) was possible since Galvani's experiment of the late eighteenth century. However, its use to enable a person to stand on a paralyzed leg was first demonstrated by Liberson and colleagues[1] and by Kantrowitz[2] in 1960 and 1961.

Since then, FES has been applied to enable paraplegics with traumatic (complete) upper motor neuron lesions of the spinal cord to stand and to take steps (unbraced) with walker support. All control and initiation of limb functions (standing up, taking right and left steps, sitting down) was either manual or done with foot switches (in certain hemiplegics, in some patients with partial paralysis, or in those with some pelvic control). Furthermore, all adjustments of the stimuli to compensate for muscle fatigue were also manual.

The need for a patient-responsive nonmanual control to respond to the patients' intentions and automatically adjust the stimuli for fatigue is obvious, not only because of psychological satisfaction but also because the patient needs to concentrate on balance and posture; his concentration should not be diverted to fingers or hands. Furthermore, just when the patient may lose balance due to fatigue, he can least afford to manipulate knobs in order to make manual adjustments of the stimuli. EMG-based control that eliminates this manual activation or initiation of limb functions and manual adjustments of stimuli levels is described in the next sections of this chapter.

It was developed by the first author and his colleagues in laboratories at Illinois Institute of Technology in Chicago and at the University of Illinois at Chicago since early 1981. It has been studied and applied to paraplegic patients at the Rehabilitation Medicine Department of Michael Reese Hospital and Medical Center in Chicago since 1981 in cooperation with the second author, who is Chairman of the Department of Rehabilitation Medicine of Michael Reese Hospital and Medical Center.[3-6] It is presently used by several such patients at the same department, under a joint research project of the University of Illinois at Chicago and Michael Reese Hospital and Medical Center. This program is based solely on use of noninvasive (surface) stimulation and surface EMG signals.

*This chapter is based on research at the University of Illinois at Chicago and at the Michael Reese Hospital and Medical Center, Chicago, IL under the support of the National Science Foundation, Washington, DC (contract No. 8616402) and under a grant to Michael Reese Hospital by Mr. Ted Field of Los Angeles, CA.

ABOVE-LESION EMG CONTROL OF ELECTRICAL STIMULATION

The activation of the various electrically stimulated limb functions (standing up, right step, left step, and sitting down) in coordination with the patient's intention of executing any of these functions is probably the most challenging control problem in FES. Not only is manual control by hand or finger manipulation not psychologically satisfying and not only does it involve distraction of the patient's concentration from his posture, but also finger control may initiate a step when his posture is inadequate, thus precipitating a fall because he has no sensation.

Control that necessitates inserting electrodes in the spine or in the brain is not technically feasible, especially not for daily walking. Also, this is unacceptable to patients, who would not walk around with such implants. Since the patient lacks sensation, this approach may also lead to loss of balance due to lack of coordination with the patient's posture. Keeping these facts in mind, we decided to utilize the surface EMG taken from the patient's upper trunk above the level of the lesion. From this area the mapping of contractions of the upper trunk muscles is performed by computerized signal processing and analysis. Such mapping of the contractions of the upper trunk above the lesion yields information on the only part of the body in which muscle contractions are, at least partly, naturally correlated with intentional major changes in body posture and also with major intentional limb functions. Specifically, if a T8 complete paraplegic is to attempt standing up from a chair, he will try to lift himself by the arms in the hope that eventually (via FES) the quadriceps muscles will contract to extend the knee and allow standing up. The natural upper trunk muscle movements involved in this elevation by means of the arms allow computer discrimination of their contraction pattern via their respective surface EMG patterns, even under the most natural and untrained attempt to stand up. Hence, once the computer discriminates this unique EMG signal pattern, it sends a control command to the FES stimulator to stimulate the quadriceps to have the patient stand up immediately with the contractions of his own quadriceps. Similarly, when a patient who stands with walker support under FES attempts to take a right or left step, he must shift body balance and move the walker in preparation for that step using the upper trunk (namely, all

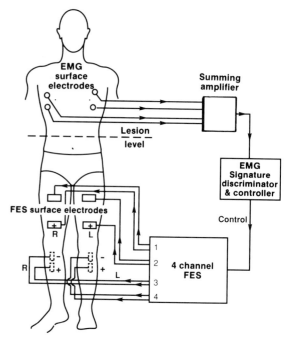

Figure 21–1. Schematic of above-lesion EMG control of FES.

that the patient can naturally use). This natural change in upper trunk contraction pattern in preparation for a step produces its own unique EMG pattern. Again this can be detected by the EMG control computer, which immediately sends the appropriate FES stimuli in order to produce a right (left) step, and so on. Figure 21–1 illustrates the schematics of this above lesion FES control.

The Mathematical Algorithm

The surface EMG signal is the cumulative electrical response of hundreds of muscle fibers to the firings of many motor units. The firings of above-lesion motor units can be viewed as trains of unsynchronized impulses, which thus have a statistical Poisson distribution. These trains of impulses are passed through muscle fibers and tissues, which act as a low-pass filter on their input, to yield a low-pass filtered Poisson process. This can be shown to be almost a Gaussian signal [8,9] and is the surface EMG signal (Fig. 21–2).[6-8] This EMG signal is denoted as y_k, where k is an integer (k = 0, 1, 2 ...) denoting discrete time. It can, by its near-Gaussian nature, be rigorously described in terms of a linear autoregressive (AR) time series (signal) model as follows[9]:

$$y_k = a_1 y_{k-1} + a_2 y_{k-2}$$
$$+ \ldots a_n y_{k-n} + w_k \quad (1)$$

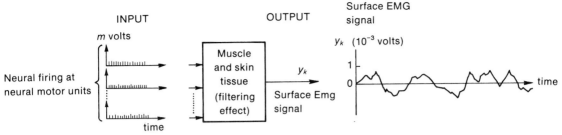

Figure 21–2. The mathematical model of the surface EMG signal.

where a_i is a set of AR parameters, with n being the model's order, and w_k being discrete white noise satisfying

$$E[w_k] = 0 \qquad (2)$$
$$E[w_k w_p] = 0 \; \forall \; k \neq p \qquad (3)$$
$$E[w_k w_p] = W \; \forall \; k = p \qquad (4)$$

with this white noise being inaccessible,[8] representing the stochastic forcing function of y_k to make the model of equation (1) mathematically rigorous.

The EMG signal's pattern is thus[4–8] reduced, via equation (1) is a set of n parameters a_1, a_2 to a_n. Once the EMG signal y_k of equation (1) is passed to the above-lesion EMG control computer via upper trunk surface electrodes, the parameters a_1 to a_n are rapidly added by this computer. A signal identification algorithm[9] is used that is fast to converge (namely, an algorithm requiring as few sample values of y_k as is possible). Noting considerations of convergence, convergence rate, and computational speed, the identification algorithm presently employed is a near least square gradient-lattice algorithm[6] that is described in detail in Chapter 7 of ref. 9. However, the details are beyond the scope of this discussion. Identification of a_i is made on the basis of 150 to 180 data points, when y_k is sampled at a rate of 580 samples per second, and where a model on order of n = 4 is considered. The considerations of model order are those of discrimination between patterns relating to different intended limb functions, noting that the higher n is, the more data points are required for convergence. However, for a sequence of more than 200 data points, the model of equation (1) becomes strongly nonstationary such that its identification becomes meaningless. (It no longer represents the muscle contraction pattern that it must detect.) Since our task is pattern discrimination[6,7] rather than signal reconstruction, and since n = 4 yields as good or better discrimination than does a higher n, we chose n = 4. Consid-

erations of sampling rate are also those of discrimination rather than of signal reconstruction. For pattern discrimination purposes, the discriminant information is contained in frequencies up to 300 Hz, to yield the sampling rate of approximately 600 samples per second.[6]

Presently real-time above-lesion EMG control is accomplished via a control computer based on a CMOS Motorola 68000 microprocessor. The whole FES stimulator and control computer hardware is presently battery operated in a patient-borne size. The stimulator employs 8 AA batteries.

BELOW-LESION RESPONSE EMG CONTROL OF FES LEVELS

When muscles that are stimulated by FES undergo fatigue, the common practice (when transcutaneous stimulation is employed) is to increase stimuli levels or stimuli pulse-width, thus increasing the stimuli's average current flow. Switching between stimulation sites has been attempted but has not yet proved effective. Manual adjustments of FES levels when the patient's knee starts to collapse require the patient to divert attention away from his posture to his hands at the worst possible time. Most devices that measure knee angle are cumbersome and bulky. Furthermore, they respond only when the knee angle changes, which is too late. The employment of the response EMG, as obtained at the stimulation site in response to the stimulus, can circumvent this difficulty, using surface electrodes similar to the ones used for above-lesion EMG pick-up. We anticipate the possibility of being able to use the stimulation electrodes themselves for this EMG pick-up. In contrast to the upper trunk above-lesion EMG, which is stochastic by its relation to hundreds of unsynchronized firings of CNS-activated motor neurons, the response EMG at below the lesion is a determining signal. It resembles the accumulation of hundreds of fully synchronized single-unit action potentials (which is exactly what it is, as seen in Figure 21–3), since all action potentials are the consequence of one and the same stimulus, i.e., the FES.

However, the shape of the response EMG changes with muscle fatigue and with neural fatigue (neural threshold changes that switch off action potentials of several units). These changes in shape, as shown in Figure 21–3, occur gradually and are reflected in changes in the second peak of the signal of Figure 21–3. Note that the first peak is the artifact of the stimulus itself, which, being 1000 times stronger than the response FES, has not been totally filtered out. The changes in shape are thus recognized by the control computer even before any visible change in knee angle appears. (The second trace of figure 21–3 corresponds to early fatigue, before a visible change occurs in knee angle). Thus, response EMG provides predictive control, so that stimuli adjustments do not come too late.[6] A system using this response EMG–based FES level control has been constructed and tested in our laboratory. Its schematic description is given in Figure 21–4.

EVALUATION OF ABOVE- AND BELOW-LESION EMG-CONTROLLED FES

Above-Lesion EMG Control

Both above- and below-lesion EMG control has been tested repeatedly on paraplegics at Michael Reese Hospital in Chicago. As of this writing eight patients have performed primitive walking under above-lesion control; the first patient used an experimental-response EMG control system (Fig. 21–5). Above-lesion EMG control can be implemented only after the patient's posture and balance (when standing and taking steps via FES) is considered adequate. The patient is then encouraged to attempt standing up, taking steps, and sitting down in a manner that is most natural for him. The a_i parameters of equation (1) are learned by the control computer and stored for the most natural contractions that are convenient for the patient in a given limb function (right step, left step, and so on).

Experienced above-lesion EMG-walking patients may have one misactivation per 100 steps or less. When the computer fails to rec-

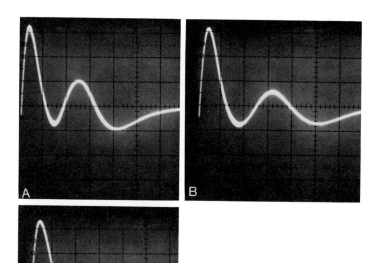

Figure 21–3. Response EMG at quadricep of paraplegic patient while standing and its progression with muscle fatigue.

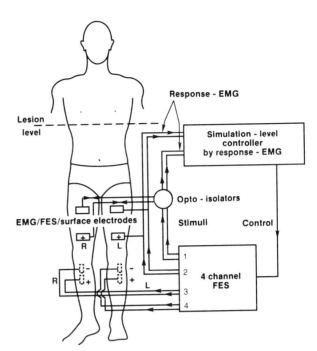

Figure 21–4. Schematic of below-lesion response EMG control of FES levels.

ognize a certain function immediately, the patient occasionally may have to prolong his upper-trunk contraction for a few more seconds. However, this situation is improving with experience. According to simulation studies, an improved identification algorithm[10] that is presently being implemented should further improve the computer's speed of recognition of upper-trunk contraction patterns. We note that when the patient intends to perform a certain limb function to take a certain step under above-lesion EMG control while his posture is inadequate, no such step will be taken, so that the patient's safety is not jeopardized. This yields an inherent safety feature to the EMG control. If, however, the patient's posture is adequate for the step that he wishes to take while the control computer does not execute one, then no harm is done to the patient. The sitting down function is the one that requires the greatest care, since if it is activated when the patient does not intend to sit, he may fall. Hence, this function is implemented with failsafe provisions. When activating the sitting down function, both of the patient's quadriceps are fully contracted and no step can be recognized for a given time interval or until the patient shuts down the system once he is seated. The same function is also activated when the patient wishes to open a door or grasp an object while standing, to avoid the remote possibility of the control computer's mistak-

enly activating a step while the patient has only one hand on the walker. Typical AR parameters (a_i) of equation (1) for the various walk functions are given in Table 21–1. Presently, as we have determined, experienced FES patients

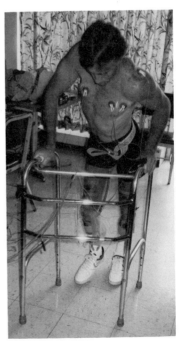

Figure 21–5. Complete paraplegic under EMG-controlled FES.

TABLE 21–1. Typical AR Parameters of Above-Lesion EMG Signal*

AR PARAMETERS Set #		RIGHT ELECTRODES					LEFT ELECTRODES				
		a_1	a_2	a_3	a_4	V	a_1	a_2	a_3	a_4	V
	14	.64	1.2	1.27	.57	.027	3.9	−.93	−.49	−.4	2.2
	15	1.48	.791	.518	.695	.035	4.29	−2.69	.666	−.69	6.25
Decision R											
	16	3.81	−.67	−.87	.16	1.76	.939	.55	1.14	0	.001
	17	4.27	−1.49	−.35	−.31	1.77	1.64	0	0	0	.001
Decision L											
	18	1.39	.254	−.42	−.533	.001	4.31	1.71	.156	−.6	6.51
Decision R											
	19	4.11	−1.62	.549	−.67	.18	1.24	0	0	0	.001
	20	5.01	−2.4	−.244	.322	5.97	1.2	.35	1.21	.363	.001
Decision L											
	21	4.08	−.854	.48	−.8	.602	3.3	−2.01	1.29	−1.0	.424
	22	2.83	−.098	−1.95	−.935	.323	2.98	−.92	.51	−.27	.185
	23	3.94	.87	.035	−.61	.59	3.38	−.33	.139	−.17	.104
	24	5.15	−1.85	−.17	−.48	5.57	3.24	−.03	−.04	−.21	.098
Decision L											
	25	1.25	1.11	.443	0	.014	4.57	2.62	.52	−.543	6.32
Decision R											
	26	4.82	−1.99	.08	−.51	4.54	1.38	1.01	−1.26	.89	.002
Decision L											
	27	2.32	−1.03	2.42	0	.061	5.2	−2.37	.66	.06	1.92
	28	2.54	.094	.695	0	.06	4.34	−1.82	.19	−.57	4.42
Decision R											
	29	4.89	−1.6	−.87	.31	3.65	3.11	.67	0	0	.355
Decision L											
	30	2.21	.031	.434	.551	.031	4.4	−2.30	.3	−.26	2.50
Decision R											
	31	4.27	.67	−1.51	.7	6.55	.96	.92	.557	.25	.016
	32	4.57	−1.51	−.137	.63	4.19	.322	1.44	1.42	0	.001
Decision L											

Key: R: Right step executed; L: Left step executed; V: Sample variance of y_k (EMG signal).

*EMG parameters' printout for a continuous walk sequence during a section from a 250 step walk by PM (T8 lesion)

Comment: These parameters are those to which the identifier converged after 160 samples at each identification run. Hence, each two lines of the table are separated by 160 samples at 550 samples/sec., i.e., by 0.291 sec. Convergence is unsatisfactory at below 160 samples (iterations). After each step taken by the patient, sampling is stopped for 0.8 sec. to allow the patient to recover his posture/balance. This results in a fastest inter-step interval of 0.8 + 0.291 sec. = 1.091 sec., which appears adequate for the patients and yields fast-flowing, smooth-looking walks. The recovery interval is adjustable according to the patient's needs. (Piece-wise stationarity of parameters is assumed over the 160-sample identification interval of 0.291 sec.)

carry about 95 to 98 per cent of their body weight on their legs while standing with FES.

Below-Lesion Response EMG Control

Response EMG control of stimulation levels has so far been tested in full on only one patient. It was applied to four patients for one leg only (while standing under manual control of the other leg). In all cases the duration of standing was extended by a factor of 4 to 20 via the automatic response-EMG control of FES levels, relative to not adjusting FES levels.

CONCLUSIONS

We believe that, for the wide acceptance of FES, nonmanual control that is automatically responsive to the patient's intent is essential. A system is only as good or as acceptable as is its control. Response-EMG control can be implemented independent of above-lesion EMG control. Hence it can be used also in conjunction with manual activation of standing and walking functions. The control is not specific to transcutaneous FES and is therefore applicable also to FES with implanted electrodes.

We see FES as the best means of getting the patient on his feet and out of the wheelchair for at least half an hour once or twice daily. Walking by FES with walker support (we do not foresee it without some support) is a better exercise and psychologically more satisfying than just standing. The merits of FES are thus beneficial psychologically and for the cardiovascular system. A positive effect can be expected on the occurrence of pressure sores. The upright posture and muscle action will improve not only circulation but also bowel and bladder activity. All these effects should be systematically studied, as they presently reflect only our observations on a limited number of patients. Such studies would require the evaluation of FES exercise in upright posture in an increasing number of paraplegics.

REFERENCES

1. Liberson WT, Holmquest HJ, Scott D, et al: Functional electrical stimulation of the peroneal nerve synchronized with the upswing phase of gait of hemiplegic patients. Arch Rehab Med 42:101, 1961.
2. Kantrowitz A: Electronic physiologic aids. Proc. IBM Symposium, 1960.
3. Graupe D, Kralj A, Kohn KH: Computerized signature discrimination of above-lesion EMG for stimulating peripheral nerves of complete paraplegics. Proc IFAC Symp Prosthesis Control, Columbus, OH, 1982.
4. Graupe D, Kohn KH, Basseas S, Naccarato E: Electromyographic control of functional electrical stimulation in selected patients. Orthopedics 7:1134, 1984.
5. Graupe D, Kohn KH, Basseas S: Evaluation of EMG posture-mapping–based control of electrical stimulation of paraplegics. Proc. IEEE Conf. on Frontiers of Engineering and Computers in Health Care, pp. 271–274, 1985.
6. Graupe D, Kohn KH, Basseas S: Above- and below-lesion EMG pattern mapping for controlling electrical stimulation of paraplegics to facilitate unbraced walker-assisted walking. J Biomed Eng 10:305, May 1988.
7. Graupe D, Salahi J, Zhang, DS: Stochastic analysis of myoelectric temporal signatures for multifunctional single-site activation of prostheses and orthoses. J Biomed Eng 7:18, 1985.
8. Graupe D, Cline WK: Functional Separation of EMG Signals via ARMA Identification Methods for Prosthesis Control Purposes, IEEE Trans. on Systems, Man & Cybernetics, Vol. 5, pp. 252–259, 1975.
9. Graupe D: Time Series Analysis, Identification and Adaptive Filtering, Malabar, RE Krieger Publishing Co, 1984.
10. Moser AT, Graupe D: Applicability of Kalman filtering theory to the identification of time series with nonstationary covariance structures. Int J Sys Sci 20:91, 1989.
11. Sigfried J, Lazorthes Y, et al: Electrical spinal cord stimulation for spastic movement disorders. Appl Neurophysiol 44:77, 1981.
12. Walker JB: Modulation of spasticity, prolonged suppression of a spinal reflex by electrical stimulation. Science 216:203, 1982.

Physiologic Response to Tissue Injury

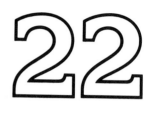

WILLIAM M. STAHL, M.D.

Tissue injury can be caused by physical disruption due to accident or during the operative procedure, by thermal damage (as in burns, electrical injuries, and frostbite), and by destruction from invading sepsis. Local changes initiated by the injury are designed to allow remodeling and healing of the local wound. Local events also occur which alter the general status of the patient by neurogenic and humoral means. In this chapter we will discuss the local responses of injured tissues, the neurogenically mediated systemic effects, and the humorally mediated changes that constitute the acute phase response.

Local trauma initiates a consistent sequence of events which includes early transient vasoconstriction that tends to control acute hemorrhage. Following this, vasodilatation occurs with opening of the microvascular beds in the injured tissue. This allows humoral and cellular elements to reach damaged cells. Permeability increases with transudation of protein-rich fluid into the tissue site. Hageman factor (XII) is activated and the clotting cascade is initiated. Platelet aggregation and degranulation occur.[1,2] Histamine, serotonin, and bradykinin are involved in this response. Both the vasoconstrictor arachidonic acid metabolites such as thromboxane A_2 and the vasodilator eicosanoids are implicated in the response.[3]

Neutrophils are the first cells to arrive at the scene of injury, playing a role in attacking microorganisms by phagocytosis and lysing devitalized tissue by the release of protease. Opsonins and antibodies leak from the altered vessels and assist the white cells in controlling local infections. Lymphocytes arrive in the wound shortly thereafter.[4] The role of these lymphocytes is not well defined and wounds appear to heal satisfactorily in lymphocyte-depleted animals.

The next cells to arrive are tissue macrophages and circulating monocytes, which differentiate into macrophages.[5] Macrophages appear to play a key role in a variety of events that occur in and around the early wound. Early on, macrophages release interleukin-1 (IL-1), a peptide which has many functions in initiating the acute phase response. Later in the initial days of wound activity macrophages secrete a substance known as angiogenesis factor that is believed to be a chemoattractant for mesothelial and vascular endothelial cells.[6,7]

Endothelial cells form capillary buds at the wound surface, and if the wound edges are approximated these capillaries bridge the wound. The dense surface layer of new blood vessels combined with fibroplasia produces granulation tissue. As long as the wound remains somewhat hypoxic, granulation tissue continues to proliferate. With closure of the wound remodeling of the capillaries occurs as epithelialization proceeds.

Fibroblasts appear in the wound approximately two days after injury and are stimulated by another factor secreted from macrophages. Collagen synthesis then follows. Fibronectin appears to play an important role in this constructive process.[8] Epithelialization then occurs by migration of epithelial cells from adjacent tissue.

Wound strength increases by the production of collagen fibers within the wound and by the remodeling of these fibers to provide a mature healed scar. In clean wounds the rate of collagen synthesis is maximal in the first two weeks, with collagen deposition maximal at three to four weeks. Vitamin A and zinc are factors that can moderate the collagen phase of healing. Vitamin A appears to restore the inflammatory stimulus required to generate healing factors, and zinc is a cofactor in a number of enzyme systems including RNA and DNA polymerases.[9]

NEUROENDOCRINE RESPONSE

The neuroendocrine response to tissue injury varies with the degree of injuries sustained. It is mediated through nerve impulses from the injured area and is blocked by denervation or spinal anesthesia. The stress response is characterized by elevated plasma catecholamine and cortisol levels, moderate decreases in thyroid hormone concentrations, and in angiotensin-converting enzyme activity.[10] The increase in plasma catecholamines is immediate and persists during the first hours after injury, with return toward normal levels after 24 hours. The magnitude of the reaction seems to be related in a general way to the magnitude of injury.[11] In a similar manner plasma cortisol levels are elevated early after injury, with return toward normal levels in 12 to 24 hours.[12,13] Other early effects involve an increase in glucagon and changes in insulin metabolism.[14,15] These hormonal changes cause major increases in hemodynamic activities, with a rise in cardiac index and an increase in peripheral circulation, provided that adequate fluid support is available. Major metabolic alterations are caused by these hormonal changes, namely, hyperglycemia, hyperinsulinemia, decreased ketone body concentration, and increased alanine and aromatic amino acid levels with a decrease in the level of branched-chain amino acids.[16,17] The net effect of hormone interactions produces an increase in serum glucose levels, an increased level of fat mobilization, and an increase in protein catabolism in the muscles to provide carbon skeletons for hepatic gluconeogenesis.

While blockade of transmission of impulses from the injured area to the central nervous system blunts the responsiveness of epinephrine and cortisol, the metabolic effects resulting in catabolism of protein and the development of negative nitrogen balance do not seem to be affected by neural blockade.[18] It is evident from the increased hemodynamic demands and increased metabolic requirements of the acutely injured patient that support of fluid volumes and cardiovascular function and the provision of metabolic substrates are vital to survival in the early period following severe injury.

In recent years, knowledge has accumulated concerning the role that macrophages play in the production of a variety of monokines which are key to the the postinjury state. The most important stimulatory monokine is interleukin-1 (IL-1). This monokine is released from monocytes activated in the area of injury by local injury, microbial action, or other inflammatory responses. Interleukin-1 has a wide variety of actions: it induces fever through its action on the hypothalamus, an action mediated by prostaglandin synthesis; the bone marrow is stimulated to produce neutrophils; neutrophils are activated to become degranulated; and fibroblasts are stimulated to produce collagen. A major activity of IL-1 is to stimulate hepatocytes to synthesize acute phase proteins at the expense of albumin synthesis. These acute phase proteins appear to have positive actions in the traumatized person. Such substances include C-reactive protein, haptoglobin, transferrin, α_1-antitrypsin, ceruloplasmin, and metalothionines, which sequester iron and zinc. The effect of these substances is to reduce the plasma levels of minerals and hemoglobin, an action that has a beneficial effect in limiting bacterial proliferation.[19,20] Interleukin-1 also participates in the metabolic alterations following injury, in that it appears to cause breakdown of muscle protein, with release of amino acids into the plasma.[21]

IMMUNE RESPONSE

It has been clearly shown that trauma produces a decrease in function of the immune system for many days following the insult. There is a decrease in total numbers of circulating T-cells (CD3), with reduction in helper/suppressor ratios (CD4/CD8). There is also a decrease in the ability of the lymphocytes to proliferate in response to standard in vitro stimuli (PHA, Con A). These effects persist up to one week following severe injury and are thought to increase the vulnerability of the patient to invasive sepsis. Stimulation of lymphocytes by IL-1 is a vital part of host defenses. This activity is carried out through the production of secondary lymphokines. The most important of these is interleukin-2 (IL-2), which is released from T-cells when stimulated by the presence of IL-1. Interleukin-2 is the most potent lymphocyte-stimulating factor known.

Under IL-2 stimulation, T-cells proliferate, with an increase in CD4/CD8 ratios and an enhancement of response to mitogens.

It has been difficult to reconcile the known facts concerning the stimulating effect of IL-2 on cellular immunity with the equally well documented clinical suppression of host defense after injury. It has become increasingly clear that activated macrophages produce other mediators in addition to IL-1. One of these is prostglandin E_2 (PGE$_2$), an arachidonic acid–derived eicosanoid which is produced via the cyclo-oxygenase pathway. Evidence is accumulating that PGE$_2$ is the suppressor arm of macrophage activation. It has been known for some time that serum from patients with severe burns or severe trauma suppresses normal lymphocyte activation in vitro and that this suppression is related to PGE$_2$ content.[22] The pathway by which PGE$_2$ suppresses cellular immunity appears to be that of suppression of IL-2 production.[23,24] This effect may be mediated by the generation of CD8 suppressor cells, which then inhibit IL-2–producing cells.[25] However, there may be other factors at work beyond the involvement of IL-2 suppression.[26]

Knowledge of some of the pathways that produce immunosuppression has suggested the possibility of immunomodulation in order to maintain immunocompetence in the trauma patient. Several classes of drugs have been considered, including cyclophosphamide, histamine, H$_2$ antagonists, and agents that inhibit the cyclo-oxygenase pathway and thus reduce production of PGE$_2$. These include the nonsteroidal anti-inflammatory agents such as ibuprofen and indomethacin.[27] One human study has shown an improvement in lymphocyte function in vitro following administration of indomethacin.[28] Whether this type of immunomodulation will improve clinical results and reduce septic complications has not yet been documented.

The physiologic response to tissue injury can thus be understood as a complex reaction involving local tissue remodeling and reconstruction, local defenses against invading microorganisms, and locally generated humoral messenger molecules that drastically alter total body function. These alterations induce cardiopulmonary and metabolic stress and reduce systemic immunity. Care of patients with major trauma requires knowledge of these ongoing changes and of their necessary supportive therapy.

REFERENCES

1. Ryan GB, Majno G: Acute inflammation (a review). Am J Pathol 86:183, 1987.
2. Majno G, Palade GE: Studies on inflammation. 1. The effect of histamine and serotonin on vascular permeability: an electron microscopic study. J Biophys Biochem Cytol 11:571, 1961.
3. Orgill D, Demling RH: Current concepts and approaches to wound healing. Crit Care Med 16:899, 1988.
4. Fishel R, Barbul A, Beschorner W, et al: Lymphocyte participation in wound healing. Ann Surg 206:25, 1987.
5. Diegelmann RF, Cohen IK, Kaplan AM: The role of macrophages in wound repair. A review. Plast Reconstr Surg 68:107, 1981.
6. Dinarello CA: Interleukin-1 and the pathogenesis of the acute-phase response. N Engl J Med 311:1413, 1984.
7. Banda MJ, Knighton OR, Hunt TK, et al: Isolation of a non-mitogenic angiogenesis factor from wound fluid. Proc Natl Acad Sci USA 79:7773, 1982.
8. Saba TM, Jaffe E: Plasma fibronectin (opsonic glycoprotein): its synthesis by vascular endothelial cells and role in cardiopulmonary integrity after trauma as related to reticuloendothelial function. Am J Med 68:577, 1980.
9. Chvapil M: Zinc and wound healing. In Zederfeldt B (ed): Symposium on Zinc. Lund, Sweden, AB Tika, 1974.
10. Chernow B, Alexander R, Smallridge RC, et al: Hormone responses to graded surgical stress. Arch Intern Med 147:1273, 1987.
11. Davies CL, Newman JF, Molyneux SG, Grahame-Smith DG: The relationship between plasma catecholamines and severity of injury in man. J Trauma 24:99, 1984.
12. Mohler JL, Michael KA, Freedman AM, et al: The serum and urinary cortisol response to operative trauma. Surg Gynecol Obstet 161:445, 1985.
13. Barton RN, Stoner HB, Watson SM: Relationships among plasma cortisol, adrenocorticotrophin and severity of injury in recently injured patients. J Trauma 27:384, 1987.
14. Gann DS, Lilly MP: The neuroendocrine response to multiple trauma. World J Surg 7:101, 1983.
15. Wilmore DW: Hormonal responses and their effects on metabolism. Surg Clin North Am 56:999, 1976.
16. Kirkpatrick JR: The neuroendocrine response to injury and infection. Nutrition 3:221, 1987.
17. Cerra FB, Siegel JH, Border JR: Correlations between metabolic and cardiopulmonary measurement in patients after trauma, general surgery, and sepsis. J Trauma 19:621, 1979.
18. Fohring U, Reinhart K, Schafer M, Dennhardt R: Epidural anesthesia does not modify metabolic response to major surgery. Crit Care Med 14:329, 1986.
19. Dinarello CA: Interleukin-1 and the pathogenesis of the acute phase response. N Engl J Med 311:1413, 1984.
20. Pepys MB, Baltz ML: Acute phase proteins with special reference to C-reactive protein and related proteins (pentaxins) and serum amyloid A protein. Adv Immunol 34:141, 1983.
21. Clowes GHA Jr, George BC, Villee CA Jr, Sararis

CA: Muscle proteolysis induced by a circulating peptide in patients with sepsis or trauma. N Engl J Med 308:545, 1983.

22. Ninneman JL, Stockland AE: Participation of prostaglandin E in immunosupression following thermal injury. J Trauma 24:201, 1984.

23. Faist E, Mewes A, Baker CC, et al: Prostaglandin E2 (PCE2)—dependent supression of interleukin 2 (IL-2) production in patients with major trauma. J Trauma 27:837, 1987.

24. Abraham E, Regan RF: The effects of hemorrhage and trauma on interleukin 2 production. Arch Surg 120:1341, 1985.

25. Chouaib S, Chatenoud L, Keatzmann D, Fradelezi

D: The mechanism of inhibition of human IL2 production. II. PGE$_2$ induction of suppressor T lymphocytes. J Immunol 132:1851, 1984.

26. Abraham E, Tanaka T, Chang YH: Effects of hemorrhagic serum on Interleukin-2 generation and utilization. Crit Care Med 16:307, 1988.

27. Hansbrough JF, Zapata-Sirvent RL, Peterson V, et al: Modulation of suppressor cell activity and improved resistance to infection in the burned mouse. J Burn Care Rehabil 6:270, 1985.

28. Faist E, Ertel W, Cohnert T, et al: Immunoprotective effects of cyclooxygenase inhibition in patients with major surgical procedures. Surg Forum 39:114, 1988.

Paralysis Secondary to Abdominal Aortic Aneurysm

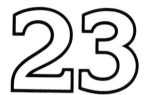

BOK Y. LEE, M.D. _____

Spinal cord ischemia occurring as a complication of intra-abdominal arterial reconstructive procedures is a rare complication,[1] the outcome of which is partial or complete paraplegia. The occurrence of this complication has been associated with the level and duration of aortic occlusion, intraoperative hypotension, inadequate intraoperative anticoagulation, atheromatous emboli, and occlusive arteriosclerosis of the spinal cord arteries. We present a review of the incidence, clinical factors, and vascular anatomy of the spinal cord. Additionally, we present a report of a patient with spinal cord ischemia with paraplegia secondary to the presence of an abdominal aortic aneurysm in the absence of any surgical procedure.

INCIDENCE

Elliott et al[2] cite 51 published cases of spinal cord ischemia secondary to surgery of the abdominal aorta. Perhaps the largest review of the incidence of this complication at a single institution comes from the Henry Ford Hospital.[2-4] In a total of 3445 surgical procedures involving the abdominal aorta, including 1861 abdominal aortic aneurysms (259 ruptured and 1602 elective), aortoiliac occlusive disease in 1188 procedures, and renal or mesenteric arterial occlusive disease in 396; only eight cases (0.2 per cent) were associated with spinal cord ischemia. All instances of complications occurred during surgery for abdominal aortic aneurysms.

In a recent report from the University of Rochester,[1] seven patients were reported with spinal cord ischemia following 744 abdominal aortic procedures (0.9 per cent): three occurred during surgery for aneurysmal disease and four during surgery for aortoiliac occlusive disease.

CLINICAL FEATURES

Elliott et al[2] have summarized the clinical features of 51 published cases. Of these 51 cases, 23 (45 per cent) occurred following repair of a ruptured abdominal aortic aneurysm and 17 (33 per cent) followed elective resection. In the series from Henry Ford Hospital,[2] five of 259 repairs of ruptured abdominal aortic aneurysm (1.9 per cent) were associated with spinal cord ischemia compared with three of 1602 elective resections (0.2 per cent). Of the 51 published cases, 10 (19.6 per cent) occurred following aortoiliac reconstructive procedures; there were none in the series from Henry Ford Hospital.

With the addition of the recent report from the University of Rochester,[1] the number of published cases becomes 58. The types of aortic lesions and mortality in these 58 cases is summarized in Table 23–1.

Examination of the published cases of spinal cord ischemia following abdominal aortic procedures does not yield any specific clinical features that would indicate why certain patients sustain spinal cord injury. The anatomic features of the blood supply to the spinal cord may be an important precipitating factor.

TABLE 23–1. Types of Aortic Lesions and Mortality in 58 Reported Cases of Spinal Cord Ischemia Following Surgery on the Abdominal Aorta

TYPE OF AORTIC LESION	REPORTED CASES		DEATHS	
	No.	Percentage	No.	Percentage
Ruptured abdominal aortic aneurysm	24	41%	12	40%
Elective abdominal aortic aneurysm	19	33%	9	30%
Occlusive aortoiliac disease	14	24%	9	30%
Occlusive renal disease	1	2%	0	0%
TOTAL	58	100%	30	100%

SPINAL CORD VASCULAR ANATOMY

The vascular anatomy of the spinal cord can be divided into a proximal or extraspinal division, an intermediate division, and a terminal distribution system.[2]

The proximal or extraspinal division is composed of the vertebral, ascending cervical, deep cervical, intercostal, and lumbar arteries. Collateral interconnections are plentiful in the cervical and sacral regions and less so in the thoracic region. Thus, interruption of the blood supply in the thoracic region cannot be compensated for through collateral pathways as well as in the cervical and sacral regions.

The intermediate division is composed of the spinal radicular arteries connecting the branches of the aorta to the terminal distribution system of blood vessels lying on the spinal cord. In the adult, radicular arteries are few and usually include up to two cervical, three thoracic, two lumbar, and those supplying the sacral spinal cord. The great radicular artery (Adamkiewicz) is usually located at the T–9 to T–12 level and is considered the main feeder of the anterior spinal artery in the distal thoracolumbar spinal cord.

The terminal distribution system is composed of the anterior spinal artery and paired posterolateral spinal arteries. The anterior spinal artery is the largest, extends the full length of the spinal cord, and is fed by branches of the two vertebral arteries. In the region lacking radicular blood vessels, the anterior spinal artery is the sole source of blood.

From the foregoing review of the vascular anatomy of the spinal cord, one can see that the spinal cord, particularly the thoracic cord, is highly vulnerable to any interruption of its blood supply. Elliott et al[2] point out the relative lack of a collateral circulation between branches of the intercostal arteries in the thoracic area as opposed to the cervical, lumbar, and sacral areas, the limited communication among the three spinal arteries, the small number of anterior spinal radicular arteries, and the variability of the level of origin of the great radicular artery.

CASE REPORT

A 63-year-old white man, paraplegic from the level of T10, was admitted from a community hospital. The patient had a history of stroke from which he had recovered, generalized arteriosclerosis, myocardial infarction, hypertension, and hypothyroidism. Over the past few years, the patient had developed progressive spastic paralysis. An extensive neurologic examination was inconclusive; the consensus was the presence of ischemic myelitis secondary to the presence of an abdominal aortic aneurysm. The aneurysm had not been resected.

At the time of admission, physical examination revealed a thin, cachectic man in no obvious distress. The patient's vital signs were stable, rales were noted at the base of the lungs, and his heart showed a regular rhythm. The patient's neck revealed scars from previous bilateral carotid endarterectomies and his abdomen was soft with a palpable abdominal aorta. A neurologic examination revealed marked wasting of

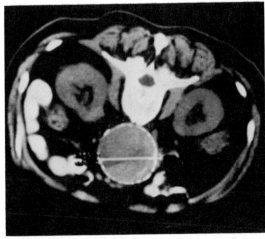

Figure 23–1. Computed tomography of the abdomen showing dilated abdominal aorta (5 cm) with a calcified wall and thrombus.

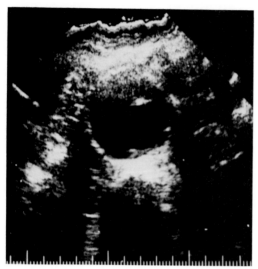

Figure 23–2. Ultrasound scan showing an aneurysmal sac measuring 11 cm × 5 cm at umbilicus level.

the muscles, particularly evident in the distal muscles of the hands and the muscles of the legs and hips. No fasciculations were visible and there were marked flexion contractures of the lower extremities with spasticity. Previous computed tomography of the abdomen (Fig. 23–1) had revealed a dilated abdominal aorta measuring 5 cm at the largest diameter proximally with a calcified wall. An area of low attenuation within the lumen was thought to be representative of thrombus. A large aneurysm was noted beginning at the level of the renal arteries and extending to the bifurcation. The presence of thrombi within the aneurysm was suggested by areas of low attenuation. The aneurysm measured 6 cm × 6.5 cm (anterior-posterior × transverse). Ultrasound of the abdominal aorta done almost eight months later revealed an aneurysmal sac measuring 11 cm in length and 5 cm anterior-posterior at the level of the umbilicus (Fig. 23–2). The patient's condition remained stable and unchanged since admission.

COMMENT

The case report demonstrates that the thoracic spinal cord is particularly vulnerable to interruption of its blood supply during surgical intervention, blunt abdominal trauma, or in the presence of a dissecting abdominal aortic aneurysm. As discussed previously, the thoracic spinal region is relatively poor in collateral circulation, thus limiting the extent of compensatory blood supply through other routes. Additional complications include the limited intercommunication of the anterior spinal artery and the long length and narrow diameter of the great radicular artery. An additional complicating factor during surgical intervention is the variable origin of the great radicular artery.

In conclusion, steps may be taken to limit the occurrence of spinal cord ischemia following intra-abdominal surgical procedures. The occurrence of spinal cord ischemia, as the case report demonstrates, and spontaneous paralysis due to abdominal aortic aneurysm embolization to the great radicular artery in the absence of surgical intervention is unpreventable but is an extremely infrequent source of morbidity.

REFERENCES

1. Picone AL, Green RM, Ricotto JR, et al: Spinal cord ischemia following operations on the abdominal aorta. J Vasc Surg 3:94, 1986.
2. Elliott JP, Szilagyi DE, Hageman JH, et al: Spinal cord ischemia: Secondary to surgery of the abdominal aorta. In Bernhard VM, Towne JB (eds): Complications in Vascular Surgery, 2nd edition. Philadelphia, Grune & Stratton, 1985, pp 291–310.
3. Szilagyi DE, Hageman JH, Smith RF, Elliott JP: Spinal cord damage in surgery of the abdominal aorta. Surgery 83:38, 1978.
4. Elliott JP, Szilagyi DE, Hageman JH, Smith RF: Spinal cord damage secondary to surgery of the abdominal aorta. In Bernhard VM, Towne JB (eds): Complications in Vascular Surgery. Philadelphia, Grune & Stratton, 1980, pp 407–426.

24 Spinal Cord Injury Rehabilitation

GARY M. YARKONY, M.D.

In 1945 Sir Ludwig Guttman stated that "Rehabilitation after spinal injuries seeks the fullest possible physical and psychological readjustment of the injured person to his permanent disability with a view to restoring his will to live and working capacity."[1] This comment is still poignant today as improvements in acute care and long-term medical management have resulted in increasing life spans for individuals with spinal cord injury. Although research continues toward a cure for the conditions resulting from spinal cord injury, these individuals must not let this hope interfere with their reintegration into society.

Although estimates of the exact number of spinal cord injuries per year vary, there are approximately 10,000 persons annually who survive these injuries and are hospitalized.[2,3] The prevalance of spinal cord injury is estimated to be 906 spinal injuries per million persons at risk. Because this population is young, with most injuries occurring in the 16 to 30 age group (mean age = 29.7, median = 25.0), the importance of rehabilitation and reintegration into the community is crucial.[4] Recent studies indicate that the life span postinjury is increasing.[5]

Vital to rehabilitation after spinal cord injury is an interdisciplinary team[6] functioning in an appropriate facility.[7,8] Comprehensive units with skilled therapists capable of providing all aspects of care for spinal cord injured persons are essential. The concept of specialized spinal cord injury units was first developed in the United States by Munro[9] and in England by Guttman.[10] Care of spinal cord injuries in these units should provide for a coordinated system of care with decreased secondary complications and lifelong follow-up. A comprehensive rehabilitation program, which provides a full range of services and maximum patient participation, enhances the likelihood of achieving favorable outcomes, promotes the resumption of meaningful life roles, and facilitates the opportunities for community reintegration.[8]

ASPECTS OF REHABILITATION IN THE ACUTE CARE PHASE

The most important aspects during the acute care phase are related to saving the life of the traumatized patient. Efforts to prevent further damage to the spinal cord include immobilization of the spine, correction of the deformity, steroids and maintenance of the cardiovascular and other biological parameters. It is essential that, while these complex problems are being managed, efforts are made to prevent secondary complications that will interfere with rehabilitation.[11] Two of the most essential complications to be prevented are pressure sores and joint contracture. Consideration must also be given to the presence of concomitant head injury[12] and its effect on further rehabilitation and urological management.

Joint range of motion can be maintained by range of motion (ROM) exercises and splinting. As the patient is initially flaccid, ROM exercises performed daily may be all that is necessary. Joints affected by local trauma or edema may require more. The best guide is careful reassessment and upgrading of the program if loss of range of motion occurs. As spasticity develops, ROM exercises may be necessary two or three times daily. Splinting of the wrist in a functional position of extension with the web space of the thumb maintained in abduction is a useful adjunct. Splinting of the ankles at 90 degrees may be necessary if plantar flexion contractures develop. Studies on contracture development after spinal cord injury show a decreased incidence of contracture development in a specialized system of acute care.[13]

Although ROM exercises are generally in the domain of the therapist, it is essential that the nursing staff be able to perform these exercises. Frequently, family members can assist in these activities if they will not interfere with life support equipment. This not only prevents deformity but gives family members the satisfaction of contributing to the care of their loved one. Particular care should be given to the shoulder, as a quadriplegic suffering from adhesive capsulitis of this joint may have a more difficult and prolonged rehabilitation. Contractures most commonly occur in the acute care phase in the hip, knee, and ankle.

Prevention of pressure sores is best accomplished by frequent turning and careful skin inspection. The patient should be turned initially every two hours. Skin should be kept clean and dry. Shearing forces, particularly during transfers, should be avoided. Particular care should be exercised when using the RotoRest bed that the bed is not stopped frequently, defeating its usefulness. Pressure sores in the sacral area[4] are the most common during the acute care phase of rehabilitation, but one must also be careful to protect the heels and other bony prominences.

Optimal urological management in the acute care phase is often limited by the need to closely monitor fluid and electrolyte balance. An indwelling catheter may be the most practical method in these situations. When the patient is stabilized intermittent catheterization should be considered. Because catheterizations should be performed every four hours initially and volumes maintained at less than 450 cc, it is essential that there be sufficient staff to manage the program. It is better to leave an indwelling catheter in place than to have a poorly managed intermittent catheterization program. Recent studies have shown that early intermittent catheterization does not produce any long-term advantages to spinal cord injured patients in terms of urinary infection rates, upper tract pathological abnormalities, or ultimate bladder drainage method. Urethral complications may be increased with long-term indwelling catheterization (>3 months) and these patients may benefit from suprapubic trocar cystostomy if rehabilitation will be delayed.[14]

Head trauma is a common problem that coexists with spinal cord injury. Up to 60 per cent of patients may have concurrent head injury. It is important to assess this during the acute care phase because further medical intervention may be needed and the patient's initial ability to comprehend his disability and cooperate with therapy may be limited.

THE REHABILITATION TEAM

A physician trained in spinal cord injury care coordinates the rehabilitation team and manages medical complications that may result from the spinal injury. This physician must also be responsible for the lifelong care of the patient. In the United States this physician is generally a physiatrist. Consultants in urology, orthopedic surgery, neurologic surgery, plastic surgery, psychiatry, and internal medicine may assist the physiatrist because of the complex nature of the problems the patient may develop. However, it remains the responsibility of the primary physician to coordinate this care and make all decisions with the patient's input and consent. Particular medical issues common or unique to spinal cord injury are addressed later in this chapter.

The rehabilitation nurse[15] in a spinal injury unit has numerous responsibilities beyond providing basic nursing care. Nurses work closely with the physician and collaborate with the management of skin lesions and the neurogenic bowel and bladder. The nurse also assumes a major role in patient and family teaching. This teaching includes performance of catheterization and bowel management techniques, skin inspection, and medication and its side effects. Prevention and management of complications such as autonomic dysreflexia, deep venous thrombosis, pulmonary embolism, and urinary tract infection are key areas of an educational program that enhances the quality of life and prevents long-term medical costs. The rehabilitation nurse collaborates with the therapists in ensuring that skills learned in therapy are practiced on the nursing unit.

Occupational therapists[16] provide training in activities of daily living including dressing, feeding, writing, and homemaking. They may provide splints to maintain range of motion or dynamic splints that assist in the performance of functional skills. Occupational therapists should be able to evaluate and train spinal cord injured individuals in the use of environmental controls if needed to enhance their interaction with the environment. This is particularly important for the high-level quadriplegic. Occupational therapists often collaborate with nurses in training and modification of equipment necessary for self-catheterization and bowel management.

The physical therapist's[17] primary role is enhancement of mobility skills. Teaching may begin with basic tasks such as balance, sitting, and turning in bed and then progress to more complicated skills. The physical therapist can teach wheelchair use and safe transfers, instructing family members to assist or perform these tasks if necessary. In turn, patients are taught to instruct care providers in the safe performance of these skills. Gait training with braces, canes, crutches, or other devices as needed is provided. Equipment such as wheelchairs and shower and bathroom equipment are recommended by the therapist and obtained through durable equipment firms in the patient's community.

Rehabilitation engineering is an important part of a comprehensive spinal cord injury rehabilitation center. The rehabilitation engineer may assist in the design and construction of special wheelchair modifications to improve seating posture and prevent pressure sores, and construct and modify environmental controls or other electronic and mechanical aids such as computers and electric wheelchairs.

Vocational rehabilitation counselors assist in the patient's return to work or school. They may guide the patient into new careers or work with the former employer to return patients to their former jobs. The counselor works with job placement specialists and representatives of the state offices of rehabilitation services. Driver education is an important component of vocational rehabilitation. Improvement of vocational outcomes in patients undergoing spinal cord injury rehabilitation is still needed. Employment status of spinal cord injured persons has been described.[18]

Social workers assist the team and the patient throughout the rehabilitation stay and coordinate discharge planning. They work closely with the psychologist to manage any psychosocial problems that may arise. The social worker is the main link between the patient's family and the rehabilitation team.

The clinical psychologist provides counseling services to the patient and family members. These services must be available to all spinal cord injured patients, as adaptation to this degree of injury has many difficulties. The interaction of each patient with a psychologist is therefore crucial. In addition, the psychologist should be able to provide neuropsychologic assessment to assist in the rehabilitation of the patient with concurrent brain injury or when necessary for vocational evaluation and planning. The psychologist may assist team members in management techniques to deal with patients who are having problems adapting to the rehabilitation unit.

Therapeutic recreation adds a dimension to rehabilitation far beyond a diversion for the hospitalized patient. Recreation therapists may assist the patient to return to preinjury areas of interest or to develop new interests such as wheelchair sports. Activities may occur on the nursing unit, in special recreation areas, or in the community as permitted by the patient's medical condition.

The assistance of speech pathologists and audiologists may also be required. This is most often the case when swallowing problems or concurrent brain trauma is present.

Although the rehabilitation team has been described as a group of individuals with distinct responsibilities, the key to a successful rehabilitation of the spinal cord injured person is collaboration among all team members. This is necessary for such activities as community reentry programs and wheelchair seating clinics that must be interdisciplinary. Therapists must be aware of each others' skills and limitations to achieve solutions to problems that arise as a result of the unique needs of the individual. Collaboration will yield the unique solutions necessary to foster maximum independence.[6,19]

FUNCTIONAL LEVELS AND REHABILITATION OUTCOMES

The classification system of the American Spinal Injury Association is used to define levels of injury and enhance communication for patient care and research.[20] The level of injury is defined as the last (most caudal) level with normal sensory function in all modalities and motor strength of grades 3 to 5 (fair strength) or better. The zone of partial preservation is three segments below that level, with a complete lesion defined as the absence of motor sensory function below the zone of injury. An incomplete lesion is defined as any sensory or motor function below the zone of partial preservation. This includes sacral sparing, and a patient with rectal sensation only below the

TABLE 24–1. Classification of Level After Spinal Cord Injury/Standards of the American Spinal Injury Association[2]

LEVEL	MUSCLE
C4	Diaphragm
C5	Elbow flexors
C6	Wrist extensors
C7	Triceps
C8	Flexor digitorum profundus
T1	Intrinsic musculature of hand
T2–L1	Sensory Level
L2	Iliopsoas
L3	Quadriceps
L4	Tibialis anterior
L5	Extensor hallucis longus
S1	Gastrosoleus
S2–S5	Sensory Level

From the American Spinal Injury Association: Standards for Neurological Classification of Spinal Injury Patients. Chicago, American Spinal Injury Association, 1989.

zone of partial preservation is considered to have an incomplete lesion. However, patients may have some motor or sensory function just below the last normal level of injury but within the zone of injury and their lesions will be considered complete, e.g., a C5 quadriplegic may have trace or poor wrist extension but have no motor function below C6 (considered C5 complete). The key muscles for each myotome of this classification are described in Table 24–1 and dematomes are illustrated in Figure 24–1.

Quadriplegic is defined as damage of neural elements within the cervical segments of the spinal canal. Paraplegia is defined as damage to the thoracic, lumbar, or sacral segments within the spinal canal including conus medullaris and cauda equina. These definitions exclude root avulsion and peripheral nerve injury outside the spinal canal.

The Frankel classification[20] may be used to classify injuries to the spinal cord as well. A complete lesion is Frankel Class A. Preserved sensation only, Class B, includes the presence of any sensation without the presence of spared motor function in an incomplete patient. Preserved motor nonfunctional, Class C, is defined as the presence of motor function that has no functional value in an incomplete patient. Class D is defined as the presence of useful motor function in an incomplete patient. A patient who has complete return of normal motor and sensory function throughout has a Frankel Class E lesion. These patients may have brisk reflexes. The classification of injuries based on the anatomy of the spinal cord is described in Figure 24–2.

Sensory Dermatomes
Front View

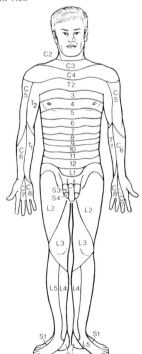

Sensory Dermatomes
Back View

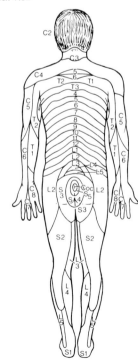

Figure 24–1. Sensory levels, standards of the American Spinal Injury Association. (Reproduced with permission of the American Spinal Injury Association, Chicago, Ill., 1989.)

Anatomical Classification

Central Cord Syndrome: Dissociation in degree of motor weakness with lower limbs stronger than upper limbs and sacral sensory sparing.

Brown-Sequard Syndrome: Modified hemisection of cord. Homolateral paralysis and contralateral sensory loss.

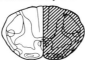

Figure 24–2. Spinal cord injury syndromes. (Reproduced with permission of the American Spinal Injury Association, Chicago, Ill., 1989.)

Anterior Cord Syndrome: Motor paralysis with hypesthesia, hypalgesia and preservation of posterior column sensory function.

Posterior Cord Syndrome: Motor paralysis with loss of posterior column sensory function. (Very rare).

Mixed Syndrome: Unclassifiable combination of above.

A

Conus Medullaris Syndrome: Injury through sacral cord (conus) and lumbar nerve roots traversing the neural canal with areflexic bladder, bowel and lower limbs.

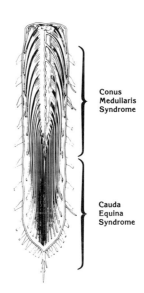

Conus Medullaris Syndrome

Cauda Equina Syndrome

Cauda Equina Syndrome: Injury below the conus to lumbosacral nerve roots within the neural canal with areflexic bladder, bowel and lower limbs.

B

FUNCTIONAL OUTCOMES AFTER SPINAL CORD INJURY REHABILITATION

Prediction of functional abilities that can be achieved following rehabilitation can generally be guided by the degree of residual muscle function.[21–24] Patients at all levels of injury will benefit from rehabilitation. Skills that the patient cannot perform must be taught through rehabilitation so the patient can guide others in the performance of these skills. An educational program for these patients, their families, and their caregivers is an essential component of the rehabilitation program. All concerned must be trained to recognize and prevent the medical and physical complications that may occur after spinal cord injury.

Skills learned in the rehabilitation setting must be generalized to the home environment and community prior to discharge to enhance reintegration into society after discharge. This can be accomplished through therapeutic weekend passes and community activities conducted during the rehabilitation stay. It is important to individualize the rehabilitation program for each patient. Patients who are motivated, if given the opportunity, may achieve goals expected for patients with greater motor skills. Allowing the patients to attempt a complex skill and determine on their own if it is feasible is more valuable than an explanation by a staff member that is often interpreted by the patient as a denial of an opportunity to achieve greater independence. Patients benefit from spinal cord injury rehabilitation at all ages.[25] Paraplegic patients who are older will have difficulty performing more complex mobility and skills required for activities of daily living. After discharge patients can be expected to maintain the ability to perform functional tasks learned during the initial rehabilitation period.[26] A description of functional outcomes and rehabilitation and equipment considerations at different levels of injuries is provided. This is intended to serve as a guide for the various levels and is not to be interpreted as a complete description of all equipment available and skills performed.

C1–C4 Quadriplegia

Rehabilitation of high quadriplegics requires sophisticated electronic equipment and a staff trained in dealing with the respiratory problems that may develop. Patients with lesions at C1 and C2 may have sparing of the phrenic nerve and be managed with implanted phrenic nerve pacemakers. (Pacing of the diaphragm may be simultaneous or intermittent.) These patients have a lesser need for equipment than do ventilator-dependent patients and are often easier to manage and discharge from the rehabilitation environment. They may also have their tracheostomies plugged or discontinued if secretions are not a problem. Patients with lesions above C4 who are ventilator-dependent participate in rehabilitation programs similar to those of the phrenic nerve pacemaker patients, although the equipment, respiratory circuitry, and tracheostomy interfere with communication and lead to greater discharge problems. Patients with lesions at the C4 level will often be free of respiratory equipment beyond the initial acute care stage but require similar functional aids to the respiratory dependent injuries.

A major component of rehabilitation in these individuals is the use of technical aids such as environmental controls.[16,27] Cooperation between an occupational therapist and rehabilitation engineer is often necessary to modify commercially available equipment for the individual patient. Equipment that may be necessary includes call systems, telephones, page turners, door openers, and environmental control units. Environmental control units may access these devices or they may be prescribed individually. Environmental control units may be simple devices that access a few appliances or complex systems activated from a remote wheelchair unit. Control options include breath control (sip and puff), mouth sticks, or mechanically activated systems. Simple systems are available commercially as well but often require significant hand function. Voice-activated systems are rarely prescribed due to financial limitations. Computers may be accessed through devices such as the Microdec,[16] which enhances word selection by selecting letters and words most likely to be selected on the basis of the letters already chosen.

Electric wheelchairs are essential at these levels of injury. They may be controlled by breath control, chin control, voice activation, or by hand control in patients with spared function. These chairs may be reclined by head-activated switches to perform pressure reliefs. A manual wheelchair will be necessary as well because the electric wheelchair may not be accessible to all environments, is not easily transportable, and may be in need of charging and repair. Lifts may be necessary for transfers as patients are dependent at this level.

C5 Quadriplegia

Patients with lesions at the C5 level have functional deltoids and/or biceps. The presence of functional biceps and appropriate splinting allows for significant improvements in functional abilities.[28] These patients may initially require use of a balanced forearm orthosis for arm placement during activities of daily living such as feeding and typing (Fig. 24–3). This device is particularly useful for patients with partial C4 lesions with inadequate elbow flexors. A long opponens orthosis provides wrist stability and utensil slots and pen holders to allow these patients to perform activities such as feeding, writing, and typing. Other less commonly used devices include the cable-driven orthosis or the electrically powered orthosis, or the ratchet orthosis that provides tenodesis similar to that used by a C6 quadriplegic. With these assistive devices, C5 quadriplegics will be able to feed with food cut up, perform oral facial hygiene with equipment set up, and assist with dressing.

Electric wheelchair propulsion may be performed with a hand control. Patients may propel a manual wheelchair with oblique projections indoors and occasionally on unlevel surfaces for short distances.

C6 Quadriplegia

Active wrist extension and the presence of the C6 component in the proximal musculature enhances functional independence. Wrist extensor recovery is common, although its return can be delayed.[29] Tenodesis, opposition of the thumb to the index finger with wrist extension, is used for functional activities. The RIC tenodesis orthosis (Fig. 24–4) is easily fabricated for tenodesis training during the early phases of training. Many patients are provided with wrist-driven flexor hinge orthosis (Fig. 24–5) to perform tasks requiring increased pinch strength such as catheterization and

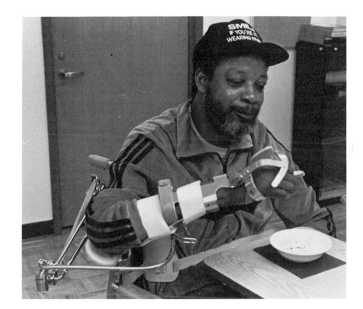

Figure 24–3. The balanced forearm orthosis.

feeding. Patients at this level often use short opponens orthosis with utensil slots and writing splints with simple D ring velcro handles to assist in performing feeding, writing, and oral facial hygiene. C6 quadriplegics usually feed with food provided, perform their oral facial hygiene, execute upper extremity dressing, and assist or are independent with lower extremity dressing. They may catheterize themselves and perform their bowel program with assistive devices.[30]

Manual wheelchair propulsion is independent on level surfaces and is enhanced on rough terrain. Vertical wheelchair projections may be required in conjunction with wheel-

chair gloves. Some patients may require electric wheelchairs for work and school. Transfers may be independent or assisted from bed to wheelchair with a sliding board.[17]

C7–C8 Quadriplegia

The addition of functional triceps at C7 greatly enhances transfer and mobility skills. C7 quadriplegics may also benefit from en-

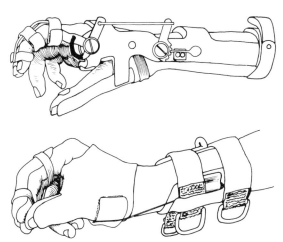

Figure 24–4. *Top,* Wrist-driven flexor hinge splint; *bottom,* RIC tenodesis splint.

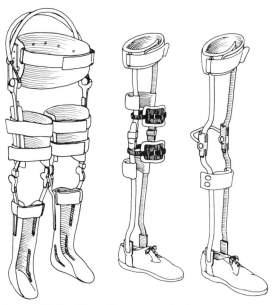

Figure 24–5. Three designs of orthosis for ambulation *(right)* Scott-Craig orthosis *(center)* standard knee ankle foot orthosis *(left)* reciprocating gait orthosis (LSU-RGO).

hanced finger extension. Tenodesis splints may be used to assist in activities of daily living, most of which are independent at this level. Wheelchair and transfer skills are markedly enhanced and wheelchair propulsion is improved on rough terrain and slopes.[23] Our center has reported a case of a C7 quadriplegic who was able to walk a short distance with a specially modified walker.[19] Although this is far from the norm, it is an example of the importance of allowing a patient to attempt functional skills far beyond that predicted at a given level of musculature functioning.

C8 quadriplegics have flexor digitorum profundus. Although hand function is not normal, there is the opportunity for total independence from a wheelchair level. C8 quadriplegics may be able to balance their wheelchairs on the rear wheels (wheelies) and independently transfer their wheelchairs into their cars. A van may no longer be necessary.[17] Homemaking tasks are more easily performed.

Thoracic Paraplegia

The T1 level is the first level with normal hand function. Because thoracic levels proceed caudally, intercostal and abdominal musculature is present leading to enhanced respiratory function and trunk balance. Patients at all thoracic levels may be independent from a wheelchair level and able to manage their bowel and bladder function. Variable outcomes at the thoracic level are often described based on various levels of injury within the thoracic spinal cord. Our studies in a large series of thoracic patients show that this is not generally true. Patients at all levels should attempt complex transfers, standing, and ambulation because most descriptions based on thoracic levels are artificial.[31]

Lumbar Paraplegia

Hip flexion is present at the L2 level, knee extension at L3, and dorsiflexion at L4. The L5 level adds the extensor hallucis longus and the S1 level adds the gastrocnemius and soleus muscles. Lumbar patients may all be independent from the wheelchair level and ambulation is common. Community ambulators generally have proprioception at the hips and ankles, good pelvic control, hip flexors, and a quadriceps muscle on one side. Lack of hip extension and abduction could be compensated for by canes or crutches and loss of ankle control with ankle foot orthosis.

Orthotic Devices

There are numerous orthotic devices that have been developed for paraplegic ambulation;[32] Figure 24–5 depicts three such devices. The standard metal upright knee ankle foot orthosis generally has upper and lower thigh bands, drop locks, a calf band, and a single action (Klenzak) or double action ankle joint. A pelvic band and hip joint are rarely added except in children as they add increased weight and energy requirements and are not necessary because patients can extend at the hips using the ligaments of the hip to stabilize.[33] The Scott-Craig[34] design with a bale lock at the knee, a patellar tendon strap, and a rigid ankle support provides a lighter weight orthosis. The knee is eccentrically placed and lower thigh and calf band closures are eliminated. Improved donning and doffing, standing, and more efficient ambulation results. There are two recent designs of orthoses that attempt to restore a reciprocating gait pattern, the reciprocating gait orthosis (RGO) or Louisiana State University orthosis (LSU),[35] and the adult hip guidance orthosis (Parawalker, HGO).[36] The RGO uses a Bowden cable system commonly used in prosthetic devices that allows alternate hip flexion as the hip is lifted and forces are transferred from the weight bearing side via extension. Although this system yields a more esthetic gait pattern, it is less efficient than the Scott-Craig orthosis and more cumbersome and expensive.[37] The Parawalker combines a pair of rigid leg braces and a rigid pelvic brace articulating with ball-bearing hinges. Hybrid systems with this brace or the RGO and functional neuromuscular stimulation have demonstrated the possibility of ambulation combining these two techniques.[38]

In spite of the development of numerous orthotic systems it is uncommon for paraplegics to ambulate at the community level.[39–42] Numerous studies have shown that with the six determinants of gait loss the energy requirement per unit distance is at least six times that of normal levels.[29,43,44] As in other disabilities, gait slows to a more tolerable level. The rejection of KAFOs for functional ambulation is therefore common.[39,40,45,46] Patients may however use their braces for other purposes. Standing for short periods to reach objects at home or work or for short exercise periods during the day is found to be of value by many. Many paraplegics exercise with their KAFOs in home with parallel bars or with a walker or crutches. Brief periods of ambulation may be necessary in environments that are not wheelchair accessible. Many patients report enhanced bowel function from these periodic standing or walking times.

There are numerous approaches recommended in dealing with the paraplegic person who would like to ambulate.[32] Although we advise our patients of the difficulties associated with ambulation—the high energy requirements and the dangers of falling—the decision to attempt ambulation lies with the patient. Temporary KAFOs are available; therefore, custom fitting is not necessary. Patients can discover on their own if ambulation is feasible and not feel that they were denied their chance to walk. The patient must first learn the necessary prerequisite skills from the wheelchair level prior to the trial of gait training. This often enhances cooperation in these areas in individuals whose only stated goal is to "walk out of here." The trial of gait training often prevents patients from seeking out other rehabilitation facilities to obtain this goal and allows them to focus on more appropriate goals without feeling imposed upon.

AUTONOMIC DYSREFLEXIA AND AUTONOMIC DYSFUNCTION

Autonomic dysreflexia (AD)[47–50] has been reported to occur in 48 per cent of patients with complete lesions above T6 and in 85 per cent of quadriplegics. It is often referred to as autonomic hyperreflexia (AHR) and generally occurs in patients with lesions at or above T6. The syndrome develops secondary to a noxious stimulus below the level of injury. The afferent signals from this stimulus are transmitted via the spinothalamic tracts and dorsal columns to the sympathetic fibers in the lateral horns. An exaggerated sympathetic response results with increased levels of norepinephrine resulting in hypertension, piloerection, nasal congestion, and sweating.

The most common symptoms are pounding headache caused by the reflex dilatation of cranial vessels, sweating, and cutaneous vasodilation. The common signs are hypertension, bladder or bowel distension, and tachycardia. Although reflex bradycardia is not commonly observed in this syndrome, it may occur. The diagnosis should not be excluded in the absence of bradycardia. Morbidity and mortality result from the effects of the hypertension. Mental status changes, seizures, and death caused by intracranial hemorrhage have been reported.[47,51]

The first step in management of AD is prevention and patient and family education. Patients with adequate bladder and bowel management who follow their prescribed programs are less likely to develop these complications. They should be instructed to monitor their fluid intake, especially if they are on intermittent catheterization, to avoid overdistension or to catheterize more frequently if fluid intake will be increased. Prescribed bowel regimens should be followed with proper diet and use of stool softeners as needed. Patients should be aware of the danger of AD and be knowledgeable of inciting factors such as tight clothing or urinary drainage leg bags, plugged or kinked catheters, pressure sores, urinary tract infections, or ingrown toenails.

Management of the acute episode rarely requires pharmacologic intervention. The patient should be sat up, tight clothing loosened, and a cause sought. Most often bladder distension is the causative factor and can be relieved by straight catheterization, unkinking or changing a blocked catheter, or draining a full urine collection bag. If a distended bladder is ruled out, fecal impaction should also be ruled out. An anesthetic ointment should be used to decrease the risk of aggravating the dysreflexia. Removal of the impaction will often result in resolution of the symptoms.

If hypertension persists, pharmacologic intervention may be indicated. Nitrates and nifedipine are easy to use and may be effective. Nitrates may be given as amyl nitrate, sublingual nitroglycerin, or nitropaste. The cutaneous preparation is useful because it can be easily removed when the inciting stimulus resolves or the episode spontaneously ceases. Antihypertensives may be necessary when the aforementioned measures fail. Hydralazine, which may be given IM or IV, is probably the most practical drug, particularly if venous access is difficult. Diazoxide and nitroprusside are effective intravenous medications but diazoxide is given via IV push, and nitroprusside is usually given in intensive care units.

Patients with recurrent AD may require prophylaxis with α-blocking agents. These should be reserved for those cases in which the etiologic factor is unknown or not controllable. Patients with AD that is predictable such as episodes associated with the bowel program may require nitrates for use at those times. Phenoxybenzamine, an α-blocker, is effective, and often only 10 mg to 30 mg is required daily.[52] Many patients use a single daily dose; some are reluctant to use this medication because phenoxybenzamine has been associated with malignancy in laboratory animals. Other effective α-blocking agents include mecamylamine, guanethidine, prazosin, and clonidine. Clonidine has recently been reported to decrease spasticity and may be particularly advantageous.[53,54]

Regular medical follow-up may identify and eliminate problems such as renal and bladder stones or ingrown toenails that may eventually cause AD. These problems should also be investigated in patients with recurrent episodes.

Sweating may be a manifestation of a noxious stimulus similar to that of AD. A cause should be sought prior to initiating treatment. Bladder stones are a common cryptic cause of sweating. Post-traumatic syringomyelia may cause sweating in the absence of other signs or symptoms. Recommended medications for sweating are mecamylamine or atropine.[52] There have been anecdotal case reports of propoxyphene decreasing idiopathic sweating.[55]

Orthostatic hypotension often interferes with remobilization after spinal cord injury. As the acute care stays have been shortened it is less of a problem. Patients should be sat up slowly in bed prior to transferring. Support hose and an abdominal binder are worn. If 90 degree sitting position in the wheelchair is not tolerated, a recliner chair is used. The tilt table may help restore postural reflexes. If physical measures are not successful, sodium chloride may be used alone or in combination with ephedrine. In rare cases use of mineral-corticoids is necessary. Long-term use of these medications is rarely needed.

Abnormalities of thermoregulation may interfere with community and other activities. Patients with lesions above T8 may be poikilothermic.[10] Precautions must be taken during temperature extremes to prevent hypothermia or hyperthermia. Patients will often report febrile episodes after being in a warm environment. This should be assessed prior to initiating a medical workup for a source of infection.

HETEROTOPIC OSSIFICATION

Heterotopic ossification is also known as ectopic bone or para-articular osteoarthropathy.[56,57] It is bone that forms in abnormal locations most often around the hips and knees after spinal cord injury. The bone is true bone as opposed to dystrophic calcification. The incidence has been estimated to be from 16 per cent to 53 per cent.[58]

There are numerous clinical presentations of heterotopic bone. It is often found on routine radiographs when it has not been clinically suspected. It may present as swelling around a joint or may first present as loss of range of motion. Heterotopic ossification may present with findings similar to a deep venous thrombosis with proximal hip swelling and distal edema resulting from vascular compression. It is crucial to rule out a deep venous thrombosis that may be life-threatening and not to assume that when heterotopic bone formation is present that a deep venous thrombosis is excluded.[57,59]

Diagnosis is made most often by plain x-ray or bone scan. Suspected heterotopic ossification with positive clinical findings may present with negative x-rays initially. Radionuclide triple-phase bone scan will often be positive in these situations.[60] Bone will be identified on the initial angiographic phase in these instances. Alkaline phosphatase may be elevated as well, but by itself is of little diagnostic value because most spinal cord injured patients have healing fractures or have undergone recent orthopaedic surgery.

Etidronate disodium (Didronel) may be used prophylactically to decrease the amount but not the incidence of heterotopic ossification.[58] Recommended dosages are 20 mg/kg daily for two weeks followed by 10 mg/kg for 10 weeks in a single dosage. The most common side effects are gastrointestinal and when they occur the dosage may be split. In the presence of heterotopic ossification, Stover recommends continuing etidronate disodium for six months to one year.[57]

Range of motion exercises are of utmost importance for joints affected by heterotopic ossification.[61] A joint not receiving ROM exercise will ultimately lead to ankylosis. The best guideline to frequency of ROM exercises is the clinical response.

Surgical resection should be considered only for a clinical benefit to the patient. The mere presence of the bone is not sufficient reason to operate. The bone should be removed if a clinical problem exists, such as joint ankylosis with decreased functional abilities or pressure sores resulting from poor positioning. Surgical complications include infection, hemorrhage, and recurrence of the ossification. Bone should generally be present from one to two years and have a mature appearance on x-ray and decreased uptake on serial bone scans. Etidronate disodium is given prophylactically prior to surgery and continued for one year.[57]

PAIN

The incidence of pain after spinal cord injury has been reported to be as high as 100 per cent. A useful classification system has been described:[62]

1. cauda equina (radicular)
2. visceral
3. mechanical (myofascial)
4. psychic
5. spinal cord (dyesthetic)

Dyesthetic pain syndrome, pain distal to the injury often described as central pain or phantom pain, may be extremely disabling. Patients often describe this pain as "cutting, burning, piercing, radiating, or tight."[63]

As with any medical problem that develops, a history and physical should be taken and any local or medical cause ruled out. Patients may have abdominal visceral complications, post-traumatic syringomyelia, or suffer from tendinitis, bursitis, or a similar condition that may occur in the general population.

Management of dyesthetic pain syndrome is difficult.[64] When the condition exists it must be explained adequately to the patient. Pharmacologic intervention should be avoided unless pain interferes with activities, sleep, or mood state. The patient should be reassured as to the nature of the pain problem and the fact that it is not a sign of a medical problem. Therapy should be initiated with the most benign medications possible. Acetaminophen or nonsteroidal anti-inflammatory drugs should be attempted initially. Transcutaneous nerve stimulation benefits a small number of patients in our clinical experience. Of the centrally acting drugs used such as phenytoin, carbamazepine, and amitriptyline, amitriptyline appears to be the most effective. Amitriptyline acts centrally to decrease reuptake of serotonin and norepinephrine. A once-daily dosage at bedtime also enhances sleep.

SPASTICITY

Spasticity is a common complication of spinal cord injuries. It is defined as "a motor disorder characterized by a velocity-dependent increase in tonic stretch reflexes (muscle tone) with exaggerated tendon jerks, resulting from hyperexcitability of the stretch reflex, as one component of the upper motor neuron syndrome."[65] Spasticity is variable but in general, initially follows a flexor pattern after the termination of spinal shock, followed by extensor spasticity in patients with lesions above the conus medullaris.[66,67]

Spasticity may interfere with positioning functional activities and can cause discomfort or safety concerns. Therapeutic intervention should be initiated with a specific goal in mind. The mere presence of spasticity is not an indication for its treatment. The patient should be made aware of the beneficial effects of spasticity such as maintenance of muscle bulk and decreased lower extremity edema prior to initiating treatment.

The basis of control of spasticity is appropriate medical and nursing management. A patient's complaints of increased spasticity may indicate a urinary tract infection, a pressure sore, or insufficient ROM exercises. Spasticity often improves when these problems are treated. Frequently, patients awakening with increased spasms may require ROM exercises in the morning, before beginning their daily routine. If this fails and bladder stones, bowel impactions, and other noxious stimuli are not found, pharmacologic intervention may be necessary.

Baclofen, diazepam, dantrolene, and most recently clonidine are most commonly used to treat spasticity. Use of these agents for long-term management is considered "justifiable if the drug produces a notable reduction in painful or disabling symptoms and permits increased function by the patient, perhaps with a need for less intensive nursing care."[64] Care must be taken not to decrease useful spasticity that may serve as an aid for transfers. The minimal effective dosage should be used and should be tapered gradually if the medication(s) are discontinued.

Baclofen is considered by many to be the treatment of choice for spasticity after spinal cord injury. Its major site of action is the spinal cord and it is equally effective in complete and incomplete lesions. Baclofen is given in dosages from 10 mg to a maximum of 80 mg daily, although there are reports of dosages beyond the maximum recommended by the manufacturer. The most common side effect is transient drowsiness, and sudden discontinuance may cause hallucinations.[67,68]

Diazepam[66-68] is a centrally acting benzodiazepine useful in management of spasticity resulting from spinal cord injury. It may be used alone or in combination with baclofen and dantrium. Use of diazepam is limited primarily by its tranquilizing properties. Recommended dosage is 2 mg b.i.d. slowly increasing, if necessary, to 15 mg to 20 mg daily. Dosages greater than this may be tolerated by some patients but most find them oversedating.

Dantrolene[66,67,69] differs from the previously described medications in that it is peripherally acting. It suppresses the release of calcium from the sarcoplasmic reticulum decreasing the activity of the contractile apparatus. Dantrium's usefulness is limited by its side effects. It may produce drowsiness, lightheadedness, or confusion. The potential for hepatic toxicity, particularly in females and patients older than 35, or in those on estrogen, limits its usefulness. Liver functions should be repeated regularly, making its usage difficult in outpatients in whom follow-up is often inconsistent due to transportation and other difficulties. Dosage begins with 25 mg twice a day and may be slowly increased to 100 mg four times a day. Dosages as high as 200 mg four times a day are rarely necessary.[66,69]

Clonidine[53,67] is an antihypertensive agent that has recently been shown to be useful in spasticity management. Clonidine's primary action is as a central α-adrenergic blocker. It may be given orally or through a transdermal delivery system. Dosage is in the range of 0.1 mg to 0.5 mg daily. Major side effects are dry mouth, drowsiness, and sedation. Hypotension may occur and the drug should be withdrawn slowly.

Invasive procedures may be necessary in patients whose condition is intractable to basic medical management and pharmacologic intervention. Motor point blocks with phenol[67,70] may selectively decrease spasticity in muscle groups that are causing particularly functional difficulties or problems with hygiene. Examples of this are local blocks to spastic hip adductor muscles or wrist flexors interfering with tenodesis.[9,67] The duration of their effectiveness is variable from months to more than one year. Although more aggressive uses of phenol such as intrathecal are possible, they convert the bladder from upper motor neuron to lower motor neuron and are rarely indicated.

Surgical procedures most commonly performed are tendon lengthening procedures, peripheral neurectomy, and rhizotomy.[71,72] The tendons most commonly lengthened are the heel cords and adductors. Posterior rhizotomies may be performed as an open surgical procedure or as a percutaneous radiofrequency rhizotomy. The procedure is often effective but recurrence of spasticity is a problem.[71]

The need for destructive rhizotomies and myelotomies may soon be replaced by continuous intrathecal baclofen.[73,74] A "baclofen pump" is placed in the abdominal wall and attached to a lumbar subarachnoid catheter. Dosages as high as 650 mg/day are programmed externally by a computer and radiofrequency transmitter. This technique described by Penn may allow for lower doses of baclofen to be used because they are delivered to the site where needed with markedly enhanced control of spasticity.[73,74]

NEUROGENIC BLADDER MANAGEMENT

There are numerous classification schemes for abnormalities of bladder and sphincter control after spinal cord injury or other nervous system trauma. The simplest classification for management in spinal cord injured persons is upper and lower motor neuron lesions.[75,76] An upper motor neuron (UMN) bladder may be described as a spastic or reflexic bladder. The isolated bladder maintains its contractile function and may contract and attempt to empty spontaneously. This action may be coordinated with sphincter relaxation, a synergic pattern or uncoordinated sphincter contraction, a dysynergic pattern. Patients with UMN bladders will have an intact bulbocavernosus reflex on physical examination. Lower motor neuron (LMN) bladders are flaccid because of the distal cord involvement. They are generally found with more distal cord lesions but may be seen with high cervical and thoracic lesions with associated lumbar fractures.

Management options for bladder dysfunction are numerous. Of major consideration in selection of a management technique is the patient's life style and preferences in cooperation with the optimal medical situation to decrease renal and bladder complications. Although a technique may be optimal medically, it should not be chosen if it will require significant assistance or require the patient to become homebound for proper and consistent performance. The performance of surgical procedures such as suprapubic catheterization on a routine basis as the preferred method of management is not justified. Several management techniques are described below. Although intermittent catheterization may be the preferred method, its practicality in each patient must be considered.

Intermittent catheterization decreases the

risks of infection and stones caused by the presence of an indwelling catheter.[45,77-81] Although some C6 quadriplegics can perform self-catheterization, it generally requires good hand function and the ability to manage lower extremity clothing in an efficient manner. The patient must be well motivated to perform the procedure on a regular basis and have adequate facilities available when away from the home environment. For patients with UMN bladder with a synergic pattern, this technique is often used until satisfactory voiding with low residuals (generally less than 100 cc) is obtained. Patients may use this technique in conjunction with medications that inhibit voiding such as oxybutynin (Ditropan) or propantheline bromide (Pro-Banthine), or with external (condom) catheters. Intermittent catheterization techniques may take advantage of the safe emptying interval as described by Wu[82] to prevent and treat urinary tract infections.

External catheters are generally used in spinal cord injured males who void between catheterizations or who have developed a balanced bladder. Patients who have contractile bladders but void with a dysynergic pattern may undergo external sphincterotomy and become free of an indwelling catheter or intermittent catheterization.[73,83-86] Patients should be aware of the difficulties associated with the usage of external catheters, such as local irritation or breakdown of the penis, and leakage and improper tight fitting leading to infection and upper tract abnormalities.[87]

Suprapubic catheters[88] offer many advantages over indwelling catheters. Complications such as penile-scrotal fistulas and urethral injury are diminished. The catheter is easy to change and long-term studies in small series of patients have not shown any major adverse long-term effects.[78]

Indwelling catheters although not ideal from the medical standpoint[76] are preferred by many patients. Ease of management and the absence of need for a surgical procedure are two advantages. Disadvantages are risks of infection, bladder stones, urethral damage, fistulas, and a reported increased incidence of bladder carcinoma. On the other hand many patients have found that this secure leak-free method allows for their easier reintegration into society and return to work. The ileal conduit should be reserved for patients with progressive hydronephrosis not managable by other means.[89]

Long-term follow-up of patients with neurogenic bladders is essential. There are three methods commonly used. Intravenous pyelo-

grams (IVP) were traditionally performed on an annual basis. This technique is invasive and may be unsafe in patients with impaired renal function or dye allergy. Poor compliance often results from the discomfort associated with the procedure. Renal ultrasound is a viable replacement for IVP.[90,91] It is noninvasive and offers diagnostic capabilities similar to those of the IVP. Renal scintography has been proposed as a more accurate diagnostic technique.[78]

Pharmacologic intervention may assist in management of the neurogenic bladder. Bethanechol (Urecholine) may stimulate bladder contraction, although its usefulness in UMN lesions has been questioned.[92] It may enhance dysynergia in high level patients by stimulating the sympathetic ganglions as well. Pro-banthine and Ditropan discussed earlier may be useful to decrease bladder contractability in patients with a spastic bladder, or in patients who prefer not to void between intermittent catheterizations. Alpha-adrenergic agents such as phenylpropanolamine or ephedrine may be both helpful and harmful after spinal cord injury. In patients with high level lesions who void spontaneously, they may stimulate the internal sphincter and inhibit voiding and enhance autonomic dysreflexia. In patients with lower level lesions, these sympathomimetic agents may be used to prevent voiding. Phenylpropanolamine (Ornade Spansule Capsules) may be conveniently administered for this purpose.

GASTROINTESTINAL FUNCTION

Abnormalities resulting in impaired defecation follow neurologic patterns similar to that of the neurogenic bladder. The goal of a bowel program is to develop a predictable time of elimination that is most effective, most convenient, and least expensive for the patient.[15]

A proper diet is essential in management of the neurogenic bowel. Sufficient fluid and fiber intake is essential. Dietary instruction and awareness of foods with high fiber content such as bran should be instituted as soon as feasible. Patients may often be asked to make a major dietary change after their injury. Stool softeners such as docusate sodium (Colace) or bulk softeners such as psyllium (Metamucil) are the most commonly used supplements. A mild laxative such as casanthranol may be used in combination with docusate sodium (Peri-Colace) when motility is a problem.

There are two general patterns of bowel regulation.[93] Patients with upper motor neuron neurogenic bowel are generally regulated with suppositories and/or digital stimulation on a daily or every other day basis. A schedule that can easily be incorporated into a person's life style should be determined. Lower motor neuron lesions are more difficult to regulate and may require manual removal. Patients often tend to decrease the frequency of their bowel program performance which may lead to fecal impaction and diarrhea. This is often misinterpreted as a primary problem and antidiarrheal agents are used that compound the problem. Specific bowel management procedures have been described by Matthews.[15]

WHEELCHAIR CONSIDERATIONS

Proper seating in a wheelchair is of utmost importance.[16,94] The seating system must allow the individual to propel the chair properly and should not contribute to spinal deformity or pressure sore development. A high back and head support may be needed for patients who cannot propel their wheelchair manually. Patients who propel their chair require freedom of movement and the back of the wheelchair should be below the scapula. A lumbar support that will maintain the lumbar lordosis or a firm back support may be necessary. The seat should be inclined to prevent forward sliding and a firm seat will prevent the sling effect and decrease abnormal positioning and pressure sore development. Trunk and arm supports may be necessary in higher levels. Difficult positioning problems may require custom molded seating systems.

Cushions will help to decrease pressure and the incidence of pressure sores. A common misconception regarding wheelchair cushions is the erroneous conclusion that they eliminate the need for pressure reliefs. Pressure reliefs every 10–15 minutes must be continued on all seating surfaces. Considerations in choosing cushions include effect on posture, transfer skills, heat, and moisture.

SEXUAL DYSFUNCTION

Sexual dysfunction in spinal cord injured males varies with the location and extent of the lesion.[95,96] Erections are more common in injured patients with upper motor neuron lesions as compared to those with lower motor neuron lesions, particularly if the lesion is more cranial in location. Reflex erections occur with an intact sacral cord and psychogenic erections that are cerebrally mediated in lower motor neuron lesions. Ejaculation increases in frequency if the lesion is caudal and is more common in partial lower motor neuron lesions. Males with incomplete lesions have better erectile and ejaculatory function.

Sexual dysfunction must be approached from two aspects. Psychological counseling, training, and education is the first component.[96,97] The second component is provision to the person of technological advances that may enhance erectile or ejaculatory function.

Restoration of erections may be mechanical, pharmacologic, or surgical. There are two commonly used external aids for the restoration of erections. Both use a vacuum system to cause tumescence of the penis. The ErecAid system[98,99] consists of a plastic cylinder and a vacuum pump after which a constrictive band is placed at the base of the penis. This is left in place for 30 minutes and decreases blood flow to the penis. The Synergist system uses a condom-like device which remains in place during intercourse. A small tube that is wrapped around the base of the device after use allows the creation of a vacuum.

Numerous medications have been used for restoration of erection.[100–103] The most common are papaverine and phentolamine each used alone or in combination. In clinical practice most patients respond to papaverine alone in dosages of 3 mg to 80 mg.[102] Use of one agent as opposed to a combination may produce less side effects. An injection is given in the proximal third of the penis in the midline of the lateral aspect.[101] Pressure and massage is then applied for several minutes. A tourniquet may be applied during this period. The major side effect is priapism and, as a result, a low test dosage should be used on the first visit. This is particularly important in patients with UMN lesions and reflex erections that are present but transient and are too brief for sexual intercourse.

Surgical management for restoration of erections involves the use of semirigid or inflatable penile prosthesis. Semirigid protheses[42,104,105] may be used for sexual intercourse and for maintenance of external urinary appliances. Spinal cord injured patients are at greater risk due to sensory loss, vasomotor abnormalities, and the associated pressure from the implant. Complications include extrusion and infection. An inflatable penile prosthesis decreases the risk of erosion; mechanical breakdown is the major problem.[106] The choice of the technique to enhance erectile function depends on patient preference and experiences with the various techniques. Patients will often choose the method they find to be most natural or simple to use. Nonsurgical treatment should be explored before using surgical means.

Fertility after spinal cord injury has been estimated at 5 per cent.[95,96] Techniques under development may increase this severalfold.[107] More caudal incomplete lesions generally have the best prognosis. The earliest technique to stimulate ejaculation was intrathecal neostigmine, which was described by Guttman.[108] This technique is not in common usage, and deaths have been reported. Recently, injection of subcutaneous physostigmine has been proposed as an alternative of choice.[19] The most commonly used techniques at this time are vibratory ejaculation and electroejaculation.

Vibratory ejaculation is noninvasive with few side effects.[74,109] It requires intact thoracolumbar sympathetics from T11 to L2 and an intact conus medullaris cauda equina reflex. The technique has been well studied by Brindley and by Sarkarati and others.[109,110] The Ling 201 vibrator at approximate 80 Hz and 2.5 mm peak to peak amplitude appears to be the most effective. Other vibrators may be used but response is variable. If success is obtained with the Ling vibrator, we attempt use of other commercially available vibrators that can be used at home. Vibration is applied to the lower ventral surface of the glans penis for 3½ minutes followed by a 1½ minute pause for four cycles, totalling 20 minutes. Vibratory stimulation usually fails within the first six months. It is usually successful if the hip flexion response is present; the hip flexes when the sole of the foot is scratched. There are contradictory reports as to whether semen quality improves with repeated attempts.

Rectal probe electroejaculation may be attempted when vibratory ejaculation is not successful. There are several devices being used for this technique.[65,110–113] Seminal emission results when the right or left obturator point is found. Patients must be monitored for autonomic dysreflexia. Pain may limit this procedure's utility in patients with incomplete lesions, and rectal mucosal damage is a possible complication. This technique causes emission by stimulating sympathetic efferent fibers. Fertility may be enhanced at all levels by decreasing scrotal temperature. A simple technique of sitting with the legs abducted in the wheelchair may be satisfactory.[22]

Normal menstruation lost after a spinal cord injury usually returns within several months to a year if affected. Fertility is usually unimpaired. Potential problems during labor include autonomic dysreflexia. Studies on sexual functioning in females after spinal cord injury are limited by small series with varying levels of injury. Sexual relationships for females with spinal cord injury may be enhanced by appropriate training and counseling.[96]

RESPIRATORY DYSFUNCTION

Respiratory problems are a significant cause of morbidity and mortality after spinal cord injury. The diaphragm is often the only functional muscle with the intercostals and abdominal muscles paralyzed. Vital capacity is diminished generally by one-third and expiratory reserve volume is markedly diminished. Rehabilitation efforts should be directed toward improving vital capacity chest mobility and cough.[15,59,114]

There are numerous methods to enhance vital capacity. Incentive spirometry encourages chest expansion. Inspiratory training devices that have variable resistance to inspiratory force are available and may enhance maximum inspiratory pressure and endurance. Exercise programs should be instituted to strengthen the remaining muscles of respiration. Diaphragmatic strengthening is an important component of this as well as strengthening of the remaining accessory muscles in the neck. Glossopharyngeal breathing[17] uses the muscles of the mouth, pharynx, and larynx to swallow air into the lungs. This technique enhances vital capacity, promotes chest expansion, and assists in weaning from the ventilator. An abdominal corset will support the abdominal contents when erect and allow for a more normal positioning of the diaphragm. This enhances diaphragmatic excursion from the erect position. Chest mobility is maintained by methods described previously such as incentive spirometry and glossopharyngeal breathing. The chest may be stretched manually as well once or twice a day to maintain or increase range of motion.

Enhancement of active expiration and cough is crucial to maintain bronchial hygiene. The clavicular portion of the pectoralis major is a muscle of active expiration in tetraplegic patients. Potentially strengthening this muscle may improve cough effectiveness and long-term respiratory outlook. Assistive cough is performed by applying pressure inwardly and upwardly to the upper abdomen. This technique enhances peak flow during cough and assists in clearing of secretions.

PSYCHOLOGICAL COUNSELING AND LIFELONG FOLLOW-UP

The clinical psychologist is a vital member of the rehabilitation team.[97,115,116] Psychological services should be routinely available to all patients. Additional support should be available from peer visitors who can share their experiences with the newly injured person. Group sessions help patients to better adjust to their disabilities and gain insight into their situation. The psychologist may be active in sexual and family counseling and in helping the team to develop strategies to foster a more successful rehabilitation outcome.

Comprehensive follow-up services of the rehabilitation team should be available to all patients. An annual history, physical, and urological workup is mandatory. Services that may not have been appropriate initially, such as vocational rehabilitation, may benefit outpatients who are ready to reach their maximum rehabilitation potential.

REFERENCES

1. Guttmann L: New hope for spinal cord injury sufferers. Paraplegia 17:6, 1979.
2. Anderson DW, McLaurin RL: The national head and spinal cord injury survey. J Neurosurg 53:S1, 1980.
3. Young, JS, Burns PE, Bowen AM, et al: Spinal Cord Injury Statistics: Experience of the Regional Spinal Cord Injury Systems. Phoenix, AZ, Good Samaritan Medical Center, 1982.
4. Stover SL, Fine PR: Spinal Cord Injury: The Facts and Figures. Birmingham, University of Alabama, Birmingham, 1986.
5. Geisler WO, Jousse AT, Wynne-Jones M, et al: Survival in traumatic spinal cord injury. Paraplegia 21:364, 1983.
6. Fordyce WE: On interdisciplinary peers. Arch Phys Med Rehabil 62:51, 1981.
7. Bedbrook GM: Spinal injuries with tetraplegia and paraplegia. J Bone Joint Surg 61–B:267, 1979.
8. Yarkony GM, Roth EJ, Heinemann AW, et al: Benefits of rehabilitation for traumatic spinal cord injury: Multivariate analysis in 711 patients. Arch Neurol 44:93, 1987.
9. Freed ML: Traumatic and congenital lesions of the spinal cord. In Kottke FJ, Stillwell GK, Lehmann JF (eds): Krusen's Handbook of Physical Medicine and Rehabilitation, 3rd ed. Philadelphia, WB Saunders, 1982, pg 643.
10. Guttmann L: Spinal Cord Injuries Comprehensive Management and Research, ed. 2. Boston, Blackwell Scientific Publications Inc, 1976.
11. Steinberg FU: The Immobilized Patient. New York, Plenum, 1980.
12. Davidoff G, Morris J, Roth E, et al: Closed head injury in spinal cord injured patients: Retrospective study of the loss of consciousness and post-traumatic amnesia. Arch Phys Med Rehabil 66:41, 1985.
13. Yarkony GM, Bass LM, Keenan V III, Meyer PR Jr: Contractures complicating spinal cord injury: Incidence and comparison between spinal cord centre and general hospital acute care. Paraplegia 23:265, 1985.
14. Lloyd LK, Kuhlemeier KV, Fine PR, Stover SL: Initial bladder management in spinal cord injury: Does it make a difference? J Urol 135:523, 1986.
15. Matthews PJ, Carlson CE: Spinal Cord Injury: A Guide to Rehabilitation Nursing. Rockville, MD, Aspen, 1987.
16. Hill JP: Spinal Cord Injury: A Guide to Functional Outcomes in Occupational Therapy. Rockville, MD, Aspen, 1986.
17. Nixon V: Spinal Cord Injury: A Guide to Functional Outcomes in Physical Therapy Management. Rockville, MD, Aspen, 1985.
18. DeVivo MJ, Fine PR: Employment status of spinal cord injured patients three years after injury. Arch Phys Med Rehabil 63:200, 1982.
19. Yarkony GM, Jones R, Hedman G, O'Donnell A: Jones-Hedman walker modification for C7 quadriplegic patient: Case study in team cooperation. Arch Phys Med Rehabil 67:54, 1986.
20. American Spinal Injury Association: Standards for Neurological Classification of Spinal Injury Patients. Chicago, American Spinal Injury Association, 1989.
21. Bergstrom EMK, Frankel HR, Galer IAR, et al: Physical ability in relation to anthropometric measurements in persons with complete spinal cord lesion below the sixth cervical segment. Int Rehabil Med 7:51, 1985.
22. Brindley GS: Deep scrotal temperature and the effect on it of clothing, air temperature, activity posture, and paraplegia. Br J Urol 54:49, 1982.
23. Bromley I: Tetraplegia and Paraplegia: A Guide for Physiotherapists, ed 2. New York, Churchill Livingstone, 1981, p 37.
24. Woolsey RM: Rehabilitation outcome following spinal cord injury. Arch Neurol 42:116, 1985.
25. Yarkony GM, Roth EJ, Heinemann AW, Lovell L: Spinal cord injury rehabilitation outcome: The impact of age. J Clin Epidemiol 41:173, 1988.
26. Yarkony GM, Roth EJ, Heinemann AW, et al: Functional skills after spinal cord injury: Three-year longitudinal followup. Arch Phys Med Rehabil 69:111, 1988.
27. Voda JA, Gordon RE: Environmental control and augmentative communication program for nonverbal physically disabled persons. Arch Phys Med Rehabil 63:511, 1982.
28. Yarkony GM, Roth E, Lovell L, et al: Rehabilitation outcomes in complete C5 quadriplegia. Am J Phys Med Rehabil 67:73, 1988.
29. Ditunno JF, Sipski ML, Posuniak EA, et al: Wrist extensor recovery in traumatic quadriplegia. Arch Phys Med Rehabil 68:287, 1987.
30. Yarkony GM, Roth EJ, Heinemann AW, Lovell L: Rehabilitation outcomes in C6 tetraplegia. Paraplegia 26:177, 1988.
31. Yarkony GM, Roth EJ, Meyer PR, et al: Rehabili-

tation outcomes in complete thoracic spinal cord injury. Am J Phys Med Rehabil 69:23, 1990.

32. Merritt JL: Knee-ankle-foot orthotics: long leg braces and their practical applications. *In* Redford JB (ed): Physical Medicine and Rehabilitation: State of the Art Reviews, Vol 1. Hanley and Belfus, Philadelphia, 1987, p. 67.

33. Warren CG, Lehmann JF, deLateur BJ: Pelvic band use in orthotics for adult paraplegic patients. Arch Phys Med Rehabil 56:221, 1978.

34. Lehmann JF, Warren CG, Hertling D, et al: Craig-Scott orthosis: A biomechanical and functional evaluation. Arch Phys Med Rehabil 57:438, 1976.

35. Douglas R, Larson PF, D'Ambrosia R, McCall RE: The LSO reciprocation-gait orthosis. Orthopaedics 6:834, 1983.

36. Patrick TH, McClelland MR: Low energy cost reciprocal walking for the adult paraplegic. Paraplegia 23:113, 1985.

37. Merrit JL, Miller NE, Houson TJ: Preliminary studies of energy expenditure in paraplegics using swing through and reciprocating gait pattern. (Abstract). Arch Phys Med Rehabil 64:510, 1987.

38. McClelland M, Andrews BT, Patrick JH, et al: Augmentation of the Oswestry Parawalker Orthosis by means of surface electrical stimulation: gait analysis of three patients. Paraplegia 25:32, 1987.

39. Coughlan JK, Robinson CE, Newmarch B, Jackson G: Lower extremity bracing in paraplegia—a follow-up study. Paraplegia 18:25, 1980.

40. Heinemann A, Magiera-Planey R, Schiro-Geist C, Gimenes G: Mobility for persons with SCI: An evaluation of two systems. Arch Phys Med Rehabil 68:90, 1987.

41. Mikelberg R, Reid S: Spinal cord lesions and lower extremity bracing: An overview and follow-up study. Paraplegia 19:379, 1981.

42. Rossier AB, Fam BA: Indication and results of semirigid penile prosthesis in spinal cord injury patients: Long-term followup. J Urol 131:59, 1984.

43. Fisher SV, Gullickson G: Energy cost of ambulation in health and disability: A literature review. Arch Phys Med Rehabil 59:124, 1978.

44. Merkel KD, Miller NE, Merritt JL: Energy expenditure in patients with low-, mid-, or high-thoracic paraplegia using Scott-Craig knee-ankle-foot orthoses. Mayo Clin Proc 60:165, 1985.

45. Nanninga JB, Wu Y, Hamilton B: Long-term intermittent catheterization in the spinal cord injury patient. J Urol 128:760, 1982.

46. O'Daniel WE, Hahn HR: Follow-up usage of the Scott-Craig orthosis in paraplegia. Paraplegia 19:373, 1981.

47. Erickson RP: Autonomic hyperreflexia: Pathophysiology and medical management. Arch Phys Med Rehabil 61:431, 1980.

48. Kurnick NB: Autonomic hyperreflexia and its control in patients with spinal cord lesions. Ann Intern Med 44:678, 1956.

49. Kursh ED, Freehafer A, Pursky L: Complications of autonomic dysreflexia. J Urol 118:70, 1978.

50. Lindan R, Joiner E, Freehafer AA, Hazel C: Incidence and clinical features of autonomic dysreflexia in patients with spinal cord injury. Paraplegia 18:285, 1980.

51. Yarkony GM, Katz RT, Wu Y: Seizures secondary to autonomic dysreflexia. Arch Phys Med Rehabil 67:834, 1986.

52. Halstead LS, Claus-Weker J: Neuroactive Drugs of

53. Donovan WH, Carter E, Ross CD, Wilkerson MA: Clonidine-effect on spasticity: A clinical trial. Arch Phys Med Rehabil 69:193, 1988.

54. Maynard FM: Early clinical experience with clonidine in spinal spasticity. Paraplegia 24:175, 1986.

55. Tashjian EA, Richfor KJ: The value of Propoxyphene Hydrochloride (Darvon)® for the treatment of hyperhidrosis in the spinal cord injured patient: An anecdotal experience and case reports. Paraplegia 23:349, 1985.

56. Kewalramani LS, Ortho MS: Ectopic ossification. Am J Phys Med Rehabil 56:99, 1977.

57. Stover SL: Heterotopic ossification. In Bloch RF, Basbaum M (eds): Management of Spinal Cord Injuries. Baltimore, Williams & Wilkins, 1986, p 284.

58. Finerman G, Stover SL: Heterotopic ossification following hip replacement or spinal cord injury. Two clinical studies with EHDP. Metabol Bone Dis Relat Res 4&5:337, 1981.

59. Venier LH, Ditunno JF: Hetrotopic ossification in paraplegic patient. Arch Phys Med Rehabil 54:475, 1971.

60. Freed JH, Hahn H, Menter R, Dillon T: The use of the three phase bone scan in the early diagnosis of heterotopic ossification and in the evaluation of Didronel therapy. Paraplegia 20:208, 1982.

61. Stover SL, Hataway CT, Zeiger HE: Heterotopic ossification in spinal cord injured patients. Arch Phys Med Rehabil 56:199, 1975.

62. Donovan WH, Dimitrijevic MR, Dahm L, Dimitrijevic M: Neurophysiological approaches to chronic pain following spinal cord injury. Paraplegia 20:135, 1982.

63. Davidoff G, Roth E, Guarracini M, et al: Function-limiting dysesthetic pain syndrome among traumatic spinal cord injury patients. A cross sectional study. Pain 29:39, 1987.

64. Davidoff G, Guarracini M, Roth E, et al: Trazadone hydrochloride in the treatment of dyesthetic pain in traumatic myelopathy: A randomized double-blind placebo-controlled study. Pain 29:151, 1987.

65. Brindley GS: Electroejaculation and the fertility of paraplegic men. Sexuality and Disability 3:223, 1980.

66. Davidoff RA: Antispasticity drugs: Mechanisms of action. Ann Neurol 17:107, 1985.

67. Merritt JL: Management of spasticity in spinal cord injury. Mayo Clin Proc 56:614, 1981.

68. Young RR, Delwaide PT: Drug therapy spasticity. N Eng J Med 304:28, 1981.

69. Young RR, Delwaide PT: Drug therapy: spasticity. New Eng J Med 304:96, 1981.

70. Wood KM: The use of phenol as a neurolytic agent: A review. Pain 5:205, 1978.

71. Herz DA, Parsons KC, Pearl L: Percutaneous radio frequency foramenal rhizotomies. Spine 6:729, 1983.

72. Kosdon DL, Lathi ES: A prospective study of radio-frequency chizotomy in the treatment of post-traumatic spasticity. Neurosurgery 15:526, 1984.

73. Penn RD, Krois JS: Continuous intrathecal baclofen for severe spasticity. Lancet 2:125, 1985.

74. Penn RD, Kroin JS: Long-term intrathecal baclofen infusion for treatment of spasticity. J Neurosurg 66:181, 1987.

Choice in Spinal Cord Injury. Houston, The Institute for Rehabilitation and Research, 1980.

75. Bedbrook GM, Sedgley GY: The management of spinal injuries: Past and present. Int Rehabil Med 2:45, 1980.

76. Borkin M, Dolfin D, Herschorn S, et al: The urologic care of the spinal cord injury patient. J Urol 129:335, 1983.

77. Guttmann L, Frankel H: The value of intermittent catheterization in the early management of traumatic paraplegia and tetraplegia. Paraplegia 4:63, 1966.

78. Kuhlemeir KV, Lloyd LK, Stover SL: Long-term follow-up of renal function after spinal cord injury. J Urol 134:510, 1985.

79. Maynard FM, Diokno AC: Urinary infection and complications during clean intermittent catheterization following spinal cord injury. J Urol 132:943, 1984.

80. Maynard FM, Glass T: Management of the neuropathic bladder by clean intermittent catheterization: 5-year outcomes. Paraplegia 25:106, 1987.

81. McGuire E, Savastano JA: Long-term followup of spinal cord injury patients managed by intermittent catheterization. J Urol 129:775, 1983.

82. Wu YC: Total bladder care for the spinal cord injured patient. Ann Acad Med Singapore 12:387, 1983.

83. Golji H: Urethral sphincterotomy for chronic spinal cord injury. J Urol 123:204, 1986.

84. Jameson RM: The long-term results of transurethral division of the external urethral sphincter in the neuropathic urethra with reference to potency. Paraplegia 20:299, 1982.

85. Morrow JW, Bogaard TP: Bladder rehabilitation in patients with old spinal cord injuries with bladder neck incision and external sphincterotomy. J Urol 117:164, 1977.

86. Schellhammer PF, Hackler RH, Bunts RC: External sphincterotomy: rationale for the procedure and experiences with 150 patients. Paraplegia 1A:5, 1979.

87. Newman E, Price M: External catheters: Hazards and benefits of their use by men with spinal cord lesions. Arch Phys Med Rehabil 66:310, 1985.

88. Grundy DJ, Fellows GJ, Gillett AP, et al: A comparison of fine-bore suprapubic and an intermittent urethral catheterization regime after spinal cord injury. Paraplegia 21:227, 1987.

89. Hackler RH: When is an ileal conduit indicated in the spinal cord injured patient? Paraplegia 16:257, 1978.

90. Calenoff L, Neiman HL, Kaplan PE, et al: Ultrasonography in spinal cord injury patients. J Urol 128:1234, 1982.

91. Rao KG, Hackler RH, Woodlief RM, et al: Real time renal sonography in spinal cord injury patients: Prospective comparison with excretory urography. J Urol 135:72, 1986.

92. Awad SA: Clinical use of bethanechol. J Urol 133:523, 1981.

93. Comarr AE: Bowel regulation for patients with spinal cord injury. JAMA 167:18, 1958.

94. Zacharkow D: Wheelchair posture and pressure sores. Springfield, IL, Charles C Thomas, 1984.

95. Bors E, Commorr AE: Neurological disturbances of sexual function with special reference to 529 patients with spinal cord injury. Urol Survey 10:191, 1960.

96. Sha'ked A: Human Sexuality and Rehabilitation Medicine: Sexual Functioning Following Spinal Cord Injury. Baltimore, Williams & Wilkins, 1981.

97. Trieschmann RB: Spinal Cord Injuries, Psychological, Social and Vocational Adjustment. New York, Pergamon Press, 1980.

98. Nadig PW, Ware JC, Blomoft R: Noninvasive device to produce and maintain an erection like state. Urology 27:126, 1985.

99. Witherington R: External aids for treatment of impotence. J Urol Nurs 6:1, 1987.

100. Am Sidi A, Cameron JS, Duffy LM, Lange PH: Intracavernous drug-induced erections in the management of male erectile dysfunction: experience with 100 patients. J Urol 135:704, 1986.

101. Brindley GS: Pilot experiments on the actions of drugs injected into the human corpus cavernosum penis. Br J Pharmacol 87:495, 1986.

102. The Medical Letter on Drugs and Therapeutics: Intracavernous injections for impotence 29(751):95, 1987.

103. Wyndaele JT, deMeyur JM, deSy WA, Clossens H: Intracavernous injection of vasoactive drugs for treating impotence in spinal cord injury patients. Paraplegia 24:271, 1986.

104. Golji H: Experience with penile prosthesis in spinal cord injury patients. J Urol 121:288, 1979.

105. Iwatsubo L, Tanaka M, Takahoshi K, Akatso T: Non-inflatable penile prosthesis for the management of urinary incontinence and sexual disability of patients with spinal cord injury. Paraplegia 24:307, 1986.

106. Light JK, Scott FB: Management of neurogenic impotence with inflatable penile prosthesis. Urology 26:341, 1981.

107. Brindley GS: The fertility of men with spinal injuries. Paraplegia 22:337, 1984.

108. Otani T, Kondo A, Takita T: A paraplegic fathering a child after an intrathecal injection of neostigmine: Case report. Paraplegia 23:32, 1985.

109. Brindley GS: Reflex ejaculation under vibratory stimulation in paraplegic men. Paraplegia 19:299, 1981.

110. Sarkarati M, Rossier AB, Fam BA: Experience in vibratory and electroejaculation techniques in spinal cord injury patients: A preliminary report. J Urol 138:59, 1987.

111. Brindley GS: Electroejaculation: Its technique, neurological implications and uses. J Neurol Neurosurg Psychiatry 44:9, 1981.

112. Halstead LS, VerVoort S, Seager SWJ: Rectal probe electrostimulation in the treatment of nonejaculatory spinal cord injured man. Paraplegia 25:120, 1987.

113. Martin DE, Warner H, Crenshaw T, et al: Initiation of erection and semen release by rectal probe electrostimulation (RPE). J Urol 129:637, 1983.

114. Haas A, Pineda H, Haas F, Axen K: Pulmonary Therapy and Rehabilitation: Principles and Practice. Baltimore, Williams & Wilkins, 1979, p. 92, 133.

115. Bracket TO, Condon N, Kindelan KM, et al: The emotional care of a person with a spinal cord injury. JAMA 252:793, 1984.

116. Tucker SJ: The psychology of spinal cord injury: patient-staff interaction. Rehabil Lit 41:114, 160, 1980.

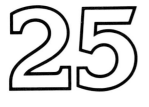# Management of Coping Problems in Spinal Cord Injury Rehabilitation

WILLIAM REINBOLD, M.D.

INTRODUCTION

Even the best adjusted spinal cord injured patient or clinician will be able to identify with the disturbed coping in spinal cord injury rehabilitation focused on in this chapter. In this discussion there will be no attempt to cover successful adaption in spinal cord injured patients.

Problems in adaption can be expected when the initial rehabilitation threatens to extend beyond six months for paraplegics or nine months for quadriplegics. A systematic mental health consultation should be done in such cases. The aforementioned timetable does not imply a finite end to the psychic recovery process. The integration of a disability into the psyche and social systems is a lifelong and dynamic process.

The clinical environment in which I acquired my experience with spinal cord injured patients is composed of staff and patients, similar in many respects to any hospital setting where spinal cord injured patients are rehabilitated. Once the context is established, observations and priorities in treatment will be presented. Requirements and expectations of staff and the patient's significant others, the patient's perspectives, and the interaction of these systems are discussed.

I hope to develop a perspective that will help clinicians who find themselves thwarted by "impossible" treatment situations. This chapter will emphasize that, despite the obvious priorities of enhancing self-accountability and

self-worth in the inordinately helpless or unmotivated patient, working for change may have to begin in the social system.

Peer support and confrontation are extremely valuable in getting patients to acknowledge how their individual ways of functioning affect the attitudes and responses of others. The staff have turned negative patient behavior into an object of study rather than viewing such incidents as unpleasant aspects of their care. This makes it easier to support patients who are extremely rejecting. Remarkably enough, defensive and distrustful patient behavior seems to lessen in the face of realistic support. How this realistic support is given to challenging patients is described in the sections that follow.

UNIT STRUCTURE

The Special Treatment Unit for Spinal Cord Injury at the Long Beach Veterans Administration Medical Center is a 10-bed individually housed unit of the 150-bed Spinal Cord Injury Service. The clinical staff includes 14 nursing staff personnel (nurses and nurse's aides), a head nurse, a psychiatric social worker, a case manager, a primary medical physician, and a psychiatrist coordinator.

The unit has accepted a mandate to treat two populations that initially appear quite different. One group includes self-motivated patients who have identified a need to address a problem with substance abuse, anxiety, pain, depression, or disruption of family or work. The other group is physician-referred. Chemical dependencies to legal or illegal substances are well represented in both categories. The unit staff, in consultation with the referring physician, determines whether patient's noncompliant, disruptive, or self-defeating behaviors warrant transfer to the unit. There is vigorous attempt to disturb maladaptive behavior styles while administering medical care. This constitutes nothing more or less than helping to make the patients more aware of how their actions and attitudes are perceived by others and how they affect the actions of others.

Avoidance is confronted by the insistence on involvement in certain activities (communal lunch, community meeting, and community outing). Provocative or attention-seeking behavior is defeated by the staff's refusal to interact with patients on their terms. For example, threats from a patient to leave against medical advice if demands are not met do not stir much overt staff interest.

There are a variety of social contexts in which the patients experience one another and the staff. The nursing staff provides 24-hour care. Other elements of the unit activity include patient and staff community meetings, psychotherapy group meetings, extramural outings, communal lunches, and staff conferences with individual patients. Material from any elements of the program may be brought into the patient conference for consideration by all members present. The clinical vignettes discussed in this chapter focus on particular observations that are covered within such patient conferences.

Treatments organized on an individual basis are individual psychotherapy, Alcoholics Anonymous step study, journal writing, and couples or family therapy. Despite my initial skepticism, some patients have benefited from family therapy with their own parents.

SAFETY

A primary goal of the program is to provide for the safety of patients and staff. The safety sought is more than protection from physical harm. Staff ability to contain provocative, violent, or masochistic behavior without loss of composure helps patients feel more comfortable expressing themselves.[1]

The patient who has come to feel that no one really cares may have become extremely hesitant to reveal certain personal feelings that may be too desperate, uncertain, or negative. Many spinal cord injured patients whose relationships are impaired suffer from the frustration of not feeling that they are really heard or understood. These patients, who may successfully interact with other patients and staff, may come to find that communications within their personal relationships are restricted.

Membership in a peer group of spinal cord injured patients and involvement with staff who are well experienced with rehabilitation provide special benefits to patients on the unit. These patients have an opportunity to interact with others in an environment in which their injury is not the most unique thing about them.

Many troubled patients have come to attribute to their injury whatever difficulty they have with others. Problems in establishing or sustaining vocational or avocational goals may be blamed too easily on the injury. Conflict within a relationship may become less resolvable when either party concludes that the injury is the problem. Yorke discusses psychoanalytic treatment in physically disabled patients whose physical disability "becomes a physical coathanger on which to put a whole psychopathological wardrobe."[2,3]

Patients and staff on the unit do not treat spasms or bowel and bladder accidents as crises. There is no need for communication to stop when such events occur. These things may happen to any of the patients and are handled matter-of-factly. Furthermore, there is no substitute for peer confrontation when one patient feels that another is overplaying the debilitating role of the injury in intergroup relationship problems.

DIAGNOSIS

When the possibility of psychiatric problems exists, an accurate psychiatric diagnosis is crucial. This minimizes unnecessary frustration for patients and staff. Ensuring that performance expectations of both patients and clinicians are realistic is very important. Overlooking a psychotropic medicine that might be indicated or raising unrealistic expectations of cognitively impaired patients are pitfalls for both patients and staff that can be avoided with effective consultation. It is convenient to consider four major categories: psychotic syndromes (such as manic depressive illness, schizophrenia, or major affective disorder); an organic syndrome (acute or chronic and transient or fixed); anxiety disorders; and character disturbances. A more comprehensive breakdown of these categories is purposefully left to other sources, since psychiatric differential diagnosis is beyond the scope of the chapter. A fifth possiblity, which can leave the referring clinician feeling empty handed, is a patient for whom no psychiatric label applies.

In fact, the point at which psychiatric consulation is requested may lead to collective disappointment. Utilizing a psychiatric consultant as a final approach to a frustrating clinical situation can raise unrealistic expectations. When, for example, no new diagnosis is made or no changes of medicine are indicated, there may be the feeling that the consulation was worthless. Depending upon the consultant's familiarity with the particular treatment environment, he may also feel that the contribution has been limited. It does take a rather thorough knowledge of the treating environment to engineer new approaches that might involve the whole social system of clinicians and significant others.

Any inpatient or outpatient facility serving spinal cord injured patients may need to cultivate mental health resources. There may need to be a way of recognizing limitations for both parties in the consultation. The mental health consultant may need to become comfortable with not being able to effect much change in a difficult clinical situation while working with the patient alone. Equally important are expectations that the primary caregivers place on the consultant. Care providers may be told, for example, that no clearly defined disorder exists that is treatable and that a violent patient may be more appropriately dealt with by the legal system. Likewise, observations and comments on the interactions of staff may be seen as more threatening than helpful.

There is another source of reluctance in calling mental health consultations that bears further discussion. The clinician may think that calling a psychiatrist is a recognition of clinical failure. He may consider the consultation request an extremely unkind thing to do to the patient and a further risk to an already strained relationship. Even patients with a clear sense of their own mental suffering and a desire for help usually are threatened by a psychiatric consultation. Who would expect an individual adjusting to the profound challenge of spinal cord injury to be any less wary of criticism than any patient whose mental fitness is being questioned? Calling consultations sooner when trouble is suspected rather than later when crisis is at hand could do much to mutually enhance each party's sense of clinical competence.

DEMANDS ON CAREGIVERS

The 30 minutes of each weekday staff meeting are crucial in the maintenance of clinical perspectives and priorities emphasized throughout this chapter. This regularly occurring forum provides mutual support to caregivers and helps guarantee respect for the burdens placed on the individual team members. It helps the treatment team reach consensus, minimizes splitting by the patients, and is the principal mechanism through which limits on undesirable behavior are achieved.

Any remarkable patient behavior is reported. Throughout the day, team members list on a blackboard any negative events such as noncompliance with turning for skin pressure relief, medication refusals, unsafe cigarette smoking, verbal or physical threats to other patients or staff, leaving the unit without permission, and clinical signs of substance use. Staff members' responses to such activities and considerations of the overall state of each patient's treatment are considered. Issues of patient and staff safety are evaluated and restrictions may be applied.

The restrictions in an increasing order of severity are: 24-hour ward restriction; time-limited radio or TV restriction for the bedridden; smoking restriction when applicable; and discharge for substance users who are medically able to leave. Substance users whose medical condition prohibits discharge may be placed on ward restriction until medically fit to be discharged.

Staff consensus is particularly important in deciding when a patient conference may be needed. Some of the aforementioned restrictions are delivered to the patients after the staff meeting. However, when a more long-standing or dangerous pattern exists, a patient conference may be called.

For example, a patient began to jeopardize his renal function by seriously limiting his fluid intake. He received neither restrictions nor extra solicitation to drink from nursing staff. Instead, at a patient conference he was told the natural history of impending renal failure in the hospital. It was explained that at any point he could experience clouding of consciousness, he could be declared incompetent, and emergency procedures such as a central line placement could be performed without his consent. He then became accountable for his own fluid intake and proceeded to interact with the staff in less dangerous ways.

The approach of conducting the patient conference with members of all disciplines attending conveys concern for the patient and dictates limits within which the team will be engaging the patient around the specific conflict. Many patients who are inordinately helpless, frightened, lonely, or aloof attempt to interact with nursing staff in regard to elements of nursing care. Such patterns are quickly discerned and evaluated in the half-hour staff meeting. When indicated, staff assistance for meals, hygiene, or dressing may be time-limited. The patient is then encouraged to have his emotional needs met through the psychotherapy group, through spending less-structured time with peers, or through more traditional verbal interchanges with nurses and other staff. An added benefit of a patient's learning to consolidate and organize his care is his help in making it easier for attendants to care for him.

The non-nursing staff, who lead the psychotherapy groups, know from the staff meetings how each patient is relating to nurses. The group therapists are able to emphasize priorities discussed in the staff meeting that immediately precedes the group. Furthermore, the non-nursing staff in the staff conference can support nurses in the very difficult role of setting limits.

For example, a patient may complain in a group meeting that none of the nurses really cares about him or want to help him. Attention might then be drawn to pervasive patterns of his relating to others on whom he depends in or out of the hospital. Such a patient may have been through multiple changes of attendants in recent history, or his family and friends may have actually abandoned him because of his neediness. Group members can share their observations of his functioning and challenge the utility of his approach to nurses. Fellow patients, after all, are receiving care from the same staff and are present 24 hours a day to observe their peer's functioning.

The unit staff strives to standardize all aspects of care. Special treatment is conscientiously avoided. Requests for care to be postponed until a particular staff member is available for its delivery are regularly denied. Each patient is assigned a primary nurse. The primary nurse is the agent through whom any changes in care plans are made. Patients who require assistance with bowel and bladder care or showering cannot expect such help during treatment program hours. Requests for repositioning or transferring in or out of bed are expected to occur on a two-hour interval set for each patient. This is the interval at which patients are turned for skin pressure relief.

In summary, the staff holds as a major priority the maintenance of a consistent and predictable system of care delivery. For purposes of staff and peer observation, how each patient functions within the system then reflects more his individual style than a random collection of personality clashes with caregivers and peers. A benefit beyond the data thus generated is that nurses have a priority other than trying to please the patient on his terms. They concentrate their efforts on creating a standardized care environment, providing a system with which the patient can begin to make compromises.

CONFLICT ENGAGEMENT

One suggestion for managing patients with behavioral difficulty is to assess as thoroughly as possible the avenues of conflict expression. Some clinicians have difficulty discussing with members of other disciplines their sometimes disparate priorities. This may frequently involve difficulty with thinking about a problem patient from even a greater number of frustrated perspectives than one's own. Clinicians, especially those less experienced, may have trouble being candid about frustrations that difficult patients may evoke.

An example of conflict avoidance can be in the chronic administration of anxiolytic or hypnotic agents. Despite their toll on short-term memory and therefore learning, benzodiazepines are often administered on an ongoing basis to spinal cord injured patients. Changes of dose or specific chemicals within this class of drug often mediate conflict on the clinical scene.

It takes practice to stop doing for others what they can do for themselves. This is a major nursing priority on the unit that often takes a period of adjustment for new nursing personnel. This is true not only in the physical realm such as assisting in transfers, dressing, and eating but also in keeping to schedules and commitments or even making important decisions.

Patients on the unit must specifically request any assistance that they require any time that they may require it; a morning routine is not developed by the nursing staff *for* the patient. The absence of a set routine gives the patient practice in directing others who are required to help and forces mental and verbal effort by the patient in efforts to relate to others. Furthermore, it eventually becomes impossible for patients to hide attitudes toward caretakers from fellow patients and the staff when nothing occurs automatically without the patient's involvement.

Two ways of coping with intense feelings of negativity in a social context are to split them off or act them out. Either route constitutes a covert action, an act of denial. "Splitting" as a way of organizing one's interpersonal world consists of rigid differentiation between those people whose loyalty and good intentions can be trusted and those who operate in bad faith. Choosing one individual or a group of people to hate and choosing to idealize others is one way of avoiding contaminating feelings of despair, envy, humiliation, contempt, and exploitation. One then imagines that such problems can be avoided by avoiding such negative people. In patients, this usually motivates requests to be cared for by only one or two staff members. Staff refusal to cooperate on the patient's terms undermines the success of this approach. To act out feelings is to act in ways that give expression to attitudes about others without acknowledging them verbally or even consciously. Excessive demands for staff attention is a frequently encountered problem for staff dealing with difficult patients. It may become the subject of a patient conference. It may be pointed out to such a patient how he involves staff and even other patients in himself only through requests for assistance. He may require support in broadening his avenues of approaching others.

NARCISSISTIC INJURY

Narcissistic injury to patients refers here to disillusionments experienced by patients with themselves or their treatment. Narcissistic injury to clinicians refers to a sense of failure in providing relief of suffering and problems of overidentification with patients. To overidentify is to be thrown off course by the patient's behavior. That is, the clinician may become so overwhelmed by "putting himself in the patient's shoes" that he does not listen to the patient, thereby clouding professional judgment.

Patients who have experienced intense deprivation or isolation from satisfying human contact often develop significantly negative views and expectations. That is, it is preferable to be prepared for the worst than caught by surprise by a successful manipulation or exploitation at the hand of one who has been carelessly trusted. A cautiousness develops in the patient. Finding that people are merely being nice could interfere with expectations and leave the patient feeling baffled by contradictory feelings.

Consider the case of Diego. In his late fifties, this street-wise alcoholic became quadriplegic when as a pedestrian he was struck by a car. One attitude that was extremely prominent throughout months of staff conferences was Diego's expressed alienation from any useful people. Anything that was being accomplished in his rehabilitation was by his long suffering alone. The staff were regularly portrayed in his staff conferences as ogres who were impeding his progress. The staff continued to feel remarkably unappreciated, despite their constant care and concern. When his impaired breathing capability necessitated their helping him cough by pressing on his stomach they restricted him from smoking. They also implemented the benzodiazepine (Valium) detoxification required of all patients entering the program on chronic treatment with such agents. In order to force development of workable portions of his upper extremities, they insisted that he use a manual wheelchair rather than an electric one. They also repositioned him every two hours to prevent the development of pressure sores.

One reaction to suddenly being in the crisis of having to experience more negativity, emotional confusion, and uncertainty about the future than one can handle is to split the load among significant others. Frequently in the treatment unit the staff and fellow patients are really all the individual has left.

In a patient/staff conference well into his clinical course, the staff agreed that progress had been made when he began to articulate the view that the nurses were merely carrying out their responsiblities. Although there was still a measure of contempt for their loyalty to the doctor, his negativity toward them began to lessen.

The 1950 film "The Men" accurately depicts episodes of narcissistic rage in both the spinal cord injured patient and his physician. There are a number of scenes in which the recently injured Marlon Brando becomes enraged when fellow patients, nurses, physicians, or his fiancée persist in attempts to interact with him when he would much prefer being left alone. His physician, who ordinarily handled a variety of responsibilities to patients, families, and staff, the morning after the loss of one of his patients to infection blasts his ward of patients for their passivity and expectations of him to perform magical cures.

The physician's outburst had most to do with his expectations of himself. Whether he saw himself as having to keep death away, provide perfect protection from suffering, or never act as though he had ever been adversely affected by suffering, any such magical expectations may have been at stake. (In the film, the physician does suppress his distress rather quickly as he moves on to the next patient.) One very helpful support to any clinician is the sense of not having to manage the treatment by himself. Integrating fully members of all disciplines involved helps share the burden of seeing spinal cord injured patients through their difficult rehabilitation.

ARTIFICIAL SOCIAL SYSTEM

Drawing attention to the artificial nature of the staff and patient milieu may serve a variety of aims. In the initial patient conference with staff, the patient is usually asked to consider the luxury of never having to see any fellow patient or staff member again once treatment is complete. This is said with the hope that the patient might feel less obligated by preset expectations of people well known to him or with whom he expects to have ongoing contact. Projections may become more readily subject to contradiction by actual peer and staff performance in areas emotionally sensitive for the patient. Furthermore, the risks of experimenting with new methods of interaction with others in one's emotional world may be lessened within the context of this interested but temporarily assembled collection of others.

Birk, in writing about integrating types of psychotherapy (individual, marital, group, milieu), draws attention to the usefulness and completeness of information about patient functioning that can be generated by following the therapeutic process in more than one modality.[4]

A fundamental problem seen in many spinal cord injured patients who complain of feeling isolated from family members or others pertains to the patient's perception of what others can tolerate. Many such patients avoid conflict to a degree that important interpersonal difficulties are merely tolerated but are never resolved. The psychotherapy group provides an opportunity for honest feedback as to how others are affected by revelations of distress, unhappiness, discouragement, and irritation.

An unfortunate number of spinal cord injured patients with impaired coping seem to be operating at the perceived limits of others' patience and understanding. It is as though there is no room for further risk within important relationships. The identified patient's family will often complain that their loved one never speaks up over distress or gives fair opportunity for resolution of conflict.

There are a number of possible ways to encourage experimentation with one's peer group. Patient and staff community meetings on a regular basis can provide a forum for the acknowledgment of differences and the support for valued ideas and activities of others. This can serve as a remarkably powerful antidote to isolation and feelings of helplessness in being able to influence anything positively. A community meeting can provide highly articulate feedback from peers and staff. Like a psychotherapy group, it permits new opportunity to risk engaging others in previously untried emotional areas.

Such opportunity need not be limited to patients. Staff can also benefit and grow in their comfort in supporting patients beset with significant coping difficulties. For example, a patient who is extremely negative and rejecting of others (such as Diego) might be affecting staff and peers similarly. It can be very difficult to be realistically supportive of a person who is functioning in a highly rejecting way. When staff members find patients experiencing similar frustration with one of their peers, they may feel much less inadequate in the face of "impossible" patient demand. In this way the patients can even identify with the clinician's frustration and thereby provide a measure of support to the caregiver.

Hospital Fairy Tale vs Extramural Reality

A perspective frequently overlooked in treatment planning around difficult spinal cord injured patients (recurring pressure sores, socioeconomic failure, chemical dependency) is the integration of intramural and extramural realities of patients while they are in the hospital. The clinician's view may become so restricted or desire to effect positive change may be so profound that short-term obtainable clinical goals may be substituted for more comprehensive possibilities.

One particular group of responses, "symptom chasing," falls into this category. Treating a good night's sleep as too high a priority may be distracting attention from learning the nature of sources of intrapsychic turmoil that might be keeping the patient awake or helping the patient to resolve daytime problems in structuring physical and/or mental activity that naturally fatigue him. Chronic use of sleeping medication only further distorts the natural biology of sleep rhythms and invites, particularly with increasing doses, a degree of daytime sluggishness. However, patient and clinician may tacitly agree to the mutual expectation that the doctor may be doing something helpful.[5] Even when the physician believes that a reliable mental health resource exists in which the patient can work out difficulty, the undermining effect of one or another medication may be underestimated.

Similar problems exist in attempts to treat anxiety chemically or to remove all sources of anxiety while in the hospital. Expecting upset family members to go easy on the patient or to take over some of his responsibilities or decision-making while he is an inpatient may temporarily remove him from problems but may only further insulate him from potential resolutions. In the earlier section on conflict engagement, methods through which staff and patient began to cooperate in embracing rather than fleeing from or insulating each other from the patient's turmoil are discussed.

A crucial piece of clinical data emerged around one quadriplegic man named Edward, through observation of his behavior within the unit's artifical social system when it included or lacked his wife's presence. After some weeks on the unit, Edward's chronic grimacing and focus on abdominal pain gave way to periods of enjoyment in interacting with other patients and staff. Feeding time became obviously more pleasurable. He entered into the psychotherapy group and there are in photographs that document his joyful participation in relay races on one of the community outings.

However, his wife's visits always seemed to precipitate his presenting symptoms of marked suffering with pain. It seemed that the couple had fallen into a rigid pattern for coping with his situation of being injured. He suffered and consequently she felt sorry for him.

Furthermore, he was denied the opportunity to create social encounters that did not include her, despite his capability of getting around the community independently in his electric wheelchair. Although his wife may have complained to the staff about her husband's pain, she was not willing to permit Edward's experimentation in interacting with others in his situation as he had for a time on the unit. He felt that he was in no position to disagree with her.

DRUGS

Use of neuroleptics and larger doses of antidepressants is best left to a psychiatrist. However, in this section some drugs are discussed that have unique usefulness in spinal cord injury. Some of the drugs or uses included here are not necessarily commonly prescribed by psychiatrists.

Spasms

Baclofen (Lioresal), an analog of gaba-butyric acid, has an inhibitory effect on spasms through its effect on the nervous system. Most patients are not bothered by possible adverse effects of drowsiness, insomnia, or confusion. It is important to determine whether, for any reason, there has been a precipitous withdrawal from this otherwise rather innocuous drug. If a more orderly withdrawal cannot be instituted (whether the patient is suddenly NPO or suddenly uncooperative), a neuroleptic may be required to control such psychotic symptoms as hallucinations or disorganized thought processes.

Dantrolene (Dantrium) is a peripherally acting muscle relaxant. Although there seems to be advantages to its not having much effect on the central nervous system, its usefulness is limited by the nonspecificity of the muscle relaxation. That is, help with spasms is achieved at the price of having decreased use of all skeletal muscle.

Benzodiazepines have previously been introduced in the section on conflict engagement. I regularly include in an educational module for newly injured patients some words about "symptom chasing." That is, attempting to treat anxiety, spasms, or sleeplessness chronically with benzodiazepines can easily evolve into a treatment that is ultimately worse than the original set of problems. Specifically, tolerance for the desired primary effects of the drug, relative withdrawal between doses with rebound spasms, anxiety or sleeplessness, and the inevitable short-term memory impairment further debilitate the individual. Tolerance refers to an increasing dose requirement for accomplishment of a desired effect. To continue indefinitely increasing a benzodiazepine daily dose leaves the patient vulnerable to increasing impairment of memory and consequently learning.

The clinician should take into account the endpoint of benzodiazepine use when committing a patient to use of such agents. The majority of patients referred to the unit for problems of noncompliance or inordinate helplessness either are currently or have at some point been given ongoing benzodiazepine treatment.

Memory impairment can usually be demonstrated in the sometimes subtle yet clear impairment in concentration that lead to a lost interest in reading or other tasks requiring retention of ideas, such as watching a movie and following the story. This subtle sign of cognitive impairment may be too easily lost in a clinical impression of depression. I believe that the diagnosis of depression tends to be overused by clinicians who have not had extensive experience with spinal cord injured patients. It may be easy for the clinician to turn episodes of sadness or irritability into a full-blown clinical depression warranting antidepressant use.

Pain Associated with Spasms

Low-dose antidepressants (Tofranil, Elavil, and Sinequan at 25 mg–50 mg t.i.d.) may be useful for pain and/or anxiety. A single trial dose helps establish whether the patient can use the drug without oversedation. Sedating side effects often lessen within a few days of use. Narcotics may work well but cannot be used chronically for the profound level of tolerance that develops to pain relief.

CONCLUSION

An effort has been made to share some treatment strategies and perspectives with clinicians who face problems of inordinately helpless, violent, chemically dependent, or self-defeating spinal cord injured patients.

Acknowledgment

At the exclusion of many dedicated clinicians, the author gives special thanks to Gail Capone, Mary Martin, RN, and Marta Perez, MSW. These three individuals have contributed in special measure the combination of bullheadedness and sensitivity required for the unit's success.

REFERENCES

1. Reinbold W: Drug intoxication, psychiatric crisis and assaultive spinal cord injury patients. In Eltorai, Ibrahi M (ed): Emergencies in Chronic Spinal Cord Injury Patients. Washington, DC, Eastern Paralyzed Veterans Association, 1984, p 177.
2. Castelnuovo-Tedesco P: Psychological consequences of physical defects: a psychoanalytic perspective. International Review of Psychoanalysis 8:145, 1981.
3. Yorke C: Some comments on the psychoanalytic treatment of patients with physical disabilities. Int J Psychoanal 61:188, 1980.
4. Birk L: Behavioral/psychoanalytic psychotherapy within overlapping social systems: a natural matrix for diagnosis and therapeutic change. Psychiatric Annals 18:296, 1988.
5. Hartmann E: The Sleeping Pill. New Haven, CT, Yale University Press, 1978.

26 A Changed World: Socioeconomic Problems of Spinal Cord Injured Patients

CARLETON PILSECKER, M.S.S.W.

A spinal cord injury seldom creeps up on you. Occasionally a disease process gradually impinges on one's mobility and feeling; symptoms associated with spinal cord injury increasingly appear. But ordinarily paraplegia or quadriplegia strikes in a moment and the world once known—the world that one could easily traverse and manipulate and interact with in long-established, sometimes automatic ways—is instantaneously gone. Even everyday language no longer fits. "The next step" is literally impossible. Your well-wishers say: "Cross your fingers and hope for the best," but you can't do the former, and so you wonder about the latter. And what does the greeting card's "Get Well Soon" message mean to you?

Society can be largely indifferent to the fact that the world has changed drastically for spinal cord injured persons, thus leaving most of the responsibility for "adjusting"—that complex, challenging, often frustrating process that begins in the unfamiliar, frightening, pain-producing, sometimes supportive environment of a hospital—to the injured themselves. Actually, for a significant period of time immediately post injury, the hospital constitutes the patient's world. It is here that the newly injured person first learns the meaning of the new label "disabled," fights against some of its portents, succumbs to others, and comes to more or less "accept" the fate that has been inflicted. Along the way, hospital staff assists or impedes the patient's progress.

Primary intentions of hospital staff are to assist the injured patient. Physicians diagnose and treat the conditions associated with the injury expertly. Nurses provide care and comfort humanely and well. Therapists manipulate immobile limbs, teaching and encouraging knowledgeably. Psychologists offer meaningful counseling. Dietitians specify and advocate health-inducing food choices. Vocational counselors give realistic guidance concerning the world of employment. Social workers provide plentiful opportunities for evaluating the patient's present and future options and open the door to a variety of significant community resources. One of these patients' first substantial social tasks, postinjury, is to decide how to partake of this largesse—how to chart their own course, how to establish some measure of control over events, when, still unsure of the duration and ultimate extent of personal limitations, they are given a welter of orders, directions, suggestions, advice, and information by staff. A significant contribution, then, that staff can make to the patient's successful negotiation of this task is, whenever possible, to "speak with one voice." Multidisciplinary planning for and with the patient is essential.

Even with sound multidisciplinary planning and good intra-staff communication, this task may be complicated for some patients when they have a different rehabilitation goal from that of staff. The staff members who engage in the explicit development of goals for patients are predominantly well imbued with the American ethic of maximizing one's independence. This becomes the underlying theme of the program they provide. Many patients accept such

291

a goal and strenuously pursue it in spite of being frustrated and discomforted at times. Some patients, however, have different definitions of personal fulfillment; maximum comfort, sympathy, or service from others may be what is primarily sought. Then the patient quickly becomes labeled "non-compliant," "unmotivated," and "manipulative," and staff are tempted to diminish their efforts on the patient's behalf.

Independence is both important to and functional for patients. In our society its pursuit can and should undergird the rehabilitation program. Staff therefore need to acknowledge, as nonjudgmentally as possible, the existence of individual variance from traditional staff determined goals and, when it occurs, to try to minimize adverse reaction.

At times, even when strongly committed to the goal of independence, patients may stray from the course prescribed for them by staff. If the patient is mostly cooperative, compliant, and personable, this noncompliance is tolerated. If not, the pejorative labeling process may be generated. To avoid this—since it helps neither patient nor staff—it is well to recognize that the patient who is moderately noncompliant in the hospital is often the one who proves most adept at achieving maximum independence in the world.

SOCIAL RELATIONSHIPS

Soon after injury the patient must begin to deal with its impact on significant social relationships. Anxious family members and friends appear at the bedside and each party wonders and worries about the future. Obvious changes arise in relationships: spouses seek divorce; parents are unable to accept the unhappy new reality and discontinue significant contact with their disabled son or daughter; friends no longer find themselves having something in common with the spinal cord injured person; and the patient, on the basis of more-or-less-accurate reality testing, terminates meaningful relationships. But such events, especially when it comes to family members, are the exception rather than the rule. Usually important people remain important to the injured person, who must assess which aspects of relationships will remain unchanged and which must be different.

This concern cannot be completely resolved while the patient is hospitalized. Time back in society—perhaps considerable time—is necessary before all the strands of significant relationships are once again in place. Nevertheless, the task begins early on, so the rehabilitation program needs to provide a variety of methods for patients to experience and to explore how their relationships are now to be constituted. Encouragement of family members' attendance at therapy sessions can enable all concerned to understand the patient's possibilities, limitations, and struggles. Patient/family education programs and consumer-oriented books and pamphlets about spinal cord injury also contribute to this goal. Individual counseling sessions between social worker or psychologist and the patient or family members, in family counseling sessions, and in group counseling can help clarify options for all parties. When the patient is physically able, day passes, weekend passes, and days of residing with family in the rehabilitation unit's special patient-family living area are crucial experiments whose teaching value needs to be optimized through individual and group opportunity to discuss them afterward with staff.

One special area of social relationships that generates much question and concern is the sexual, both in terms of the injured person's ability to be satisfied and to satisfy a partner, as well as the ability to produce offspring. Patients, because of their anxiety about their sexuality and in spite of their usual eagerness to reestablish themselves as sexual beings, cannot be rushed into trying out their sexual capabilities. A follow-up study of 30 spinal cord injured men who had been rehabilitated at the Long Beach, California VA Medical Center, reported that six months following discharge, 16 had not been sexually active since their injury. Twenty-nine of the 30 reported being sexually active before injury; 8 of the now sexually inactive 16 were married and living with their wives.

How one will be accepted into the wider community is also a matter of concern following spinal cord injury. Important words of advice that spinal cord injured patients rehabilitating for a considerable time pass on to their more recently injured compatriots is that "the rehabilitation hospital staff is used to you; the world is not." And the converse is true: the patient, since injury, has related almost exclusively to hospital personnel within the official and unofficial rules of an institutional setting. The reintegration into the outside world can be made easier with the experience provided by passes and by outings. It is also beneficial to hear from and interact with "old injury" people through panel discussions, formal peer counseling programs, and use of a roster of spinal cord injury people from the local community, and to take part in the social networks on the wards, lunch rooms, and day rooms of the hospital. The formal rehabilitation program can also assist by providing social skills training: educational sessions involving discussions, videotapes, and role playing focused on the social opportunities and dilemmas an injured person can expect to encounter and positive ways of reacting to them.

FINANCES

Financial concerns are considerable in the spinal cord injured and his family as they begin to wonder about their debts to the hospital and its care providers. If the patient has been the primary wage earner, concerns center on basic living expenses and the adjustments that will be necessary; also whether alternative resources are available. Until the time comes when the injured person can return to significant employment—if it comes at all—the means of putting food on the table and paying bills becomes a central issue. The knowledgeable social worker will give crucial assistance as these concerns surface.

If it were possible to look ahead to the time of their spinal cord injury, perhaps the injured person would do one of three things: (1) sign up for a comprehensive insurance policy that not only would pay all medical and hospital costs but also provide a considerable ongoing income; (2) plan to be injured in such a manner that someone else—more likely, someone's insurance company—would have to come up with a seven-figure payoff; or (3) enlist in the armed forces and become injured by some means other than their own dereliction. In the latter case the person would have a fairly substantial, tax-exempt lifetime income. Many people who become spinal cord injured but do not have either adequate medical coverage or plentiful financial resources to fall back on will need to rely on society's "safety net" programs: Medicaid, Social Security Disability, Supplemental Security Income, Aid to Families with Dependent Children, Workmen's Compensation, or Veterans Administration Pension, until and unless they resume employment. The benefits of these programs are far from gener-

ous and, with the added burden of ongoing personal and health care costs, the injured person will likely wind up in difficult financial straits. Almost regardless of the eventual outcome, however, it is important for the patient and family to learn early what immediate resources are available and that there are long-term options with which the social worker can assist.

EMPLOYMENT

As rehabilitation progresses, the possibility of the injured person returning to former employment will become increasingly clear, although the matter may not be fully resolved until the injured person attempts to return to and function at work following hospital discharge. During the past few years considerable strides have been made in devising altered work environments and modified tasks for the spinal cord injured employee and, occasionally, some employers have adopted flexible work hours to accommodate the injured person's new capabilities. Computers have created a world of work that can be uniquely adaptable to even severely injured people. Buildings, sidewalks, and transportation have become significantly more wheelchair accessible, making employment possibilities considerably better than they once were. Vocational counselors, both in the rehabilitation setting and in state agencies, have a correspondingly enlarged opportunity to provide a service with a concrete payoff for their clients. However, some previously employed spinal cord injured people will not return to work because the rewards of whatever work is available will not outweigh the difficulties their injuries have created. Others will find themselves sufficiently well compensated for their injury that employment is no longer necessary. Some choose not to work because it would mean losing the financial benefits they receive with uncertain prospects of earning enough additional money to make it worthwhile and of being able to sustain substantial employment.

Vocational planning may require attention to renewed, revised, or newly generated educational endeavors. Visits to nearby college campuses during rehabilitation can give clear evidence of their accessibility and, with assistance from the Handicapped Students' Coordinator, of the college's interest in making further education a viable and rewarding pursuit. And, if nothing else, such visits are a useful way for getting young people who are injured into contact with young people who are not.

HOUSING

The prospect of discharge from the rehabilitation setting requires attention to the matter of housing. Only the rare individuals whose mobility is scarcely impaired can think of returning to their former home completely comfortably. Most will have to attend to at least the placement of ramps, widening of doorways, and altering of the bathroom so it is both accessible and useable. In this, as in many aspects of the new altered lifestyle, the amount of money available will be a key factor. Some patients will be unable to return to their previous housing, and the challenging task of locating affordable, wheelchair accessible living quarters must begin. A consideration for a number of patients will be the availability of Dial-a-Ride or wheelchair accessible public transportation that provides contact with the patient's important locales. Dial-a-Ride services, in some areas, have very limited span and problematic, if any, transferability from one jurisdiction to another.

Wheelchair accessible housing has been increasing in recent years, partly in response to state and local legislation mandating that a certain percentage of new apartments accommodate disabled people. These are not yet easy to find, however, unless a person has more than usual financial assets. The federal government, through the Department of Housing and Urban Development (HUD), has a program that partially subsidizes rents for disabled people. These "Section 8" funds are limited, however, and it is not unusual in some cities for applicants to wait several years before a subsidized apartment becomes available for them.

AIDES

A crucial question for many patients approaching discharge from the rehabilitation hospital is: Who will be providing necessary assistance? For some this will mean someone to do household chores and for others someone also to provide personal care. Our society tends to assume that the spouses will take on most, if not all, assistance duties. However, even the most dutiful spouse will occasionally need help and many patients will need to hire someone regularly or occasionally as their aide. Some

limited state monies are available to partially defray the costs of assistance for low-income disabled as are some Veterans Administration funds for veterans who meet certain eligibility criteria.

Not all devoted spouses choose to make themselves available for the patient's care—opting, for example, to continue or take up employment to provide a reliable income. Not all spouses are physically capable of providing care, even with all available equipment. Some are willing to take on part, but not all, of the patient's care. Bowel care is an area that often is the most difficult for the spouse to accept. Likewise, some patients refuse to let their spouse provide bowel care, fearing an adverse effect on their overall relationship and, at times, on their sexual relations. Others decide that the spouse will be called on for this critical service only in emergencies or when they are traveling and their customary arrangements are not possible.

Both the amount and kind of care needed and the availability of "natural" helpers (spouse, parents, other family) will determine the extent to which community resources will have to be enlisted. The person with limited personal care needs will likely find the necessary help to be available from a home health agency (e.g., visiting nurse association); in some of these situations Medicare may assist with or meet the costs. The person who requires a live-in attendant, on the other hand, will probably discover it to be a substantial challenge to meet the care requirements. In recent years there has been a welcome increase in community training programs for people interested in working as aides for the severely disabled. However, there is still an insufficient supply of well-trained, reliable attendants. The patient needs someone who is knowledgeable and stable; whose personality fits comfortably with that of the patient; and who will perform sometimes arduous, unpleasant tasks at all hours of the day and night for less than substantial wages. It is small wonder that this challenge is not easily met! For this reason, patients sometimes unwisely agree to be cared for by too-willing family members who are not capable of handling the responsibility, or they sometimes coerce reluctant family members into taking it on. In both cases the arrangement seldom persists profitably for long.

Hiring an attendant is a new experience for almost all recently injured patients. Staff can be helpful by assisting the patient to think carefully about which care needs must be met, about the time intervals that various kinds of assistance will be necessary, the time off duty that the aide will have, the house rules that should be formulated (e.g., whether drinking is allowed), and how patient and attendant will interact apart from the carrying out of care needs (e.g., whether they will eat together, watch TV together, or share social occasions). Some disabled people have found it difficult to be both employer and friend. Some attendants have been overwhelmed by being expected to meet the social and emotional needs as well as the physical needs of their employer. For some patients it can be helpful to have a chance in advance to "role play" the interview with a prospective attendant. In addition, social skills training can usefully include a segment on how to interact successfully with an aide.

LEISURE TIME

A spinal cord injury may well require a change in some of the patient's leisure activities. What was once comfortable and enjoyable may now be impossible or take more effort than it is worth. Some rethinking and experimenting in this area will occur in the patient's free moments during rehabilitation. The matter may not be fully settled until long after rehabilitation is complete. However, evidence of the possibilities available even to the severely disabled needs to be widely shared during the rehabilitation period. Until fairly recently even spectator sports were mostly inaccessible to wheelchair-bound people. Not only has that changed for the better, but both individual and competitive sports once thought out of reach for the spinal cord injured person are now commonplace. "Disabled" no longer necessarily equates to "inactive," unless the injured person so chooses.

LENGTHY HOSPITALIZATION

Hospitalization for most people is a brief experience. Although it may be a severe disruption, the patient is usually shielded from life-in-the-world problems while in the hospital. In contrast, hospitalization following spinal cord injury may last for several months. During this time, an array of socioeconomic emergencies can occur requiring the patient's attention: family members can become seriously ill or die; spouses bring news that a son has been suspended from school and a daughter is illegiti-

mately pregnant; homes left uninhabited are broken into and ransacked; and pets are left unattended. As a consequence, the patients' energies may be diverted from their rehabilitation program until these difficulties are attended to. At times a patient may need to leave the hospital briefly to bring about a resolution.

Isolation from the ongoing life of one's family and community can also interfere with one's concentration on rehabilitation. To miss the spouse's birthday party, the parents' silver wedding anniversary, the birth of a child, the daughter's prom, or the son's graduation may leave the patient wondering about ever again being part of the once familiar and gratifying social network. Such thoughts can be enervating, making it difficult to find the energy necessary to maximize therapy.

The length of hospitalizaton also contributes to a possible relationship dilemma for some patients and staff. The patient is wondering how much now has to be subtracted from life and how much attraction, if any, the patient still holds for other people. As a young man who formerly prided himself on his success at winning affection from young women—what can he expect now? As a middle-aged man who before injury was struggling with whether or not he could still interest women—is there any hope left? As a young woman who enjoyed flirting with and receiving appreciative attention from young men—will anyone look or respond now? Staff are the people who, for months, the patient interacts with most. Therefore, the natural tendency is for the patient to try to get the answers from them, especially when these caregivers are in close physical contact: the nurses who provide personal care and the therapists who touch and prod and move limbs. This means that staff have to be clear both about what is prompting patient behavior and what their own relationship boundaries are in order to minimize the possibility of misleading patients about what can be expected from them.

LIFE IN THE WORLD AFTER REHABILITATION

Once rehabilitation is over, full-time life in the "real world" begins. Then the process of testing one's old and new social roles gains momentum. Some will be fortunate enough to be able to pick up—as spouse, parent, employee, friend, hobbyist, church member, student— pretty much where they left off. Others, by virtue of the extent of their injury or the particular choices they make about how to cope, will considerably recast their daily activites. The former breadwinner may become the stay-at-home parent. The former patrolman may become a police dispatcher. The person whose once favorite activity was dancing may transform into a ham radio operator. The weekend camper and vacation traveler may turn into the house-bound invalid. The person who, before injury, never imagined having artistic ability may emerge as a talented painter. Quickly for some and more slowly for others the questions—What do I now expect of myself? and, What do others now expect of me?—will be answered, and then asked again and reanswered.

After living in the world for a while, spinal cord injured people often report an acceleration of the awkward experiences they began encountering early in their disability: "People stare at me," "Children ask ridiculous questions about me," "Some jerks think I'm totally helpless." They tell of embarrassing moments when their chair tipped over or when they had an involuntary bowel movement. They report surprises: "My neck gets sore from looking up all the time." "People have a hard time understanding what I can and can't do." Nevertheless, their surprise mostly comes from discovering that, in general, other people are both kind and appropriately helpful.

Maintaining consistent attendant care often proves to be the most formidable task for the severely disabled. Even devoted spouses get tired and need a vacation now and then or have a personal or family emergency that requires them to have to abandon their care responsibilities temporarily. Recognizing this, some hospitals offer respite care programs that enable the injured person to be admitted for a limited period of time while the spouse rests or attends to other duties.

Quadriplegics needing to hire attendant care frequently must adjust to a series of caretakers. Not since their mother was their care provider have they required such personal attention from others. Fidelity can scarcely be expected or demanded when the burden is heavy and compensation is low. Attendants who can find other employment options will likely take them. Those for whom there are no options may be incapable of providing good care and the disabled person will, in frustration, terminate employment. Turnover is high and the search for a good aide recurs often. Occasionally its lack of success leads the injured person, reluctantly, to enter a nursing home for a pe-

riod of time. A nursing home bed can usually be found for a cooperative spinal cord injured person. However, if substance abuse, hostile behavior, or psychiatric illness complicates heavy care needs, the prospect of locating a willing nursing home may become quite dim. The ventilator-dependent quadriplegic who has managed to corral the extensive resources necessary to live in the community will probably be particularly disadvantaged should care attendant(s) become unavailable. Nursing homes will not accommodate this patient and even hospitals may decline to admit. Specialized facilities for ventilator-dependent people are both rare and very expensive.

PRUDENT/NONPRUDENT LIFESTYLES

Being back in the world means encountering the full range of socioeconomic problems that beset everyone, plus a variety that are mostly reserved for disabled people. The way they play themselves out in the lives of the spinal cord injured illustrates a noteworthy fact concerning this population: there is a continuum with injured people whose overall behavior can be characterized as prudent on the one end and those whose overall behavior can best be described as imprudent on the other.

Some people become spinal cord injured essentially by accident. They conduct themselves reasonably, cautiously, and prudently, but fate inflicts an automobile accident or a fall. After a period of adjustment to their injury they basically return to their former prudent lifestyle, not immune to socioeconomic difficulties. A Social Security check gets lost in the mail; an attendant becomes ill. They may need temporary assistance with the financial or care emergency that is generated. Sometimes temporary assistance is not easy to locate. If housing is the problem, for example, very few missions—the community's housing resource of last resort—can accommodate people confined to a wheelchair. Thus the prudent person may be severely frustrated.

On the other end of the continuum are the people who conduct their lives impulsively, recklessly, and nonprudently. They drive too fast on their motorcycles; they dive into shallow water; they get behind the wheel of an automobile while under the influence of alcohol or drugs; they attempt to hold up a convenience store. For them, socioeconomic emergencies are just one facet of their emergency-inducing way of living. One day a large, lasting result of their lifestyle manifests as a spinal cord injury. Their approach to life will probably not change, so when they return to society from a rehabilitation hospital, they choose friends and housemates who will take financial advantage of them. They select aides who cater to their vices, who will be co-indulgers with them in their self-destructive habits, and who are impulsive and in need of immediate gratification and therefore provide unreliable, inconsistent, or inadequate care.

The lifestyles of many spinal cord injured people fall in between the two extremes on the prudent-nonprudent continuum. Their lives are more or less emergency-inducing and impulsively conducted. However, the fact that nonprudent people tend more often than prudent people to become spinal cord injured means that emergencies, chaos, and disruptiveness will be more evident in a spinal cord injured population than in the general population. Hospital staff, therefore, have to beware of stereotyping and of inaccurately painting all or most spinal cord injured patients with the same unflattering brush.

AGING WITH A SPINAL CORD INJURY

A critical impetus to the development of comprehensive treatment and rehabilitation programs for spinal cord injured people came from the large number of such injuries created during World War II. Veterans from that era still remember being told that they had a life expectancy of six months, or one year, or, at best, two years. However, that picture has changed remarkably so that the spinal cord injured, now with an essentially normal lifespan, are experiencing, along with many others in our society, the pleasures and problems of aging. However, these problems are additions to what the disabled already struggle with. Re-

tirement from work and withdrawal from social and recreational activities may come earlier than planned or desired. Increasing care may be needed at the same time that the spouse is gradually losing care-providing ability. Finances may well become tighter as additional hired assistance and equipment are needed. The nursing home, which few spinal cord injury people opt for early in their injury career no matter how disabled they are, looms larger as a possible necessity.

CONCLUSION

Generally speaking, people who have been spinal cord injured for several decades are neither nostalgic nor bitter about the years since their trauma. They do not romanticize their experience (e.g., few describe the injury as making them a better person), they continue to wish they had not been injured, and they talk of adjustment to rather than acceptance of the injury. There is grateful approval of the changes that have occurred in society: improved accessibility, better transportation, and overall more enlightened attitudes in the general public. Some express appreciation bordering on amazement for the devoted care they have received from spouses. Life has not been easy since injury and most would not want to do it again, but even for the most severely disabled there have been rewards as well as burdens, accomplishments as well as deprivations. They remember clearly the circumstances of their injury; it was the moment the world changed dramatically for them.

Acknowledgment

The author expresses appreciation to Marc Sisman, MSW, Spinal Cord Injury Social Worker, VA Medical Center, Long Beach for his contribution to the development of this chapter.

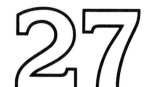

Human Analog Representation in Biomechanics and Biodynamics as Related to Spinal Cord Injury Management and Assessment

PAUL H. FRISCH, M.S., and GEORG D. FRISCH, M.S.

Spinal cord injuries resulting in a loss of motor and/or sensory function constitute one of the most catastrophic medical conditions known. A patient's life is permanently altered as a result of the severe and permanent limitations in physical function. The data presented by Kraus[1] report that the majority of spinal cord injuries result from transport-related causes, primarily motor vehicle collisions. However, minimal data exist on the specific details of the crash/impact event as related to resulting neurologic damage. Researchers attempting to identify injury mechanisms associated with transitory acceleration and crash/impact scenarios commonly utilize human analog surrogates to simulate the biodynamic response of humans to these environmental conditions. These analogs have included cadavers, nonhuman primates, and manikins. As documented by Frisch,[2,3] computer simulations have been utilized to model human interactions with the said environment. However, strong dependency on a database of human response for validation and verification limits the

application to specific areas in which extensive human data exist.

The use of manikins for test and evaluation of escape systems (ejection seat), restraint systems, physiological acceptability, and injury potentials is well documented by both the military and automotive communities. However, in the past, extensive sensors and instrumentation requirements, necessary to provide the six degree of freedom information required to precisely define the time history of selected points that correlate anatomically, required large volumes to be dedicated for instrumentation mounting. These large volumes and rigid mounting structures have limited the deformation characteristics of the manikin, thereby minimizing the degree of biofidelity attainable.

This chapter focuses on the research, development, and application of a modified state-of-the-art Hybrid III manikin, fully instrumented, supporting 96 analog data channels, coupled with a microprocessor-based data acquisition and storage system. The transducers measuring injury that correlate to manikin response parameters are incorporated to provide sufficient fidelity to enable direct comparison between dummy-based data and known human response to shock and acceleration environments. This manikin test article is self-contained, is exportable to various test facilities, and enables a consistent experimental protocol to be maintained.

The spine is a mechanical structure in which vertebrae articulate with one another through a complex arrangement of joints, ligaments, and levers, stiffened by the rib cage. The spinal stability is a result of neuromuscular control. This structure provides physiologic motion between the head, body trunk, and pelvis, transferring the weight and bending movements of the head and body to the pelvis. Determination of the mechanisms of injury is crucial in understanding spinal trauma and selecting the appropriate management techniques. In order to characterize the mechanism of injury, it is necessary to establish a quantifiable and repeatable test platform, enabling measurement of the forces and movements at various locations at the head, neck, and spinal column. This platform must also exhibit a response approximating that of its human counterpart to a driving function acceleration or shock.

Attempts to quantify the dynamic response of the human body (primarily head, neck, and spine) and the associated injury potential of high acceleration environments have been limited because of experimental protocols and hazardous environment. Human volunteer tests, through necessity, impose limitations on the acceleration levels investigated; however, these data create a quantifiable database of known response mechanism as a function of acceleration input, enabling the validation of various human analogs. The use of cadavers and live nonhuman primates affords the possibility of approaching the acceleration environment of interest; however, the significant differences in human response based on this type of human analog have not resolved the problems of assessing and correlating the injury mechanisms to their human counterparts.

The use of instrumented biodynamic manikins, with sensors measuring injury that correlate to response parameters, incorporating sufficient biofidelity to enable direct comparison between this type of human analog data and known human response to the shock and acceleration environments, has been widely investigated and utilized by the military. Accelerations resulting from emergency egress (aircraft ejection) and crash/impact events introduce a variety of head, neck, and spinal injuries. The development of this type of instrumented human analog (manikin), designed to exhibit human biodynamic and mechanical properties, has enabled the correlation of test data to human response data, and provides a method of quantitatively measured accelerations and forces at various locations that anatomically correlate.

In the design and development of a biodynamic manikin, three separate and interrelated areas need to be addressed:

1. Biomechanical requirements of the manikin
2. Instrumentation requirements of the manikin
3. System requirements of the manikin (data acquisition)

The manikin must maintain all biodynamic and mechanical properties necessary to exhibit the biofidelity to approximate the three-dimensional human response. Additionally, the manikin must provide a mounting platform housing all instrumentation and system components, enabling the measure of acceleration, loads, and forces at various anatomic locations.

MANIKIN DEVELOPMENT

The earliest recorded testing involving an anthropometric dummy was conducted by Start and Roth (1944) of the Dornier Werke in the development and testing of an ejection seat for the D0335 aircraft. This dummy was a simple wooden form used primarily for ballasting the seat with representative body weights. Today's GARD-CG dummies, typically employed for escape system testing, serve more as an instrument platform than a test article to quantify seat-occupant interaction. For dynamic tests, they provide a convenient structure to mount instrumentation and telemetry packages and serve as ballast to alter seat acceleration profiles. They are used to represent typical anatomic segment cross sections subjected to windblast and to detect deficiencies in clearance envelopes provided.

The Hybrid III manikin, chosen by the Navy to update testing protocols dealing with escape and safety equipment, is illustrated in Figure 27–1. It is a state-of-the-art manikin for which test data is available, and has been standardized as a test article that has been used by var-

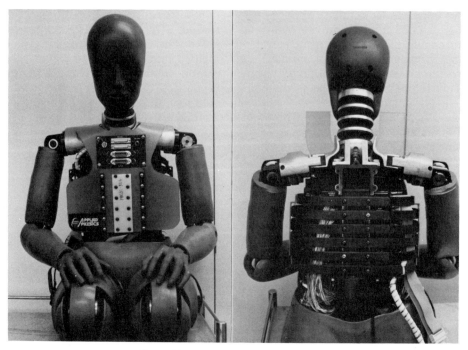

Figure 27–1. The Hybrid III manikin.

ious laboratories with promising results. Furthermore, it is a flexible manikin capable of three-dimensional response to an omnidirectional input and consequently exhibits realistic interaction with the restraint systems employed.

The development of Hybrid III by General Motors can be traced back to 1971 (Hybrid I). Its history, objectives, and attributes closely parallel the advances attempted in attaining a high degree of repeatability and improved biofidelity. Attributes that drove the performance and engineering specifications concentrated on standardization of parts, interchangeability and ease of repair, designated instrumentation locations, improved test reproducibility, incorporation of biomechanically based geometry, weight distribution, and segment moment of inertia.

The Hybrid III head consists of an aluminum shell covered by constant-thickness vinyl skin over the cranium. The neck exhibits a one-piece biomechanical bending and damping response in flexion and extension. Three rigid aluminum vertebral elements are molded in butyl elastometer, which provides high damping characteristics. Aluminum and plates attach the segment to the head and thorax, with a steel cable running through the center of the neck. The thorax of Hybrid III consists of six ribs connected to a welded steel spine. The whole assembly is ballasted for correct weight and center of gravity location. This spine provides for attachment of the neck, clavicles, ribs, and lumbar spine.

The lumbar spine is a curved polyacrylate elastometer with molded endplates for attachment to the thorax and pelvis. Two steel cables run through the central section. The lower body has correct weight distribution and is ordinarily cast in a seated position. The hip joint is a working joint and the gluteal and abdominal cast has been modified to allow for leg extension under parachute opening loads. A detailed description of the Hybrid III can be found in reference 4.

INSTRUMENTATION REQUIREMENTS

The manikin instrumentation must be considered as an integral part of any manikin development or modification effort. Proof of biofidelity will rest on the caliber and quantity of data gathered, accuracy and compatibility (in comparison with biomechanics database) of responses measured, and possible effects of sensors on the response of the manikin itself. Consequently, in addition to the structural evolution indicated, instrumentation capabilities were expanded and incorporated into the design to measure orthogonal linear acceleration components of the head and chest, the sagittal plane reactions (axial and shear forces and bending moment) between the head and neck at the occipital condyles, chest deflection, and axial femur shaft loads. For the aviation environment, this instrumentation capability has to be expanded to address injury locations and modalities that are unique, as well as to provide a capability to relate monitored human surrogate test data to biomechanics and biodynamic response data obtained in controlled laboratory experiments as well as to historical accident investigations and reconstructions.

The most recent and comprehensive review of acceleration related injuries (1972 to 1980) in the helicopter environment is that of Shanahan.[5] The distribution of spinal fractures was primarily in the T11 to L4 region, with the highest incidence, by far, occurring at L1. Naval ejection seat related injuries (1969 to 1979), as reported by Guill,[6] are concentrated in the T6 to L1 region, with principal modes at T7 to T8 and L1. Cervical injuries, concentrated at C2, were also evident, attributable primarily to parachute opening shock, canopy penetration, parachute riser entanglement, and possible aerodynamic lift created by the helmeted head during high airspeed ejections. As described by Frisch,[7] the latter aspect was in fact indicated in a recent 600 KEAS ejection test utilizing a Hybrid III manikin. Consequently, monitored manikin responses from these areas that correlate anatomically must be obtained, in sufficient degrees of freedom, to make possible an effective injury analysis and prediction. The minimum instrumentation requirements are shown in Figure 27-2. Both angular and linear acceleration components must be available to fully define the dynamic response of any rigid anatomical segment, such as pelvis, first thoracic vertebral body (T1), and head. Additionally, since compression, flexion, extension and rotation, and the associated forces and moments will be utilized to gain insight into injury mechanisms, inclusion of such measures at critical locations was also considered a basic instrumentation requirement. The

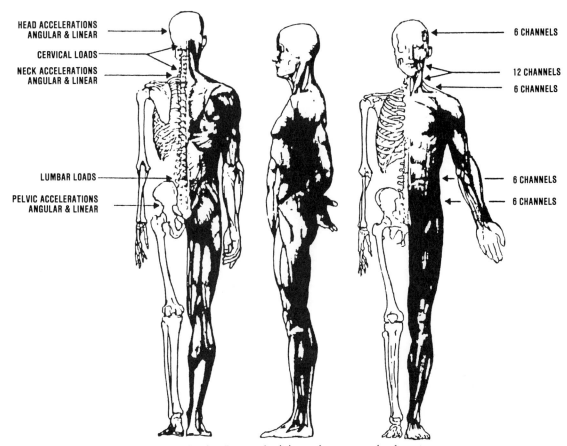

HEAD ACCELERATIONS ANGULAR & LINEAR

CERVICAL LOADS

NECK ACCELERATIONS ANGULAR & LINEAR

LUMBAR LOADS

PELVIC ACCELERATIONS ANGULAR & LINEAR

6 CHANNELS

12 CHANNELS

6 CHANNELS

6 CHANNELS

6 CHANNELS

Figure 27-2. Proposed minimum instrumentation layout.

minimal manikin supporting instrumentation system consists, therefore, of 36 channels of information. Since the driving functions of the seat must also be known to determine input-output relationships, an additional six channels are warranted.

With the sensor arrangement shown, the dynamic response of the respective segments of interest is completely defined at locations corresponding to a high incidence of injury. Additionally, transmission of forces up the spine, emanating from the pelvis and terminating at the head, can also be used to evaluate seat-man interaction and restraint efficacy, since the three-dimensional acceleration time history and relative displacement of the individual segments are known or can be calculated. In most applications, data have to be translated to points other than those directly instrumented, either to obtain estimates of responses that cannot be directly monitored or as an independent measure used as a cross check to establish accuracy of monitored values. In manikin tests, as an example, one might want to calculate accelerations or torques at the head pivot and only the head center of gravity (CG) acceleration measurements are available. Similarly, in the case of human runs, monitored "head" accelerations may have to be translated from the instrumentation mounting platforms to the head CG or the occipital condyles, since one cannot directly monitor responses at those lo-

cations. Correlation between the instrumentation coordinate system and the anatomic coordinate reference system is illustrated in Figure 27–3. The transformation of the linear and angular accelerations at the instrumentation coordinate system to their corresponding value at the anatomical coordinate system is easily accomplished by the use of direction cosine transformation matrixes documented by Frisch.[8] Body referenced inertial acceleration of a point fixed in a moving rigid body is expressed as a function of triaxial accelerations, angular rates, and angular accelerations about the respective orthogonal axes (Fig. 27–4). The sensor configurations selected to measure these responses have been detailed by Frisch[9] and consist of subminiature linear accelerometers, angular rate sensors, and angular accelerometers. They are state-of-the-art and have a history of successful utilization in both human biodynamic research and escape system and crashworthy seat testing. Their miniaturized designs are ideal for manikin applications, since they are lightweight and easily incorporated into the manikin segments for response analysis. All are commercially available, off-the-shelf items that have been proven to be dependable, require little or no maintenance, and are in keeping with performance capabilities of the data acquisition, storage, and telemetry systems.

In addition to the inertial instrumentation,

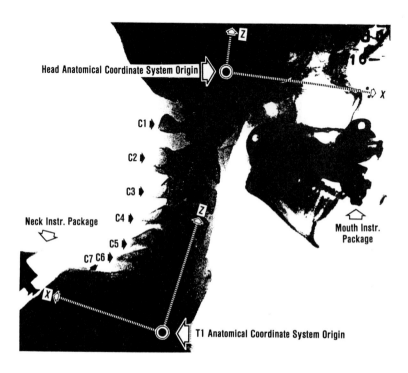

Figure 27–3. Definition of head and neck anatomic coordinate systems. Note the location of mouth and neck instrumentation packages.

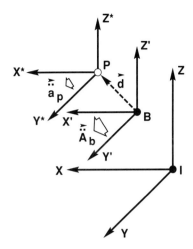

Figure 27–4. Variables required to define 6 DF of motion.

$$\textcircled{1} \quad \ddot{\vec{A}}_p = \ddot{\vec{A}}_b + \ddot{\vec{a}}_p + 2\textcircled{\times}\vec{w}_b \textcircled{\times} \vec{v}_p + \vec{w}_b \textcircled{\times} (\vec{w}_b \textcircled{\times} \vec{d}) + \dot{\vec{w}}_b \textcircled{\times} \vec{d}$$

If system P fixed relative to System B then:

$$\ddot{\vec{a}}_p = 0$$

$$\ddot{\vec{v}}_p = 0$$

$$\textcircled{2} \quad \ddot{\vec{A}}_p = \ddot{\vec{A}}_b + \vec{w}_b \textcircled{\times} (\vec{w}_b \textcircled{\times} \vec{d}) + \dot{\vec{w}}_b \textcircled{\times} \vec{d}$$

$$\textcircled{3} \quad \begin{array}{l} \ddot{A}_{xP} = \ddot{A}_{xB} + w_{pB}(w_{rB}d_y - w_{pB}d_x) - w_{yB}(w_{yB}d_x - w_{rB}d_z) + \dot{w}_{pB}d_z - \dot{w}_{yB}d_y \\ \ddot{A}_{yP} = \ddot{A}_{yB} + w_{yB}(w_{pB}d_z - w_{yB}d_y) - w_{rB}(w_{rB}d_y - w_{pB}d_x) + \dot{w}_{yB}d_x - \dot{w}_{rB}d_z \\ \ddot{A}_{zP} = \ddot{A}_{zB} + w_{rB}(w_{yB}d_x - w_{rB}d_z) - w_{pB}(w_{pB}d_z - w_{yB}d_y) + \dot{w}_{rB}d_y - \dot{w}_{pB}d_x \end{array} \left. \begin{array}{l} \\ \\ \\ \end{array} \right\} \begin{array}{l} \text{NEED:} \\ \ddot{\vec{A}} \\ \vec{A} \\ \vec{w} \text{ or } \dot{\vec{w}} \\ \vec{d} \end{array}$$

six axis load cells are also incorporated at the head-neck, neck-thorax, and lumbar spine–pelvis junctions. Figure 27–5 demonstrates the monitored data in the head-neck area. The inertial instrumentation at the manikin head CG (shown on the left) provides the angular and linear acceleration components around the head coordinate system axes. With this information, and knowing the relative location of the head pivot, torques around the atlanto-occipital (primarily a hinge joint) and atlanto-axial junction (primarily a rotating joint around the odontoid process) can be estimated. The six axis load cells, measuring flexion, extension, lateral bending moments, and shear forces, as well as axial and lateral compression and extension loads, provide independent measures of the calculated values. Similar ar-

guments can be made for the neck-thorax (N) and lumbar spine–pelvis junctions.

SENSOR CONFIGURATIONS

There are basically four instrumentation options available to quantify the six degrees of freedom motion of the segments monitored (Fig. 27–6). The first is a combination of three linear accelerometers (measuring the X, Y, Z responses) and rate gyros measuring the angular velocities around the respective axes. Differentiation of the angular velocities provides the estimates of angular accelerations required to solve the equations of motion. In the second option, angular accelerations are monitored directly and the data are integrated to obtain an-

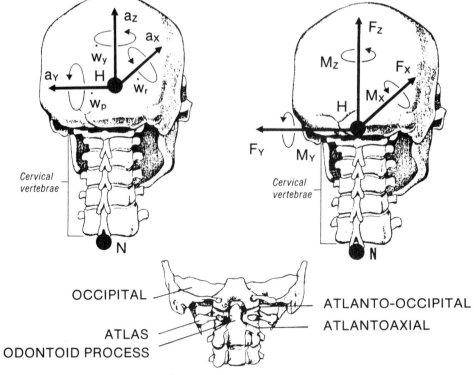

Figure 27–5. The monitored data in the head-neck area.

gular velocity estimates. Option 3 uses an array of six accelerometers, where angular accelerations are derived from differences in the respective linear accelerations measured, divided by the distance separating them. It should be noted that the cross terms involving the angular velocities are derived from the angular acceleration terms in the previous time step. Consequently, derivations conducted at time "t" are directly dependent on existing conditions at time "t–1." This has some solution stability implications, and instrumentation packages based on such an array should not be employed in long pulse duration events. Finally, under the last option (option 4), a cluster of nine accelerometers can be used to obtain separate estimates for both the angular accelerations and angular velocity cross terms (equations not shown), and these estimates are functions solely of differences between respective linear acceleration terms existing at time "t." This provides for increased stability over option 3 but still suffers under the experimental run time constraint, making it unappealing for ejection seat testing covering the catapult, rocket, and parachute opening shock phases.

SIGNAL CONDITIONING REQUIREMENTS

Because of the many advantages associated with digital techniques, continuous time signals (x(t)) are usually processed using analog to digital (A/D) conversion. Two questions arise immediately: first, the choice of sampling period (Δt); second, the quality of the sampled signal when compared with the continuous time signal (reconstruction error). The sampling theorem predicts that if the power of x(t) is limited to a band less than $\Delta t/2$ Hz, then sampling at the interval Δt enables unique reconstruction of the function x(t). This, of course, assumes that the power spectral density (PSD) exists and that the PSD, Gx(f) = 0 for all f greater than B where B is the bandwidth (folding frequency).

A problem arising from sampling data is undersampling of a waveform. If a sinusoid of frequency higher than $\Delta t/2$ Hz is sampled at a rate of $1/\Delta t$ samples per second, then the sinusoid will appear as a lower frequency. This aliasing is directly related to the sampling frequency, and since there is no guarantee that one is always dealing with band-limited signals,

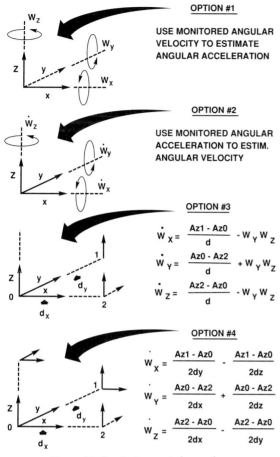

OPTION #1

USE MONITORED ANGULAR
VELOCITY TO ESTIMATE
ANGULAR ACCELERATION

OPTION #2

USE MONITORED ANGULAR
ACCELERATION TO ESTIM.
ANGULAR VELOCITY

OPTION #3

$$\dot{W}_X = \frac{Az1 - Az0}{d} - W_Y W_Z$$

$$\dot{W}_Y = \frac{Az0 - Az2}{d} + W_Y W_Z$$

$$\dot{W}_Z = \frac{Az2 - Az0}{d} - W_Y W_Z$$

OPTION #4

$$\dot{W}_X = \frac{Az1 - Az0}{2dy} - \frac{Az1 - Az0}{2dz}$$

$$\dot{W}_Y = \frac{Az0 - Az2}{2dx} + \frac{Az0 - Az2}{2dz}$$

$$\dot{W}_Z = \frac{Az2 - Az0}{2dx} - \frac{Az2 - Az0}{2dy}$$

Figure 27–6. Instrumentation options.

low-pass filters must be introduced to reduce the effective bandwidth to within tolerable error. In such cases, the selected filter characteristics influence the minimum acceptable sampling rate. The sharper the filter rolloff characteristics, the lower the required sampling frequency. An ideal step function would include no attenuation in the passband and infinite attenuation in the stopband. This, of course, is impossible and filtering becomes the objective. The higher the sampling rate (multiples of fc), the slower the acceptable rolloff; and the slower the rolloff, the higher the frequencies folded back onto the spectrum of interest. This is graphically depicted in Figure 27–7. If one samples at four times the desired cutoff frequency (4ω; 2000 Hz) then the folding frequency becomes 2ω (1000 Hz) and aliasing onto the spectrum of interest ($0-\omega$; 0–500 Hz) would occur at $3\omega-4\omega$ (first alias) and from $4\omega-5\omega$ (second alias). Providing attenuation of -40dB at the folding frequency (40 dB/octave

rolloff) will reduce the energy in the frequency folded back onto the passband to approximately -63 dB (less than 0.1 percent amplitude). This is shown as the shaded area in Figure 27–7. For a given attenuation level, sharper filter rolloff characteristics will allow smaller sampling rates.

In addition to the aliasing problem, analog to digital converters (ADC) introduce a type of error known as quantization noise, a relationship between the input quantity (voltage) and output counts. It can be shown that for a fixed range of the function being digitized, the power spectral density of the quantization noise decreases exponentially with the number of bits in the quantization word. For large N, say N greater than 10, the quantization noise tends to be negligible. Consequently, ADC should employ a minimum of 10 bit resolution to eliminate this source of errors. Choosing 12 bit ADC resolution, as we have done, has some implications on the filtering utilized. As was previously indicated, in order to attentuate the aliasing spectrum to a minimum of 0.1 per cent amplitude at 3w (1500 Hz), a minimum of -40 dB/octave rolloff was required. For 12 bit ADC, -72 dB attenuation at 1500 Hz and above is required in order to ensure that the foldback content is smaller than the ADC resolution. This corresponds to a -45 dB/octave rolloff (see Fig. 27–6). Consequently, the requirements (12 bit A/D resolution, sampling frequency of 4fc, band limiting fc = 500 Hz, 96 channels, 12 seconds experiment time) result in 3.5 Mbytes of memory to be incorporated into the manikin.

ACQUISITION SYSTEM REQUIREMENTS

From the previous discussion, it is obvious that a variety of sensors are employed and both the excitation voltages as well as sensor outputs can vary appreciably. Consequently, variable gain amplification of sensor output is required for effective analog to digital conversion (A/D). Additionally, anticipated worse case sampling rates per channel must be estimated to determine memory requirements to support 96 channels of information for experiment durations of 12 seconds. Again, using the head-neck system as an example, work by Gurdjian[10] has indicated that for the head, important first, second, and third modes are found near 300 Hz, 560 Hz (antiresonance), and 900 Hz (reso-

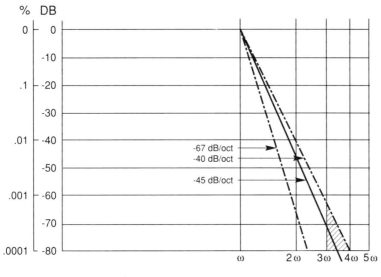

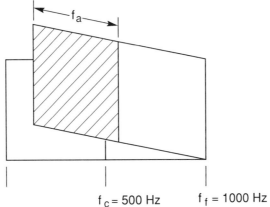

Figure 27–7. Minimal rolloff for elimination of aliasing (upper). Folding frequency with increased sampling rate (lower).

nance). In the antiresonance mode, maximum mechanical impedance (force/velocity) was found to occur, with acceleration amplification on the occiput greater than the frontal input acceleration by a factor of 3. In the resonance mode, minimal mechanical impedance occurs in which only that part of the head adjacent to the driving point is moving under the action of a vibratory force. This implies that for impacts lasting 4 ms or greater, predominantly rigid body acceleration of the skull will occur up to the energy level necessary to produce concussion. At short duration pulses (less than 3 ms), in addition to the acceleration effects, there will be added deflection patterns altered by the resonant modes of bending of the skull. Therefore, acceleration measures, relative to the head anatomic coordinate system, are only meaningful below 250 Hz when the skull moves as a rigid body. At higher frequencies, the location and not the accelerometer will influence the values obtained. Although the dummy head

may have higher frequency response, correlating that to known biomechanics of injury is tenuous at best. Since helmets are usually worn in the aerospace environment, even 250 Hz inputs are highly unlikely.

Therefore, for dummy-mounted instrumentation it would seem reasonable to bandlimit sensor information to 250 Hz. It must be remembered, however, that the dummy-based data acquisition system will also be used to monitor and store seat and/or aircraft based sensors, in which high frequency response can be anticipated. Because the proposed manikin is designed to meet tri-service requirements, system resolution is based on respective testing and data analysis specifications. The Army's use of the Eiband curve (Eiband [1959])[11] indicates that pulse durations of 2 ms must be considered in assessing seat performance. In order to quantify transient pulse durations lasting 2 ms, one must have a resolution of 500 Hz. The signal conditioning for the accelerometer channels was therefore designed to be variable up to a cutoff frequency of 500 Hz.

Given the fact that on-board storage was to be a primary design parameter, experimental run times would also have to be realistically assessed to estimate memory storage requirements to be incorporated into the manikin proper. Under tri-service applications, the longest anticipated experimental run time is 12 seconds, corresponding to high airspeed ejections. In this worst case situation, the elapsed time from escape initiation to touchdown under a stable parachute should not exceed this time duration. Consequently, the overall characteristics of the system were defined as 96-channel capacity, on-board storage, umbilical and/or PCM transmission, and 12-second experimental run time capability.

DATA ACQUISITION SYSTEM

The microprocessor-based data acquisition and storage system (DASS) is illustrated in Fig-

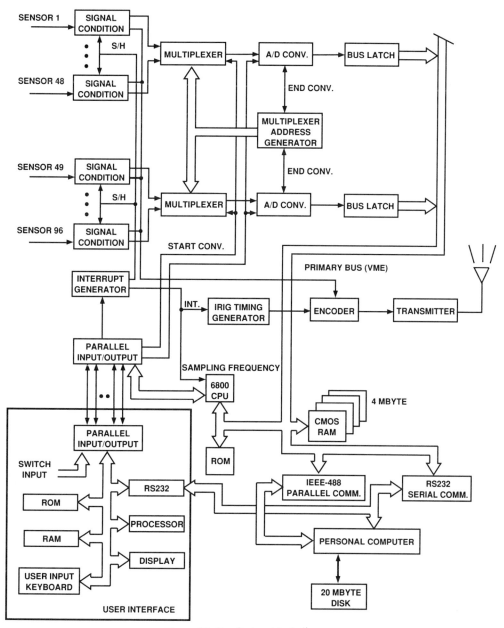

Figure 27–8. System block diagram.

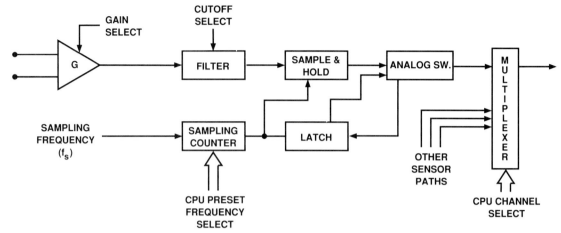

Figure 27–9. Dedicated analog signal conditioning path.

ure 27–8. The system consists of the primary unit integrated into the manikin chest and contains the processor, memory, power supply, and all analog and digital circuits to interface with the sensors. The user interface provides test-dependent data (sampling frequency, number of channels, and the like) to the primary system and is also used to extract and offload all data onto a mass storage device for processing and analysis.

The DASS internal to the manikin utilizes a 68000 series CPU, addressing 4 Mbytes of RAM memory, and houses all analog sensor input signal conditioning, ADC circuitry, timing and interrupt logic, RF circuits necessary to maintain long-range communication and timing signals, and local communications electronics to interface with the field personal computer (PC) (IBM or IBM compatible portable

PC). Each channel contains a dedicated analog signal conditioning path as illustrated in Figure 27–9 and supports a differential instrumentation amplifier with a variable, CPU programmable, sampling frequency and gain, maintaining a full-scale signal at the ADC. Connected to the amplifier is an antialiasing filter, providing a CPU adjustable (60–20,000 Hz) cutoff with a rolloff characteristic of −45 dB/octave. The filter is coupled to a dedicated sample and hold (S/H) circuit, time synchronized with all other channels. The aforementioned signal conditioning circuitry has been hybridized to harden the system, minimize space allocation, maximize reliability and interchangeability of parts, and control component errors, since all circuitry is deposited on a common substrate and subjected to uniform temperature fluctuations. This hybrid chip

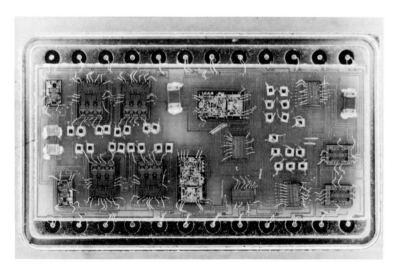

Figure 27–10. The Hybrid chip.

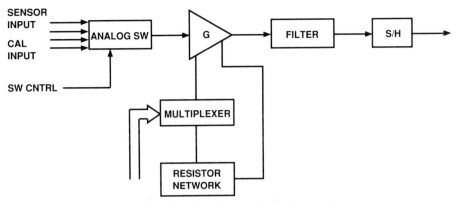

Figure 27–11. Block diagram for the Hybrid chip.

(supporting two channels) and associated block diagram are shown in Figures 27–10 and 27–11. The analog channels are multiplexed to provide multiple parallel analog input paths to four ADCs. The ADCs are high speed, bipolar input converters, maintaining 12 bit resolution. The converter function and multiplexer addressing (selection of sensor input) is under processor control. The parallel ADC paths provide a packed 6 byte data package (12 bits/channel) maximizing RAM utilization, which is crucial due to size, power, and density constraints. The system contains a stable clock oscillator, countdown circuitry and logic to provide interrupts, hold signals, and latching to support a variable data sampling frequency. Additionally, the system is designed to include the logic and RF circuits to generate, transmit, and receive long-range communications and timing signals to time lock supporting experiment equipment and verify system operation. Finally, the instrumentation system houses hardware and software to support parallel input/output lines (interprocessor communication) and RS232 asynchronous serial communication interface as well as an IEEE 488 parallel interface to maintain communications with the field unit and other external instruments or systems.

The integrated system is shown in Figure 27–1. The chest cavity contains all controls for system power-up ports for programming test parameters (number of channels, sampling rates, sensor sensitivities) and for post-test offload of all calibration and test data. The DASS unit itself (shown in the middle) is bolted onto the thoracic spine (as is the rib cage) and supports all analog circuitry, microprocessor, communication and memory boards, sensor inputs, and circuitry to switch

from external to internal power. The transmitter, for remote communication, is shown incorporated into the baseplate of the flexible lumbar spine. The encoder for the PCM system is located in the pelvis.

The field unit PC interfaces and communicates with the DASS 68000 primary. The user enters test dependent data from the keyboard, specifying to the DASS the sampling frequency, number of channels utilized (used to optimize RAM based on sampling frequency and experiment time), and sensor characteristics. A variable default mode is also provided that automatically sets all the aforementioned parameters and needs only to be changed when sensor configurations are altered. The PC also provides the desired operational mode, such as calibration, diagnostics, or acquisition. Additionally, calibration and diagnostic information appear on the PC for user system evaluation. The PC maintains a mass storage medium to offload calibration and experimental data from the DASS and supports the analysis, editing, restructuring, and loading of new or modified assembly language software routines into the 68000 based primary unit. The DASS unit is self-contained and totally powered by rechargeable batteries, housed within the manikin. The batteries provide sufficient power to maintain system operation and data integrity for four hours. The system supports a power switching network to facilitate use of external DC power for system checkout and maintenance, precluding an unnecessary drain on the on-board battery prior to testing. Figure 27–12 illustrates the manikin and associated instrumentation and data acquisition and storage system, interfaced to an IBM compatible (Compac) for a pretest verification, setup, and calibration procedure.

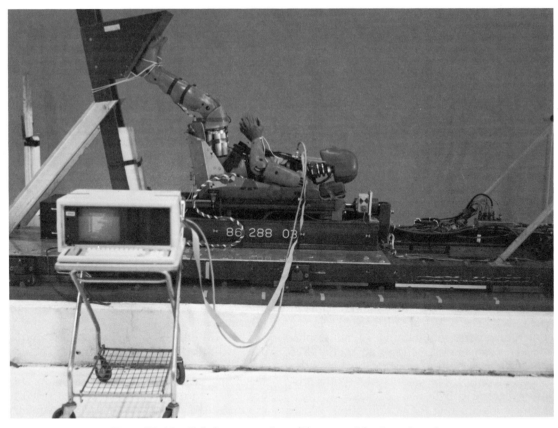

Figure 27–12. Fully instrumented manikin prepared for dynamic testing.

SYSTEM OPERATION

DASS system functions are defined by the assembly language operating software and are divided into seven phases (pretest, calibration, diagnostic and test, data offload/transfer, communications, acquisition, and system monitor). Upon power up, the system enters a pretest mode updating all status registers, memory pointers, communications ports, and hardware latches. The pretest software establishes communications with the remote user interface, determining the variable experiment-dependent characteristics such as sampling frequency, number of channels, and the sensor characteristics. Software developed on both processors (primary and remote) will perform a handshake and relay the required data to the requesting processor. Upon completion of pretest functions, the DASS primary returns to the system monitor, awaiting function mode selection from the remote user interface or PCM telemetry.

The calibration software provides a means of measuring the errors introduced from the sensor through all components of the system. The system supports two modes of calibration: automatic and manual. In the automatic mode, the processor will shunt each sensor with a known resistive load, measuring the sensor output at the ADC and storing results. The system provides for multiple, load-resistor selection, enabling measurement through a range of sensor outputs. In the manual mode, the calibration software provides a voltage substitution scheme, simulating the range of analog input into each channel and measuring a minimum of four samples per channel. The system maintains the capability to perform both pre- and post-test calibrations. The calibration results appear simultaneously on the user interface unit to verify sensor/channel operation. System calibration and status can be additionally accomplished via a PCM RF communication link for cases when remote interaction with the acquisition system is necessary. It does, however, imply that the design of the instrumentation system must be frozen for all anticipated applications, so that this reballasting procedure has to be undertaken only once.

The data acquisition software is based on an interrupt architecture, where an interrupt pulse is generated at the desired data sampling frequency. The interrupt-based acquisition is enabled by the start of an experiment signal and provides the hold signal to the sample and hold circuits, time synchronizing all channels. The number of channels is variable to a maximum of 96 and user selectable, optimizing acquisition performance and memory utilization. Each interrupt-triggered acquisition cycle starts the ADC process and subsequently enters data from the four parallel converters, storing the packed six bytes sequentially into memory. Each sampling iteration blocks all channel data with preceding elapsed-time data and a post-data separator. Acquisition terminates and returns to the system monitor automatically when either the maximum experiment time or available memory has been exceeded. The system software provides diagnostics and self-test capabilities to verify system hardware and software operation. Sensor and signal conditioning circuits are tested using a procedure similar to that detailed for calibration. The software will check selected portions of the complete RAM memory, writing data to each location and successfully retrieving the data. The timing (interrupt, sample, and hold) signals are verified prior to experiment, as are the communications with the remote user interface and the offload device.

The communications software provides the link between the DASS primary unit and remote interface via a series of parallel and serial I/O ports, shared by both processors. Each processor operates asynchronously, transmitting and receiving ASCII characters identifying operation mode status and system configuration. The remote user interface transmits a code to specify operational mode (i.e., diagnostic, acquisition, and so on). The DASS transmits ASCII codes to user interface to identify process results, system status, and data quality.

The data offload or transmit software offloads the entire content of experiment memory (system status, pre-/post-test calibrations, diagnostic information, and test data) onto the PC or other remote mass storage device. The software adheres to all protocols (XON, XOFF, and the like) specified by these bus and communications specifications. The PC maintains software to unpack the interleaved binary data and convert the binary into either/or both analog voltage levels of scientific unit data representation. The data are formatted on disk for storage and availability to the system CRT and/or hard copy record. Additionally, the PC acts as a development resource for the DASS

acquisition processor. It enables display, editing, and generation of assembly language programs. The modified or newly developed software can be downloaded into a predetermined RAM block, and modification of the program counter will enable the DASS to function under the new temporary software for evaluation and testing.

CONCLUSIONS

The manikin-based system, as described, has undergone detailed tests to verify all functional aspects and structural integrity under high G load conditions. A complete experimental prototype (fewer number of channels and memory supported) has previously been tested on the Naval Air Development Center horizontal accelerator up to 37 G (peak) and 1720 G/sec onset rates. These tests were conducted to verify robustness and feasibility of approach prior to further hardening of the system through microchip technology. Furthermore, the analog signal conditioning subsystem, employing linear and angular accelerometers discussed and integrated into the PC telemetry system, has been ejection tested up to 600 KEAS, sustaining 30 G (X), 20 G (Y), and 25 G (Z) inertial loading simultaneously.[12] Consequently, considerable confidence has evolved in the overall approach taken.

Although the system is fully incorporated into the manikin, the addition of the DASS into the chest and supporting battery power into the pelvis and legs has altered the individual manikin segment weight distributions, CG locations, and moment tensors. Before complete integration can be claimed, the individual manikin segments affected will have to be reballasted. This is not anticipated to be a major stumbling block, since the DASS and battery weight does not exceed the overall weight of the presenting utilized lead and steel ballasting provided in the manikin.

It is anticipated that from the manikin performance analysis, specific deficiencies in the resultant biofidelity will be isolated and resolved.

Acknowledgment

This chapter is dedicated to the memory of the late Georg D. Frisch, who died on August 29, 1989. His dedication and commitment to and accomplishments in the field of biomechanics and dynamics are a matter of record and are well documented. He will be missed by the research community, fellow workers, and especially by me.

REFERENCES

1. Kraus JF: Epidemiological aspects of brain and spinal cord injuries. *In* Sances, A (ed.): Mechanisms of Head and Spine Trauma. Goshen, NY, Aloray Publisher, 1986, pp. 49–68.
2. Frisch GD, D'Aulerio LA: Instrumentation Requirements for Assessing Occupant Response to Three Dimensional High Acceleration Environments. NATO-AGARD Conference Proceedings No. 322 (Impact Injury Caused by Linear Acceleration: Mechanisms, Prevention and Cost), 1982.
3. Frisch GD: Simulation of occupant-crew station interaction during impact. *In* Ewing, CL (ed.): Impact Injury of the Head and Spine. Springfield IL, Charles C Thomas, Publisher, 1982.
4. Foster JK, Kortge JO, Wolanin MJ: HYBRID III— A Biomechanically Based Crash Test Dummy. Proceedings of the 21st Stapp Car Crash Conference, Ann Arbor, MI, 1977.
5. Coltman JW, Van Ingen C, Selker F: Crash-Resistant Crewseat Limit—Load Optimization Through Dynamic Testing with Cadavers. USAAVSCOM Report TR-85-D-11, Fort Eustis, VA, 1986.
6. Guill FC: Aircrew Automated Escape Systems (AAES), Data Analysis Program Symposium. Volumes 1–4, Naval Air Systems Command, Naval Weapons Engineering Support Activity. (Symposium held at Naval Safety Center, Norfolk, VA). U.S. Dept. of Navy, Washington, D.C., 1981.
7. Frisch GD, Whitley PE, Wydra G, Holdaway D: High Speed Ejection Tests of a Modified HYBRID II Manikin. Proceedings of the 23rd Annual Symposium of the SAFE Association, Van Nuys, CA, 1985.
8. Frisch PH: Inertial Reference System to Measure Blast Induced Displacements. U.S. Army Final Report, Contract DAAA15-86-C-0075, 1988.
9. Frisch GD, Frisch PH: The Development of a Dynamic Response Sensing and Recording System for Incorporation into a State of the Art Manikin. Proceedings of the 21st Annual Symposium of the SAFE Association, Van Nuys, CA, 1983; and SAFE Journal 14(1):13–20, 1983.
10. Gurdjian ES, Hodgson VR, Thomas LM: Studies on mechanical impedance of the human skull: Preliminary report. Journal of Biomechanics 3: pp. 239–47, 1970.
11. Eiband AM: Human Tolerance to Rapidly Applied Accelerations: A Summary of the Literature. NASA Memorandum 5-19-59E, National Aeronautics and Space Administration, Washington, DC, 1959.
12. Frisch GD, Whitley PE, Frisch PH: Structural Integrity Tests of a Modified HYBRID III Manikin and Supporting Instrumentation System. Proceedings of the 22nd Annual Symposium of the SAFE Association, Van Nuys, CA, 1984; and SAFE Journal 15(2):20, 1985.

28 The Omentum in Spinal Cord Injury

HARRY S. GOLDSMITH, M.D.

Spinal cord injuries have been observed since man has recorded history. Hippocrates reported the inevitability of the disaster of spinal cord trauma and recommended that no medical treatment be offered these unfortunate people. In spite of great strides taken in the recent treatment of spinal cord injuries, a sense of futility is still felt by many medical professionals related to experimental treatment procedures for spinal cord injuries. I believe that clinical improvement will eventually be expected in a significant number of these patients and that the greater omentum, or its components, may prove to be an instrumental factor in accomplishing this therapeutic achievement.

PATHOPHYSIOLOGY OF CNS INJURY

There appear to be two major factors causing paralysis following spinal cord injury: (1) the force of the impact delivered to the spinal cord, and (2) the cascade of pathobiological events that begins shortly after injury. Although there is no way to influence the degree of spinal cord impaction causing the trauma, interest continues in many laboratories to devise new experimental strategies to lessen the secondary tissue effects that occur within the spinal cord following injury.

It has been observed that a major factor, if not *the* major factor, responsible for the irreversible damage that can occur after spinal cord injury results from the rapid development of vasogenic edema within the spinal cord.[1] An observer who follows the histologic progression of changes that occur within the spinal cord following trauma will be impressed by the centrifugal flow of vasogenic edema fluid that rapidly moves from the central gray matter toward the periphery of the spinal cord. The spinal cord swelling that results from this expanding volume of vasogenic edema occurs within the firm dural covering and the rigid vertebral canal (Fig. 28–1). This condition in which there is a rising spinal cord tissue pressure developing within the nonyielding bony compartment surrounding the cord, can cause an inversely lower perfusion pressure within capillaries located in and immediately adjacent to the site of spinal cord impact (Fig. 28–2). Fluid dynamics allow some vasogenic edema to move longitudinally up and down the spinal cord;[2] but a rising spinal cord tissue pressure can ultimately be reached whereby a halt of capillary perfusion pressure occurs which leads to irreparable spinal cord damage if the ischemic situation is not corrected within four to six hours.

Various surgical procedures have been evaluated over the years in the attempt to lower the elevated tissue pressure that can develop at the impaction site of an injured spinal cord. Myelotomy and decompression laminectomy have both been tried for this purpose, but the unpredictability of clinical benefits arising from these procedures has failed to justify their routine performance. These surgical procedures are believed to have been less successful because simply lowering spinal cord tissue pressure caused by vasogenic edema is apparently not the only mechanical factor that must be corrected in order to prevent permanent spinal cord damage. A secondary condition that appears crucial is the absorption of edema fluid that accumulates within and around the traumatized spinal cord.[3] Unfortunately, the spinal cord itself can add little to the necessary absorption because of its lack of lymphatics. Observations in our laboratory have strongly indicated that if the edema fluid surrounding an injured spinal cord is not quickly removed, the

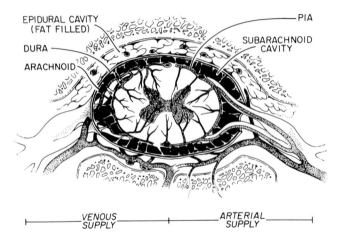

Figure 28–1. Illustration showing that as the injured spinal cord swells from vasogenic edema within the dural sac and vertebral canal, the venous outflow from the cord becomes compromised leading to increased venous pressure and further edema formation.

fluid itself becomes instrumental in the early development of fibrosis, which has a constricting effect on underlying spinal cord capillaries. This pathologic situation can result in progressive ischemia to the recently damaged spinal cord. This leads to a decreased opportunity for neurologic improvement because of diminished circulation at the injury site caused by progressively constricting scar formation (Fig. 28–3). The absorption of vasogenic edema, which limits fibrosis from developing around an injured spinal cord is therefore considered to be extremely crucial to the ultimate neurologic outcome following such an injury.

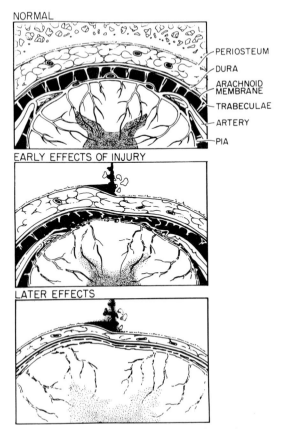

Figure 28–2. Illustrations showing how increasing vasogenic edema formation in the spinal cord leads to a decreasing capillary perfusion pressure.

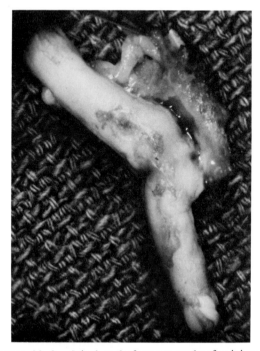

Figure 28–3. Spinal cord of cat two weeks after injury. Note persistent edema and herniation of cord at laminectomy site. Fluid and fibrosis are present above injury site and constricting scar is obvious at level of trauma.

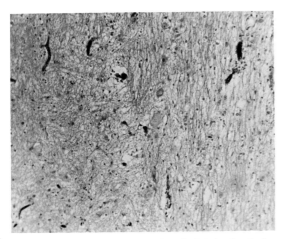

Figure 28-4. Note presence of India ink in deeply located spinal cord capillaries in a dog. Omental–spinal cord preparation was removed intact and the dye marker injected in vitro into an omental artery.

OMENTAL TRANSPOSITION TO THE CNS

For a quarter of a century, our laboratory has been involved in evaluating the experimental and clinical uses of the omentum, especially as it applies to the central nervous system.

Vascularization

It was first reported in 1973 that placing the omentum directly upon the brain would result in the development of vascular connections at the omental-cerebral interface.[4] Subsequent studies in the dog[5] and in the monkey[6] showed that vascularization between the omentum and the brain was sufficient to prevent cerebral infarction following middle cerebral artery occlusion.

The experimental success of the omentum in revascularizing the brain stimulated parallel interest in identifying any effects that the omentum might have in revascularizing the spinal cord.[7] Studies showed that blood vessels developed at the omental-spinal cord interface and that a dye marker (India ink) flowed through these blood vessels and could be identified in deeply positioned spinal cord capillaries (Fig. 28-4). It was further demonstrated that the omentum allowed blood vessels to grow in a longitudinal manner through a complete spinal cord transection site (Fig. 28-5), a phenomenon that was felt might be important if the longitudinal growth of axons through the spinal cord could be developed. The histologic observation that blood vessels developed between the omentum and normal spinal cord within 72 hours was of particular importance and was subsequently confirmed.[8] More recently it has been observed that omental-spinal cord revascularization develops even faster when the spinal cord is injured.[3] An additional observation from our laboratory that we believe to be of major importance is the ability of the omentum to develop blood vessels that penetrate directly and deeply into the central nervous system (Fig. 28-6).

Omental Absorption

It is known clinically that the omentum can absorb edema fluid from peripheral areas of the body.[9] What is generally not appreciated, however, is the enormous absorptive capacity of the omentum. This fact can be easily demonstrated by simply placing an intact piece of an animal's omentum into a beaker filled with dye (India ink) and saline. The dye will be seen almost instantaneously in omental lymphatics (Fig. 28-7). Additional evidence exists in a study reporting that 30 per cent of the entire

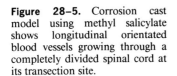

Figure 28-5. Corrosion cast model using methyl salicylate shows longitudinal orientated blood vessels growing through a completely divided spinal cord at its transection site.

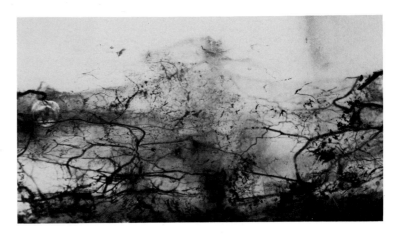

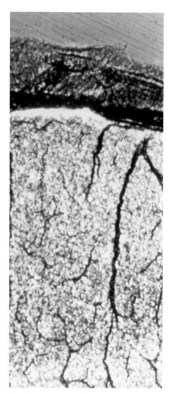

Figure 28–6. Omentum lying on brain. Note deep vertical penetration of omental blood vessels into underlying cerebral tissue; the blood-brain barrier is broken.

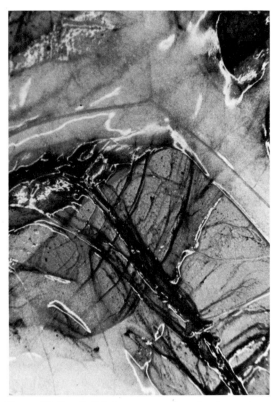

Figure 28–7. Pedicled omentum of cat has been placed for 30 seconds in a beaker filled with saline and India ink. Dye marker rapidly becomes apparent within omental lymphatics.

cerebrospinal fluid reservoir can be absorbed through the intact omentum.[8]

Spinal cord swelling caused by vasogenic edema persists in the experimental animal and in the human for many weeks after injury, during which time a severe fibrotic reaction can develop at the site of trauma (Fig. 28–3). It has been observed in our laboratory, however, that little or no fibrotic reaction occurs when the omentum is placed on the spinal cord shortly after injury (Fig. 29–8). This observation has led to the hypothesis that the failure of scar tissue to form around a traumatized spinal cord results from the omentum's ability to absorb the vasogenic edema that follows injury.[3] A dynamic equilibrium apparently develops between the production of vasogenic edema from within the spinal cord and its rapid absorption by the contiguously placed omentum. Scar tissue formation that normally develops after spinal cord injury may result within days from the activation of fibrinogen, a component of the plasma-derived vasogenic edema fluid, to fibrin; the initiation is probably stimulated by blood in the area.[10] Absorbing vasogenic edema

fluid after spinal cord injury would therefore be expected to decrease the presence of fibrinogen in the area, thereby lessening the opportunity for fibroblast proliferation at the site of spinal cord impaction. An alternative to this hypoth-

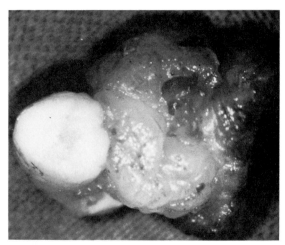

Figure 28–8. Omentum placed on injured spinal cord two weeks previously. Note firm omental-cord adherence with complete absence of edema formation.

esis is that the omentum itself has biologic substances within its tissues that are antifibrotic in activity. This possibility is reasonable given the variety of biologic material presently being found in omental tissue.

OMENTAL TRANSPOSITION— EXPERIMENTAL STUDIES

The concepts presented in this chapter pertaining to acute spinal cord injuries are (1) vasogenic edema develops shortly after spinal cord injury and can, in the area of impact, result in a very high tissue pressure with an inversely lower to absent capillary perfusion pressure, and (2) fibrosis in the area of spinal cord injury can occur within days if vasogenic edema fluid resulting from the trauma is not absorbed. With this hypothesis in mind, the physiological properties of the omentum would strongly indicate that the earlier this structure is placed on the spinal cord after injury, the greater the opportunity for post-traumatic recovery as measured by improved motor and neuroelectrical activity.

In order to test this theory, a series of experiments were performed in cats.[3] All animals in these studies were subjected to a 450 gm/cm injury to their spinal cords using the standard weight dropping technique described by Allen.[11] Final motor and neuroelectrical evaluations were made 30 days after injury, at which time the animals were sacrificed.

Omental Placement

Controls (11 Cats)—No Omental Application

Eleven cats acted as the controls in this study by having the dura excised over the site of spinal cord injury exactly three hours after trauma. Nine of these animals had persistent paralysis of the hind limbs at the time of death. Of the two remaining cats in this control group, one could walk and the other could push up on its hind legs. Positive somatosensory evoked potentials (SEPs) returned in 25 per cent of the hind legs in this control group (5/20 [1 animal died]).

Early (3 Hours) Omental Application—11 Cats

Five cats who had the omentum placed directly on the spinal cord exactly three hours after injury had varying degrees of walking ability at the time of death. Two additional cats could push up on their hind limbs but not ambulate. The additional four cats in this group were permanently paralyzed at the time of death. Positive SEPs returned in 82 per cent (18/22) of the hind limbs of the animals.

Late (6–8 Hours) Omental Application— 14 Cats

All animals in this group were permanently paralyzed at the time of death. Positive SEPs returned in 4 per cent (1/28) of the hind limbs of the cats in this group.

These experiments supported the hypothesis that omental transposition to the spinal cord within hours of injury is a major factor in the subsequent return of motor and neuroelectrical activity. (Statistically significant differences were observed between the control and experimental groups. P values ranged from 0.005 to 0.05 using the Mann-Whitney Test.)

The requirement to transpose the omentum surgically within three hours after experimental trauma places severe time restrictions on the use of this procedure for clinical evaluation. This consideration motivated additional experiments in our laboratory to determine if the omentum could be placed on an injured spinal cord later than three hours after trauma with subsequent neurological improvement in the animals. This was done by use of pharmacologic agents that were administered after spinal cord injury but prior to omental transposition to the spinal cord. These experiments initially involved the use of dexamethasone, methylprednisolone, and banamine, but these agents proved unsuccessful in our studies. However, when dimethyl sulfoxide (DMSO) in conjunction with omental transposition was evaluated in animals with spinal cord injury, a statistically significant difference was noted in comparison with the control animals in preventing paralysis ($P < 0.02$) and in the differences between the return of positive SEPs ($P < 0.04$).[12] The DMSO was given intravenously in a 40 per cent solution as a bolus one hour after injury; the omentum was applied six hours after the trauma. Further experimentation is necessary to learn whether DMSO administered at various time intervals, or continuously, will allow several more hours of surgical delay after a spinal cord injury before the omentum must be applied to the spinal cord with the expectation of improved neurological function.

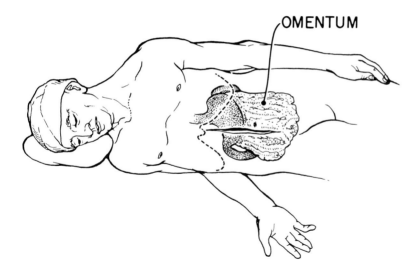

OMENTUM

Figure 28–9. It is extremely important that the patient be placed with right side down on the operating table. This allows spleen to fall toward operating area rather than retract into left upper quadrant where a bleeding short gastric vessel can become dangerously difficult to see and control.

OMENTAL TRANSPOSITION— CLINICAL STUDIES

On the basis of our experimental data, it appears that the greatest clinical benefit following omental transposition to the injured spinal cord should occur when the omentum is applied as shortly after spinal cord trauma as possible. A well-organized and dedicated spinal cord trauma team will be required to accomplish this. If such investigation has not already begun, it is expected that exploration in this important area of clinical investigation will be forthcoming.

Interest continues to increase throughout the world in the use of omental transposition onto the spinal cord of patients who had sustained a cord injury many months to years prior to surgery. I have performed the procedure on 18 patients (paraplegic and quadraplegic), with most having been injured two or more years prior to surgery. One third of these patients have shown postoperative improvement in various aspects of their motor, sensory, bladder, rectal, and thermoregulatory mechanisms.[13,14] Other investigators have reported comparable results.[15,16] However, such series are anecdotal and, until strict control studies of cord injured patients are undertaken and reported, the value of personal clinical series remains questionable.

The operative steps in performing omental transposition to the human spinal cord are initiated by entering the abdominal cavity (Fig. 28–9) and removing the omentum from the transverse colon and from a major portion of the greater curvature of the stomach (Figs. 28–10 to 28–12). If a cervical cord injury is being treated (Fig. 28–13), the lengthened omentum is brought to the cervical laminectomy site through a subcutaneously developed tunnel along the chest wall (Fig. 28–14), over the shoulder (Fig. 28–15), and then down to the spinal cord that has had the overlying dura removed (Fig. 28–16). The omentum is then fixed to the spinal cord by careful suturing of the omentum to the cut edges of the dura (Figs. 28–17 to 28–18). The overlying muscles and fascial layers are carefully and individually approximated (Fig. 28–19). When the injury is in the thoracolumbar area, the omentum is brought subcutaneously around the flank to the back, where it is placed on the spinal cord

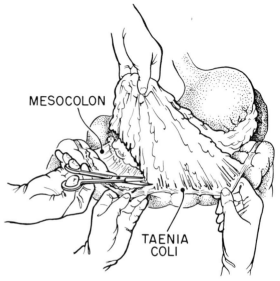

MESOCOLON

TAENIA COLI

Figure 28–10. Omentum being freed from transverse colon. The plane of dissection is practically avascular.

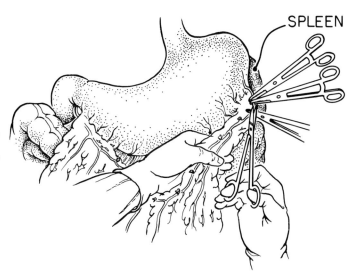

Figure 28–11. Omentum removed from stomach along greater curvature, leaving gastroepiploic vessels within omental apron. Right gastroepiploic vessels remain intact to supply omental pedicle.

that has been exposed at the appropriate laminectomy site. As more operative experience is gained, anterolateral surgical approaches to the spinal cord will likely be developed that may prove superior to the posterior approach.

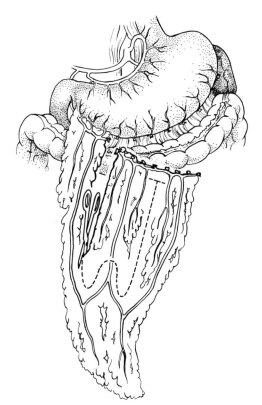

Figure 28–12. Omentum being extensively lengthened by dividing structure, with care being taken to maintain arterial supply primarily along its periphery.

INDICATIONS FOR THE FUTURE

There is no question that clinical improvement has occurred in some patients who have had the omentum transposed to their spinal cord years after injury. The question raised by this finding is why any neurologic changes should have occurred in these chronic patients, with vasogenic edema not being a factor as it is in acute spinal cord injury. I believe that the major factor responsible for any degree of postoperative improvement in such patients with chronic spinal cord injury is probably due to the additional blood supply and neurochemicals delivered to the spinal cord by the omentum. This hypothesis was strengthened when it was discovered that the omentum is the source

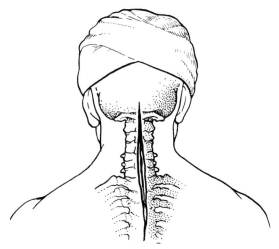

Figure 28–13. Midline cervical incision for posterior laminectomy procedure.

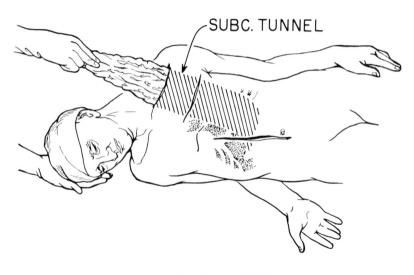

Figure 28–14. Omentum sufficiently lengthened to allow its placement in subcutaneous tunnel developed between incisions along chest.

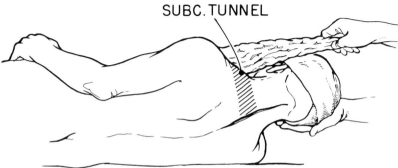

Figure 28–15. Omentum brought through the subcutaneous tunnel, then placed beneath fascia of posterior neck muscles down to spinal cord.

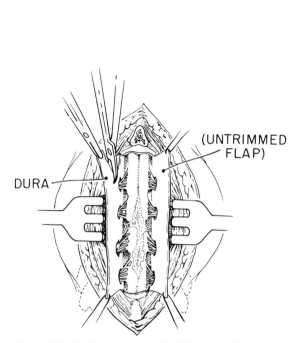

Figure 28–16. Dura opened with bilateral excision of a portion of dural flaps.

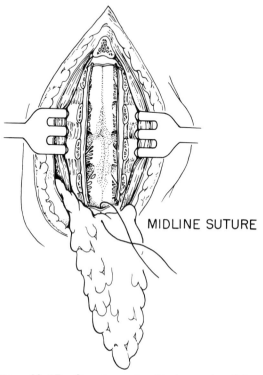

Figure 28–17. Omentum sutured to lower edge of dura for firm fixation.

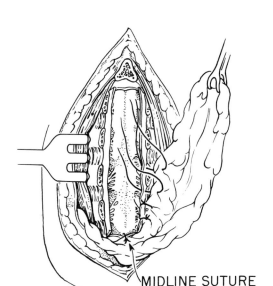

Figure 28–18. Further fixation of omentum accomplished by suturing to both edges of cut dura.

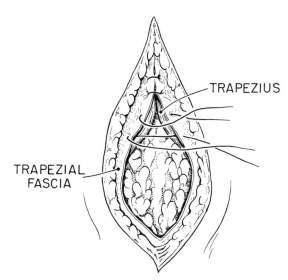

TRAPEZIUS

TRAPEZIAL FASCIA

Figure 28–19. Wound closed with careful approximation of individual muscle and facial layers.

of a potent angiogenic factor.[17,18] A more recent finding from our laboratory, equally if not even more important than the presence of an omental angiogenic factor, was the discovery of neurotransmitters within omental tissue.[19,20] Whether the omentum synthesizes these neurotransmitters or simply concentrates them from the circulation is still unknown. Perhaps it is these neurochemicals, omentum-derived nerve growth substances[21], or other, as yet unidentified, omental neurotrophic substances that may eventually explain the favorable neurologic changes that have occurred following

omental tranposition to chronically abnormal areas of the central nervous system.[22–25]

Axonal Regeneration

The question that has remained unanswered over the years is whether the spinal cord is an organ that has the potential to heal itself. The belief among many neurobiologists is that the spinal cord lacks this capacity. This belief thereby raises an alternative question that also remains unanswered: Why should the central nervous system, the most exquisite of all the organ systems in the body, be preferentially denied the opportunity to heal? In order to test the possibility that the spinal cord does have the capacity to heal itself, an experimental model in cats was devised in which a piece of spinal cord was totally excised and the ends of the transected spinal cord apposed without tension; fixation in that position was accomplished by rigid vertebral stabilization.[26]

The surgical procedure involved required the development of three separate operative steps.

1. Surgical Excision—A 5 mm section of ice-hardened spinal cord was removed using an ultra sharp stainless steel blade (Fig. 28–20). In

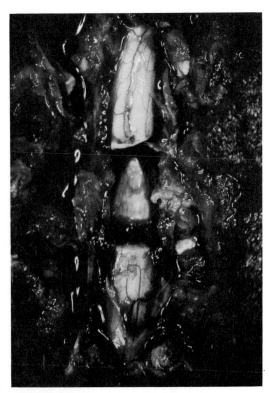

Figure 28–20. Large spinal cord defect after complete excision of a 5 mm segment with subsequent cord retraction.

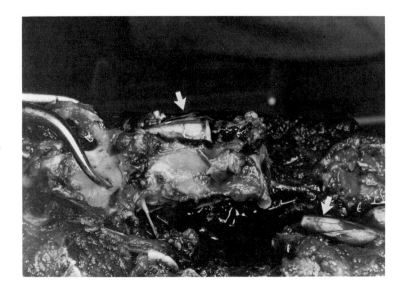

Figure 28–21. Arrows point to cut ends of spinal cord. Removal of L2 vertebra allows for extensive mobility of cord. Clamp holds proximal cord segment.

order to prevent axons from growing from dorsal root ganglia into the healing spinal cord, spinal nerves were divided outside the dural sheath but flush with the cord so that ganglia were widely separated from the spinal cord.

2. Vertebral Column Stabilization—In order to allow the severed ends of the spinal cord to be placed in apposition without tension, a lumbar vertebra was removed (Fig. 28–21). The proximal and distal vertebral bodies were then solidly secured by the insertion of stainless steel plates and screws (Fig. 28–22).

3. Spinal Cord Reapproximation—After entering the abdomen, the omentum was lengthened and brought through a subcutaneous tunnel developed around the flank to the location of the divided ends of the spinal cord. The di-

vided dura at both ends of the transected cord was then reapproximated below (anterior to) the spinal cord with several interrupted sutures. Two small (2 cm) closely parallel incisions were made in the omentum allowing a small slip of omental tissue to be placed between the approximated dura and the anterior surface of the divided spinal cord. The divided ends of the spinal cord were then carefully brought together without tension and laser-welded along the edges of the spinal cord using a CO_2 laser. This laser-fusing required only 1 to 2 watts of energy, with the laser beam being carefully directed under microscopic control to the transection site (Fig. 28–23).

After reconstructing the spinal cord by this laser technique, the pedicled omentum, except

Figure 28–22. Spinal cord apposition without tension. Note firm orthopedic stabilization below the level of spinal cord transection.

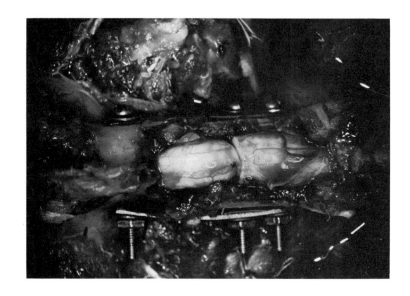

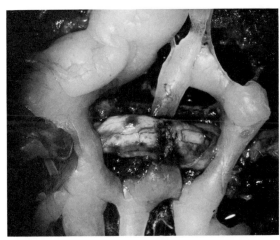

Figure 28–23. Spinal cord has been fused together by a low-energy laser beam. Physical limitation of laser injury as evidenced by charring at the transection site has been shown to be less than 0.2 mm in depth. Note piece of intact omentum below the fused spinal cord.

for the small piece previously placed below the spinal cord, was now folded back over the posterior surface of the cord, resulting in its complete envelopment by the omentum. The omental tissue is considered critical for the immediate absorption of edema fluid and subsequent revascularization at the transection site. Spinal cord immobilization was completed by fixing two long stainless steel plates along the dorsal spinal processes (Fig. 28–24).

The results of this experimental operation showed that positive postoperative SEPs (reproducible tracings) returned within two months after surgery in 7 of 15 animals who were long-term survivors of the procedure

(Figs. 28–25 A and B, 28–26 A and B). The spinal cords of the animals were carefully studied at autopsy and histologic evidence of healing and the presence of axons at the spinal cord repair site were observed (Figs. 28–27 and 28–28). Positive SEPs and the presence of axons at the transection site did not occur in control cats.

None of the animals in this experiment had any motor function return at the time they were sacrificed (45 days after surgery). This operative experiment involving the excision and reapproximation of the spinal cord has absolutely no bearing at the present time in the treatment of spinal cord injuries. The experiment simply showed that the spinal cord, like all tissues in the body, has the capacity for repair.

Omental-Collagen Preparation

Once it was known that the spinal cord had the ability to heal, attempts were made to repeat this finding but with a simpler surgical technique. The new technique employs a spinal transection model in the cat in which a collagen matrix gel is used to bridge the gap that develops between the divided ends of the spinal cord immediately following complete transection. To increase blood flow to this area in order to create a favorable environment for axonal regeneration, the pedicled omentum was transposed to cover the collagen matrix and the proximal-distal cord stump regions.[27]

The cats had complete transection of their spinal cord and dural covering, which resulted in a cord separation of 6 mm. The spinal cord

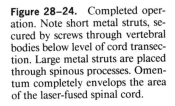

Figure 28–24. Completed operation. Note short metal struts, secured by screws through vertebral bodies below level of cord transection. Large metal struts are placed through spinous processes. Omentum completely envelops the area of the laser-fused spinal cord.

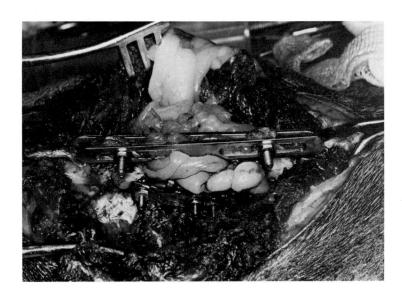

Cat #14656

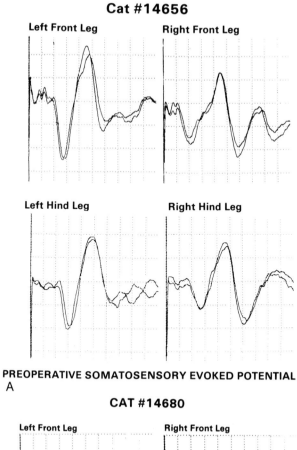

PREOPERATIVE SOMATOSENSORY EVOKED POTENTIAL

A

CAT #14680

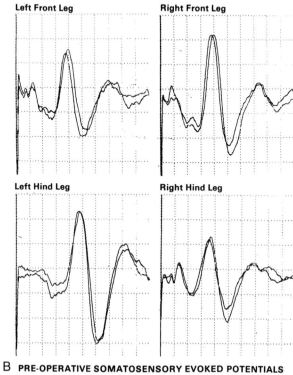

B PRE-OPERATIVE SOMATOSENSORY EVOKED POTENTIALS

Figure 28–25. *A* and *B*, Preoperative somatosensory-evoked potentials of all limbs showing normal wave patterns. Stimulation pulses of 100-microsecond duration were generated at a rate of 5 stimuli/second with a sweep speed of 10 milliseconds/grid. Amplitude is 10 microvolts/grid.

Cat #14656

Left Hind Leg

Right Hind Leg

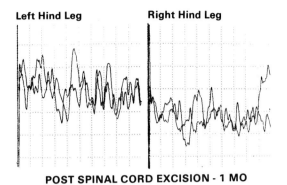

POST SPINAL CORD EXCISION - 1 MO

Left Hind Leg

Right Hind Leg

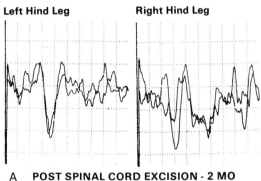

A   **POST SPINAL CORD EXCISION - 2 MO**

Cat #14680

Left Hind Leg

Right Hind Leg

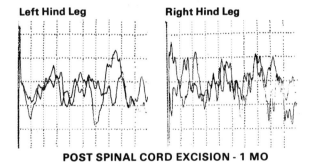

POST SPINAL CORD EXCISION - 1 MO

Left Hind Leg

Right Hind Leg

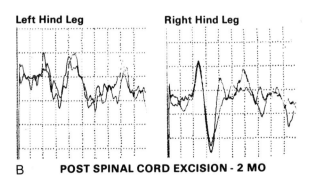

B   **POST SPINAL CORD EXCISION - 2 MO**

Figure 28–26. *A* and *B*, Upper tracings showing SEP of hind limbs one month postoperatively with no detectable responses. Lower tracings show SEPs two months postoperatively with reproducible positive and negative waves. SEP parameters are identical to parameters of Figure 28–25 *A* and *B* except amplitude is 4 microvolts/grid.

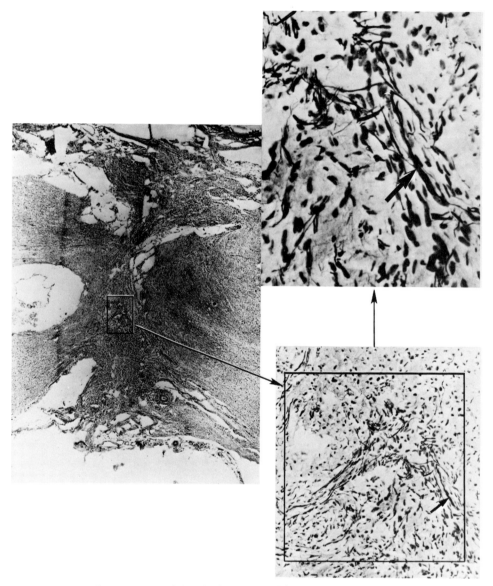

Figure 28–27. *Left,* Macrophoto of site of spinal cord excision and reapproximation of cat #14656 (Fig. 28–26*B*) showing areas of solid bridging at transection site. *Right,* Black arrows in successive photo enlargements point to one of many axons observed at transection site. (Original magnification, right lower position, 250×; Bodian silver)

stumps were irrigated with a polyvinyl alcohol and chlorpromazine solution in order to reduce axoplasmic extrusion which routinely follows spinal cord transection.

Animals were randomly separated into three groups with the gap between the divided spinal cord stumps being filled with (Group A) collagen matrix (COL), (Group B) gelfoam (GEF), and (Group C) collagen matrix plus predicted omentum (COM). The material was placed

posteriorly over the preparation. All animals were sacrificed at 90 days.

RESULTS

The vascular contribution delivered by the omentum in Group C (collagen plus the omentum) resulted in an increase of 65 per cent and 83 per cent, respectively, in blood flow to the

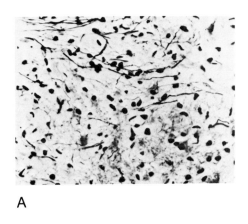

A

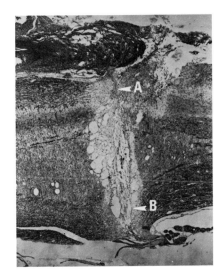

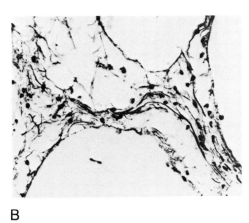

B

Figure 28–28. *Left,* Macrophoto of site of spinal cord excision and reapproximation of cat #14680 (Fig. 28–26A). Arrow A points to area of posterior columns showing solid glial union; arrow B shows spinal cord connections composed of trabecular tissue. *Right, A* shows multiple axons crossing solid tissue bridge; *B* shows one of many axons crossing trabecular bridge. (Original magnification, *A* and *B*, 250×; Bodian silver)

divided spinal cord when compared with groups A and B (Fig. 28–29). Blood vessel density counts in the collagen matrix of Group C showed a 3 to 1 increase as compared with the number of blood vessels in Groups A and B. Of particular interest was the presence in Group C of immunoreactive catecholaminergic axons that grew through the collagen matrix bridge and continued into the distal cord stump (Fig. 28–30). The blood supply from the omentum to the collagen matrix is believed to be the primary factor in the development of the tyrosine hydroxylase immunoreactive axons that were found in abundance in Group C as compared

with their sparsity or nonexistence in the other two groups. Another possibility for this axonal regeneration is that the omentum might be supplying needed circulating proteins,[28] or angiogenic[17] or neurotropic factors[19,20,21] to the sprouting nerve fibers.

Over the past decades, a great deal of experimental work has been centered on the injured spinal cord. It is now no longer just hoped, but fully expected, that treatment programs in the future, based on solid scientific foundations, will prove effective in improving the clinical status of patients who have experienced a spinal cord injury. The probability is now present

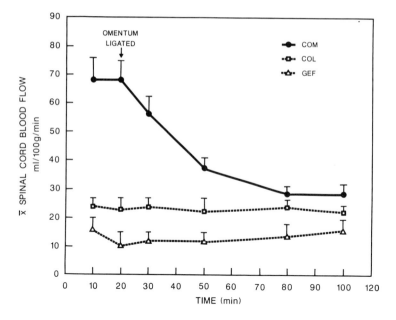

Figure 28–29. Mean averages of six serial blood flow measurements using a hydrogen clearance technique comparing COM, GEF, and COL animals. Microelectrodes placed 6 mm distal to spinal cord transection site 90 days after surgery. Analysis of variance comparing blood flow increases of COM to COL and GEF was P <0.0001 and P <0.001, respectively.

that the omentum, or its components, may prove important in such improvement.

Acknowledgment

I wish to thank Earl Steward, who has managed my laboratory for almost a decade. His untiring efforts have made possible many of the projects discussed in this chapter. He has my fondest hope and fullest expectation for success in his future career as a Doctor of Medicine.

REFERENCES

1. Goldsmith HS, Steward E, Chen WF, Duckett S: Application of intact omentum to the normal and traumatized spinal cord. *In* Kao CC, Bunge RP, Reir RJ (eds): Spinal Cord Reconstruction. New York, Raven Press, 1983.
2. Nemecek ST, Peter R, Suba P, et al: Longitudinal extension of oedema in experimental spinal cord injury. Acta Neurochir 37:7, 1977.
3. Goldsmith HS, Steward E, Duckett S: Early application of pedicled omentum to the acutely traumatized spinal cord. Paraplegia 23:100, 1985.
4. Goldsmith HS, Chen WF, Duckett S: Brain vascular-

Figure 28–30. Tyrosine hydroxylase immunofluorescent fibers are seen growing through the spinal cord (with omentum-COM groups) into the collagen bridge. Axonal regeneration continued into the distal spinal cord segment.

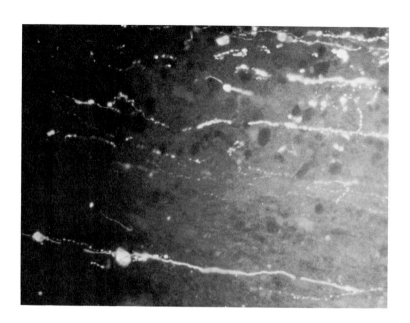

ization by intact omentum. Arch Surg 106:695, 1973.

5. Goldsmith HS, Duckett S, Chen WF: Prevention of cerebral infarction in the dog by intact omentum. Am J Surg 130:317, 1975.

6. Goldsmith HS, Duckett S, Chen WF: Prevention of cerebral infarction in the monkey by omental transposition to the brain. Stroke 9:224, 1978.

7. Goldsmith HS, Duckett S, Chen WF: Spinal cord vascularization by intact omentum. Am J Surg 129:262, 1975.

8. Levander B, Zwetnow NN: Bulk flow of CSF through a lumbo-omental pedicle graft in the dog. Acta Neurochir 41:147, 1978.

9. Goldsmith HS, de los Santos R, Beattie EJ: Relief of chronic lymphedema by omental transposition. Ann Surg 166:573, 1967.

10. Ryan GB, Grobety J, Majno G: Postoperative peritoneal adhesions. Am J Pathol 65:117, 1971.

11. Allen AR: Surgery of experimental lesions of spinal cord equivalent to crush injury of fracture-dislocation of spinal cord. JAMA 57:878, 1911.

12. Goldsmith HS, Steward E, Duckett S: Use of DMSO and omentum in acute spinal cord injury. Submitted for publication.

13. Goldsmith HS, Neil-Dwyer G, Barsoum L: Omental transposition to the chronically injured human spinal cord. Paraplegia 24:173, 1986.

14. Neil-Dwyer G, Goldsmith HS, Barsoum L: Treatment of chronic spinal cord injured patients by omental transposition. Presented at the First International Omental Congress, Research Triangle Park, North Carolina, October 28–November 1, 1988.

15. Abraham J, Paterson A, Bothra M, et al: Omento-myelo-synangiosis in the management of chronic traumatic paraplegia. Paraplegia 25:44, 1987.

16. Zou XW: Omental transposition in the surgical treatment of spinal cord injuries. Chin J Neurosurg 1:107, 1985.

17. Goldsmith HS, Griffith AL, Kupferman A, Catsim-

poolas N: Lipid angiogenic factor from omentum. JAMA 252:2034, 1984.

18. Goldsmith HS, Griffith AL, Catsimpoolas N: Increased vascular perfusion after administration of an omental lipid factor. Surg Gynecol Obstet 162:579, 1986.

19. Goldsmith HS, McIntosh T, Vezina RM, Colton T: Vasoactive neurochemicals identified in omentum. Br J Neurosurg 1:359, 1987.

20. Goldsmith HS, Marquis JK, Siek G: Choline acetyltransferase activity in omental tissue. Br J Neurosurg 1:463, 1987.

21. Siek GC, Marquis JK, Goldsmith HS: Experimental studies of omentum-derived neurotropic factors. In Goldsmith HS (ed): The Omentum—Research and Clinical Applications. New York, Springer-Verlag, 1990, pp. 85–96.

22. Zhu ZC, Wu WL, Mo YZ: Omental transposition to the brain for cerebrovascular occlusive disease. Chung Hua Wai Ko Tsa Chih 20:11, 1982.

23. Ni MS, Zou XW, Xie KM, et al: Free omental autotransplant to brain surface in ischemic cerebrovascular disease. Chin Med J 96:787, 1983.

24. Liu JF, Wang ZZ, Liu YT, et al: Intracranial transposition of pedicled omentum in the management of ischemic cerebrovascular disease (Chinese). J Nerv Ment Dis 6:321, 1980.

25. Miyamoto S, Kikuchi H, Karasawa J, et al: Study of the posterior circulation in moyamoya disease. J Neurosurg 65:454, 1986.

26. Goldsmith HS, Steward E, Kemper TL: Spinal cord excision and reapproximation followed by histologic and neuroelectrical restoration. Submitted for publication.

27. de la Torre JC, Goldsmith HS: Increased vascularity enhances spinal axon regeneration. Ann Neurol 22:141, 1987.

28. Kiernan JA: An explanation of axonal regeneration in peripheral nerves and its failure in the central nervous system. Medical Hypotheses 4:1, 15, 1978.

Nutrition in Spinal Cord Injured Patients

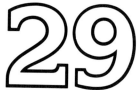

NANAKRAM AGARWAL, M.D., F.R.C.S., F.A.C.S., and
BOK Y. LEE, M.D., F.A.C.S.

Approximately 10,000 persons sustain spinal cord injuries in the United States each year. Through technologic advances, these patients can live out near-normal life spans (30 to 40 years after the injury). The leading causes of death in spinal cord injured patients are pneumonia (20.5 percent), heart disease (15 per cent), accidents (9.7 per cent), infections (8.8 per cent), and pulmonary complications (8.5 per cent).[1] One of the major problems, however, continues to be infection, leading to repeated hospitalizations.

Malnutrition is a significant covariable in the occurrence of infection and prognosis of the spinal cord injured patient. Studies on hospitalized patients show that malnutrition contributes to an increased incidence of morbidity and mortality[2] and is a significant factor in the development of acquired immune deficiencies,[3] defective wound healing,[4] pressure sore formation,[5] cardiac[6] and respiratory insufficiency,[7] and infectious complications.[8] The preservation of nutritional status would, therefore, appear to be a major factor in improving the prognosis in these patients. Fortunately, most patients are healthy and well-nourished before their injuries. A better understanding of the physiology of trauma, the prevention of malnutrition and appropriate treatment when present, and the provision of adequate amounts of nitrogen and fuel based on the patient's nutritional requirements are essential in achieving this goal.

METABOLIC RESPONSE TO SPINAL CORD INJURY

Many of the metabolic changes seen in spinal cord injury are nonspecific and are seen subsequent to the trauma. O'Connell and Gardner[9] have divided the clinical course of spinal cord injury into two major periods: the stage of flaccidity, or "spinal shock," and the return of reflex activity. The stage of flaccidity averages six weeks after the initial transection of the spinal cord and is characterized by an acute vasodepression and fall in basal metabolic rate roughly proportional to the degree of shock. Nitrogen balance becomes negative from day one[10] and can reach a peak of up to 25 grams per day, two to four weeks after injury.[11] There is a negative fluid balance in the initial three to four weeks, orthostatic hypotension is severe, and gastrointestinal function can be either hypoactive or hyperactive.[12]

The return of reflex activity is associated with abnormal loss of nitrogen, progressive weight loss, increased proportion of body fat, and decreased lean body mass.[13] There is a drastic loss of potassium that is more pronounced in quadriplegia than in paraplegia. Although the decrease in total body water parallels the loss in body weight, sodium is retained, resulting in a relative increase in extracellular water.[14] There is a decrease in muscle blood flow, and atrophied muscle cells are eventually replaced by connective tissue.[13] Hypercalciuria and hyperphosphaturia induced by immobilization and inactivity occur in the early stages of the disease and remain until mobilization occurs.[9,14]

NUTRITIONAL ASSESSMENT

Controversy still exists over methods of identifying or classifying malnutrition.[15] Currently available methods range from simple clinical judgment to highly sophisticated and expensive tests for estimating body composition. Some form of objective data is generally required for documenting the type and degree of nutritional depletion. Objective information also provides a means of monitoring the efficacy of therapeutic interventions. Most importantly, serial objective measurements enable early identification of the high-risk patient and early institution of aggressive nutritional support to reduce morbidity and mortality.

A comprehensive nutritional assessment consisting of a complete clinical and dietary history, physical examination, anthropometric measurements, and biochemical, hematologic, and immunologic tests[16] is far more valuable than individual measurements.

Body Weight

Body weight, a simple and valuable gross measurement of body composition, is measured inexactly and infrequently. In the trauma setting, Kinney and associates[17] have demonstrated that there is a high risk of death with a 25 per cent weight loss. The percentage of ideal body weight is determined with reference to weights for age, sex, and height using Metropolitan Life Insurance tables. Mild protein-calorie malnutrition is defined as a body weight of 80 to 90 per cent of ideal body weight, moderate malnutrition as 70 to 80 per cent of ideal body weight, and severe malnutrition as less than 70 per cent of ideal body weight.[18] It is far more valuable, however, to assess the percentage of usual body weight or percent weight change over a given period of time. A loss of 1 per cent to 2 per cent of body weight in one week, 5 percent in one month, or 10 per cent in six months is considered clinically significant.[19]

The interpretation of changes in body weight requires careful consideration of various factors. A gain or loss of greater than 0.2 kg/day is uncommon. Rapid changes in body weight (10 per cent of body weight in two weeks or less) most likely reflect changes in total body water as seen with overhydration, dehydration, ascites, pleural effusion, or edema.[19] From a practical standpoint, daily measurements of body weight provide valuable diagnostic and therapeutic information.

After the initial weight loss over the first three to four months after injury, there should be very little change in the patient's body weight. However, chronic spinal cord injured patients have a tendency toward weight gain, with weight changes seen in individual patients

related to changes in fat content.[20] Peiffer suggests that ideal body weight of spinal cord injured patients should be maintained at 4.5 kg and 9.0 kg below calculated ideal body weight for paraplegics and quadriplegics, respectively.[21]

Body Fat

In clinical practice, body fat mass is most commonly assessed by measuring the triceps skinfold thickness with Lange skinfold calipers. A mean of three readings taken from the back of the nondominant arm, midway between the acromial process and the olecranon process of the ulna, is usually expressed as a percentage of the standard (50th percentile) value. Severe depletion is indicated by a value less than 60 to 80 per cent of the standard value.[19] Certain precautions are needed in interpreting body fat measurements: individual observer variation, position of patient, duration and amount of pressure, presence of edema or subcutaneous emphysema, or change of site by more than 1 cm can result in a significant variation.[22]

Muscle Mass or Somatic Protein Mass

The size of the skeletal muscle mass varies considerably according to the physical condition of the body, presence or absence of disease, and disuse.[23] Skeletal muscle mass represents 4 to 6 kg of the body's total 10 to 12 kg of protein and serves as the major source of protein during periods of starvation and stress. Alterations in work capacity are also related to muscle mass. Of the various methods described in the literature for assessing muscle mass, anthropometry and 24-hour urinary creatinine levels are commonly used.[19]

Midarm Circumference and Midarm Muscle Circumference

The midarm circumference is measured at the same site as the triceps skinfold thickness. The midarm muscle circumference (MAMC) is derived from the midarm circumference (MAC) and the triceps skinfold (TSF): MAMC = MAC − (0.314 × TSF). Both values are also expressed as a percentage of standard. Severe protein-calorie malnutrition is indicated by a value less than 60 per cent of standard.[19] Anthropometric measurements, though simple, quick, noninvasive, and inexpensive, have limited accuracy because they measure individual muscle groups rather than total muscle mass and are subject to all the errors mentioned for triceps skinfold measurements.

24-hour Urinary Creatinine

The 24-hour urinary excretion of creatinine is a simple, inexpensive, and noninvasive index of muscle mass.[24] A significant relationship has been demonstrated between muscle mass and urinary creatinine excretion in both adults and children. As compared with a mean creatinine excretion of 23 mg/kg/day in healthy men, 24-hour urinary creatinine excretion in chronic spinal cord injured patients is decreased. There is a greater decrease in quadriplegics (11.81 ± 3.53 mg/kg) than in paraplegics (17.06 ± 5.21 mg/kg) and the decrease correlates with the level of spinal cord injury.[25] In this manner, 24-hour urinary creatinine excretion has the potential for being used in monitoring muscle mass in spinal cord injured patients.

Visceral Protein Mass

Visceral protein mass, the second component of body cell mass, accounts for approximately 2 kg of the total protein in a healthy adult man. It is generally measured by albumin, transferrin, retinol-binding protein, and thyroxine-binding prealbumin. The levels of these plasma proteins are more sensitive measuring criteria for protein-calorie malnutrition than are anthropometric measurements. In the presence of stress secondary to surgery, trauma, or sepsis, profound deficiencies in visceral proteins occur before any significant decrease in anthropometric measurements is seen.[19] Their fall represents decreased liver biosynthesis and turnover, and their rise parallels nutritional recovery. Besides malnutrition, other factors known to influence the levels of visceral proteins include the rate of metabolic utilization, excretion, intravascular-extravascular transfer, hydration, and type of resuscitation fluid.[26]

Albumin

Serum albumin is still the most widely studied objective measurement and is considered by some to be the most useful indicator of malnutrition.[27] An albumin level of 3.0 to 3.5 gm/dL is suggestive of mild malnutrition; a level between 2.1 and 2.9 gm/dL suggests moderate malnutrition; and a level of 2.0 gm/dL or less suggests severe malnutrition.[19]

Transferrin

Serum transferrin, a more sensitive visceral protein, has a shorter half-life (8.8 days) and a smaller plasma pool (5.29 gm) than does albumin.[28] Thus, serum transferrin levels more rapidly reflect changes in visceral protein. Actual serum transferrin values are measured by radioimmunodiffusion. However, because this technique is not readily available, transferrin values are generally calculated from the total iron-binding capacity (TIBC):[19] transferrin (mg/dL) = (0.8 × TIBC) − 43. A value between 151 and 175 mg/dL suggests mild malnutrition; a value between 100 and 150 mg/dL suggests moderate depletion; and value less than 100 mg/dL suggests severe malnutrition.

Immunologic Assessment

The importance of immunocompetence to the survival of patients who have had surgery or sepsis has been recognized for the past decade. In many patients, the competence of the immune system is clearly related to nutritional status,[3,8] but in others this relationship may not be as direct. An immunologic assessment includes a total lymphocyte count, a delayed cutaneous hypersensitivity test, serum complement levels, and tests for other cellular immune functions.

Total Lymphocyte Count

Total lymphocyte count, readily available in most patients within hours of admission, has been described as a "poor man's" assessment of immunocompetency[29] and predictor of postoperative sepsis.[30] The count, derived by multiplying the percentage of lymphocytes in peripheral smear by the white blood cell count, is considered abnormal if it is less than 1,500/mm³ and is suggestive of severe malnutrition if less than 800/mm³.

Delayed Cutaneous Hypersensitivity

Delayed hypersensitivity is determined by intradermal injections of 0.1 mL of four recall antigens: mumps, *Candida albicans,* purified protein derivative of tuberculin, and trichophytin. The skin test is considered positive if there is an induration with a diameter of 5 mm or greater at either 24 or 48 hours. Persons are classified as normal if they have test results with two or more positive readings, relatively anergic if only one test is positive, and anergic if all tests are negative.

Nutritional Status of Spinal Cord Injured Patients

An unexpectedly large percentage of patients with spinal cord injury show characteristics of malnutrition. Using a multiple isotope dilution technique for determining body composition, Shizgal et al[31] found that of 12 quadriplegics 58 per cent had a body composition characteristic of malnutrition. The nutritional state of quadriplegic patients in their study correlated significantly with the level of spinal cord injury and not with the duration of quadriplegia. Similarly, nutritional assessment of 17 otherwise healthy paraplegic men revealed that none of the patients had normal values for all four objective measurements (albumin, transferrin, total lymphocyte count, and cutaneous hypersensitivity). Mild malnutrition was evident in 47 per cent of patients, 53 per cent demonstrated some index of moderate malnutrition, and a large majority (82 per cent) were immunodeficient.[32]

ENERGY REQUIREMENTS

Guidelines for the energy needs of spinal cord injured patients are not available, and caloric requirements of these patients are not well understood. It is suggested that, from the time of injury, patients appear to have a reduction in their energy needs proportional to the amount of muscle that has been denervated.[33,34] Measurement of basal metabolic rate and total energy expenditure correlated with the level of lesion and is significantly less than that predicted by standard formulas based on normal population. This decrease in energy expenditure is, however, most marked in quadriplegics, with individual paraplegics exhibiting significant variations in their measured resting energy expenditure ranging from 82 to 125 per cent of predicted values.

Spinal cord injured patients have a tendency toward weight gain and become obese on uncontrolled diets. Obesity and loss of weight are the result of an imbalance between caloric intake and energy output. In a study of 17 paraplegics,[32] significant differences in energy expenditure were observed: only 29.4 per cent were normometabolic with a measured resting energy expenditure (MREE) of 90 to 110 per cent of predicted resting energy expenditure (PREE), 35.3 per cent were hypermetabolic with an MREE more than 110 per cent PREE, and 35.3 per cent were hypometabolic with an MREE less than 90 per cent PREE. Although caloric intake of the three metabolic groups was identical, none of the patients in the hypermetabolic group were overweight, since caloric intake was identical to measured energy expenditure. In contrast, the hypometabolic patients were consuming significantly more calories than were expended, and obesity (weight > 110 per cent ideal body weight) was maximum in hypometabolic patients (83.3 per cent). Thus, contrary to general belief, paraplegics do not have uniformly reduced energy needs.

Energy costs of ambulation and even simple activities are higher in spinal cord injured patients than are those of a normal person. In their extensive literature review, Fisher and Gullickson[35] found that a normal person walks at a rate of about 83 meters/min with an energy expenditure of 0.063 Kcal/min/kg. The disabled person walks more slowly to avoid incurring an increase in energy expenditure per minute. The more disabled the person, the more slowly he walks and the less efficient he becomes in terms of energy expenditure/Kcal/unit distance. Clinkingbeard et al[36] have shown that paraplegics consume nine times the energy per meter expended by a normal person walking at his comfortable walking speed. Furthermore, patients with a lumbar lesion walked five times faster than those with a thoracic lesion and used 320 per cent less energy expenditure per unit distance. Proper prescription braces in paraplegics reduce energy consumption, but no matter how well prescribed and fitted the braces are, a severe loss of function still exists that causes a very large energy expenditure of ambulation. Energy expenditure for propelling a wheelchair is not significantly less than that used in walking at corresponding speeds but requires nine per cent more Kcal/min than normal ambulation. Energy expenditure during wheelchair locomotion is directly related to speed and is also greater with use of upper extremities than with use of lower extremities.[35]

The activity level of quadriplegics with high-level lesions is profoundly decreased by their motor deficits. The activity level of quadriplegics with low-level lesions and paraplegics varies widely on the basis of physical abilities, individual personality, motivation, and interest. Not surprisingly, total energy expenditure and caloric needs in quadriplegics with high-level lesions are significantly less than in quadriplegics with lower lesions and in paraplegics. In contrast, total energy expenditure in many paraplegics may exceed the energy expenditure of normal patients.[33]

The significant variation in energy expenditure of spinal cord injured patients explains why nutritional guidelines in the literature are at times incomplete and often contradictory. These patients, in general, should be given a low caloric diet. Cox et al[34] have demonstrated that stable, rehabilitating patients require 23.4 Kcal/kg/day, with quadriplegics requiring 22.7 Kcal/kg/day and paraplegics requiring 27.9 Kcal/kg/day. Optimal calorie intake should be established according to the patient's previous state of nutrition and metabolic status. Some may benefit from weight loss, while a few may require higher levels of caloric intake.

PROTEIN REQUIREMENTS

Spinal cord injured patients require more protein as they experience increased nitrogen loss. Albumin elimination rates are increased in paraplegics,[37] protein loss through pressure sores is directly related to the size of the sore,[5] and the negative nitrogen balance is accentuated by the presence of infection or stress of surgery. Although it has not definitely been proved, increased protein intake does help in increasing lean body mass. All the aforementioned factors should be taken into account when calculating the amount of protein required to keep the patient in a positive nitrogen balance. The recommended intake of protein is 1.5 to 2.0 gm/kg/day with a ratio of nonprotein calories to nitrogen approximately 100 calories per gram of nitrogen. Sources of protein that contain the highest percentage of essential amino acids (fish, egg, milk) are more efficiently utilized than are plant proteins.

CONCLUSION

A multidisciplinary approach is required for optimal care of spinal cord injured patients. They are at significant risk nutritionally, and successful management requires close attention to their nutritional status, tailoring of nutritional therapy to their needs, early intensive treatment, aggressive physical therapy, and early ambulation.

REFERENCES

1. Stover SL, File PR: Spinal Cord Injury: The Facts and Figures. Birmingham, AL, University of Alabama (Birmingham), 1986.
2. Mullen J, Buzby GP, Matthews DC, et al: Reduction of operative morbidity and mortality by combined preoperative and postoperative nutritional support. Ann Surg 192:604, 1980.
3. Law DK, Durdrick SJ, Abdou NI: The effects of protein-calorie malnutrition on immune competence of the surgical patient. Surg Gynecol Obstet 139:257, 1974.
4. Greenhalgh DG, Gamelli RL: Is impaired wound healing caused by infection or nutritional depletion? Surgery 102:306, 1987.
5. Mulholland JH, Tui C, Wright AM, et al: Protein-metabolism and bed sores. Ann Surg 118:1015, 1943.
6. Viart P: Hemodynamic findings during treatment of protein-calorie malnutrition. Am J Clin Nutr 31:911, 1978.
7. Askanazi J, Weissman C, Rosenbaum SH, et al: Nutrition and the respiratory system. Crit Care Med 10:163, 1982.
8. Newmann CG: Interaction of malnutrition and infection—a neglected clinical concept. Arch Intern Med 137:1364, 1977.
9. O'Connell FB Jr, Gardner WJ: Metabolism in paraplegia. JAMA 153:706, 1953.
10. Kaufman HH, Rowlands BJ, Stein DK, et al: General metabolism in patients with acute paraplegia and quadriplegia. Neurosurgery 16:309, 1985.
11. Cooper IS, Hoen TI: Metabolic disorders in paraplegia. Neurology 2:332, 1952.
12. Claus-Walker J, Halstead LS: Metabolic and endocrine changes in spinal cord injury. II. Partial decentralization of the autonomic nervous system. Arch Phys Med Rehabil 63:576, 1982.
13. Claus-Walker J, Halstead LS: Metabolic and endocrine changes in spinal cord injury. I. The nervous system before and after transection of the spinal cord. Arch Phys Med Rehabil 62:595, 1981.
14. Cardus D, McTaggart WG: Body sodium and potassium in men with spinal cord injury. Arch Phys Med Rehabil 66:156, 1985.
15. McLaren DS, Meguid MM: Nutritional assessment at the crossroad. J Parenteral Enteral Nutr 7:575, 1983.
16. Agarwal N: Nutritional and metabolic assessment and monitoring in trauma. Trauma Q 3(3):64, 1987.
17. Kinney JH, Duke JH Jr, Long CL: Tissue fuel and weight loss after injury. J Clin Pathol (Suppl) 4:65, 1978.
18. Grant JP, Custer PB, Thurlow J: Current techniques of nutritional assessment. Surg Clin North Am 61:437, 1981.
19. Blackburn GL, Bistrain BR, Maini BS, et al: Nutritional and metabolic assessment of the hospitalized patient. J Parenteral Enteral Nutr 1:11, 1977.
20. Greenway RM, Houser HB, Lindan O, Weir DR: Long-term changes in gross body composition of paraplegic and quadriplegic patients. Paraplegia 7:301, 1969.
21. Peiffer SC, Blust P, Leyson JF: Nutritional assessment of the spinal cord injured patient. J Am Diet Assoc 78:501, 1981.

22. Hull JC, O'Quigley J, Giles GR, et al: Upper limb anthropometry: the value of measurement variance studies. Am J Clin Nutr 33:1846, 1980.

23. Moore FD, Oleson KH, McMurphy JD, et al: The body cell mass and its supporting environment. *In* Body Composition in Health and Disease. Philadelphia, WB Saunders, 1963, p 485.

24. Heymsfield SB, Arteaga C, McManus C, et al: Measurement of muscle mass in humans: Validity of the 24 urinary creatinine method. Am J Clin Nutr 37:478, 1983.

25. Agarwal N, Lee BY, DelGuercio LRM: Urinary creatinine excretion in spinal cord injured patients. Nutrition 3:192, 1987.

26. Godan MHN, Waterlow JC, Picun D: Protein turnover, synthesis and breakdown before and after recovery from protein-energy malnutrition. Clin Sci Mol Med 53:473, 1977.

27. Agarwal N, Acevedo F, Leighton LS, et al: Predictive ability of various nutritional variables for mortality in elderly people. Am J Clin Nutr 48:1173, 1988.

28. Awai M, Brown EB: Studies of the metabolism of I-131 labeled human transferrin. J Lab Clin Med 61:363, 1963.

29. Seltzer MH, Bastidas JA, Cooper DM, et al: Instant nutritional assessment. J Parenteral Enteral Nutr 3:157, 1979.

30. Lewis RT, Klein H: Risk factors in postoperative sepsis: significance of preoperative lymphocytopenia. J Surg Res 26:365, 1975.

31. Shizgal HM, Rosa A, Leduc B, et al: Body composition in quadriplegic patients. J Parenteral Enteral Nutr 10:364, 1986.

32. Lee BY, Agarwal N, Corcoran L, et al: Assessment of nutritional and metabolic status of paraplegics. J Rehabil Res 22:11, 1985.

33. Mollinger LS, Spurr GB, El Ghatit AZ, et al: Daily energy expenditure and basal metabolic rates of patients with spinal cord injury. Arch Phys Med Rehabil 66:420, 1985.

34. Cox SAR, Weiss SM, Posuniak EA, et al: Energy expenditure after spinal cord injury: An evaluation of stable rehabilitating patients. J Trauma 25:419, 1985.

35. Fisher SV, Gullickson G Jr: Energy cost of ambulation in health and disability: A literature review. Arch Phys Med Rehabil 59:124, 1978.

36. Clinkingbeard JR, Gersten JW, Hoehn D: Energy cost of ambulation in the traumatic paraplegic. Am J Phys Med 43:157, 1964.

37. Ring J, Seifert J, Lob G, et al: Elimination rate of human albumin in paraplegic patients. Paraplegia 12:139, 1974.

Index

Page numbers in *italics* refer to illustrations; page numbers followed by t indicate tables.